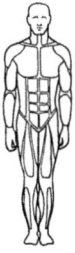

A Practical Approach to Strength and Conditioning

5th Edition

Matt Brzycki

Assistant Director of Campus Recreation, Fitness
Department of Athletics
Princeton University

Part-Time Lecturer
Department of Kinesiology and Health
Rutgers University

ISBN: 9780983575436

Cover design by Laurel Masten Cantor

Book packaged by Wish Publishing

Printed in the United States of America
10 9 8 7 6 5 4 3 2 1

To my son, Ryan; my sister, Mickey, and her sons, James and Jordan; and my brother, Mark, and his sons, Cory and Brendan. I'm very fortunate to have you as family.

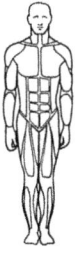

Acknowledgements

Sincere thanks to the following individuals, without whom this book wouldn't have been possible:

Laurel Masten Cantor (Princeton, New Jersey) who designed the front and back covers.

Holly Witten Kondras of Wish Publishing (Terre Haute, Indiana) who designed the interior of the book and acted as the project manager.

Raymundo Abayon, Bobbi Augustyn, Tony Alexander, Dan Bennett, Ralph Biddle, Ryan Bonfiglio, Jim Bryan, Brendan Brzycki, Ryan Brzycki, Anita Carley, Crista Collins, Nickolas Conte, Marguerite Cutchey, Roger Doobraj, David Durell, Patty Durell, Charity Fesler, Alexa Fornicola, Fred Fornicola, Jason Gallucci, Mark Harrison, Stevie Harrison, Troy Harrison, Dave Hauger, Dave Heebner, Kris Heebner, Sharon Henderson, Curt Hillegas, Jane Hunter, Vanessa Jones, Charles Kruger, Jake Marcin, Eliza Martinez, Kate O'Rourke, Tom O'Rourke Jr, John Quigley, Paul Quigley, Marty Riehm, Linda Salonek, Peter Silletti, Kurt Siudzinski, Michael Snaer, Illiana Stoilova-Rogers, Zach Turcotte, Shikha Uberoi and Lauren Woods whose photographs appear throughout the book.

Mark Asanovich, Ryan Bonfiglio, Michael Bradley, Margaret Bryan, Mark Brzycki, Luke Carlson, Patty Durell, Fred Fornicola, Lori Fornicola, Greg Fried, Greg Hammond, Mark Harrison, Stevie Harrison, Troy Harrison, Pilar Martinez, Mike McLaughlin, Tom Nowak, John Quigley, Melanie Silletti, Peter Silletti, Chris Stone, Ken Stone, Shikha Uberoi and Karl Wright who took or provided photographs that appear throughout the book.

Cybex International, Incorporated, for providing the artwork that appears on the first page of each chapter and in Figures 1.1 and 1.2.

The US Department of Agriculture for providing the MyPlate icon that appears in Chapter 19.

The US Food and Drug Administration for providing the Nutrition Facts panels that appear in Chapter 19.

The US Marine Corps for providing a photograph that appears in Chapter 25.

Images from the following sources appear in Chapters 8, 9 and 10: Calvert, A. 1902. US Patent 702,356; Chiosso, J. 1855. *The gymnastic polymachinon. Instructions for performing a systematic series of exercises on the gymnastic & calisthenic polymachinon.* London: Walton & Maberly; Health-Lift Company. 1876. *The Health-Lift reduced to a science: cumulative exercise, a thorough gymnastic system in ten minutes once a day.* New York: Health-Lift Company; Levertin, A. 1893. *Dr. G. Zander's medico-mechanical gymnastics: Its method, importance and application.* Stockholm: PA Norstedt & Sons; Ling, PH, and H Ling. 1893. *A collection of gymnastic positions, issued by the Royal Gymnastic Central Institute, Stockholm.* Stockholm: PA Norstedt & Sons; Narragansett Machine Company. 1905. *Catalogue of gymnastic apparatus made by the Narragansett Machine Co.* Providence, RI: Narragansett Machine Company; Windship, GB. 1865. US Patent 46,413.

Except as noted here or elsewhere, all photographs were taken by or provided by Matt Brzycki.

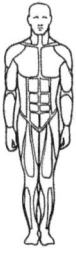

Table of Contents

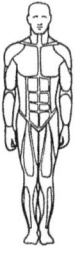

1 Basic Anatomy and Muscular Function

Before discussing any type of physical training, it's necessary for you to gain a basic understanding of your muscles and how they work. Essentially, any physical activity is a series of movements that are made by your muscles acting on your skeleton. (Their combined efforts are reflected in the term musculoskeletal system.)

More to the point, your body is basically a system of levers. Movement of these levers – your bones – is produced by your muscles which are anchored to your bones by tendons. (Tendons link muscle to bone; ligaments link bone to bone.) Perhaps the most well-known and noticeable tendon in your body is the Achilles tendon which fastens your calf muscles to your heel bone.

MUSCLE: TYPES AND STRUCTURE

There are three different types of muscle tissue: cardiac, smooth and skeletal. Cardiac muscle is found in the walls of your heart; smooth muscle is found in the walls of your blood vessels; and skeletal muscle acts across your joints to produce movement.

Your muscles are comprised of muscle fibers (muscle cells; aka myofibers) which, in turn, are comprised of myofibrils. (To get an idea of this arrangement, picture a cable that has hundreds of wires.) Within myofibrils are sarcomeres, the functional units of muscle fibers. Sarcomeres contain two protein filaments (or myofilaments) that possess contractile properties: thinner filaments made mostly of actin and thicker filaments made mostly of myosin. Muscular contraction occurs at this level. (Myofibrils have a number of other protein filaments that contribute to muscular contraction, including nebulin, titin, troponin and tropomyosin. However, the only contractile filaments are actin and myosin; titin, for example, is an elastic filament.)

TYPES OF MUSCULAR CONTRACTIONS

In normal dialogue, contraction means a process of becoming smaller or shorter. But when contraction is used in the context of muscle, this definition doesn't always hold true. Here, contraction refers to a process in which a muscle produces force. (Tension is a force that's *produced by* a muscle; load is a force that's *applied to* a muscle. So, tension and load are opposing forces.)

There are three types of muscular contractions: concentric, eccentric and isometric. Let's take a closer look at the characteristics of each type.

A concentric contraction is one in which a muscle shortens against a load (or resistance). The load moves in a direction away from the earth or opposite the direction of gravity. Examples of concentric contractions are raising a weight, ascending from a squat position, walking up stairs and running uphill. In a concentric contraction, the tension is more than the load. (This is to say, the force that's produced by a muscle is more than the force that's applied to it.) Because the load moves in the same direction as the force that's produced, the mechanical work – calculated as force multiplied by distance – is positive. This is why a concentric contraction is sometimes referred to as the positive phase of a movement or repetition.

An eccentric contraction is one in which a muscle lengthens against a load (or resistance). The load moves in a direction toward the earth or in the direction of gravity. Examples of eccentric contractions are lowering a weight, descending into a squat position, walking down stairs and running downhill. In an eccentric contraction, the tension is less than the load. (This is to say, the force that's produced by a muscle is less than the force that's applied to it.) Because the load moves in the opposite direction as the force that's produced, the mechanical work is negative. This is why an eccentric contraction is sometimes referred to as the negative phase of a movement or repetition.

Finally, an isometric (or static) contraction is one in which a muscle shortens against a load (or resistance) while the tendon lengthens by the same amount that the muscle shortened thereby producing no change in the overall length of the muscle-tendon complex and no change in the joint angle. (This observation was first made in 1938 by Dr. Archibald Vivian Hill, a British physiologist.) Examples of isometric contractions are holding a weight in the mid-range position of a repetition, maintaining a squat position and doing a plank. In an isometric contraction, the tension is equal to the load. (This is to say, the force that's produced by a muscle is equal to the force that's applied to it.) Because there's no movement during an isometric contraction, the mechanical work is zero.

Sidebar: Since mechanical work is calculated as force multiplied by distance, regardless of the amount of force that's produced by a muscle, if there's no movement – as in the case of an isometric contraction – then the distance over which the force is produced is zero and the mechanical work is zero. Of course, energy is needed in order to perform an isometric contraction. Although there's no mechanical work, there's metabolic work (which refers to the chemical reactions that occur within the cells). In a way, mechanical work can be viewed as external (outside the body) and metabolic work as internal (inside the body).

THE SLIDING FILAMENT THEORY

Though it was first met with some skepticism, the most widely accepted explanation of how muscular contraction occurs is the Sliding Filament Theory. In something that's worthy of

Ripley's Believe It or Not, the theory was proposed simultaneously in May 1954 in the same issue of *Nature* – on consecutive pages, no less – by two pairs of researchers. Each pair was led by a man named Huxley (though not related) and located in cities named Cambridge (though nearly 3,300 miles apart): Sir Andrew Huxley and Dr. Rolf Niedergerke at the University of Cambridge in Cambridge, England; and Drs. Hugh Huxley and Jean Hanson at the Massachusetts Institute of Technology in Cambridge, Massachusetts. (Fast fact: Andrew Huxley was the only one of the four researchers without a doctoral degree and a stepbrother of the esteemed author Aldous Huxley who penned the classic novel *Brave New World*.)

It was noted earlier that two protein filaments have contractile properties: actin and myosin. As the name of this theory implies, one filament is thought to slide across the other thereby shortening the muscle. But let's take a closer look at the microanatomy and dynamics of the process (minus the chemical reactions that occur).

Myofibrils are sectioned into sarcomeres which are lined up end-to-end. (Imagine a myofibril as a train and the sarcomeres as the railroad cars.) Sarcomeres house the thinner actin and thicker myosin filaments. These two filaments run parallel to one another and are arranged in what's referred to as a "hexagonal lattice" with each myosin filament interacting with six actin filaments and each actin filament interacting with three myosin filaments.

Myosin filaments are mostly composed of myosin molecules. A myosin molecule consists of three parts (or domains): a long tail, a neck and a globular head. The tails of two myosin molecules intertwine, often illustrated as something that resembles a pair of golf clubs with coiled shafts and two heads. Actin filaments are mostly composed of actin molecules. The actin molecules assemble into two strands that are wrapped around each other which form a double-helical structure, often illustrated as something that resembles a pair of twisted pearl strings.

Each myosin filament has hundreds of heads that extend toward the neighboring actin filaments. During the "power stroke," some of the myosin heads attach to the actin filaments, each head forming what's referred to as a cross-bridge. It's believed that the myosin heads then rotate (pivot) at the necks about 45 degrees in a ratchet-like fashion – much like oars in a boat – in such a way that the myosin "walks" along the actin, effectively pulling (or sliding) the actin filaments across the myosin filament. During the "recovery stroke," the myosin heads then detach (uncouple) from the actin filaments and rotate 45 degrees back to their original positions. Thus, one cycle of the process involves four steps that can be summed up as attach-rotate-detach-rotate.

The myosin heads reside at opposite ends of a myosin filament and point to a "bare zone" in the middle of the filament that's void of any heads. Cross-bridge cycling occurs at both ends, pulling the actin filaments toward the middle of the myosin filament. This shortens the sarcomere which shortens the myofibril which shortens the muscle fiber which shortens the muscle.

The process in which the myosin heads attach to and detach from the actin filaments can occur billions of times throughout a muscle in the course of a single contraction (such as during one repetition of an exercise). However, the myosin heads don't attach-rotate-detach-rotate at the same time since this would result in a series of jerks rather than a smooth movement. At any given time, the myosin heads are in different steps of the cross-bridge cycle with some involved in the power stroke and others involved in the recovery stroke.

One cross-bridge cycle moves the actin filaments about 10 or 11 nanometers. To get an idea of the microscopic milieu in which this action occurs, consider that one nanometer is one billionth of a meter. Or look at it this way: One inch is equal to 25.4 million nanometers. Taking a 10-nanometer step, then, would require *2.54 million steps to move one inch*. Taking a 10-nanometer step would also require 100,000 steps to move 0.1 millimeters which is about the thickness of this page. Not the length of the page, the *thickness* of the page. Mind-numbing, isn't it?

Sidebar: An extension of the Sliding Filament Theory was proposed by Dr. Kiisa Nishikawa and her colleagues in 2012. According to their Winding Filament Hypothesis, titin (aka connectin) – an elastic filament without contractile properties – is wound around the actin filaments by the myosin heads during the power stroke of the cross-bridge cycle. The researchers also suggest that as this happens, the myosin heads rotate the actin filaments. At the present time, however, this new twist on muscular contraction – pardon the pun – has yet to gain widespread acceptance.

JOINT JARGON

A number of terms are frequently used in the vernacular of physical training to describe the locations of muscles and their functions (or actions). Familiarity with these terms will assist you in understanding how your muscles are used.

Terms that designate locations of muscles are often used in relation to what's known as the standard anatomical position. This position is defined as the body standing erect with the feet spread about shoulder-width apart and pointed straight ahead; the arms straight and out to the sides; and the palms facing forward. In this regard, the midline of the body is an imaginary line that bisects the body into right and left halves. Common locational terms include medial (toward the midline), lateral (away from the midline), anterior (front) and posterior (back).

A handful of other terms are employed on a fairly regular basis to describe the functions of muscles. Flexion is a decrease in the angle between two bones and extension is an increase in the angle between two bones. Abduction is movement of a limb away from the midline of the body and adduction is movement of a limb toward the midline of the body. Finally, rotation is turning about the vertical axis of a bone. (In the ensuing discussions, the use of the terms backward, forward, downward and upward are based on an individual standing erect.)

THE MAJOR MUSCLES

Incredible as it may seem, there are more than 600 muscles in the human body (and about six billion muscle fibers). In fact, each one of your forearms has 19 separate muscles with such exotic-sounding names as extensor carpi radialis brevis and flexor digitorum superficialis. Don't worry, it's well beyond the scope and purpose of this book to discuss your muscles in such great detail; instead, the focus will be on your major muscles.

It's convenient to organize the major muscles into these nine areas: hips, upper legs, lower legs, torso, upper arms, lower arms, abdominals, lower back and neck. Brief notes on the location and primary function(s) of each muscle are given along with anatomical terminology that's generally accepted in discussions of physical training. (Anterior and posterior views of the muscles are illustrated in Figures 1.1 and 1.2, respectively.) Also provided are examples of activities in which a particular muscle would be used.

HIPS

Your hip region is made up of three major muscle groups: the gluteals, adductors and iliopsoas.

Gluteals

Your gluteals (or "glutes") are located on the back of your hips. They're composed of three main muscles: the gluteus maximus, gluteus medius and gluteus minimus. The largest and strongest muscle in your body is the gluteus maximus (which forms your buttocks or "butt"). The primary function of this muscle is hip extension (driving your upper legs backward). Your gluteus medius and gluteus minimus cause hip abduction (spreading your legs apart). Your gluteal muscles are involved significantly in walking, jogging/running, jumping and stairclimbing.

Adductors

Your adductor group is composed of five muscles that are found throughout your inner thigh: the gracilis, pectineus, adductor longus, adductor brevis and adductor magnus (which is the largest of the five). The muscles of your inner thigh are used during hip adduction (bringing your legs together).

Iliopsoas

The iliopsoas is actually a collective term for three muscles that are located in very close proximity on the front of your hips: the iliacus, psoas major and psoas minor. The main function of the iliopsoas is hip flexion (bringing your upper legs toward your torso). Your iliopsoas has a major role in many activities such as lifting your knees when walking, jogging/running and stairclimbing. The iliopsoas is sometimes considered with the muscles of the abdomen. (Fast fact: The psoas minor is absent in roughly half of the population; and oddly enough, some individuals only have this muscle on one side of their bodies.)

UPPER LEGS

The two major muscle groups of your upper legs (or thighs) are the hamstrings and quadriceps.

Hamstrings

Your hamstrings (or "hams") are found on the back of your upper legs and actually include three muscles. From the medial side to the lateral side, the muscles are the semimembranosus, semitendinosus and biceps femoris. Together, these muscles are involved in knee flexion (bringing your heels toward your buttocks) and hip extension (driving your upper legs backward). Your hamstrings are used extensively during jogging/running and jumping. One of the best reasons to strengthen your hamstrings is that they're quite susceptible to pulls and tears. Clearly, strong muscles on the back of the upper legs are necessary to counterbalance the powerful muscles on the front of the upper legs.

Quadriceps

Your quadriceps (or "quads") are found on the front of your upper legs. As the name implies, the quadriceps include four muscles. From the medial side to the lateral side, three of the muscles are the vastus medialis, vastus intermedius and vastus lateralis; the fourth muscle is the rectus femoris which resides on top of the vastus intermedius. The main function of your quadriceps is knee extension (straightening your legs). Your quadriceps are involved in jogging/running, kicking, jumping, biking and stairclimbing.

Sidebar: It's generally accepted that the vastus medialis is comprised of the vastus medialis longus (VML) and vastus medialis obliquus (VMO). As hinted by its name, the fibers of the VML run longitudinally, following the shaft of the femur (upper-leg bone) toward the knee; and as hinted by its name, the fibers of the VMO run obliquely, angling toward the femur near the knee. (The VMO can be identified by its teardrop-shaped appearance on a well-developed upper leg). Nevertheless, there has been much debate about whether the VML and VMO are two parts of one muscle or two separate muscles. Among other things, the fibers of the vastus medialis are positioned "in series" and change gradually from a longitudinal to a diagonal orientation, not abruptly. This suggests that the VML and VMO are, in fact, two parts of the same muscle. And on a related note, a common belief is that the VMO can be preferentially targeted with the "terminal" leg extension, an abbreviated version of the traditional leg extension in which the range of motion for each repetition is restricted to the last 10 to 15 degrees of completely straightening the leg. This notion was first advanced in 1962 by Dr. Ian Smillie – a renowned orthopedic surgeon from Scotland – who also hyped the vastus medialis as "the key to the knee." However, there's no scientific evidence that this exercise – or any other supposed VMO-strengthening exercise – is effective for isolating the VMO.

LOWER LEGS

The calves and dorsi flexors are the two major muscle groups in your lower legs.

Calves

Your calves are comprised of two important muscles that are located on the back of your

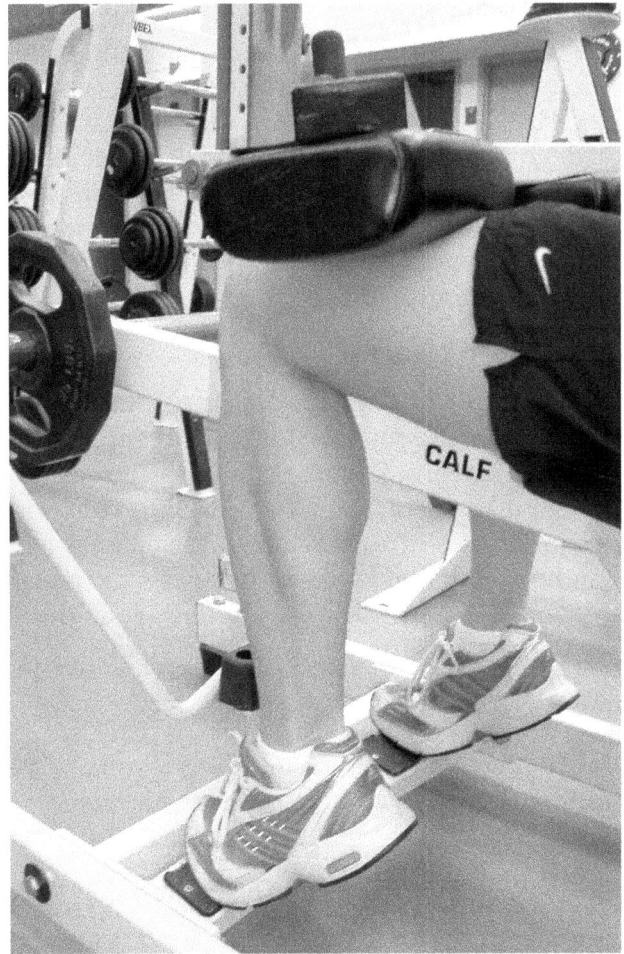

When the angle between your upper and lower legs is about 90 degrees or less, the function of the gastrocnemius is diminished and the soleus makes a greater contribution to the movement.

lower legs: the gastrocnemius (or "gastroc") and soleus. The gastrocnemius is a superficial muscle that makes up the visible bulk of the calves; the soleus lies beneath the gastrocnemius. These two muscles have a common tendon of insertion – the Achilles tendon – and are jointly referred to as the triceps surae or, more simply, the gastroc-soleus. (The "triceps" designation counts the two heads of the gastrocnemius along with the soleus. Another perspective, though less popular, includes the gastrocnemius, soleus and plantaris as the triumvirate.)

The gastrocnemius and soleus are employed in plantar flexion (aka ankle extension; straightening your ankles as in pointing your foot downward or rising up on your toes). Normally, the gastrocnemius is involved more than the soleus in plantar flexion. However, when the angle between your upper and lower legs is about 90 degrees or less – such as in the seated position – the function of the gastrocnemius is diminished and the soleus makes a greater contribution to the movement. Your calves play a major role in jogging/running, jumping and stairclimbing.

Dorsi Flexors

The front of your lower legs contains four muscles that are sometimes simply referred to as the dorsi flexors. The largest of these muscles is the tibialis anterior. The dorsi flexors are primarily used in dorsi flexion (aka ankle flexion; bending your ankles as in bringing your foot upward). It's critical to strengthen your dorsi flexors as a safeguard against shin splints.

TORSO

The three major muscle groups in your torso are the chest, upper back and shoulders.

Chest

The main muscles that surround your chest area are the pectoralis major and pectoralis minor which are collectively known as the "pecs." The pectoralis major is thick, flat and fan-shaped and the most superficial muscle of your chest wall; the pectoralis minor is thin, flat and triangle-shaped and positioned beneath the pectoralis major. Together, these two muscles pull your upper arms across your torso. The chest is involved in pushing and throwing movements. (Fast fact: In anatomical discussions, major and minor are comparative terms that signify larger and smaller, respectively; as an example, the pectoralis major is larger than the pectoralis minor.)

Upper Back

The latissimus dorsi is a long, broad muscle that comprises most of your upper back. As a matter of fact, the "lats" are the largest muscle in your upper body. Its primary function is to pull the upper arms backward. Your lats are an essential muscle in assorted pulling movements and climbing skills. In addition, developing your upper back is necessary to provide muscular balance between the anterior and posterior segments of your torso.

Shoulders

Your deltoids (or "delts") are composed of three separate parts (or heads) which surround or "cap" your shoulder: the anterior deltoid is found on the front of your shoulder and is used to raise your upper arm forward; the middle deltoid is found on the side of your shoulder and is used to lift your upper arm sideways; and the posterior deltoid is found on the back of your shoulder and is used to draw your upper arm backward when it's positioned perpendicular to your torso.

The trapezius is a kite-shaped (or trapezoid-shaped) muscle with upper, middle and lower portions. The upper portion resides at the base of your neck and across your shoulders; the middle portion covers much of your upper back; and the lower portion extends from your middle back to your shoulders. There are three primary functions of the "traps": shoulder elevation (shrugging your shoulders as if to say "I don't know") done by the upper and lower portions; neck extension (bringing your head backward) done by the upper portion; and scapulae adduction (aka scapulae retraction; pinching your shoulder blades together) done by the middle and lower portions. The trapezius is sometimes considered with the muscles of the neck. (Fast fact: In shoulder elevation, the upper and lower portions of the trapezius co-contract – pull in opposite directions – which prevents unwanted movement of the scapulae.)

Situated beneath the middle portion of the trapezius are the rhomboid major and rhomboid minor which are collectively referred to as the rhomboids. The main job of these diamond-shaped muscles is scapulae adduction.

The rotator cuff is a group of four muscles that are located deep within your shoulders. The subscapularis and teres major perform internal (or medial) rotation of the upper arm while the infraspinatus and teres minor perform external (or lateral) rotation of the upper arm. (Some sources recognize the supraspinatus as a fifth muscle of the rotator cuff, involved in external rotation.) In addition to rotating the upper arm, these muscles are also largely responsible for maintaining the structural integrity and stability of your shoulder joint. The rotator cuff is highly prone to overuse injuries. One of the most common conditions is shoulder-impingement syndrome, a general term used to describe pain that's often characterized as tightness or pinching in the shoulder.

UPPER ARMS

The two major muscles of your upper arms are the biceps and triceps.

Biceps

The prominent muscle that's located on the front of your upper arm is technically known as the biceps brachii. As the name suggests, the muscle has two separate parts. When the biceps are fully contracted, these two heads can be seen separated by a groove on a well-developed upper arm. The primary function of your biceps is elbow flexion (bending your arms). Your biceps assist your upper back in pulling and climbing movements.

Triceps

The prominent muscle that's located on the back of your upper arm is technically known as the triceps brachii. As the name suggests, the muscle has three separate parts: the long, lateral and medial heads. When the triceps are fully contracted, these three heads produce a horseshoe-shaped appearance on a well-developed upper arm. The primary function of your triceps is elbow extension (straightening your arms). Your triceps assist your chest and shoulders in pushing and throwing movements.

LOWER ARMS

The forearms are the major muscles in your lower arms.

Forearms

As mentioned previously, each one of your forearms has 19 different muscles. These muscles

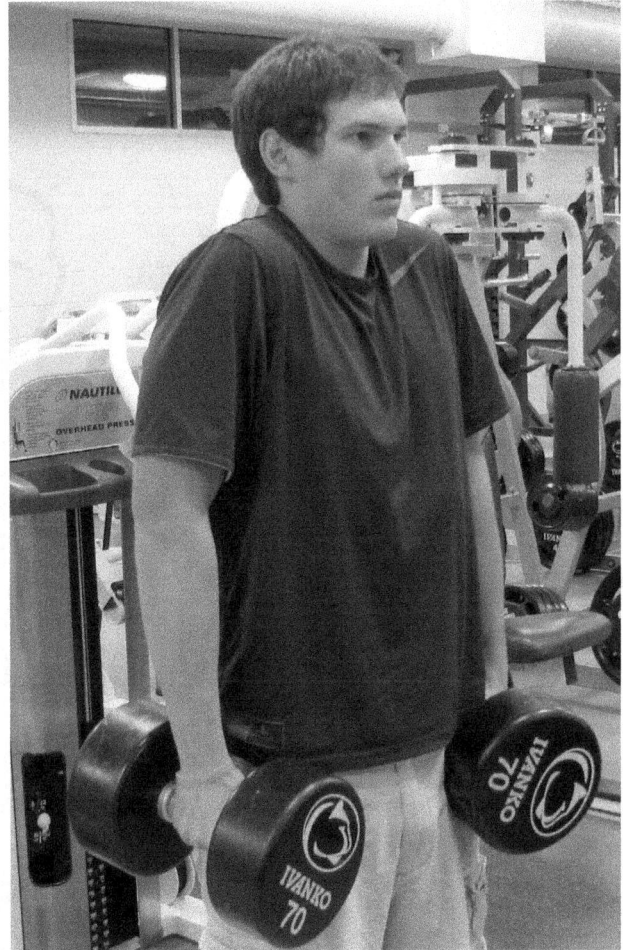

The upper portion of the trapezius is involved in shoulder elevation. (Photo by Mark Harrison.)

can be divided into two groups on the basis of their location and function. The anterior group on the front of your forearm causes wrist flexion (bending your wrist with your palm facing up) and pronation (turning your hand from a palm-up to a palm-down position); the posterior group on the back of your forearm causes wrist extension (bending your wrist with your palm facing down) and supination (turning your hand from a palm-down to a palm-up position). Since the muscles of the forearms affect your wrists, hands and fingers, they're extremely important in pulling movements, climbing skills and tasks that involve gripping. (Fast fact: An easy way to remember the difference between the functions of supination and pronation is to think of supination as "soup in" or turning your hand upward to hold a bowl of soup and pronation as

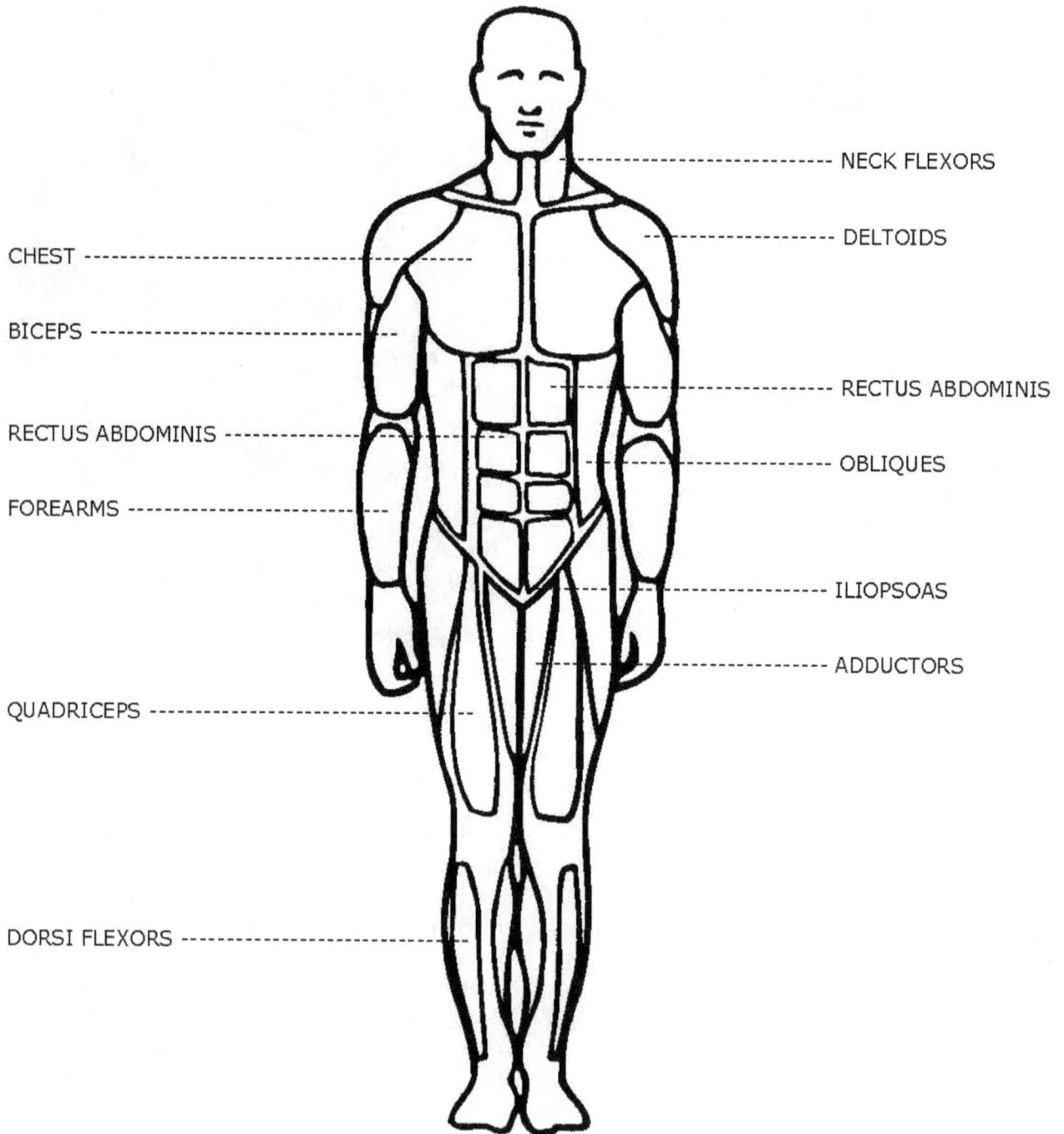

CHEST
BICEPS
RECTUS ABDOMINIS
FOREARMS
QUADRICEPS
DORSI FLEXORS

NECK FLEXORS
DELTOIDS
RECTUS ABDOMINIS
OBLIQUES
ILIOPSOAS
ADDUCTORS

Figure 1.1: Anterior view of the muscles (artwork provided by Cybex International, Inc.)

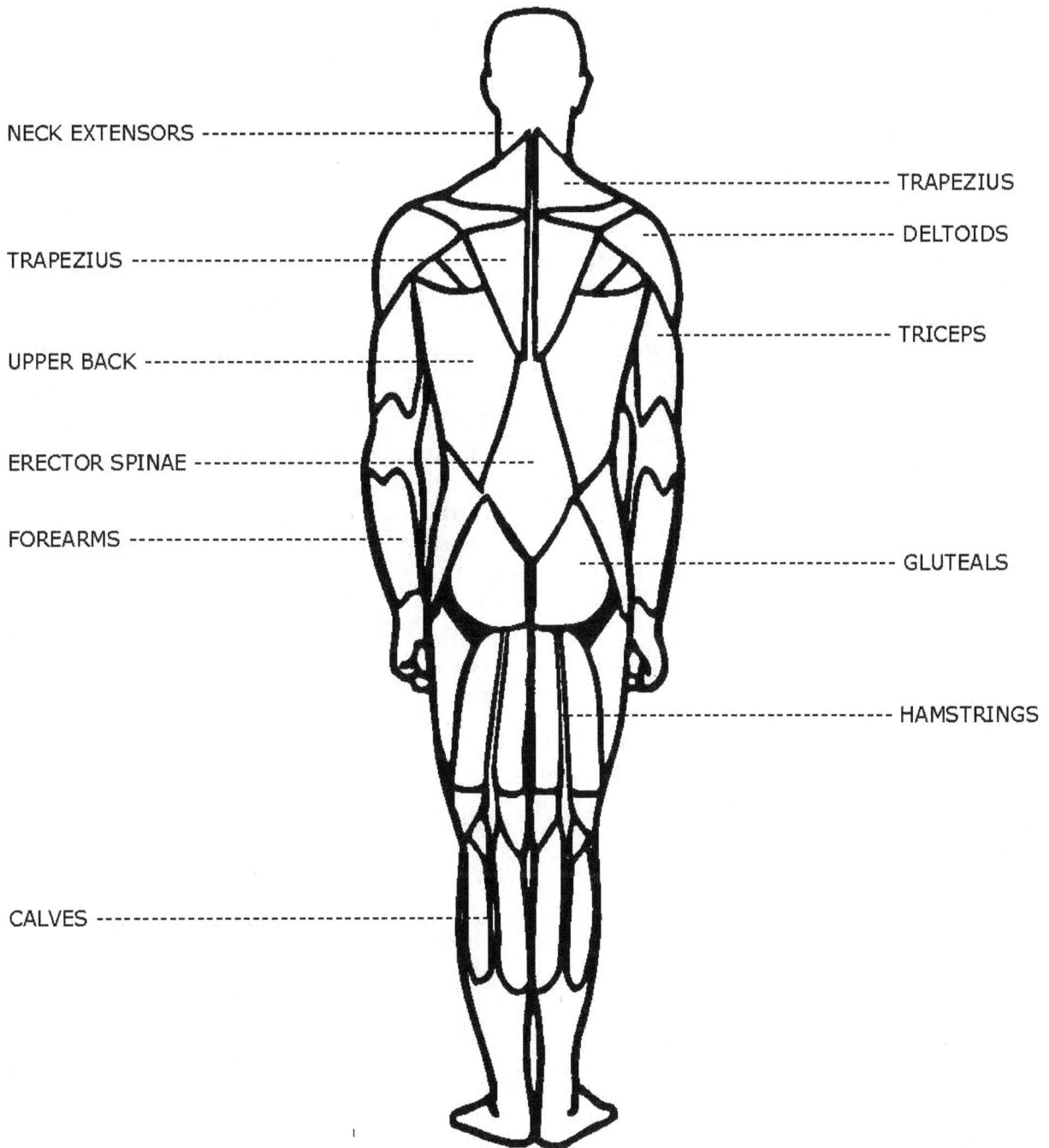

NECK EXTENSORS

TRAPEZIUS

DELTOIDS

TRAPEZIUS

TRICEPS

UPPER BACK

ERECTOR SPINAE

FOREARMS

GLUTEALS

HAMSTRINGS

CALVES

Figure 1.2: Posterior view of the muscles (artwork provided by Cybex International, Inc.)

"pour out" or turning your hand downward to empty the bowl.)

ABDOMINALS

The abdominal muscles are comprised of the rectus abdominis, obliques and transversus abdominis.

Rectus Abdominis

The muscle that comprises the outermost layer of your abdominal wall is the rectus abdominis. The fibers of this long and narrow muscle run vertically across the front of your mid-section from the lower rim of your rib cage to your pelvis. Its main function is torso flexion (pulling your torso toward your upper legs). The fibers of the rectus abdominis are interrupted along their vertical course by three horizontal fibrous bands which has inspired the term washboard abs (or six-pack abs) when describing an especially well-developed abdomen. This distinctive architecture has led to the popular but erroneous belief that the upper and lower portions of the rectus abdominis are two separate muscles. Your rectus abdominis helps to control your breathing and plays a role in forced expiration during intense exercise/activity.

Obliques

The external and internal obliques reside on both sides of your mid-section. The external oblique extends diagonally downward from your lower ribs to your pubic bone, looking somewhat like the shape of a "V." It has two main functions: torso lateral flexion (bending your torso to the same side) and torso rotation (turning your torso to the opposite side). The internal oblique – which is located immediately under the external oblique – extends diagonally upward from your pubic bone to your lower ribs, looking somewhat like the shape of an upside-down or inverted "V." It has two main functions: torso lateral flexion (bending your torso to the same side) and torso rotation (turning your torso to the same side). In a nutshell, your obliques are used during movements in which your torso bends laterally or turns. The external and internal obliques are also involved in forced expiration during intense exercise/activity.

Transversus Abdominis

The muscle that comprises the innermost layer of your abdominal wall is the transversus abdominis. The fibers of this muscle run horizontally across the front of your mid-section. The primary function of the transversus abdominis is to constrict your abdomen. Also, this muscle helps to control your breathing and, like the other abdominal muscles, is involved in forced expiration during intense exercise/activity.

LOWER BACK

The most important muscles in your lower back are the erector spinae (or spinal erectors).

Erector Spinae

Located on the posterior and lateral portion of your mid-section is a group of three muscles that are collectively known as the erector spinae (aka spinal erectors). From the medial side to the lateral side, the muscles are the spinalis, longissimus and iliocostalis. The main function of the erector spinae is torso extension (straightening your torso from a bent-over position). However, the erector spinae also assist in torso lateral flexion (bending your torso to the side) and torso rotation (turning your torso).

NECK

The major muscles of your neck include the neck flexors and neck extensors.

Neck Flexors

The muscles on the front of your neck can be collectively referred to as the neck flexors. The most prominent of these muscles is the sternocleidomastoideus. This muscle has two parts – one located on each side of your neck – that start behind your ears and run down to your sternum (breastbone) and clavicles (collarbones). When both sides of the sternocleidomastoideus contract at the same time, it results in neck flexion (bringing your head toward your chest); when one side acts alone, it results in neck lateral flexion (bending your neck to the side) or neck rotation (turning your head). Like the other muscles of the neck, your neck flexors help to stabilize your head and are used in several sports and activities, most notably soccer. (Fast fact: Humans have seven cervical vertebrae in their necks which is the same as nearly all mammals, including giraffes; each cervical vertebra of a giraffe, though, can be 10 inches long or more.)

Neck Extensors

The muscles on the back of your neck can be collectively referred to as the neck extensors. These muscles are mainly used in neck extension (bringing your head backward).

Sidebar: Perhaps the hottest topic in sports medicine is concussion awareness, prevention and management. A concussion is a traumatic injury of the brain that temporarily disrupts its normal function. According to the National High School Sports-Related Injury Surveillance System, 1.2 million injuries occurred at the scholastic level in nine sports during the 2014-15 academic year, including more than 292,000 concussions which represented 24.5% of all injuries. Although often

associated with football and other combat sports, concussions have a high prevalence in a number of other sports such as ice hockey, lacrosse and soccer. In one study, athletic trainers at 51 high schools measured the head and neck circumferences, neck length and neck strength of 6,704 athletes who played basketball, lacrosse and soccer during two different academic years. The study revealed that in comparison to uninjured athletes, concussed athletes had a smaller neck circumference; a smaller neck-to-head circumference ratio (a small neck coupled with a large head); and lower neck strength. In addition, for every one-pound increase in neck strength, there was a 5% decrease in the odds of sustaining a concussion. The researchers discovered what many have long suspected: Having a larger and stronger neck reduces the risk of concussion. Therefore, it's critical for those who participate in sports that have a high prevalence of concussions to strengthen all of the muscles that influence their necks.

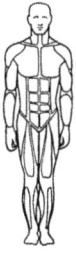

2 The Physiological Basis of Physical Training

It's beneficial for you to know how your body produces and utilizes energy during your physical training. Familiarity with these concepts will help you to understand how the physiological processes affect your physical performance. In addition, this knowledge will help you to structure your aerobic and anaerobic training in an effective manner. Also important is an understanding of the basic operations and functions of your circulatory and respiratory systems.

ADENOSINE TRIPHOSPHATE

The energy that's needed to perform muscular (mechanical) work doesn't come directly from the nutrients – the carbohydrates, protein and fat – that you consume. Instead, the energy comes from adenosine triphosphate (ATP), a molecule with a high energy yield that populates most cells, particularly muscle cells (muscle fibers). Fittingly, ATP is referred to as the energy currency of the cell. In brief, ATP liberates chemical energy that's converted into mechanical energy which is used to perform muscular work. But let's take a closer look at the process.

ATP consists of an adenosine component – made up of adenine (a nucleobase) and ribose (a sugar) – that's bonded to three phosphate groups which comprise the "business end" of the molecule. Chemical energy is stored in the two high-energy bonds that hold the phosphate groups together. When the bond between the second and third phosphate groups is broken – meaning that the outermost phosphate group is separated from the rest of the molecule – energy is released. This process yields adenosine diphosphate (ADP) and inorganic phosphate. (Fast fact: Dr. Karl Lohmann – a German physician and biochemist – discovered ATP in 1929; he initially referred to it as inosinic acid.)

THE ENERGY SYSTEMS

In order for you to perform muscular work for prolonged periods of time, a steady – and hefty – supply of ATP must be made available to your muscle fibers. How hefty? A person who weighs 154 pounds requires about 143 pounds of ATP each day. This is to say, the daily amount of ATP that's needed is almost the same as his/her bodyweight.

The problem is that the body has a limited stockpile of about 50 grams (about 1.76 ounces) of ATP. For continued exertion, then, ATP must be rebuilt by rephosphorylating ADP (that is, adding a phosphate group back to ADP). Interestingly, energy is released from the breakdown of ATP into ADP and energy is required to convert ADP back into ATP. (Fast fact: For a 154-pound individual who uses 143 pounds of ATP over the course of a day, each

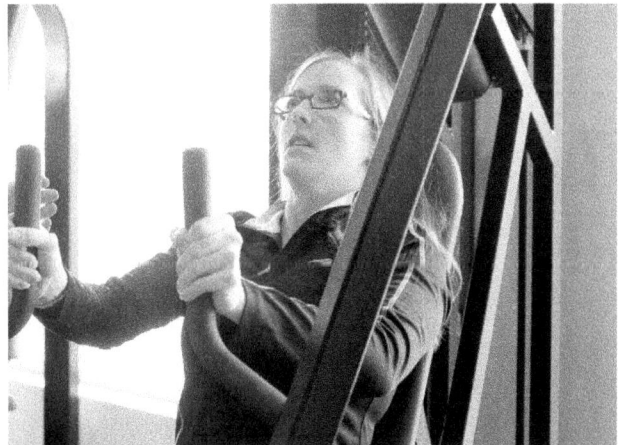

In order for you to perform muscular work for prolonged periods of time, a steady – and hefty – supply of ATP must be made available to your muscle fibers. (Photo provided by Luke Carlson.)

ATP molecule must be reassembled about 1,300 times.)

The process by which ATP is rebuilt involves the integrated efforts of three energy systems (or pathways). In essence, your energy systems have one common and primary purpose: to rebuild ATP in order to produce energy so that you can perform muscular work. Two of the energy systems can operate in the absence of oxygen and are labeled anaerobic; the other energy system can only operate in the presence of oxygen and is labeled aerobic. The two anaerobic pathways are the ATP-PC System and Anaerobic Glycolysis; the aerobic pathway is Aerobic Glycolysis.

The ATP-PC System

Your immediate, high-intensity energy system is the ATP-PC System (aka the Phosphagen System). In the ATP-PC System, ATP is rebuilt from the breakdown of phosphocreatine (PC) or, alternately, creatine phosphate (CP). Because both contain phosphate groups, ATP and PC are collectively referred to as phosphagens.

Like ATP, PC is an energized molecule that's stored in your muscle fibers. Also like ATP, PC releases energy when the bond that links the phosphate group to the rest of the molecule is broken. This process yields creatine and inorganic phosphate. The phosphate is "donated" to ADP to convert it back into ATP.

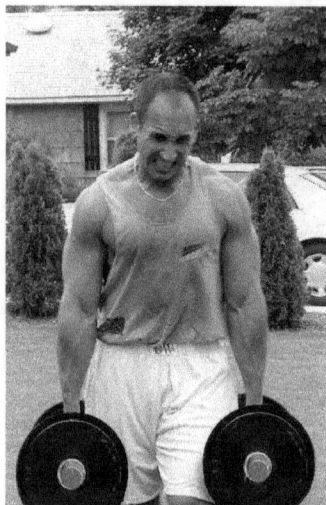

High accumulations of lactate are believed to cause feelings of heaviness in the muscles, labored breathing and fatigue. (Photo by Lori Fornicola.)

As quickly as ATP is broken down during brief, intense efforts, it's immediately and continuously reassembled until the PC stores are depleted. Ironically, PC can only be rebuilt with the energy that's released from the breakdown of ATP. (This occurs during rest or a reduced level of intensity.)

Without being rebuilt, the ATP stores in a working muscle would be spent from an all-out effort within a handful of seconds. With assistance from PC, the ATP stores in a working muscle would be spent from an all-out effort of about twice that duration.

So, the total amount of energy that's available from the ATP-PC System is very limited. Obviously, the usefulness of your stored phosphagens is in their rapid availability, not in their sheer quantity.

The ATP-PC System is mainly responsible for supplying ATP during maximum efforts that last about 10 seconds or less. This includes throwing a fastball, punting a football, spiking a volleyball, driving a golf ball and sprinting down the basketball court.

Anaerobic Glycolysis

Your short-term, high-intensity energy system is Anaerobic Glycolysis (aka the Lactic Acid System). In your body, carbohydrates are converted into glucose which can either be utilized instantly in that form or stored as glycogen in your liver and muscles for later use. The term glycolysis means to break down glucose and, as noted earlier, anaerobic means in the absence of oxygen. Therefore, Anaerobic Glycolysis literally means to break down glucose in the absence of oxygen.

It should be mentioned that the starting point of glycolysis can also be glycogen. However, glycogen must first be broken down into glucose by a process known as glycogenolysis. To be clear, glycogenolysis isn't an energy system; it's essentially an extra step that can be taken prior to glycolysis. (On a related note, the process in which glycogen is made from glucose is known as glycogenesis.)

The breakdown of glucose produces energy which is used to rebuild ATP. A complete breakdown of glucose occurs in the presence of oxygen. But because Anaerobic Glycolysis operates in the absence of oxygen, there's only a partial breakdown of glucose. This process forms pyruvate which is subsequently converted into lactate.

Sidebar: The terms are often used interchangeably but, technically, pyruvate is different from pyruvic acid; and lactate is different from lactic acid. Pyruvate and lactate are the salts of their respective acids.

When a log is burned, it leaves ash as a remnant. In this sense, lactate is the ashen remnant of Anaerobic Glycolysis. When lactate enters the blood at a greater rate than it leaves, it accumulates and becomes more concentrated. High accumulations of lactate produce an acidic environment that can irritate nerve endings and cause pain, discomfort and distress; it's also believed to cause feelings of heaviness in the muscles, labored breathing and fatigue. (Fast fact: A small amount of lactic acid is formed under resting conditions but doesn't accumulate since the rate at which it's produced equals the rate at which it's removed.)

The first minute or so of intense muscular work depends on your ability to rebuild ATP without the use of oxygen. The production of ATP is quite rapid but, in the absence of oxygen, is somewhat limited.

The ATP-PC System and Anaerobic Glycolysis are jointly responsible for supplying ATP during maximum efforts that last about 30 seconds or less. This includes sprinting about 200 meters and swimming about 50 meters. Anaerobic Glycolysis is mainly responsible for supplying ATP during maximum efforts that last between about 30 and 90 seconds. This includes running about 400 meters, swimming about 100 meters and doing a gymnastic routine on the uneven bars.

Aerobic Glycolysis

Your long-term, low-intensity energy system is Aerobic Glycolysis (aka the Aerobic System). When the anaerobic pathways are unable to keep pace with the metabolic demands of muscular work, Aerobic Glycolysis becomes the predominant energy system. Recall that the term glycolysis means to break down glucose and aerobic means in the presence of oxygen. Therefore, Aerobic Glycolysis literally means to break down glucose in the presence of oxygen.

As you can see, then, both Anaerobic Glycolysis and Aerobic Glycolysis – sometimes referred to as fast glycolysis and slow glycolysis, respectively – break down glucose. In other words, glycolytic reactions occur in both the anaerobic and aerobic realms. However, Aerobic Glycolysis can also break down fat while Anaerobic Glycolysis can only use glucose. (Protein isn't a preferred source of energy.)

Because Aerobic Glycolysis operates in the presence of oxygen, there's a complete breakdown of glucose. This process forms pyruvate which is subsequently converted into carbon dioxide and water. (Recall that during Anaerobic Glycolysis – in the absence of oxygen – pyruvate is converted into lactate.) Carbon dioxide is continually removed by the blood and transported to the lungs where it's exhaled; water is either used in the cells or excreted in the urine.

The process of rebuilding ATP aerobically occurs in specialized organelles (subunits) of muscle fibers known as mitochondria (the singular of which is mitochondrion). Given that a mitochondrion produces such a large amount of energy, it's often referred to as the powerhouse of the cell. Muscle fibers are usually very rich in mitochondria; in particular, an abundance of mitochondria resides in cardiac muscle (which is found in the walls of your heart) and slow-twitch muscle fibers.

The longer the duration of an activity, the greater the reliance on Aerobic Glycolysis. The major advantage of Aerobic Glycolysis is that it produces a relatively large amount of ATP. But the need to transport and deliver oxygen makes it a time-consuming operation. (Fast fact: Oddly enough, Aerobic Glycolysis is also the predominant energy system under resting conditions.)

Anaerobic Glycolysis and Aerobic Glycolysis are jointly responsible for supplying ATP during

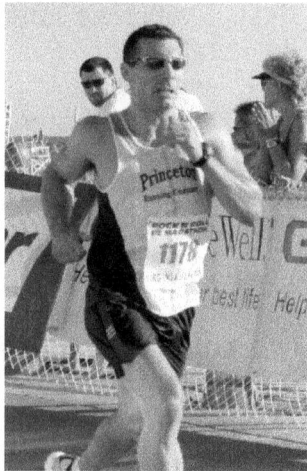

Aerobic Glycolysis is mainly responsible for supplying ATP during physical efforts that last about three minutes or more. (Photo provided by Ryan Bonfiglio.)

physical efforts that last between about 1.5 and 3.0 minutes. This includes running about 800 meters, swimming about 200 meters, rowing about 500 meters, wrestling a two-minute period and boxing a three-minute round. Aerobic Glycolysis is mainly responsible for supplying ATP during physical efforts that last about three minutes or more. This includes rowing 2,000 meters, swimming 500 meters, cycling five miles and running a marathon.

THE "ENERGY CONTINUUM"

The need for a particular energy system is determined by the time and intensity requirements of a specific activity. At one end of the energy continuum is the ATP-PC System which is the predominant energy pathway for immediate, high-intensity efforts; at the other end of the energy continuum is Aerobic Glycolysis which is the predominant energy system for long-term, low-intensity efforts. In between these two extremes is Anaerobic Glycolysis which partners with either the ATP-PC System or Aerobic Glycolysis to supply energy for short-term, high-intensity efforts. So the production of ATP can be immediate (the ATP-PC System), short term (Anaerobic Glycolysis) or long term (Aerobic Glycolysis).

Your body uses the energy system(s) that's available to meet the existing metabolic challenge. Generally, the most efficient energy system(s) is deployed to maximize the resynthesis of ATP and minimize the accumulation of lactic acid.

Blood lactate is an excellent indicator of which energy system you mainly used during your effort. A high level of blood lactate indicates that the primary energy system was Anaerobic Glycolysis; a low level of blood lactate indicates that the primary energy system was Aerobic Glycolysis.

Although one of your energy systems may serve as the principal means of supplying ATP to meet your particular needs, all three systems contribute to the performance of most sports and activities. For example, playing full-court basketball is mainly anaerobic because it involves a series of brief, all-out efforts such as sprinting, jumping and so on. But it also has an aerobic component since the anaerobic efforts are required over an extended period of time. So, energy is needed from the anaerobic pathways as well as the aerobic pathway. In fact, a blend of all energy systems is the most likely scenario for the majority of sports and activities that you might perform.

Remember that as the time of an activity increases, the energy continuum shifts away from anaerobic work toward aerobic work. It should also be noted that your energy systems operate in phases on a progressive scale. Moreover, your body doesn't shift abruptly from one energy system to another; the transition between the energy systems is very subtle. In a sense, all three energy systems overlap each other. Clearly, if you can improve the efficiency of your energy systems through physical training, then you can also improve your performance potential.

To summarize the responsibilities of the energy systems across the energy continuum: The ATP-PC System for maximum efforts of about 10 seconds or less; the ATP-PC System and Anaerobic Glycolysis for maximum efforts of about 30 seconds or less; Anaerobic Glycolysis for maximum efforts of about 30 to 90 seconds; Anaerobic Glycolysis and Aerobic Glycolysis for physical efforts of about 1.5 to 3.0 minutes; and Aerobic Glycolysis for physical efforts of about three minutes or more.

LACTIC ACID: A CLOSER LOOK

For many years, lactic acid was thought to be the primary suspect in muscular fatigue and, consequently, the root cause of the decline in performance during high-intensity activity. But a 1986 study challenged this belief and, in the process, kicked off a heated controversy about the role of lactic acid. The argument escalated in 2004 when an editorial in *Science* referred to lactic acid as "the latest performance-enhancing drug." Adding fuel to the fire was a series of highly contentious debates in at least two scientific journals in 2005 and 2006 and an article in *The New York Times* in 2006.

Scientists have taken sides and made compelling cases for their respective position. According to one tribe, conditions other than the accumulation of lactic acid cause muscular fatigue. These scientists point to research that shows lactic acid doesn't cause muscular fatigue; rather, lactic acid *delays* muscular fatigue. According to another tribe, most of the research that shows lactic acid doesn't cause muscular fatigue examined muscle fibers from animals – such as frogs and rats – in which the cell membrane had been "skinned" (removed) or from isolated non-contracting muscle. These scientists point out that the results from such studies can't be extrapolated or generalized to humans and real-life scenarios in which muscle fibers operate as a system.

So, is lactic acid a friend or a fiend? At this point in time, it's too hard to tell. Clearly, muscular fatigue is a complex biochemical process. Future research may offer definitive proof about the exact role of lactic acid (though characterizing it as a "performance-enhancing drug" seems to be quite a stretch). While scientists sort things out, it's safe to say that lactic acid might not be the main perpetrator in muscular fatigue but it's certainly a contributor. (Fast fact: Lactic acid was discovered by Carl Wilhelm Scheele – a German-Swedish chemist – in 1780; he's also credited with discovering oxygen – yes, *oxygen* – in or around 1774.)

The Lactate Shuttle Hypothesis

Related to the dispute about the role of lactic acid is the lactate shuttle hypothesis, a concept that's not without its own share of controversy. The lactate shuttle hypothesis was launched in 1984 by Dr. George Brooks at a scientific meeting in Belgium and published the next year. (In his words, "the initial reaction [to the hypothesis] was mixed.")

In 1998, Dr. Brooks modified his original hypothesis to include two types of shuttles: intracellular (within cells) and extracellular (between cells). According to the hypothesis, intracellular lactate shuttles transport lactate from the cytoplasm (the fluid within a cell) into the mitochondria where it's converted back into pyruvate; extracellular lactate shuttles transport lactate between fast-twitch fibers and slow-twitch fibers as well as to the liver where it's converted back into glucose by a process known as gluconeogenesis (which literally means the formation of new glucose). Your muscles can use this glucose to rebuild ATP.

While scientists have generally accepted the extracellular lactate shuttle, there's a good bit of disagreement about the intracellular lactate shuttle. In short, the fate of lactate is subject to debate.

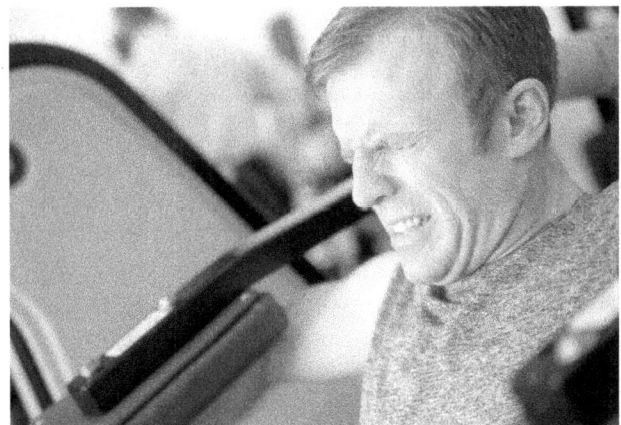

It's important for you to make your physical training progressively more challenging in order to provide an overload. (Photo provided by Luke Carlson.)

Lactate Threshold

It was mentioned earlier that a small amount of lactic acid is formed under resting conditions. However, under resting conditions, the rate at which lactic acid is produced equals the rate at which it's removed. When lactic acid – lactate – is produced at a greater rate than it's removed, it begins to accumulate in the blood. The point at which there's a sharp rise in blood lactate is known as the lactate threshold.

Sidebar: Anaerobic threshold is often used interchangeably with lactate threshold. However, use of the term anaerobic threshold – which was coined by Drs. Karlman Wasserman and Malcolm McIlroy in 1964 – has fallen out of favor, mainly because it promotes the misconception that there's a starting point (or "threshold") for anaerobic glycolysis.

You can improve your lactate threshold through training but the degree to which it can be improved is largely determined by your genetics. Being able to delay and/or tolerate the accumulation of blood lactate allows an individual to perform with a high level of intensity for a sustained length of time with less fatigue. Everything else being equal, those who have a higher lactate threshold have a greater potential to resist fatigue during prolonged activities than those who have a lower lactate threshold.

Here's an illustration: Oxygen intake – which is discussed in detail in Chapter 14 – is an excellent indicator of aerobic fitness. Consider two female athletes who have the same oxygen intake but different lactate thresholds. Suppose that Athlete A has a higher lactate threshold and, as a result, can sustain 75 to 85% of her maximum oxygen intake and Athlete B can sustain 50 to 60% of her maximum oxygen intake. Since Athlete A can perform at a higher percentage of her maximum oxygen intake than Athlete B, everything else being equal, Athlete A would have a greater aerobic potential. Or look at it this way: For the same level of effort, the point at which lactic acid rises sharply in the blood would occur much sooner in Athlete B than in Athlete A. This would put Athlete B at a huge disadvantage.

Underscoring this point further is an interesting anecdote about Lance Armstrong and lactic acid. Armstrong was a professional road-racing cyclist who won the Tour de France a record seven consecutive times from 1999 to 2005. His victories and other achievements were erased in 2012 due to his use of performance-enhancing drugs (which he had vehemently denied for many years). Nonetheless, in those days, Armstrong was one of the top endurance athletes on the planet. From 1992 to 1999, Armstrong underwent extensive physiological testing that was conducted by Dr. Edward Coyle at the Human Performance Laboratory at the University of Texas at Austin. Dr. Coyle discovered two important things about Armstrong and lactic acid: Compared to other athletes of his caliber, he accumulated less of it and tolerated more of it. When tested in January 1993, Armstrong accumulated 30 to 55% less blood lactate during exhaustive exercise (stationary cycling) than all of the other competitive cyclists who had ever been tested at the same laboratory. In addition, Armstrong had a high lactate threshold. In untrained individuals, lactate threshold occurs around 50 to 60% of maximum oxygen intake; in trained individuals, it's around 65 to 85%. When tested in November 1992, Armstrong's lactate threshold occurred at 85% of his maximum oxygen intake which on that day was 70.5 milliliters per kilogram of bodyweight per minute (mL/kg/min); in September 1993, it was 81.2 mL/kg/min. (Dr. Coyle estimated that during Armstrong's string of victories in the Tour de France, his maximum oxygen intake was at least 85.0 mL/kg/min, a value that's among the highest ever reported for any endurance athlete. Not for any competitive cyclist, for *any endurance athlete.*) In effect, his high lactate threshold enabled him to perform with a level of effort that was closer to his aerobic limits in comparison to most individuals. (Besides having a high lactate threshold and high oxygen intake, Armstrong's muscular efficiency while pedaling a stationary cycle was extraordinary. More on that point in a bit.)

Similar findings were reported on Paula Radcliffe, the current world-record holder in the women's marathon with a time of 2:15:25 which was set way back in 2003. From 1991 to 2003, Radcliffe underwent extensive physiological testing that was conducted by Dr. Andrew Jones at the University of Exeter in the United Kingdom. Dr. Jones discovered that Radcliffe – who has run three of the four fastest times ever by a woman in the marathon – accumulated roughly half as much blood lactate during exhaustive exercise (treadmill running) than other highly competitive runners. This, combined with excellent running economy and an oxygen intake that was way "off the charts" for a woman – consistently hovering around 70.0 mL/kg/min with a high mark of 80.0 mL/kg/min – gave her an enormous physiological advantage as a long-distance runner. (Fast fact: Lactate threshold, oxygen intake and economy – the amount of work that's done by the metabolic, neuromuscular and biomechanical systems in relation to the energy that's expended – are considered to be the three main predictors of success in endurance activities.)

The physiological responses of Armstrong and Radcliffe in comparison to other elite athletes in their corresponding sports are remarkably consistent with a study of 12 female cross-country skiers from Norway; six were world-class athletes and six were national-class athletes. When roller skiing at the same speed, the world-class athletes accumulated 34.7% and 50.0% less blood lactate than the national-class athletes while double poling and diagonal striding, respectively. (They also had significantly lower heart rates and ratings of perceived exertion than the national-class athletes.)

PHYSIOLOGICAL OVERLOAD

Any type of physical training – whether it's done for anaerobic, aerobic, strength, flexibility, metabolic, power or skill improvements – must incorporate what's become perhaps the most widely referenced tenet in exercise science namely, the Overload Principle. The term overload means that a targeted physiological and/or neurological system is made to work harder than it's accustomed to working by being exposed to progressively greater demands. Among other things, this suggests that your effort must surpass a threshold in order to trigger what's known as compensatory adaptation. (More information about the Overload Principle and compensatory adaptation is discussed in Chapter 4.)

Over a period of time, you'll likely find that the same activity – which was originally difficult – can be performed with less effort. As a result, it's important for you to make your physical training progressively more challenging in order to provide an overload and produce further physiological improvements in the target system (such as your musculoskeletal, respiratory and/ or circulatory system).

Because of this, it's vital that you keep accurate records of your physical performances. Maintaining records permits you to track your progress thereby making your workouts more productive and more meaningful.

THE "ULTIMATE PUMP"

A thorough discussion about the physiological basis of physical training wouldn't be complete without mention of the most important muscle in your body and primary driving force behind the three energy systems: your heart. The heart is a large, hollow, cone-shaped organ that's located just behind your sternum (breastbone). It's about 5.0 inches long, 3.5 inches wide and 2.5 inches thick, roughly the size of a man's clenched fist. The average adult male heart weighs about 10 ounces while its female counterpart weighs about eight ounces.

Your heart is the ultimate endurance muscle or "pump." It contracts about 100,000 times each day, pausing only briefly after a contraction to fill with more blood for its next contraction. This muscular pump is comprised of left and right halves. Each half of your heart consists of two chambers: an atrium and a ventricle. The atria are the recovery chambers of your heart and the ventricles are the pumping chambers.

Your blood has two routes or circuits: the systemic circuit and the pulmonary circuit. In the systemic circuit, the powerful left ventricle of your heart pumps oxygen-enriched blood to your body tissues (such as your skeletal muscles). The blood collects carbon dioxide and other metabolic wastes and returns to the right atrium of your heart. In the pulmonary circuit, the right ventricle of your heart sends oxygen-depleted blood that's laden with carbon dioxide to your lungs. The blood drops off carbon dioxide, picks up oxygenated blood and returns to the left atrium of your heart.

Normally, the right half of your heart pumps the same amount of blood as the left half of your heart. However, the left half of your heart is much stronger and better developed than the right half. This is because the left half of your heart must pump blood throughout your entire body (the systemic circuit) while the right half only has to pump blood to your lungs (the pulmonary circuit).

Heart Rate

As the blood surges out of the ventricles, it pounds the arterial wall. This impact is transmitted along the length of the artery and can be felt as a throb or a "pulse" at those points where an artery is just under your skin. The beat of your pulse is synchronous with the beat of your heart.

To a degree, the rate of the heartbeat is dependent on the size of the organism. A good rule of thumb is that the smaller the size of the organism, the faster the beat of the heart. A normal resting heart rate for humans is about 60 to 80 beats per minute (bpm). A woman's heart beats about six to eight times per minute faster than a man's. A child's heart beats even more rapidly. At birth, a baby's heart rate could be as high as 130 bpm. Animals that are larger than humans have slower heart rates; an elephant's heart rate is about 30 bpm. Animals that are smaller than humans have faster heart rates; a shrew's heart rate is more than 800 bpm. (Fast fact: The Etruscan shrew holds the distinction of having perhaps the highest heart rate ever recorded in any animal with 1,511 bpm.)

Active individuals usually have lower resting heart rates than inactive individuals. It wouldn't be unusual for a person who's highly active to have a resting heart rate of 50 bpm or less. This is especially important since a lower resting heart rate is a predictor of cardiovascular risk and mortality. Related to this is the notion that the heart is limited to a certain number of beats over the course of a lifetime. For instance, suppose that the human heart can only beat about 2.5 billion times before it simply wears out from the labors of continual usage. In this scenario, an individual who has an average resting heart rate of 70 bpm could expect to live a little less than 68 years; on the other hand, an individual who has an average resting heart rate of 60 bpm could expect to live a little more than 79 years. If there's a limit to the number of times that a heart can beat in a lifetime, a decrease in the resting heart rate of just 10 bpm would translate into more than 11 additional years of life. While this idea hasn't been proven scientifically, it's still quite intriguing. And it does underscore the importance of having a lower resting heart rate.

Blood Pressure

When your heart forces blood through your circulatory system, the fluid is under pressure. Your blood pressure is a measure of the force that's exerted by your blood against the arterial walls. Blood pressure has two measures: systolic and diastolic. Your systolic blood pressure is the maximum pressure in your arteries when your ventricles contract; your diastolic blood pressure is the maximum pressure when your ventricles recover (refilling with blood).

Blood pressure is measured in milliliters of mercury (mmHg). An example of a blood-pressure reading would be 120/80 in which the upper number (120) is the systolic pressure and the lower number (80) is the diastolic pressure.

Of no small concern is high blood pressure (hypertension). The 2017 Hypertension Clinical Practice Guidelines from the American Heart Association and the American College of Cardiology redefined the categories of resting blood pressure for adults. Normal is a systolic pressure of less than 120 *and* a diastolic pressure of less than 80; elevated is a systolic pressure of 120 to 129 *and* a diastolic pressure of less than

80; stage 1 hypertension is a systolic pressure of 130 to 139 *or* a diastolic pressure of 80 to 89; stage 2 hypertension is a systolic pressure of at least 140 *or* a diastolic of at least 90; and hypertensive crisis is a systolic pressure that's higher than 180 *and/or* a diastolic that's higher than 120. (Fast fact: The Centers for Disease Control and Prevention estimate that more than 75 million American adults – one out of three adults – have hypertension.)

Those in the latter category should consult with their physician immediately. Those who have chronic high blood pressure should consult with their physician. The same holds true for those who have chronic low blood pressure (aka hypotension). Note that if the systolic and diastolic pressures are in two different categories, the classification is based on the higher category. For instance, if the systolic pressure is 120 (elevated) and the diastolic pressure is 80 (stage 1 hypertension), the classification would be stage 1 hypertension.

THE RESPIRATORY PROCESS

Respiration is a combination of inspiration and expiration. Inspiration (or inhalation) is an active process in which your lungs inflate and air enters your body. Expiration (or exhalation) is a passive process in which your lungs deflate and air exits your body. During intense exercise/ activity, however, expiration is an active process which is referred to as forced expiration.

The primary muscle of inspiration is your diaphragm. Located in your upper abdominal cavity, the diaphragm is a large, dome-shaped sheet of muscle. Lending some assistance to the diaphragm are your external intercostal muscles (which reside between your ribs along with your internal intercostal muscles). Forced expiration involves your abdominal muscles and internal intercostal muscles.

The respiratory process is accomplished without continuous conscious effort. Actually, respiration is a rhythmic action: Inflation of your lungs during inspiration causes expiration; deflation of your lungs during expiration causes inspiration.

Your respiratory system has two major functions: to exchange gases and maintain your acid-base balance.

GAS EXCHANGE

Your diaphragm – with assistance from your external intercostals in conjunction with the natural changes of pressures within your body – produces an open exchange of oxygen and carbon dioxide. The right ventricle pumps venous blood to your lungs that's low in oxygen and high in carbon dioxide. In the lungs, your blood unloads carbon dioxide and loads oxygen. The blood returns to the left atrium as arterial blood that's high in oxygen and low in carbon dioxide.

A second exchange of gases occurs between your blood and tissues. In this case, your left ventricle pumps arterial blood to your tissues that's high in oxygen and low in carbon dioxide. In the tissues, the blood unloads oxygen and loads carbon dioxide. Essentially, this gas exchange converts arterial blood into venous blood. The venous blood returns to your right atrium where the entire process of gas exchange and transport is repeated over and over again.

Acid-Base Balance

The respiratory process also maintains harmony between the acidity and alkalinity of your blood. This is known as the acid-base balance. The inability to remove and/or buffer certain substances that form as a result of intense efforts will tip the delicate acid-base balance toward an environment that's either too acidic (acidosis) or too basic (alkalosis) and spawn a variety of physiological disturbances.

In particular, an environment that's too acidic contributes to muscular fatigue and may inhibit the biochemical reactions that are needed for energy production. Acidosis can have respiratory or metabolic causes. Respiratory acidosis results when carbon dioxide is produced at a greater rate than it leaves; metabolic acidosis results when lactate (lactic acid) enters your blood at a greater rate than it leaves.

Sidebar: A direct measure of acidity or alkalinity is pH (which stands for potential of hydrogen). In 1909, Dr. Søren Sørensen – a

Danish chemist – introduced the pH scale; it ranges from 0 to 14. A pH that's less than 7.0 is acidic while a pH that's more than 7.0 is alkaline (or "basic"); a pH of 7.0 is neutral. The lower the pH is from 7.0, the greater the acidity; the higher the pH is from 7.0, the greater the alkalinity. It's important to note that the pH scale is logarithmic in that the units differ by multiples of 10. For example, a pH of 5.0 is 10 times more acidic than a pH of 6.0 and 100 times more acidic than a pH of 7.0; a pH of 9.0 is 10 times more alkaline than a pH of 8.0 and 100 times more alkaline than a pH of 7.0. At rest, the pH of venous blood and arterial blood is about 7.35 and 7.4, respectively. The approximate pH of some common substances includes 0.0 for battery acid; 2.0 for vinegar; 2.3 for lemon juice; 2.4 for Coca-Cola® and Pepsi®; 2.8 for 5-Hour Energy™; 3.0 for Gatorade® Lemon-Lime; 3.4 for Red Bull®; 3.8 for orange juice; 4.0 for tomato juice; 4.2 for Listerine®; 5.1 for Starbucks® Regular Roast coffee; 6.5 for milk; 7.0 for distilled water; 9.0 for baking soda; 12.0 for Clorox® Regular-Bleach; and 14.0 for liquid drain cleaner.

BETTER FUNCTION = BETTER PERFORMANCE

As you improve the functional ability of your energy systems through physical training, you'll be better suited to delay and/or tolerate the accumulation of blood lactate, discard waste products and exchange gases thereby postponing muscular fatigue. Otherwise, you must abbreviate – or perhaps even terminate – your activities until you re-establish a metabolic environment that can accommodate your efforts.

Being able to resist fatigue is an absolute requirement for training, practicing and competing at high levels. It's clear that your physical performance is linked to the development and improvement of your three energy systems.

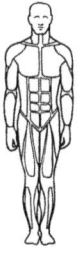

3 Genetics and Strength Potential

Genetics is the study of heredity. It's well known that people inherit a variety of physical and behavioral traits from their parents. These traits are passed along from one generation to the next by genes which are made of deoxyribonucleic acid (DNA).

MAJOR MOMENTS IN HISTORY

Early research in genetics dates back to the mid-1850s. From 1856 to 1863, Gregor (nee Johann) Mendel – an Austrian monk – conducted experiments with pea plants to learn how traits were inherited. He presented the results of his studies in 1865 and published the results the following year. Mendel is credited with identifying three principles (or laws) of heredity. For his significant contributions, Mendel is recognized as the father of modern genetics.

Mendel's work was largely overlooked until it was rediscovered in 1900, nearly four decades or so after he completed his now famous experiments (and long after his death in 1884). Later that decade, the terms genetics and gene entered scientific lingo. In 1905, William Bateson – an English biologist – coined the term genetics; and in 1909, Wilhelm Johannsen – a Danish botanist – coined the term gene.

The history of genetics is replete with important events on its timeline that pertain to DNA. In 1869, Dr. Friedrich Miescher – a Swiss physician and professor of physiology – separated nucleic acids from cells, thus isolating DNA. In 1944, an experiment by Drs. Oswald Avery, Colin MacLeod and Maclyn McCarty – all physicians and researchers – suggested that DNA was the hereditary molecule. **In 1952, a series of experiments by Drs.** Alfred Hershey and Martha Chase – both American geneticists – confirmed the role of DNA.

In 1953, Dr. James Watson and Francis Crick cemented their place in history with a discovery of epic proportions. While working at the University of Cambridge, their scientific backgrounds proved to be highly compatible: Watson was a geneticist doing post-graduate work and Crick was a physicist working on his doctoral degree in biophysics. In the April 25 issue of *Nature*, they proposed the double-helical structure – think twisted ladder – that's now readily recognized as the shape of DNA. The somewhat unassuming article – it was barely more than one page in length and accompanied by a hand-sketched diagram of DNA that was done by Crick's wife, Odile – would become a launching pad for future investigations in genetics. In this regard, it would be remiss not to acknowledge the contributions of Drs. Maurice Wilkins and Rosalind Franklin. While at King's College in London, the two co-workers provided invaluable information to Watson and Crick that contributed to their model of DNA. In 1962, Watson and Crick shared the Nobel Prize in Physiology or Medicine with Dr. Wilkins; Dr. Franklin was inexplicably snubbed. (Fast fact: Dr. Wilkins – referred to as "the third man of the double helix" in his autobiography – was a physicist who had worked on the Manhattan Project, helping to develop the atomic bomb.)

The Human Genome Project began in 1990 with the goal of sequencing and mapping all of the human genes (which are collectively referred to as the genome). This massive undertaking – billed as "nature's complete genetic blueprint for building a human being" – was completed in April 2013. At the start of the project, scientists believed that humans had as many as 100,000 genes or more. It has since been determined that humans have a mere 20,500 genes. By contrast, a tomato has more than 30,000 genes. Think

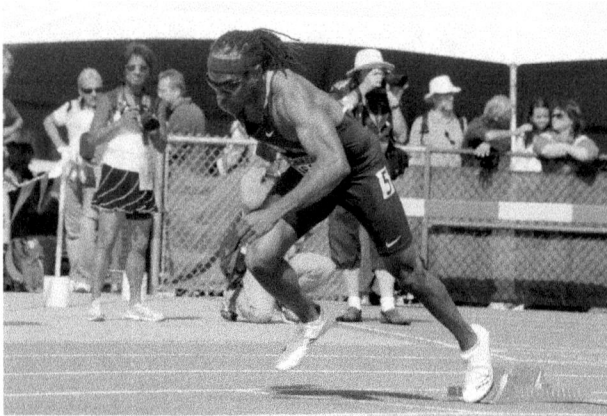

Those who have a high percentage of fast-twitch fibers include highly accomplished sprinters and others whose success is predicated on speed, strength and power. (Photo by Ken Stone.)

about this the next time that you reach for a bottle of ketchup.

Sidebar: Chimpanzees – "our closest living relatives" – have 86 genes that we lack and we have 689 genes that chimpanzees lack. All told, about 93.6% of the "gene pool" is the same between humans and chimps.

GENETIC VARIATION

The potential for genetic variation is simply enormous. These variations are most evident in physical appearance and include eye color, hair color, nose shape, hair distribution and skeletal height. (Fast fact: Genetic variation also influences handedness; roughly 10% of the population are lefties.)

Genetic variation plays an extremely important role in a person's response to strength training. Because of genetic variation, some people make superior gains in strength (and size) while others make inferior gains, even when employing the same strength program (performing the same exercises and set/repetition scheme). The fact of the matter is that each individual inherits a unique genetic profile with a unique genetic potential for improving strength (and size). This may even be true of identical twins since, according to at least one study, identical twins might not be identical.

GENETIC FACTORS

A number of genetic factors determine your response to strength training. These include the following:

Muscle Fiber Type

One of the most influential of all genetic factors is your muscle fiber type. Muscle fibers can be broadly categorized into two major types: slow twitch (ST) or Type I and fast twitch (FT) or Type II. (The term twitch refers to contraction of a single muscle fiber.) From a functional standpoint, muscle fibers differ in several ways, including speed of contraction, magnitude of force and degree of fatigability.

Relative to FT fibers, ST fibers contract slower, produce less force and have more endurance; relative to ST fibers, FT fibers contract faster, produce more force and have less endurance.

Sidebar: This isn't to say that ST fibers contract slowly. ST fibers contract quickly but not as quickly as FT fibers. The contraction time of fibers is measured in *thousandths of a second*. The time to peak force is about 50 milliseconds in FT fibers and about 100 milliseconds in ST fibers. To put this into perspective, a proverbial "blink of an eye" takes about 300 milliseconds.

Because of their fatigue characteristics, ST fibers are often referred to as being oxidative, meaning that the fibers are highly aerobic and heavily dependent on oxygen for energy; FT fibers are often referred to as being glycolytic, meaning that the fibers are highly anaerobic and heavily dependent on glucose for energy. (Fast fact: Research has also identified five intermediate or "hybrid" fiber types that possess varying characteristics of both FT and ST fibers.)

Most muscles have a blend of about 50% ST fibers and 50% FT fibers but some muscles have a higher proportion of one type or the other. For example, the soleus tends to have a greater percentage of ST fibers (as much as 85%) as do the so-called postural muscles (which include the trapezius and lower back); the triceps tend to have a greater percentage of FT fibers (as much as 70%). Regardless of the distribution, the different fiber types are intermingled throughout each muscle, arranged in a mosaic pattern.

Some individuals inherit a higher-than-average proportion of one fiber type that influences their performance potential in sports and activities that require speed, strength and endurance. It has been noted that FT fibers contract faster and produce more force than ST fibers. (The greater production of force is mainly because FT fibers have a larger diameter than ST fibers.) Everything else being equal, those who have a high percentage of FT fibers have a greater potential to exhibit speed, strength and power than those who have a low percentage of FT fibers. Examples are highly accomplished sprinters, competitive weightlifters and others whose success is predicated on speed, strength and power. Everything else being equal, those who have a high percentage of ST fibers have a greater potential to exhibit endurance than those who have a low percentage of ST fibers. Examples are highly accomplished long-distance runners, triathletes and others whose success is predicated on endurance. (Really fast fact: One study found that the percentage of fast-twitch fibers in the vastus lateralis and gastrocnemius of wild cheetahs – the fastest mammals on land with top running speeds of more than 60 miles per hour – is 75.9% and 58.5%, respectively.)

It should be mentioned that an individual's fiber-type mixture can vary from one muscle to another. And the mixture may even vary from one side of the body to the other. In one study,

for instance, there was a 26% difference in the proportion of ST fibers in the vastus lateralis of a volleyball player (73% in the right leg and 47% in the left).

Hypertrophy refers to an increase in the size of an organ or a tissue due to an increase in the *size* of cells (or fibers); atrophy refers to a decrease in the size of an organ or a tissue due to a decrease in the size of cells. Both FT and ST fibers have the potential for hypertrophy. However, FT fibers display a much greater potential for hypertrophy than ST fibers. This means that individuals who have a high percentage of FT fibers have a greater potential to increase the size of their muscles. It's interesting to note that FT fibers not only hypertrophy faster and to a greater degree than ST fibers but also atrophy faster and to a greater degree.

Incidentally, there's no scientific evidence that consistently and convincingly supports the notion that ST fibers can be converted into FT fibers or vice versa. It appears as if one type of muscle fiber may take on certain metabolic characteristics of another type but actual conversion doesn't occur. Stated differently, you can't convert one fiber type into another any more than you can convert lead into gold. Simply put, it's impossible to switch the twitch.

While on the subject, hyperplasia refers to an increase in the size of an organ or a tissue due to an increase in the *number* of cells. Hyperplasia is thought to take place by fiber splitting or

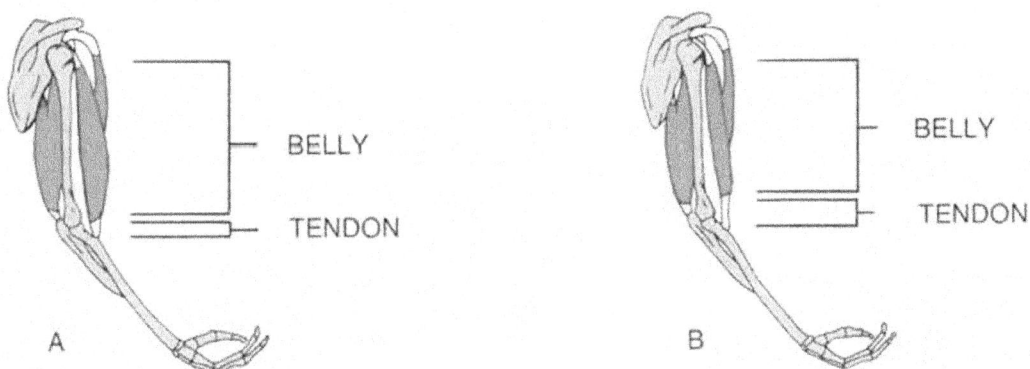

Figure 3.1: Muscle-to-tendon ratio

budding. Although hyperplasia has been demonstrated experimentally in the muscle tissue of several avian and mammalian species – including quails, chickens, cats, rats and mice – there's no definitive proof that it occurs in the muscle tissue of humans. Most likely, strength training results in the addition of protein filaments – namely, actin and myosin – not in the addition of muscle fibers. (Fast fact: In humans, certain cells do undergo hyperplasia, including those of the adrenal glands and prostate gland; other cells don't undergo hyperplasia, including those of the brain, heart and muscle.)

One last point in this regard pertains to charts that indicate how many repetitions you should strive to perform with a percentage your one-repetition maximum (1-RM; the maximum weight that you can lift one time). Because the proportion of FT and ST fibers has a major role in muscular endurance, the number of repetitions that can be done with the same percentage of a 1-RM won't be the same for everyone; individuals who have a high percentage of FT fibers aren't likely to do as many repetitions as individuals who have a high percentage of ST fibers. In effect, achieving the recommended number of repetitions could be too difficult – or outright impossible – for some and too easy for others. So, these charts are only applicable to the segment of the population that happens to have inherited a mixture of fiber types that corresponds to the suggested repetitions.

Muscle-to-Tendon Ratio

The muscle organ consists of two parts: the belly (primarily muscle fibers) and the tendon (the fibrous connective tissue). The potential for a muscle to increase in size is related to the length of its belly and tendon. Everything else being equal, those who have long bellies and short tendons have a greater potential for achieving muscular size than those who have short bellies and long tendons.

Consider two individuals who have the same bone lengths but different muscle-to-tendon ratios. Suppose that Lifter A has a long bicep muscle and a short bicep tendon and Lifter B has a short bicep muscle and a long bicep tendon. In

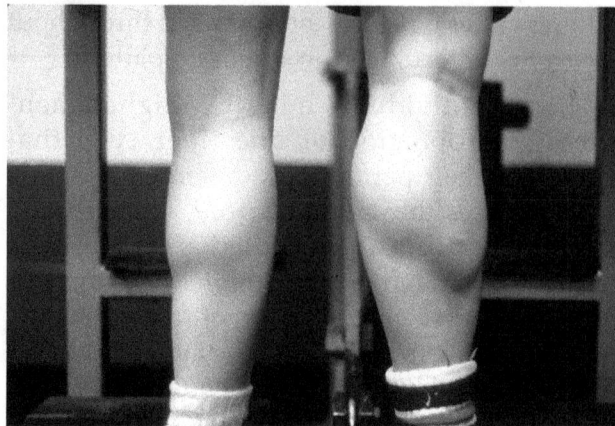

The dramatic impact of muscle-to-tendon ratios can be seen in this photograph of two individuals who are contracting their calves.

this example, as depicted in Figure 3.1, Lifter A has a greater potential to increase the size of his bicep than Lifter B.

The dramatic impact of muscle-to-tendon ratios can be seen in the photograph above of two individuals who are contracting their calves. Note that the lengths of their lower legs are roughly the same. But the lengths of their muscle bellies and tendons are very different which dictates the size of their muscles. The individual on the right has a much longer muscle belly and shorter tendon than the individual on the left. At the time of the photograph, both individuals – female collegiate gymnasts in their freshman year – were training partners who had been doing the same strength program for nearly eight months, performing the same exercises and set/repetition scheme.

But how is the muscle-to-tendon ratio associated with strength potential? To understand this better, think about the cross-sectional area of a muscle. A cross-section is a cut that's made perpendicular to a structure. If you cut down a tree in this manner and looked down at the stump, you'd see the cross-section of the tree. The size of that surface is its cross-sectional area.

Now, think about the cross-sectional area of a muscle this way. A bigger muscle has a larger cross-sectional area. A larger cross-sectional area contains a greater number of protein filaments (actin and myosin) and cross-bridges thereby

26

increasing the capacity to produce force. Therefore, a bigger muscle – in terms of its cross-sectional area – is also a stronger muscle. This means that individuals with long muscle bellies have the potential to be quite strong.

Sidebar: The amount of force that a muscle can produce per unit of cross-sectional area is known as specific tension. It's thought that the specific tension of muscle is about 29.0 to 43.5 pounds of force per square inch. So, 1.5 square inches of muscle can produce about 43.5 to 65.25 pounds of force; 2.0 square inches of muscle – a bigger cross-sectional area – can produce about 58.0 to 87.0 pounds of force. Interestingly enough, the specific tension of a muscle is about the same as the specific tension of a myosin filament only on a much smaller scale, of course.

So why, then, do so many successful runners and jumpers have long Achilles tendons and short calf muscles? Well, when the foot strikes the ground while running and jumping, the Achilles tendon stretches and absorbs the force of the impact. The force is stored as potential energy which is then immediately released as kinetic energy. This mechanism amplifies the force that's produced by the calf muscles. The end result is a more powerful – and more efficient – movement. Think of a tendon being stretched as a rubber band being stretched. Stretching a rubber band gives it potential energy which when "shot" is released as kinetic energy. Everything else being equal, a longer rubber band can stretch more – and absorb/store more – than a shorter rubber band. And everything else being equal, a longer tendon can stretch more – and absorb/ store more – than a shorter tendon. Just check out the length of an Achilles tendon in a kangaroo!

Understand, too, that a small difference in the length of a muscle makes a big difference in strength (and size) potential. In theory, the potential cross-sectional area of a muscle is equal to its length squared and the potential volume of a muscle is equal to its length cubed. To illustrate, a muscle that's three inches long would have a potential cross-sectional area of nine square inches [3 inches x 3 inches] and a potential volume of 27 cubic inches [3 inches x 3 inches x

3 inches]; a muscle that's four inches long would have a potential cross-sectional area of 16 square inches [4 inches x 4 inches] and a potential volume of 64 cubic inches [4 inches x 4 inches x 4 inches].

As with muscle fiber types, an individual's muscle-to-tendon ratio can vary from one muscle to another. It's difficult to determine the actual length of a muscle because it may be hidden by subcutaneous fat (located beneath the skin) or lie below other muscles. However, the length of the triceps, the forearms and especially the calves is usually easy to identify. The lengths of a muscle and its tendon aren't subject to change.

Testosterone Level

Although testosterone is typically associated with men, the hormone is also present in perfectly normal women. In men, testosterone is produced by the testes; in women, roughly 50% is produced by the ovaries and 50% by the adrenal glands. The secretion of testosterone is regulated by pituitary hormones.

Testosterone influences the secondary sexual characteristics. In men, for example, it lowers the voice and promotes the growth of facial and body hair. Additionally, testosterone stimulates increases in strength and muscle mass. In short, its major action is to promote growth. Everything else being equal, those who have high levels of testosterone have a greater potential to improve their strength (and size) than those who have low levels of testosterone.

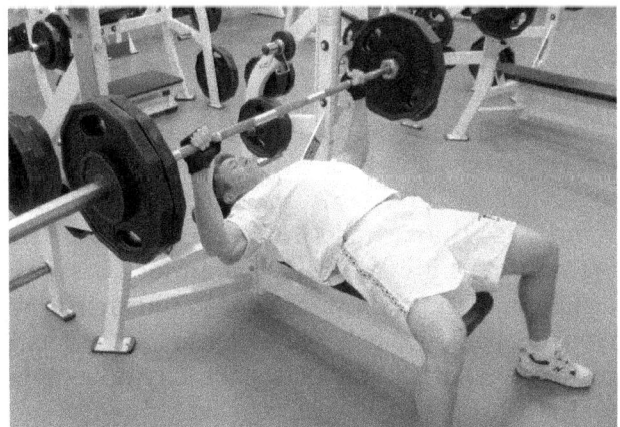

Favorable lever lengths and body proportions in the bench press are short arms and a thick chest.

Interestingly, a number of studies have also found a correlation between testosterone levels and aggressive behavior in both men and women. This isn't unique in the animal kingdom, by the way. Bull sharks are said to have the highest levels of testosterone found in any creature (land or sea) and their aggressive behavior is legendary. It is, perhaps, the most dangerous type of shark in the world.

Lever Lengths and Body Proportions

Archimedes, an ancient Greek mathematician, physicist and engineer, once said something along these lines: "Give me a place to stand and with a lever I will move the whole world." Considering the weight of the planet, that would involve quite a lever. His point, of course, was that levers can be used to lift heavy weights. And levers are a large part of genetics.

Some individuals have lever (bone) lengths and body proportions that give them greater leverage in lifting weights and a greater potential for increasing strength than other individuals. This is readily apparent in the sport of powerlifting. Competitive powerlifting consists of three movements: the squat, bench press and deadlift. Favorable lever lengths and body proportions in the squat are a short torso, wide hips and short legs; favorable lever lengths and body proportions in the bench press are short arms and a thick chest; favorable lever lengths and body proportions in the deadlift are a short torso, wide hips and short legs. (Long arms are also an asset in the deadlift; more on that point in a bit.) Everything else being equal, those who have favorable lever lengths and body proportions have a greater strength potential in certain exercises because they don't have to move the weight as far as those who have less favorable lever lengths and body proportions. The end result is that these individuals can lift extraordinarily heavy weights. In fact, a study of 68 competitive powerlifters found that they were of average to below-average height and had relatively short limbs. (Fast fact: Olympic-style weightlifting consists of two movements: the snatch and clean and jerk; at one time, the clean and press was also contested but the movement

was discontinued after the 1972 Munich Olympics.)

Here's another way to look at it: Consider two individuals who are tasked with lifting 200 pounds in the bench press. Because of lever lengths and body proportions, suppose that Lifter A has to move the weight a distance of 21 inches (1.75 feet) and Lifter B has to move the weight 24 inches. Since mechanical work is defined as force (here, weight) multiplied by distance, Lifter A must do 350 foot-pounds of work [1.75 ft x 200 lb] and Lifter B must do 400 foot-pounds of work [2.0 ft x 200 lb] to accomplish the identical task. In other words, Lifter A doesn't need to produce as much force – or do as much work – as Lifter B to raise the same weight. Everything else being equal, Lifter A would have greater leverage than Lifter B and a greater strength potential. (Fast fact: Gaspard-Gustave Coriolis – a French mathematician, mechanical engineer, scientist and educator – introduced the modern scientific definition of the term work in 1829.)

Any discussion of limb length almost always involves wingspan (aka arm span) which is the distance between the fingertips of both arms that are extended out to the sides and parallel to the ground. The average individual has a wingspan that's about the same as his or her height. The first person to note this relationship is thought to be Marcus Vitruvius, a Roman architect who lived in the first century BC. The association between wingspan and height was later popularized and immortalized in 1490 by Leonardo da Vinci with his iconic Vitruvian Man which was based on the writings of Vitruvius. Text that accompanies his fabled artwork states that "the length of the outspread arms is equal to the height of a man."

Short limbs are highly favorable in just about every exercise. (The lone exception is the deadlift.) Ironically, however, long limbs – the exact opposite – are highly favorable in just about every sport. Having long limbs, for example, is a valuable asset in baseball, basketball, boxing, football, rowing, swimming and volleyball.

Much ado was made about the wingspan of Michael Phelps, a swimmer of unmatched athletic accomplishments – winning 28 Olympic medals, 23 of which were gold – who stands 6'4" with a 6'7" wingspan, a difference of three inches. While that's certainly above average, it's not as mythical as was implied by the hubbub. (What's really remarkable about Phelps, though, is that at a height of 6'4", he has an inseam of only 32", meaning that he has short legs coupled with a long torso which is a big advantage in swimming.) Far more impressive in this area is Brittney Griner, a professional basketball player who stands 6'8" with a 7'3.5" wingspan, a difference of 7.5 inches. Given that, it's not much of a shock to learn that she blocked more shots in her collegiate career (736) than any other player – man or woman – in history. Notable in the combat sport of mixed martial arts is Jon Jones, a light heavyweight champion, who stands 6'4" with a 7'0.5" wingspan, a difference of 8.5 inches.

But the most extraordinary measure among famous athletes might belong to Sonny Liston, a heavyweight boxer who stood 6'1" with a reported wingspan of 7'0" – *nearly a one-foot difference* between his wingspan and height. Liston won the world heavyweight championship in September 1962 and held the title until February 1964. In that fight, he lost to 22-year-old Cassius Clay who soon thereafter changed his name to Muhammad Ali. By the way, Ali stood 6'3" with a 6'8" wingspan.

While short limbs are a disadvantage in most sports, it doesn't necessarily guarantee athletic mediocrity. Take boxing, for instance, where "reach" is a standard part of a fighter's physical portfolio or "tale of the tape." Mike Tyson – who became the youngest world heavyweight champion of all time in 1986 and was one of the most feared fighters to ever step inside the ring – stood 5'10 with a wingspan of 5'11", a difference of only one inch. This, of course, is barely better than average. Yet, Tyson ruled the heavyweight division, winning his first 37 fights (33 by knockout; 27 fights never went past the second round) and successfully defending his title nine times over the course of about four years. Then there's heavyweight Rocco Marchegiano who

stood 5'10.5" with a wingspan of 5'8", a difference of *minus 2.5 inches*. And no, those numbers aren't typos. In spite of his "alligator arms," Marchegiano was no palooka in the ring. Better known as Rocky Marciano – whose name and fighting style were the inspiration for the character Rocky Balboa – he retired as an undefeated heavyweight champion with a record of 49-0 (43 by knockout), winning the belt in 1952 and successfully defending his title six times over the course of about three years.

Sidebar: A related metric is the ape index which is a ratio of wingspan to height (wingspan divided by height). So, the average individual who has a wingspan that's the same as his or her height would have an ape index of 1.0. And in case you're wondering, the ape index of an ape – an average adult male gorilla with a height of about 5'9" and a wingspan of about 8'0" – is nearly 1.4. That's a 27-inch difference between height and wingspan!

Body Type

Another genetic factor that plays a critical role in strength potential is your physique or body type. In the 1940s, Dr. William Sheldon – a physician and psychologist – advanced the idea that there are three main body types: endomorph, mesomorph and ectomorph. These classifications continue to be widely used in science and academia. (Fast fact: Dr. Sheldon – being a psychologist – tried to associate body types with behavior, a belief that has long since been discredited.)

Endomorphs have a soft and round physique. They have a very high percentage of body fat without much muscle tone. An example of an endomorph is a sumo wrestler. Mesomorphs have a heavily muscled physique. They have an athletic build with broad shoulders, a large chest and a trim waist (giving them a V-shaped appearance). An example of a mesomorph is a competitive bodybuilder. Finally, ectomorphs have long limbs and a slender physique. They have a very low percentage of body fat without much muscle size. An example of an ectomorph is a long-distance runner.

Relatively few individuals can be classified as being extremes of one body type or another. Rather, most people have varying degrees of endomorphy (fatness), mesomorphy (muscularity) and ectomorphy (leanness).

The component that's present to the greatest degree indicates the dominant or "base" body type. If one of the two remaining components is present to a greater degree than the other, then it's also used to describe the body type.

For instance, those with a high degree of endomorphy have the base body type of an endomorph. If this is coupled with a moderate degree of mesomorphy, their body type is a mesomorphic endomorph. They mainly have a round physique along with some degree of muscular development. Many shot putters and football linemen are examples of mesomorphic endomorphs (as well as endomorphic mesomorphs).

Similarly, those with a high degree of ectomorphy have the base body type of an ectomorph. If this is coupled with a moderate degree of mesomorphy, their body type is a mesomorphic ectomorph. They mainly have a slender physique along with some degree of muscular development. Many 400-meter sprinters and wide receivers are examples of mesomorphic ectomorphs (as well as ectomorphic mesomorphs). Incidentally, the most common body types in sports are probably the mesomorphic ectomorph and ectomorphic mesomorph.

Others with moderate degrees of mesomorphy and endomorphy or moderate degrees of mesomorphy and ectomorphy have the body type of a mesomorph-endomorph and mesomorph-ectomorph, respectively. The mesomorph-endomorph has an equally round and muscular physique while the mesomorph-ectomorph has an equally slender and muscular physique.

Dr. Sheldon introduced the term somatotype in 1940. A somatotype is a numerical descriptor of overall physique in terms of body shape and body composition. Somatotypes are derived from a rating system in which an individual is given a score for each of the main body types. There are

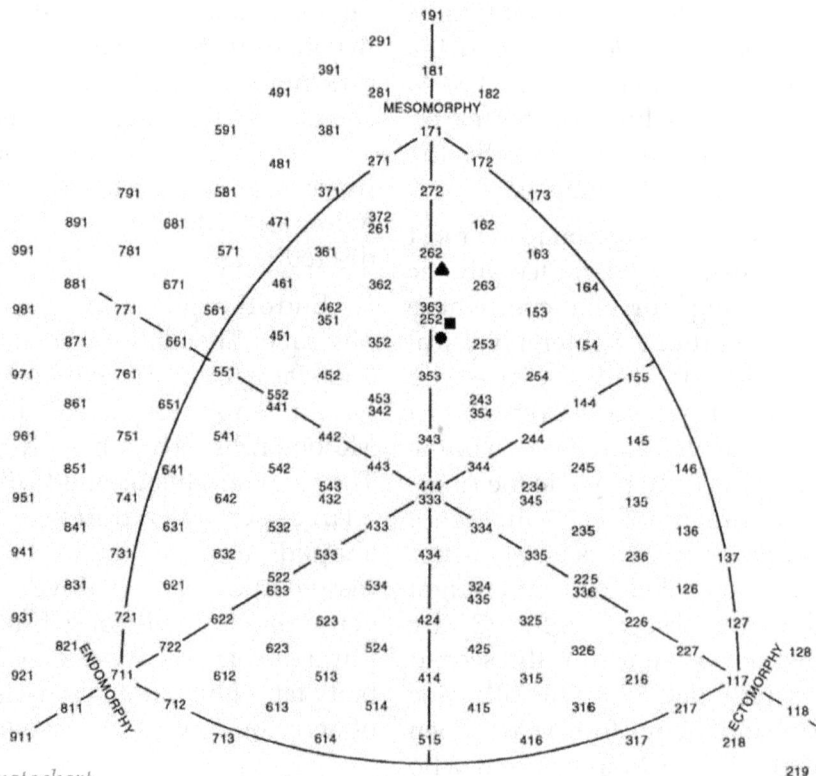

Figure 3.2: Sample somatochart

three numbers used in a somatotype: a number for endomorphy, mesomorphy and ectomorphy (always in that order).

The system that was created by Dr. Sheldon employs a scale that ranges from 1 to 7 to designate the degree of each of the three components with 1 being the least amount and 7 being the greatest. His system relied heavily on photographic (visual) assessments – which, of course, are highly subjective – and used only two anthropometric measurements (height and weight). In 1967, two researchers – Barbara Heath and Dr. Lindsay Carter – published an article on the Heath-Carter Method that uses a 9-point scale. Their system relies entirely on anthropometric measurements. The Heath-Carter Method is the most preferred means of somatotyping.

With the Heath-Carter Method, ratings of 0.5 to 2.5 are considered low, 3.0 to 5.0 moderate, 5.5 to 7.0 high and 7.5 to 9.0 very high. In this system, a somatotype of 9-1-1 (read as "nine-one-one") is an extreme endomorph, 1-9-1 is an extreme mesomorph and 1-1-9 is an extreme ectomorph.

As mentioned earlier, most people have varying degrees of endomorphy, mesomorphy and ectomorphy. When using numerical descriptors, then, somatotypes of 5-5-1 and 4-4-2 would be indicative of a mesomorph-endomorph and somatotypes of 1-5-5 and 2-4-4 would be indicative of a mesomorph-ectomorph; somatotypes of 4-6-2 and 3-5-1 would be indicative of an endomorphic mesomorph and somatotypes of 1-3-6 and 2-3-5 would be indicative of a mesomorphic ectomorph. (Fast fact: By his own estimate, Dr. Sheldon's somatotype was 3.0-3.5-5.0.)

The three-number rating can be recorded on what's known as a somatochart. The chart can be used to plot groups of specific athletes – gymnasts, rowers, weightlifters or wrestlers, for instance – where a cluster of ratings would indicate that a certain body type predominates in a particular sport. Or it can be used to examine the body type of the same person over time. In Figure 3.2, for example, the somatochart shows

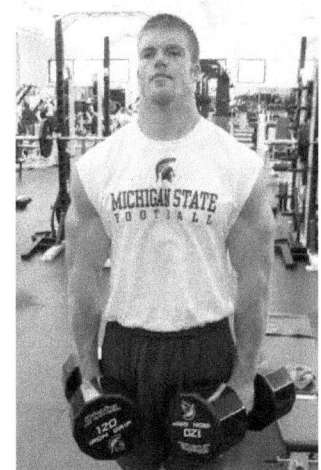

The body type that has the greatest potential to increase strength is the mesomorph. (Photo provided by Ken Mannie.)

an individual (this author) on three separate occasions: May 1982 (circle), April 2005 (square) and November 2013 (triangle). The somatotypes were 2.5-4.0-2.0 in 1982 at age 25; 1.8-4.4-2.0 in 2005 at about age 48; and 1.7-5.8-2.3 in 2013 at age 56.5. In each case, the base body type is a mesomorph. Note that over the course of 31.5 years, the rating for endomorphy changed by 0.8 units (from 2.5 to 1.7); the rating for mesomorphy changed by 1.8 units (from 4.0 to 5.8); and the ectomorphy rating changed by 0.3 units (from 2.0 to 2.3). So after more than three decades, the ratings in endomorphy and ectomorphy remained low while the rating in mesomorphy increased from moderate to high. Despite the consistency that's demonstrated by this example, body types are subject to change.

Having said all of this, how can you determine your somatotype? Well, it involves 10 anthropometric measurements: four skinfolds (triceps, subscapular, suprailiac and calf); the circumferences of your flexed arm and calf; the widths between the epicondyles of your humerus (upper-arm bone) and femur (upper-leg bone); height; and weight. Using a variety of equations, a somatotype is then calculated from these measurements with ratings in endomorphy (from the skinfolds), mesomorphy (from the muscle circumferences and bone widths) and ectomorphy (from height and weight). Needless to say, the process can be complicated. Nonetheless, you can get a general idea of your body type by simply considering your physique.

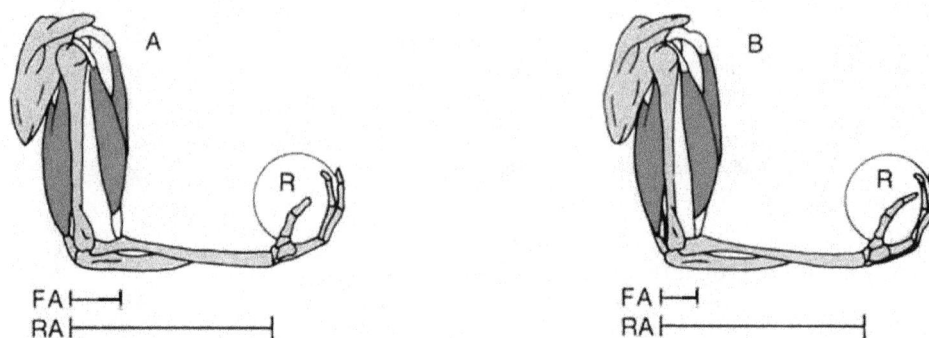

Figure 3.3: Tendon insertion

If you have a heavily muscled physique, your body type is mainly a mesomorph; if you have a slender physique, your body type is mainly an ectomorph. You get the picture.

A number of studies have related body type to physical performance and trainability. For instance, a study of 41 physical-education students found that mesomorph-ectomorphs and mesomorphs have a greater potential to improve various aspects of their aerobic fitness than mesomorph-endomorphs and ectomorphs. As you might suspect, the body type that has the greatest potential to increase strength is the mesomorph. In one study, the average somatotype of 54 male powerlifters was 4.3-8.8-0.5, showing that mesomorphy is dominant. Everything else being equal, those who have a high degree of mesomorphy have a greater potential to improve their strength than those who have a low degree of mesomorphy.

It was noted previously that body types are subject to change. This can be done through an increase/decrease of muscle mass and/or an increase/decrease of body fat; bone widths aren't subject to change.

Sidebar: Somatotyping has an insidious origin story that dates back to the late 1800s and America's fascination with posture testing. In that era, screenings for posture occurred at many high schools and universities. Around 1880, Harvard University began taking nude "posture photos" of its freshman class. This continued until about 1940 when the program was taken over by Dr. Sheldon and Dr. EA Hooten, another Harvard researcher. The two made arrangements with numerous other elite schools, taking tens of thousands of nude photographs – from the front, side and rear – of freshmen at the likes of Princeton University, Yale University, Mount Holyoke College, Radcliffe College, Smith College, Swarthmore College, Vassar College, Wellesley College and the University of Washington. The photographs were taken under the guise of postural testing but were actually used by Dr. Sheldon in his research on somatotyping. Dr. Sheldon – who personally took thousands of photographs – was able to continue this practice until 1950 when it abruptly ended following student protests at the University of Washington (though the ritual existed at some schools through the 1970s). *The New York Times* later referred to this as the Great Ivy League Nude Posture Photo Scandal.

Tendon Insertion

At one time or another, you've probably encountered individuals who were far stronger than they appeared. In fact, they may have been amazingly strong despite not having much in the way of muscular size. If strength is directly related to the size of a muscle – in terms of its cross-sectional area – how can this be? One possibility is that these individuals have favorable insertion points of their tendons. Everything else being equal, those who have tendons that insert farther from an axis of rotation (aka a fulcrum; here, a joint) have a greater biomechanical advantage and strength potential than those who have tendons that insert closer to an axis of rotation.

Consider two individuals who are tasked with holding 20 pounds in their hands a distance of 12.0 inches from their elbows while keeping their lower arms parallel to the ground and maintaining a 90-degree angle between their upper and lower arms. Suppose that Lifter A has a bicep tendon that inserts on his forearm 1.2 inches from his elbow and Lifter B has a bicep tendon that inserts on his forearm 1.0 inch from his elbow.

In this example, as depicted in Figure 3.3, the force (tension) that's necessary to maintain a resistance (load) in a static position can be calculated by using this equation: force multiplied by force arm equals resistance multiplied by resistance arm or, more simply, $F \times FA = R \times RA$. The force arm is defined as the distance from the axis of rotation – in this case, the elbow – to the point where the force is applied (the insertion point of the tendon); the resistance arm is defined as the distance from the axis of rotation to the point where the resistance is applied.

Entering the aforesaid values into the equation and solving for force reveals that Lifter A must produce 200 pounds of force to hold the 20-pound weight in a static position while Lifter B must produce 240 pounds of force to accomplish the identical task. In other words, Lifter A doesn't need to produce as much force – or make as much effort – as Lifter B to hold the same weight. Everything else being equal, Lifter A would have greater leverage than Lifter B and a greater strength potential.

This depiction of static forces is somewhat simplified. However, it still illustrates the fact that a very small difference in the insertion point of a tendon can produce a considerable amount of variation in leverage. The insertion point of a tendon can be accurately determined using magnetic resonance imaging (MRI) and X-rays.

The effect that the insertion point of a tendon has on a bone can be likened to the position of a knob on a door. Placing the knob (insertion point of the tendon) away from the hinge (the elbow) gives you greater leverage, making it easier for

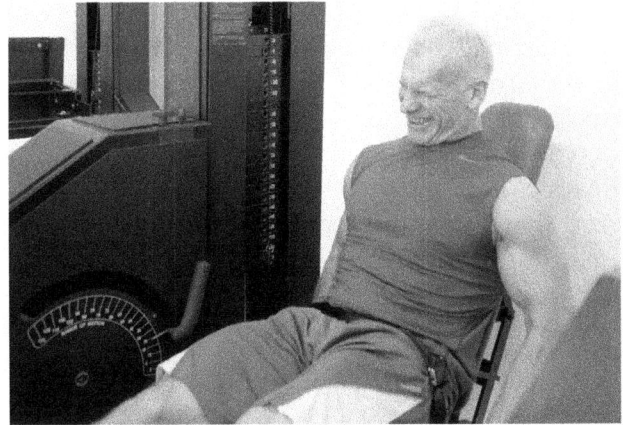

Your response to training is largely determined by your genetic profile. (Photo provided by Luke Carlson.)

you to pull the door (the bone) than if the knob was closer to the hinge.

Neurological Efficiency

One more genetic factor that has a significant role in determining strength potential deals with the nervous system; it has been dubbed neurological efficiency (or neuromuscular efficiency). This refers to an individual's inherited ability to innervate (or stimulate) muscle fibers and is another reason why some individuals are far stronger than they appear.

It has been suggested that some individuals can innervate higher percentages of their muscle fibers than others which gives them a greater potential to improve their strength. Consider two individuals who have the same amount of muscle mass. Suppose that Lifter A can innervate 40% of his muscle fibers and Lifter B can innervate 30%. Everything else being equal, Lifter A would have access to a higher percentage of muscle fibers than Lifter B and a greater strength potential.

HERITABILITY DICTATES TRAINABILITY

With due respect to Thomas Jefferson – the main author of the United States Declaration of Independence – all men (and women) *aren't* created equal. If two individuals perform the same strength program, it's highly unlikely that they'll end up having the same level of strength (and size). Each individual responds in a unique manner because everyone inherits a unique genetic profile with a unique genetic potential for improving strength (and size). Simply, some people are predisposed toward developing high levels of strength (and size) while others are not. And that's why the same strength program can result in one person who looks like Arnold Schwarzenegger and another who looks like Arnold Palmer.

So, your response to strength training isn't necessarily due to a particular program or workout. Indeed, following the routines of successful weightlifters doesn't mean that you'll attain their same level of strength; following the routines of successful bodybuilders doesn't mean that you'll attain their same level of size.

Train a chimpanzee like a gorilla and you might get a slightly stronger chimpanzee . . . but you'll never get a gorilla. The next time that you're in the fitness center, take a look at different pairs of training partners. You'll see that individuals who work out together usually have different levels of strength (and size), despite performing the same exercises and set/repetition scheme).

The truth is that heritability dictates trainability. Your response to training is largely determined by the traits that you have in your genetic portfolio. The cumulative effect of your inherited muscular, mechanical, hormonal and neural traits is what determines your strength potential. An individual who has a high percentage of FT fibers; long muscle bellies coupled with short tendons; a high level of testosterone; desirable lever lengths and body proportions; a high degree of mesomorphy; favorable insertion points of tendons; and an efficient neurological system would be incredibly strong (as well as physically impressive). Compared to the average person, this genetic marvel would be capable of almost unbelievable feats of strength. There are some men and women like that but most aren't as fortunate.

For all intents and purposes, you can't change the characteristics that you've inherited from your ancestors. And you can't travel back in time to pick your parents. However, this doesn't mean that there isn't any hope for you to get stronger; just be realistic about it. In terms of your response to strength training, the three letters in the English language that are of utmost importance are DNA. Regardless of your genetic destiny, your goal should be to achieve your strength potential.

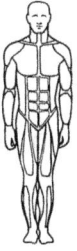

4 Strength Training

Strength can be defined as the ability of a muscle to produce force. It follows, then, that strength training is a means to improve this ability.

BENEFITS

There are many benefits of strength training. First of all, increasing your strength will improve your capacity to perform everyday tasks more easily. Strength training will also increase your muscle mass and decrease your body fat which will improve your body composition and physical appearance.

In addition, strength training can increase your bone mineral density thereby combating the destructive effects of osteoporosis. There are psychological benefits as well. This includes increased mental alertness, self-confidence and self-esteem.

For athletes, strength training can reduce the frequency and severity of injuries. If you can increase the strength of your muscles, connective tissues and bones to tolerate more stress, you'll reduce the likelihood of incurring an injury. By increasing their functional strength, athletes will also take an important step toward realizing their physical potential. Having greater strength allows them to perform their activities more easily and be more resistant to fatigue.

WHAT APPROACH?

Most fitness authorities agree that strength training can be extremely beneficial. Many, however, disagree over which approach is best for increasing strength (and size). The different approaches – and the enormous amount of conflicting advice – often leave people utterly confused.

A common practice is to adopt the strength programs of successful individuals or teams, a practice that frequently adds to the confusion. If you were to compare the strength programs of individuals who are very strong, you might be in for quite a surprise: Not only is it likely that their programs are vastly different but also that, in many cases, they offer contradictory information. Some strength programs use fast repetition speeds, others slow repetition speeds; some use mostly multiple sets of each exercise, others mostly single sets of each exercise; some use split routines, others total-body workouts; some use mainly free weights, others mainly machines; and so on.

Yet, despite these and other differences, many strength programs are highly effective. How, then, do you choose which program to follow if you're looking to improve your strength (and size)?

CHOOSING A PROGRAM

When choosing a strength program, it's important to consider scientific research. Interestingly, research has been unable to

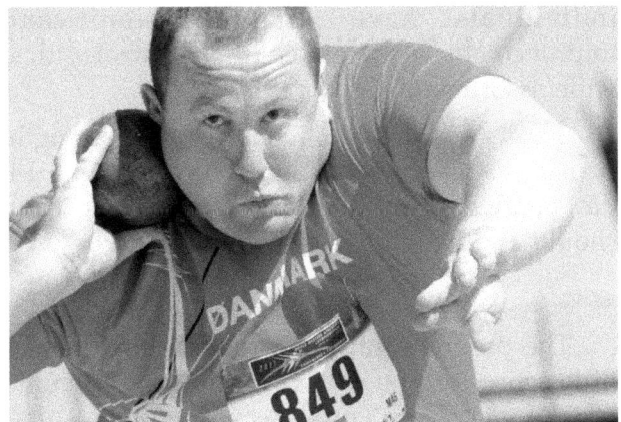

By increasing their functional strength, athletes will take an important step toward realizing their physical potential. (Photo by Chris Stone.)

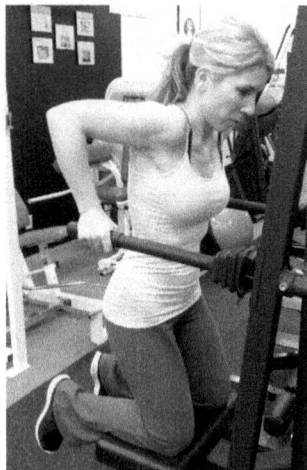

Research has shown that a variety of methods can be used to increase strength. (Photo by Fred Fornicola.)

determine that one method of strength training is superior to another. If anything, research has shown that a variety of methods can be used to increase strength. In one study, significant improvements in strength were made by nine groups that did different combinations of one, two and three sets and two, six and ten repetitions. Moreover, research has shown that a variety of equipment can be used to increase strength. In several studies, significant improvements in strength were made by groups that used free weights and groups that used machines.

When choosing a strength program, it's also important to consider anecdotal evidence. Though anecdotal reports lack the same scientific scrutiny as research studies, their sheer volume is so overwhelming in this case that they can't be discounted. The inescapable fact is that countless individuals have attained significant improvements in their strength (and size) with a wide assortment of programs.

So, it's possible that many types of strength programs can yield favorable results. In determining which program to implement, you should ask the following six questions:

Is It Productive?

The program must be productive. It makes little sense for you to invest time in a strength program if it doesn't produce meaningful results. A program will be productive as long as it's based on scientific research, common sense and deductive reasoning, not unfounded advice, wild speculation and wishful thinking.

Is It Comprehensive?

The program must be comprehensive. A strength program should address all of the major muscles in your body, not just the "showy" or "cosmetic" ones. Frequently, muscles that are often injured get ignored (such as those surrounding the knee, ankle, neck and lower back) while muscles that are often flaunted get emphasized (such as the chest, biceps, triceps and abdominals). If you happen to be a competitive athlete, a comprehensive strength program is one that's performed year-round, including throughout the off-season and in-season. Training during the season is especially critical since this is when athletes need to be at their best in terms of strength and conditioning.

Is It Practical?

The program must be practical. In other words, it must be relatively easy to understand. In some instances, strength programs are grossly overcomplicated and correspondingly confusing. The use of pseudoscientific terminology adds to the confusion. Strength training needn't be complex.

Is It Efficient?

The program must be efficient. It should produce the maximum possible results in the minimum amount of time. A strength program that requires you to lift weights for lengthy periods of time and/or more than several workouts per week isn't an efficient use of your time . . . nor is it necessary. By utilizing a program that's time-efficient, you'll have a greater opportunity to pursue other activities such as preparing for academic endeavors and, if you're an athlete, performing sport-specific skills and conditioning. And don't forget about the extra time that you could dedicate toward your personal activities and interests. You should *invest* time in the fitness center, not *spend* time.

Is It Sustainable?

The program must be sustainable. Strength training should be viewed as a long-term commitment, not a short-term fling. Adherence to a strength program is essential for producing favorable results. A program will be worthless if you abandon it after the first few weeks or months. For a program to be beneficial, it should be something that you can maintain into your thirties, forties and beyond.

Is It Safe?

The program must be safe. At first glance, many strength programs can look quite appealing. Closer inspection, however, may reveal that the programs are highly questionable in terms of safety. There's no need whatsoever to perform potentially dangerous activities or exercises in the fitness center. It's certainly true that physical activities have inherent participatory risks. But this doesn't mean that you should do physical activities that present risks to your orthopedic health.

A RECAP

In short, the program that you choose should be productive, comprehensive, practical, efficient, sustainable and safe. It's these criteria that form the underlying theme for the ensuing information.

COMPONENTS OF STRENGTH TRAINING

Unless you happen to be a competitive weightlifter or bodybuilder, there's absolutely no need for you to train like one. Competitive athletes have different goals than most of the population. Essentially, the main goal of a competitive weightlifter – a powerlifter or an Olympic-style weightlifter – is to do one repetition with as much weight as possible; the main goal of a competitive bodybuilder is to achieve the best physique possible. With no disrespect intended, neither of these goals has much relevance to the average person – or the average athlete, for that matter – who doesn't compete as a weightlifter or bodybuilder.

You can increase your strength (and size) in a manner that's productive, comprehensive, practical, efficient, sustainable and safe by incorporating these 10 components of strength training:

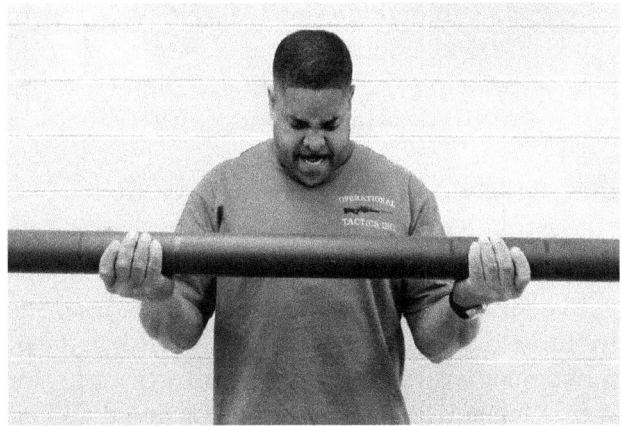

A high level of intensity is necessary for maximizing your response to strength training. (Photo by Peter Silletti.)

1. Level of Intensity

The most important factor that determines your results from strength training is your genetic (inherited) profile. This includes your muscle fiber type, muscle-to-tendon ratios, testosterone level, lever lengths and body proportions, body type, tendon insertions and neurological efficiency. However, you can't control the genetic cards that you were dealt. The most important factor that you *can* control is your level of intensity. (In strength-training parlance, intensity shouldn't be confused with a percentage of a maximum weight. Rather, intensity is another word for effort.)

A high level of intensity is necessary for maximizing your response to strength training. Here, a high level of intensity is characterized by reaching – or at least approaching – the point of muscular fatigue. In simple terms, this means that you've exhausted your muscles to the extent that you literally can't do any additional repetitions with proper technique.

The Overload Principle

If you fail to achieve an appropriate level of intensity – or an adequate level of muscular fatigue – your increases in strength (and size) will be less than optimal. Evidence for this notion is found in the Overload Principle. In 1933, Dr. Arthur Steinhaus – a physiologist and one of 11 founders of the American College of Sports Medicine – used "overload" to describe a method in which subjects "were trained to perform successfully heavier work" and then referred to it as a "principle." As a result, Dr. Steinhaus has been credited with coining the Overload Principle. It has since become what's perhaps the most widely referenced tenet in exercise science.

In regards to strength training, Dr. Roger Enoka – now a distinguished professor at the University of Colorado whose research interests include the neuromuscular determinants of movement – defines the Overload Principle this way: "To increase their size or functional ability, muscle fibers must be taxed toward their present capacity to respond." He adds: "This principle implies that there is a threshold point that must be exceeded before an adaptive response will occur."

Stated otherwise, an adequate level of muscular fatigue must be produced in order for a muscle to adapt. Your effort must be great enough to surpass this threshold to trigger compensatory adaptation. As the name of this process implies, a muscle compensates for appropriate demands (stress) that are placed on it by adapting. The way that a muscle adapts is by getting stronger (and bigger) within the scope of an individual's genetic profile. Look at it like this: In response to what amounts to an assault, a muscle reinforces itself in preparation for another incursion. (This is just one of many types of compensatory adaptation that can take place at the cellular level.)

The General Adaptation Syndrome

Make no mistake about it: In order for you to achieve optimal increases in strength (and size), you must produce an adequate level of muscular fatigue. So if you produce too little muscular fatigue, you may not have stimulated any compensatory adaptation. But if you produce too much muscular fatigue, you may not have permitted any compensatory adaptation; it may even cause a loss of strength (and size).

This becomes evident when looking at stress and how people respond/adapt to it. In 1936, Dr. Hans Selye – an endocrinologist from what was then Austria-Hungary – wrote a letter to the editor of *Nature* in which he described how animals responded to physical stress. Dr. Selye noted "a generalized effort of the organism to adapt itself to new conditions" and proposed naming this mechanism the General Adaptation Syndrome (GAS). The three-stage process can be used to describe how a muscle responds to physiological stress during strength training. In the Alarm Stage, the stress causes damage to the muscle (in the form of very small tears or micro-tears at the cellular level). This is followed by the Resistance Stage during which the body defends itself against the stress-induced damage through compensatory adaptation by increasing in strength (and size) which offers protection against a future threat. Stress that's too severe induces the Exhaustion Stage in which the demands that are placed on the muscle exceed its ability to recover and adapt.

To reiterate: In order for compensatory adaptation to occur, a muscle requires the right amount of stress. Too little and there's *no need* for a muscle to adapt; too much and there's *no chance* for a muscle to adapt.

Therefore, your level of intensity should be high . . . but it should also be appropriate. Consider this analogy: If you used a hammer on a regular basis for short periods of time you'd form calluses on your palm. Basically, the calluses are a compensatory (and protective) adaptation to frictional heat. If you hammered for a long enough period of time, however, you'd develop blisters instead. Here, the excessive demands have surpassed the adaptive ability of your tissue because the stress was too much and too frequent. In brief, you should train with a high level of intensity without overdoing it.

How do you know if the demands that you've placed on your muscles are too little or too much? You should monitor your performance in terms of the resistance that you use and the repetitions that you do. If you continue to make progress in your performance, then the demands are appropriate.

Favorable Results

The main reason why most people fail to maximize their response to strength training is simply because they don't train with an appropriate level of intensity. Simply, a sub-maximum effort yields a sub-maximum effect. Athletes should also keep in mind that "you play like you practice." If you're an athlete and do your strength training with a low level of effort, will you be able to ratchet up your intensity when needed in competition?

That being said, you must also use your judgment in deciding what level of intensity is appropriate for you. Intensity is a relative term that depends on your level of fitness. Exercise of low intensity for an active individual may be of high intensity for an inactive individual. So if you haven't been training on a regular basis or aren't in the best of shape, then you should adjust your effort accordingly. Also, some individuals may not be comfortable exercising to the point of muscular fatigue. Those who feel uneasy about training with a high level of intensity should terminate the set a few repetitions short of muscular fatigue. Remember, you can control your level of intensity when you train; your efforts can be as easy or as hard as you desire.

The fact that your results from strength training are directly related to your level of effort shouldn't come as much of a surprise. It's like anything else in life: How hard you work at your other physical training, your job and even your relationships largely determines your success at those endeavors.

2. Progressive Overload

In 1944, Dr. Thomas DeLorme – a physician and freshly minted lieutenant in the US Army Medical Corps who was assigned to the Gardiner General Army Hospital in Chicago – introduced a protocol of "heavy resistance exercise" to strengthen the muscles of soldiers who were wounded and/or injured during World War II. His protocol was based on the lessons that he had learned from his own experience. In the early 1930s, he began lifting weights in an attempt to increase his muscular strength and size in order to recover from rheumatoid fever (a very serious disease that targets children; although rheumatoid fever is rare now in the US, it was much more prevalent in the 1930s and 1940s). By 1936, he had participated as a competitive

The load that's applied to your muscles must be increased steadily and systematically throughout the course of your strength program. (Photo provided by Luke Carlson.)

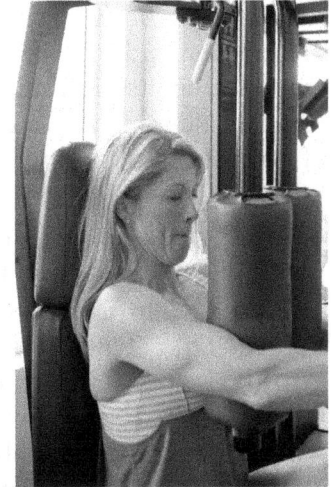

weightlifter. After the war ended, Dr. DeLorme left the Army and worked at the Massachusetts General Hospital in Boston where, in 1948, he and Dr. Arthur Watkins – a physician who headed the hospital's Department of Physical Medicine – revised the original protocol of "heavy resistance exercise" as a new protocol of "progressive resistance exercise." For his efforts, Dr. DeLorme is known as the father of progressive resistance exercise. (Fast fact: Dr. DeLorme's wife, Eleanor, supposedly suggested using the term progressive resistance exercise.)

Unfortunately, little of what's done in most fitness centers can be characterized as progressive. It's not uncommon for someone to perform the same number of repetitions with the same amount of resistance over and over again, workout after workout. Suppose that today in a particular exercise, you did 10 repetitions with 150 pounds and a month later you were still doing 10 repetitions with 150 pounds. Did you increase your strength? Probably not. On the other hand, what if you were able to do 12 repetitions with 165 pounds a month from now? In this case, you performed 20% more repetitions with 10% more resistance. That's excellent progress over the course of one month.

The Overload Principle, Revisited

Improvements in muscular strength (and size) depend on the continued application of the Overload Principle. This means that your musculoskeletal system must be overloaded or made to work harder than it's accustomed to working by being exposed to progressively greater demands. To be more specific, the load that's applied to your muscles must be increased steadily and systematically throughout the course of your strength program. This is often referred to as progressive overload.

The concept of progressive overload dates back to the sixth century BC when it was said to be used by Milo of Croton, roughly two millennia before Drs. DeLorme and Watkins first popularized their protocol of progressive-resistance exercise. Milo was a renowned Greek warrior and athlete who won a total of 32 championships as a wrestler in the four Panhellenic festivals that were held in various cities throughout Greece: the Olympic Games, Pythian Games, Isthmian Games and Nemean Games. (Women competed in the Heraean Games.) According to folklore, he periodically lifted a baby bull on his shoulders. As the bull increased in size, so did Milo's strength. This crude method of progressive overload has been credited with developing his legendary strength. (His interpretation of a calf raise may have been a bit too literal, though.)

In order to overload your muscles, every time that you train you should try to increase the resistance that you use and/or the repetitions that you do in comparison to a previous workout. This can be viewed as a double-progressive technique (with "double" referring to resistance and repetitions). Stated otherwise, you must expose your muscles to demands that they haven't previously encountered by using more resistance and/or doing more repetitions. Exposing your muscles to progressively greater demands triggers compensatory adaptation in response to the unaccustomed workload. Your muscles adapt to such demands by increasing in strength (and size). The extent to which this occurs then becomes a function of your genetic profile.

In a nutshell, here's how to implement the double-progressive technique for any given exercise: If you do or surpass the maximum number of repetitions in your prescribed repetition range – say that your repetition range is 10 to 15 and you did 15 – then in your next workout, you should increase the resistance; if

you didn't do the maximum number of repetitions in your prescribed repetition range – say that your repetition range is 10 to 15 and you did 14 – then in your next workout, you should use the same resistance and try to increase the number of repetitions.

Appropriate Progressions

Your progressions in resistance need not be in Herculean leaps and bounds. You should increase the resistance in an amount with which you're comfortable . . . but the resistance that you use must always be challenging. Fortunately, this may be accomplished much more systematically than the method that was used by Milo and his growing bull.

Progressions should be thought of in *relative* terms, not *absolute*. Always increasing the resistance by a set value of, say, five pounds can be problematic. Think about it: Making a five-pound progression from 100 to 105 pounds is an increase of 5%; making a five-pound progression from 10 to 15 pounds is an increase of 50%.

Your muscles will respond better if the progressions in resistance are about 5% or less, depending on the degree to which the set was challenging. Suppose, for example, that an exercise has a repetition range of 15 to 20. If it was fairly hard for you to do 20 repetitions, then you should make a slightly smaller progression in resistance; if it was fairly easy for you to do 20 repetitions, then you should make a slightly larger progression in resistance.

The idea behind making smaller progressions – known as micro-loading – is the fact that you'll hardly notice a slightly heavier resistance and your repetitions won't decline much if at all. In other words, it's much easier for your muscles to adapt to subtle increases in resistance. Consider this example: Imagine that an exercise has a repetition range of 15 to 20 and you did 200/20 (200 pounds/20 repetitions). If you increased the resistance by 10% (by 20 pounds) the next time you do that exercise, it's likely that you'd notice the significantly heavier weight and might do 220/15 or 220/16. Doing 16 repetitions means that you must improve the number of repetitions by 25% (from 16 to 20) before you can make your next progression in resistance which may prove to be a very daunting task. If, instead, you increased the resistance by 1.25% (by 2.5 pounds), it's not likely that you'd notice the slightly heavier weight and might do 202.5/20. Another 2.5-pound increase the next time you do that exercise may result in 205/20. Eventually, you might progress to the point where you were doing 220 pounds for at least 18 or 19 repetitions. So, you made the 20-pound increase in a number of small progressions instead of a large progression and, as a result, you allowed your muscles to adapt gradually to the resistance. And now, you'd only need to increase your repetitions by one or two in order to make your next progression in resistance. This scenario is hypothetical, of course, but it wouldn't be unusual for this to actually happen. The point is that your muscles will respond better to smaller increases in resistance than larger ones.

To make smaller progressions in resistance, you can use fractional plates or lighter barbell plates for exercises that are done with free weights and plate-loaded machines. Fractional plates weigh as little as 0.25 pounds; barbell plates weigh as little as 1.25 pounds. If lighter barbell plates aren't available, you can simply hang something from the bar (or the movement arm of the machine) such as a small ankle weight.

Selectorized machines have weight stacks with plates that are usually 10, 12.5, 15, 20 or 25 pounds. Many of these machines offer a self-contained system of making smaller progressions in resistance such as the use of a drop-down weight. With some selectorized machines, a saddle plate (or add-on weight) must be placed on the top plate of the weight stack. (Standard weights for saddle plates are 2.5 and 5.0 pounds.) Another option is to secure a fractional plate or light barbell plate to the weight stack of the machine by first inserting a selector pin through the hole in the plate and then into the weight stack. (This is often referred to as "pinning" a plate.) You can also place any object that weighs about one or two pounds on top of a weight stack as long as it won't fall off while you're using the equipment.

With dumbbells, you can use magnetic add-on weights. These weights – which can be round or hex to match the shape of the dumbbells – can be secured to the ends of the dumbbells and allow you to make increases in resistance that are much more desirable. So instead of having to jump from 25- to 30-pounders – a 20% increase in resistance – the use of 1.25-pound magnetic add-on weights can produce a pair of dumbbells that weigh 26.25 pounds. (Magnetic add-on weights can also be secured to the weight stacks of selectorized machines.) Another option for making smaller progressions with dumbbells is to employ ankle weights. Using 20-pound dumbbells with 1.25-pound ankle weights around your wrists produces 21.25 pounds of resistance.

Again, the resistance that you use must always be challenging. If you recently began a strength program or changed the exercises in your routine, it may take several workouts before you find a challenging weight. That's understandable; simply continue to make progressions in the resistance as needed.

A RECAP

For those who want to realize their physical potential, progressive overload has always been – and will always be – of utmost importance. You must place demands on your musculoskeletal system that are beyond what it's accustomed to using. If you lifted 200 pounds today for 12 repetitions, then in a future workout, you should try to increase the resistance that you used and/or the repetitions that you did.

Bottom line: Don't overlook overload.

3. Number of Sets

There's no agreement as to how many sets of an exercise should be done to achieve optimal increases in strength (and size). Most of the recommendations, though, are between one and three sets.

In determining which strength program to implement, one criterion is that the program must be productive. Research shows that doing one set of each exercise is a productive approach to strength training. In fact, the overwhelming majority of scientific evidence indicates that single-set training is at least as effective as multiple-set training. Let's take a closer look at what the research says.

In 1998, an extensive review of the literature by Drs. Ralph Carpinelli and Robert Otto of Adelphi University (NY) and later reviews by Dr. Carpinelli examined dozens of studies that compared different numbers of sets. It would be an understatement to say that their findings raised an eyebrow . . . and ruffled some feathers. In total, they found 62 studies of which five showed that multiple-set training was significantly better than single-set training and 57 that did not. This is to say, 57 of the 62 studies showed that there was no significant difference between single-set training and multiple-set training. Who saw that one coming? Drs. Carpinelli and Otto concluded that "the preponderance of evidence suggests that for training durations of 4 to 25 weeks there is no significant difference in the increase in strength or hypertrophy as a result of training with single versus multiple sets."

In one study, researchers at the University of Florida randomly assigned 42 subjects to two groups: One group did one set of 8 to 12 repetitions and the other group did three sets of 8 to 12 repetitions. Prior to the study, the subjects had done strength training for an average of 6.2 years. Both groups did the same nine exercises, performing each set to the point of muscular fatigue, and trained three times per week for 13 weeks. Both groups had significant increases in strength, endurance and body composition with no significant differences between groups.

In a more recent study, researchers in the United Kingdom randomly assigned 16 subjects to two groups: One group did one set of six repetitions and the other group did three sets of six repetitions. Prior to the study, the subjects had done the exercises that were tested for at least one year. Both groups did the same nine exercises, performing each set to the point of muscular fatigue, and trained three times per week for eight weeks. Both groups had significant increases in strength with no significant difference between groups. Also, both groups

significantly reduced the sum of seven skinfold measurements but the group that did one set had a significantly greater decrease than the group that did three sets.

It has been argued that although doing one set of each exercise might be productive for those who are inexperienced (or "untrained"), this isn't the case for those who are experienced (or "trained"). However, research shows otherwise. To quote Drs. Carpinelli and Otto: "There is no evidence to suggest that the response to single or multiple sets in trained athletes would differ from that in untrained individuals."

So, the basis for doing one set of each exercise has powerful and compelling support from research. But how is this possible? Recall that an adequate level of muscular fatigue must be produced in order to trigger compensatory adaptation. The number of sets that it takes you to produce that level of muscular fatigue really doesn't matter. This comes with a major caveat, though: For one set of each exercise to be productive, the set must be performed with an appropriate level of intensity (preferably reaching – or at least approaching – the point of muscular fatigue).

Is doing one set of each exercise for everyone? No. But it still represents a viable option.

In determining which strength program to implement, another criterion is that the program must be efficient. If doing one set produces virtually the same results as doing multiple sets, then doing one set of each exercise is an efficient approach to strength training. After all, why perform multiple sets of each exercise when you can obtain similar results from one set of each exercise in a fraction of the time? (Note that in the two preceding studies, doing three sets of each exercise compared to doing one set of each exercise – *three times as much volume* – didn't produce any better results.)

With efficiency in mind, many individuals have advocated doing one set of each exercise. This includes Dan Riley who logged 27 years as a strength coach in the National Football League (with the Washington Redskins and Houston Texans) and another eight at the collegiate level (with the US Military Academy and Penn State). Coach Riley – one of the early crusaders for safe, efficient training – states, "Your goal must be to perform as few sets as possible while stimulating maximum gains. If performed properly, only one set is needed to generate maximum gains. In our standard routines, one set of each exercise is performed."

To be clear, this isn't to say that the optimal number of sets for each exercise is one. Doing any reasonable number of sets can be productive. However, there's really no need to do more than three sets of each exercise. (An exception to this would be individuals who do low-repetition sets such as competitive weightlifters. In this case, they should perform warm-up sets prior to their low-repetition efforts to reduce their risk of injury.)

If you prefer to do more than three sets of each exercise, you should be aware of several things. First of all, simply doing a high number of sets doesn't guarantee that you've overloaded your muscles. If the resistance that you use isn't demanding enough then you won't produce an adequate level of muscular fatigue and your workout won't be as effective as possible. Remember, a large amount of low-intensity work doesn't necessarily produce an overload. So if you'd rather do more than three sets of each exercise, make sure that you're challenging your muscles with appropriate demands. In addition, keep in mind that doing too many sets (or too many exercises) can create a situation in which the demands that you've placed on your muscles have exceeded your ability to recover and adapt. Also, doing too many sets (or too many exercises) increases your risk of incurring an overuse injury such as tendinitis and bursitis. And as was indicated earlier, doing a high number of sets is relatively inefficient in terms of time. This makes it an undesirable option for many time-conscious individuals who simply don't have large gaps of free time in their busy schedules.

The point is this: Keep your sets to the minimum amount that's needed to produce an adequate level of muscular fatigue.

Strength training is an anaerobic activity that's characterized by short-term, high intensity efforts. (Photo provided by Luke Carlson.)

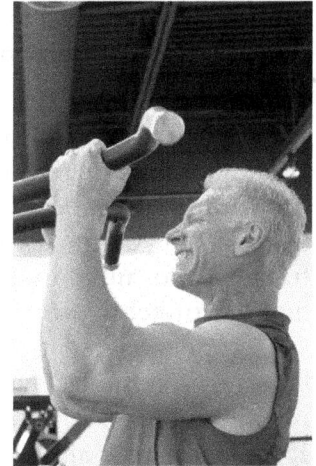

Quality v Quantity

You should emphasize the *quality* of work that's done in a strength program, not the *quantity* of work. Don't perform meaningless sets; make every set count. The most efficient program is one that produces the maximum possible results in the minimum amount of time.

4. Number of Repetitions

Determining an appropriate repetition range depends on a number of factors and, even then, has some degree of variability. Understand first that strength training isn't an aerobic activity that's characterized by long-term, low-intensity efforts; rather, it's an anaerobic activity that's characterized by short-term, high-intensity efforts. Therefore, the duration of a series of repetitions – a set – should be in the anaerobic domain. Efforts that last from a split second to several minutes are considered to be anaerobic (assuming, of course, that the level of effort is great enough to justify an anaerobic response). Intense efforts at the lower end of this time frame carry a higher risk of injury and those at the upper end have an increasingly greater reliance on the aerobic pathway. Narrowing the window of time to roughly 30 to 120 seconds represents a safe and effective range for strength training with lower durations assigned to smaller muscles and higher durations to larger ones. (Larger muscles – those in your hips and legs – should be trained for a slightly longer duration because of their greater size and work capacity.) Thus, time frames might be 90 to 120 seconds for a hip exercise, 60 to 90 seconds for a leg exercise and 30 to 60 seconds for a torso exercise.

Be that as it may, doing sets for a specified amount of time under load (TUL) or, alternately, time under tension (TUT) can be tricky and tedious. But you can use the aforementioned time frames to formulate repetition ranges. Suppose that you prefer to use a speed of movement that's six seconds per repetition. Dividing six seconds into the time frames that have been noted yields repetition ranges of 15 to 20 for your hips, 10 to 15 for your legs and 5 to 10 for your torso. (A repetition range of 8 to 10 is recommended for torso exercises that have an abbreviated range of motion.) Remember, these ranges are based on six-second repetitions. Different repetition speeds require different repetition ranges. Suppose that you prefer to use a speed of movement that's 10 seconds per repetition. Dividing 10 seconds into the time frames that have been noted yields repetition ranges of 9 to 12 for your hips, 6 to 9 for your legs and 3 to 6 for your torso. (You're encouraged to experiment with different repetition speeds and vary them based on your personal preferences and performance objectives.)

Genetic Considerations

Due to certain aspects of their genetic profile – most notably their predominant muscle fiber type – some individuals may require repetition ranges that are either a bit higher or lower than that prescribed for the general population. For example, individuals who have a high percentage of slow-twitch (ST) fibers would probably benefit more from doing slightly higher repetitions because their predominant fiber type is more suited for muscular endurance. Here, repetition ranges might be 20 to 25 for the hips, 15 to 20 for the legs and 10 to 15 for the torso. Individuals who have a high percentage of fast-twitch (FT) fibers would probably benefit more from doing slightly lower repetitions because their predominant fiber type is less suited for muscular endurance. Here, repetition ranges might be 12 to 15 for the hips, 9 to 12 for the legs and 4 to 8 for the torso.

In one study, sprinters trained with low repetitions, middle-distance runners with medium repetitions and long-distance runners with high repetitions. All three groups experienced excellent and equal gains in strength. (In all likelihood, successful sprinters have a high percentage of FT fibers and successful long-distance runners have a high percentage of ST fibers.)

Fiber types can be identified in a laboratory from a muscle biopsy. In this procedure, a needle with a hollow core is inserted into a muscle. The guillotine portion of the needle is used to snip a small plug of the tissue (about the size of a grain of rice). This sample is extracted by the needle – similar to the way that a core sample of soil is taken – and sent to a laboratory where it's analyzed under a microscope. A muscle biopsy isn't for everyone, though, since it results in the removal of tissue and most people are understandably reluctant to give away free samples. Moreover, the accuracy of muscle biopsies has also been questioned. For one thing, fiber "headcounts" are subject to different interpretations. And since the distribution of fibers varies throughout a muscle, the site from which the biopsy is taken might not be indicative of the overall fiber-type mixture. Indeed, using a single biopsy to predict fiber type for an entire muscle is somewhat akin to taking a census of those who reside in a city block and then extrapolating the results to an entire country. (Fast fact: When performing a biopsy to investigate fiber types, the muscle that's most often selected by researchers is the vastus lateralis of the quadriceps.)

One way to guesstimate your fiber types is to assess their fatigue characteristics during a test of muscular endurance. To do this, you'd determine your one-repetition maximum (1-RM; the maximum weight that you can lift one time). Then, you'd take 75% of your 1-RM and perform as many repetitions as possible using proper technique. For instance, if you find that your 1-RM is 80 pounds on the bicep curl, you'd use 60 pounds for the endurance test [80 lb x 0.75 = 60 lb]. It would be expected that 10 repetitions could be done with 75% of a 1-RM. If you do a relatively high number of repetitions with 60 pounds – more than about 10 – it's likely that your biceps have a high percentage of ST fibers; if you do a relatively low number of repetitions with 60 pounds – less than about 5 – it's likely that your biceps have a high percentage of FT fibers. But remember, since the composition and distribution of fibers can vary from one muscle to another, the results of an endurance test aren't necessarily reflective of your entire musculoskeletal system; you'd have to perform different tests for different muscles.

Muscular endurance can vary quite a bit from one individual to another. Dr. Wayne Westcott – now a professor of exercise science at Quincy College (MA) – reported data on 141 subjects who did an endurance test with 75% of their 1-RMs on a Nautilus® 10-degree chest machine. Again, it would be expected that 10 repetitions could be done with this workload. And according to the data, the subjects completed an average of about 10.46 repetitions. However, only 22 of the 141 subjects (15.6%) did exactly 10 repetitions. A little more than two thirds of the subjects were clustered in the neighborhood of 10 repetitions. More specifically, 96 of the 141 subjects (68.1%) did between 8 and 12 repetitions – a very popular repetition range, by the way – while 45 of the 141 subjects (31.9%) did either less than 8 repetitions or more than 12. At the extremes of muscular endurance, two subjects did 5 repetitions (a sprinter and a thrower) and one managed 24 (a triathlete). Interestingly, by removing five outliers – the subjects who did 17, 19 and 24 repetitions – the remaining 136 subjects completed an average of 10.15 repetitions with 75% of their 1-RM which is remarkably close to the expected number of 10 repetitions.

Muscle biopsies weren't done in this study. Nonetheless, a sprinter and thrower likely have a high percentage of FT fibers and it's reasonable to think that this is evidenced by the relatively low number of repetitions that these subjects did during the test of muscular endurance. And a triathlete likely has a high percentage of ST fibers and it's reasonable to think that this is evidenced by the relatively high number of repetitions that

this subject did during the test of muscular endurance.

Here's one more way to think about the fatigue characteristics that were displayed by these three subjects: When you're no longer able to do any repetitions with 75% of your 1-RM, it means that you've lost a little more than 25% of your maximum strength. So the two subjects who did 5 repetitions lost about 5% of maximum strength per repetition while the subject who did 24 repetitions lost about 1% of maximum strength per repetition. In other words, the two subjects who did 5 repetitions fatigued much more quickly with each subsequent repetition while the subject who did 24 repetitions fatigued much more slowly with each subsequent repetition.

An intriguing study was conducted at the University of North Dakota where researchers found wide variations in muscular endurance among 98 football players. In this study, four of the athletes had the same 1-RM in the bench press (300 pounds). When tested with 75% of this weight (225 pounds), three of those athletes completed 9, 10 and 11 repetitions which is about what would be expected. But the fourth athlete showed greater muscular endurance: He did 16 repetitions.

Muscle biopsies weren't done in this study either so there's no way to be certain that the differences in muscular endurance were related to differences in fiber types. However, even if other factors may come into play, the influence that fiber types have on muscular endurance can't be overlooked or underemphasized.

You can also make a logical guesstimate of your fiber type based on your performance in certain activities. If you're successful in activities that require muscular endurance, you probably have a high percentage of ST fibers and should perform slightly higher repetitions; if you're successful in activities that require strength, speed and/or power, you probably have a high percentage of FT fibers and should perform slightly lower repetitions.

Another way of making a reasonable guesstimate of your fiber types is to consider your muscular development. FT fibers have a much

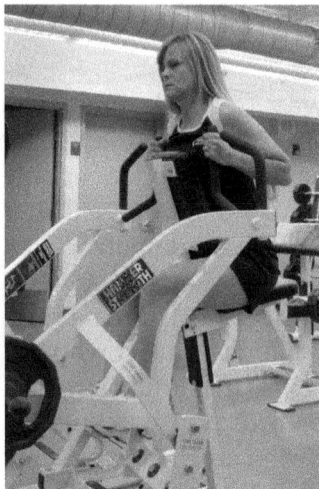

You should raise the weight in a smooth, controlled manner without any explosive or jerking movements.

greater potential to increase in size than ST fibers. Therefore, if you have a significant amount of muscular development, you probably have a high percentage of FT fibers; if you have an insignificant amount of muscular development, you probably have a high percentage of ST fibers (assuming, of course, that your lack of muscular development isn't the result of inactivity).

A final point about FT and ST fibers: The use of lower repetitions isn't suggested as a way to convert ST fibers to FT fibers. Nor is the use of higher repetitions suggested as a way to convert FT fibers to ST fibers. As noted in Chapter 3, there's no scientific evidence that consistently and convincingly supports the belief that ST fibers can be converted into FT fibers or vice versa. In other words, you can't convert ST fibers into FT fibers any more than you can convert a draft horse into a racehorse. Train a draft horse like a racehorse, you might get a slightly faster draft horse . . . but you'll never get a racehorse. Performing slightly higher or lower repetitions would be done to maximize your response to strength training based on the predominant muscle fiber type that's you have in your genetic portfolio.

Another genetic factor that has some influence on repetition ranges is lever length. In many exercises, those who have long limbs (levers) must move the resistance over a greater distance than those with short limbs and, therefore, must produce tension over a greater distance than those who have short limbs.

Everything else being equal, a long-limbed individual would probably be more fatigued after doing the same number of repetitions than a short-limbed individual. Depending on the circumstances, using a lower repetition range could keep the effort in the anaerobic domain. As a result, someone with long limbs would probably benefit more from doing slightly lower repetitions, especially in multiple-joint exercises (such as the bench press, lat pulldown and leg press) and certain free-weight exercises (such as the bicep curl) where limb length is a factor in the distance that the resistance moves.

Special Considerations

Repetition ranges of 15 to 20 for the hips, 10 to 15 for the legs and 5 to 10 for the torso will be safe and effective for most of the population. However, slightly higher repetition ranges are suggested for certain individuals. This includes younger teens and older adults along with anyone who has orthopedic issues. In addition, women who are pregnant should do slightly higher repetitions because of the increased laxity in their ligaments and joints during gestation. Slightly higher repetition ranges would also be recommended for those who have hypertension or are doing rehabilitative training.

In these cases, repetition ranges might be 20 to 25 for the hips, 15 to 20 for the legs and 10 to 15 for the torso. Doing higher repetitions requires the use of lighter weights; this, in turn, reduces the orthopedic stress that's placed on the bones, connective tissues (including tendons and ligaments) and joints.

5. Proper Technique

Most people have no understanding of – or pay no attention to – how they perform their repetitions. Yet, the repetition is the foundation of a strength program. Think about it: A program is comprised of workouts. Workouts are comprised of sets. And sets are comprised of repetitions.

So regardless of the type of strength program that you employ, a productive program begins with a productive repetition. If your repetitions aren't productive, then your sets won't be productive. If your sets aren't productive, then your workouts won't be productive. And if your workouts aren't productive, then your program won't be productive.

In order to maximize your response from strength training, it's absolutely essential that you do each repetition with proper technique. A repetition has four checkpoints: the positive (raising) phase, the mid-range position, the negative (lowering) phase and the range of motion.

Checkpoint #1: The Positive Phase

A repetition starts with raising the weight. To minimize the use of momentum, you should raise the weight in a smooth, controlled manner without any explosive or jerking movements. Raising a weight with high speeds isn't recommended for two main reasons.

First, high-speed repetitions are less productive than low-speed repetitions. Here's why: When weights are lifted too quickly, the muscles produce tension during the initial part of the movement . . . but not for the last part. In simple terms, the weight is practically moving by itself. In effect, the load on the muscles is decreased – or eliminated – and so are the potential gains in strength (and size).

This fact has been known since the experiments of Dr. Archibald (AV) Hill – a British physiologist – in 1922. According to his force-velocity curve (or relationship), the force that a muscle can produce at a fast speed is less than the force that a muscle can produce at a slow speed. In other words, an increase in speed produces a decrease in force. So if you want your muscles to produce a greater force – and you should – then you need to employ a slower speed. (Fast fact: Dr. Hill shared the Nobel prize in Physiology or Medicine in 1922 with Dr. Otto Meyerhof, a German biochemist.)

Unfortunately, the use of excessive momentum is demonstrated in fitness centers across the world on a daily basis (albeit, in most cases, unknowingly). Imagine that you raised the weight so quickly during the leg extension that the pad left your lower legs partway through the repetition. Think about it: The pad is attached to the movement arm of the machine which, in turn, is connected to the resistance by some means (such as a cable or belt). If the pad is no longer in contact with your lower legs, there's no load on your muscles. If there's no load on your muscles, there's no stimulus – or reason – for the muscles to adapt. Sure, you will obtain some benefit when your muscles were loaded during the first part of the repetition (when the pad was against your shins). However, you will not obtain any benefit when your muscles were unloaded during the last part of the repetition (when the pad wasn't against your shins). There's no question that the more momentum is used to raise a weight, the less productive will be the repetitions.

Second, high-speed repetitions carry a greater risk of injury than low-speed repetitions. Using an excessive amount of momentum to raise a weight increases the shear force that's encountered by a given joint; the faster a weight is raised, the higher this force is amplified, especially at the point of explosion. (Fast fact: Shear force acts parallel to a joint; compressive force acts perpendicular to a joint.)

In one study, three experienced male weightlifters performed the squat with 40%, 60% and 80% of their four-repetition maximum (4-RM; the maximum weight that they could lift four times) at three different speeds with a barbell and a selectorized machine. The shear forces at the knee joint were less for the slower speed of movement in comparison to the faster speed of movement at every point along the range of motion for the barbell as well as the machine. For example, when using the barbell, one of the subjects incurred a peak shear force of approximately 225 pounds when the weight was raised in about 2.13 seconds and a peak shear force of approximately 270 pounds when the weight was raised in about 0.83 seconds. (His results were typical of all three subjects.) This is clear evidence that a slower speed of movement reduces the shear force on joints. The authors noted, "At the knee, where shear is resisted primarily by the ligaments, the value of the joint shear force during any activity serves as an

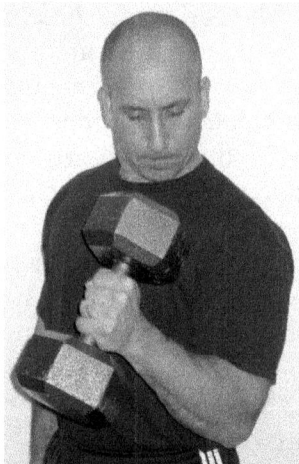

Pausing briefly in the mid-range position allows you to focus your attention on your muscles when they're fully contracted. (Photo by Lori Fornicola.)

important measure of the exposure of that joint to injury."

In another study, 10 subjects performed the clean and jerk with 40%, 60% and 80% of their 1-RM at three difference speeds with a barbell; the weights were raised in an average of about 1.55, 2.65 and 5.77 seconds. The peak compressive and shear forces at the lumbar spine were less for the slower speed of movement in comparison to the faster speed of movement. For example, when using 80% of their 1-RM, the peak compressive force was approximately 169 pounds with the slower speed and 280 pounds with the faster speed; the peak shear force was approximately 142 pounds with the slower speed and 273 pounds with the faster speed.

When the compressive and shear forces exceed the structural limits of a joint, an injury occurs to the muscles, connective tissues and/or bones. In addition, it's also possible that some injuries that occur *outside* the fitness center actually had their genesis *inside* the fitness center from employing certain techniques – such as high-speed repetitions – that weakened the structural integrity of the joint. To ensure that your repetitions are safe and productive, it should take at least one to two seconds to raise the weight.

Sidebar: In regard to speed of movement, it's interesting to consider the range of motion (ROM) through which a joint is exercised. For instance, during the bicep curl, the elbow joint has a ROM that's about 135 degrees. If you raised the weight at 60 degrees per second, it would take about

2.25 seconds to do the positive phase of this exercise. In comparison, during the lateral raise, the shoulder joint has a (safe) ROM that's about 90 degrees. If you raised the weight at 60 degrees per second, it would take about 1.5 seconds to do the positive phase of this exercise.

Checkpoint #2: The Mid-Range Position

After raising the weight, you should pause briefly in the mid-range position where the muscle is fully contracted. This brief pause – essentially an isometric contraction – should only take long enough for you to demonstrate that you're in control of the resistance.

Where's the mid-range position of a repetition? These two examples should help to make it clear: When performing a tricep extension, the mid-range position is where your arms are almost completely straight (extended); when performing a bicep curl, the mid-range position is where your arms are completely bent (flexed).

Most people are very weak in the mid-range position of a repetition because they rarely, if ever, emphasize it. Pausing briefly in the mid-range position allows you to focus your attention on your muscles when they're fully contracted. Furthermore, a brief pause in the mid-range position permits a smooth transition between the raising and lowering of the weight and helps to reduce the influence of momentum. If you can't pause briefly in the mid-range position, it's likely that you're raising the weight too quickly and literally throwing it into position.

Checkpoint #3: The Negative Phase

A repetition ends with lowering the weight. The importance of emphasizing the negative phase of a repetition can't be overstated. Numerous studies have shown that repetitions involving both concentric and eccentric contractions produce greater increases in strength (and size) than those involving just concentric contractions.

Why? Because the same muscles that you use to raise a weight are also used to lower it. In a bicep curl, for example, your biceps are used in raising and lowering the weight. The only difference is that when you raise the weight, your biceps are *shortening* against the load and when you lower the weight, your biceps are *lengthening* against the load. So by emphasizing the lowering of the weight, each repetition becomes more efficient and each set becomes more productive. Because a "loaded" muscle lengthens as you lower the weight, emphasizing the negative phase of a repetition also guarantees that the muscle is being stretched safely.

You have three levels of strength: concentric, isometric and eccentric. Your eccentric strength is *always* greater than your concentric strength in the same exercise. (Your isometric strength is ranked somewhere between your concentric and eccentric strength, varying at different joint angles.) Stated differently, you can *always* lower more weight than you can raise (again, in the same exercise).

How much greater is eccentric strength compared to concentric strength? In one study, 30 men were randomly tested for their concentric and eccentric 1-RM strength in the bench press. Prior to the study, the subjects had done the bench press for an average of at least once per week for one year or more. A mechanical hoist was used to lower the weight to the chest during concentric testing and raise the weight from the chest during eccentric testing. (During the eccentric 1-RM test, the subjects lowered the weight in three seconds; the time to raise the weight wasn't disclosed.) The researchers found that eccentric 1-RM strength (255.2 pounds) was about 24% greater than concentric 1-RM strength (205.8 pounds).

Based on the findings of this study, if the most weight that you can raise is 100 pounds, then the most weight that you can lower is about 124 pounds. It's important that these results aren't overgeneralized, however. The study involved the bench press with a barbell while taking three seconds to lower the weight; and all of the subjects were men. The results might not apply to other exercises, equipment and repetition speeds; and the results might not apply to women.

So while it's known that eccentric strength is greater than concentric strength, it's not known

by how much. Also not known is the reason why eccentric strength is greater than concentric strength. One theory is that the difference in strength is due to the role of titin, a protein filament with elastic properties. This theory aligns itself with the Winding Filament Hypothesis that was mentioned in Chapter 2. It's thought by some that when a muscle shortens during a concentric contraction, titin is wound around the actin filaments by the myosin heads. And when a muscle lengthens during an eccentric contraction – or is actively stretched – titin stiffens which results in a greater production of force.

Regardless of the reason why eccentric strength is greater than concentric strength, the fact is that negative work requires less effort than positive work. Indeed, walking down stairs is much easier than walking up stairs. And lowering a weight is much easier than raising a weight (in the same exercise). It makes sense, then, that the negative phase of a repetition should take more time to complete than the positive phase. To ensure that your repetitions are safe and productive, it should take at least three to four seconds to lower the weight.

Sidebar: Negative work also has a lower metabolic cost than positive work. More specifically, oxygen intake and caloric expenditure are lower during negative work than during positive work.

Checkpoint #4: The Range of Motion

A repetition should be done throughout the greatest possible ROM that safety allows: from a full stretch to a full contraction and back to a full stretch. But walk into most fitness centers and you'll see partial repetitions (aka half repetitions) being done on a wide variety of exercises. Classic examples include not lowering the bar all the way to the chest when doing the bench press and not fully straightening the arms when doing the chin-up, pull-up and bicep curl.

Performing your repetitions throughout a full ROM allows you to maintain – or perhaps increase – your flexibility. Researchers at the University of North Dakota randomly assigned 25 exercise science majors to two experimental groups that did either strength training or flexibility training for the same muscles and joints. (A third group acted as a control and didn't train.) After five weeks, the experimental groups significantly increased their ROM in three of four measures of flexibility and there were no significant differences between groups. (The experimental groups made a small but nonsignificant improvement in the fourth measure of flexibility.)

Moreover, performing your repetitions throughout a full ROM ensures that you're stimulating your entire muscle – not just a portion of it – thereby making the repetitions more productive. Research has shown that strength training is very angular-specific, meaning that improvements occur at or near the training angle. In one study, for example, isometric training – in which two sets of 10 repetitions were done at one joint angle – produced increases in strength that were specific to the joint angle that was trained plus about five degrees on either side of that point.

The need to perform repetitions throughout a full ROM is even more evident when considering studies of dynamic contractions which are more typical of a strength program. Researchers randomly assigned 40 men to two experimental groups: One group did repetitions of the bicep curl with a full ROM, raising and lowering the weight from 0 to 130 degrees (from a full stretch to a full contraction) and the other group did repetitions of the bicep curl with a partial ROM, raising and lowering the weight from 50 to 100 degrees. (A third group acted as a control and didn't train.) The experimental groups did two to four sets of the bicep curl two days per week for 10 weeks. The group that used a full ROM had significantly greater improvements in muscular strength (25.7% versus 16.0%) than the group that used a partial ROM. The group that used a full ROM also had greater increases in muscle thickness (9.7% versus 7.8%) than the group that used a partial ROM but the difference wasn't large enough to reach statistical significance. In short, full-range exercise is necessary for a full-range effect.

This doesn't imply that you should avoid limited-range repetitions altogether. During rehabilitative training, for example, you can exercise throughout a pain-free ROM and still manage to stimulate some gains in strength (and size). However, full-range repetitions are more productive and should be performed whenever possible.

A RECAP

It's much safer and more productive to perform each repetition with proper technique. To be more specific, you should (1) raise the weight in a smooth, controlled manner without any explosive or jerking movements; (2) pause briefly in the mid-range position; (3) emphasize the lowering of the weight; and (4) use a full ROM. These are hardly new concepts, by the way. In 1950, Drs. DeLorme and Watkins advised that "the load should be neither swung forward with a ballistic movement nor dropped under the influence of gravity." Raising the weight in at least one to two seconds and lowering it in at least three to four seconds is a good indication that momentum didn't play a significant role in the performance of the repetition.

Effectively, then, it should take at least four to six seconds to perform a repetition. Researchers at the Washington University School of Medicine assigned 13 men to an experimental group that did strength training three to four days per week for 16 weeks. (A second group acted as a control and didn't train.) Each workout consisted of one set of 14 exercises that addressed all of the major muscles. Each set was done to the point of muscular fatigue. It took six seconds to perform each repetition: Two seconds to raise the weight and four seconds to lower the weight. The subjects in the experimental group increased their maximum upper-body strength by an average of 50% in the five exercises that were tested and maximum lower-body strength by 33% in the three exercises that were tested.

Remember, *how well* you lift is more critical than *how much* you lift. Your strength program will be much safer and more productive when you perform each repetition with proper technique.

Sidebar: A classic example of *improper* technique is bouncing the barbell off your chest when doing the bench press. Yes, as a result, you can lift more weight and/or do more repetitions. But the reason why you can do this is because when the barbell crash-lands on your chest, you compress it like a coil spring and in recoiling, you literally get a boost to assist in lifting the weight. Suffice to say, this isn't advisable. For one thing, it makes the exercise less safe; cracked sternum, anyone? And it makes the exercise less productive; your muscles won't get as much out of the exercise.

6. Duration of a Workout

When it comes to strength training, more isn't necessarily better. An inverse relationship exists between time and intensity: As the time of an activity increases, the level of intensity decreases. Stated otherwise, you can't train with a high level of intensity for a long period of time. Consider this analogy: With respect to anaerobic training, compare the time (length) and intensity of a workout that consists of four 400-meter sprints to a workout that consists of eight 400-meter sprints. In doing four sprints, the time of the workout would be relatively low but the level of intensity would be relatively high; in doing eight sprints, the time of the workout would be relatively high but the level of intensity would be relatively low. So as the time of an activity goes up, the level of intensity goes down.

The fact is that you can train for a short period of time with a high level of intensity or a long period of time with a low level of intensity. But you can't train with a high level of intensity for a long period of time. In order to train with a high level of intensity, you must train for a brief period of time. If you lengthen the duration of your workout – by increasing either the number of exercises or sets that you normally perform – you must reduce your level of intensity. And, of course, using a lower level of intensity isn't desirable.

It's important to note that carbohydrates are your preferred source of energy during intense activity. Carbohydrates circulate in your bloodstream as glucose and are stored in your liver and muscles as glycogen. The liver and muscles can only stockpile a limited amount of

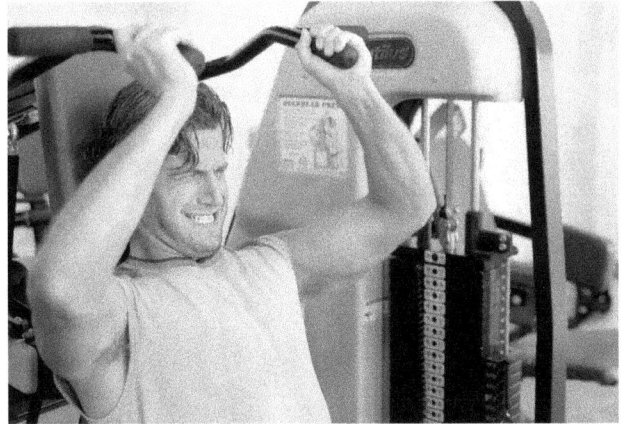

You can make your workouts more efficient – and more intense – by taking very little recovery between exercises/sets. (Photo provided by Luke Carlson.)

glycogen. For the average individual, estimates vary but seem to be around 500 grams of glycogen with about 100 grams stored in the liver and 400 grams stored in the muscles. (A negligible amount of glucose circulates in the blood.)

The rate at which you use calories is a function of your level of intensity; as your level of intensity increases, your rate of caloric expenditure increases. Now, suppose that you did strength training with a high level of intensity which required an average of 10 calories per minute. If you had 500 grams of glycogen "on tap" – 2,000 calories – you could conceivably work out for about 200 minutes or so before draining the reservoir. The amount of glycogen that's available can vary considerably among individuals. But even if you have enough glycogen to provide energy for as much as three hours, it doesn't mean that your workout has to be that long. An intense and comprehensive workout can be completed in approximately one hour or less. (Fast fact: Dr. Claude Bernard – a French physiologist – is credited with discovering and naming glycogen in 1857.)

Be advised that the duration of a workout is a critical factor in program adherence, especially among those who are new to training. Studies have shown that individuals tend to discontinue their programs when they're prescribed lengthy workouts.

The exact duration of a workout depends on several factors such as the size of the fitness

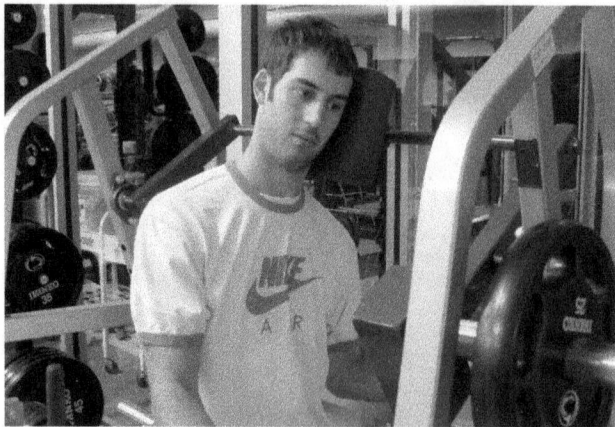

Those who participate in combat sports should include two to four exercises for their neck to strengthen and protect their cervical area against catastrophic injury. (Photo by Troy Harrison.)

center, the amount of equipment, the preparation for each exercise/set (such as adjusting seats, setting weights and so on), the number of people using the fitness center, the transition time between each exercise/set and the availability of a training partner. Generally speaking, however, you should be able to complete a comprehensive workout in no more than about one hour.

You can make your workouts more efficient – and more intense – by taking very little recovery between exercises/sets. The length of your recovery interval depends on your level of fitness. Initially, you may require several minutes of recovery between exercises/sets to catch your breath or feel that you can produce a maximum level of effort. With improved fitness, your pace between exercises/sets can be quickened. (To be clear: The *speed* with which you do your repetitions shouldn't be quickened, just the *pace* between exercises/sets.) When performed in this fashion, the shared demands that are placed on your musculoskeletal, respiratory and circulatory systems create improvements in metabolic fitness that can't be approached by traditional methods of strength training.

7. Volume of Exercises

Most individuals can accomplish a total-body workout with 14 exercises or less. The focal point for the majority of these exercises should be your

major muscles: your hips, legs and torso. Include one exercise for your hips, hamstrings, quadriceps, calves/dorsi flexors, biceps, triceps, abdominals and lower back. Because your shoulder joint allows movement at many different angles, you should perform two exercises for your chest, upper back and shoulders. You can choose any exercises that you prefer to address those body parts.

Some individuals may need to do slightly more than 14 exercises. For instance, those who participate in combat sports – such as football, rugby, boxing, judo and wrestling – should also include an additional two to four exercises for their neck to strengthen and protect their cervical area against catastrophic injury. Those who participate in sports or activities that require grip strength – such as baseball, golf and tennis – should include one exercise for their lower arms (forearms).

Once again, when it comes to strength training, more isn't necessarily better. Performing too many exercises can produce too much stress which may not permit compensatory adaptation. A total-body workout that contains 20 exercises could be metabolically devastating for someone who has a low tolerance for strength training. And the more exercises that you perform, the more difficult it will be for you to maintain an appropriate level of intensity.

This isn't to say that you can't do an extra exercise or two in order to emphasize a particular body part. As long as you continue to make improvements in your strength, you're not performing too many exercises. So if your workout consists of 20 exercises and you're making progress, then you're not overtraining. But if you plateau in one or more exercises, it's probably because the volume of your training has compromised your ability to recover.

8. Order of Exercise

The order in which you perform your exercises is essential in producing optimal improvements in strength (and size). The order of your exercises also determines which muscles you emphasize or target.

Researchers randomly assigned 48 men from the Brazilian Navy Academy into two experimental groups: One group trained their muscles from largest to smallest, doing the bench press, lat pulldown, shoulder press, bicep curl and tricep extension; the other group trained their muscles from smallest to largest, doing the same five exercises but in the reverse order. (A third group acted as a control and didn't train.) The experimental groups did three sets of each exercise and trained three times per week for eight weeks. The order in which the exercises were completed was critical in the improvements that were made. For example, gains in the bench press were 39.8% when the exercise was done first and 18.6% when it was done last; gains in the tricep extension were 74.3% when the exercise was done first and 50.0% when it was done last. In other words, doing an exercise earlier in the workout led to the greatest improvements.

As a rule of thumb, the idea is to train your most important muscles as early as possible in your workout. It stands to reason that you'd want to address those muscles while you're fresh, both mentally as well as physically. Larger muscles are generally more important than smaller muscles. In effect, then, your workout should begin with exercises that involve your largest muscles and proceed to those that involve your smallest ones.

The Lower Body

The largest and most powerful muscles are found in your lower body specifically, your hips and legs. What's the best order of exercise for training your lower body? Consider this: Multiple-joint movements that are done for your lower body – such as the leg press and deadlift – require the use of your upper legs for assistance. Your upper legs – your hamstrings and quadriceps – are the "weak link" in those exercises because they have a smaller amount of muscle mass. So if you fatigue your upper legs first, you'll weaken an already weak link thereby limiting the workload placed on the muscles of your hips. As a result, it's usually best to train your hips before your upper legs.

What would happen if you did train your upper legs immediately prior to your hips? In other words, what if you did the leg extension and then the leg press? This sequence of exercises would be very effective in fatiguing your quadriceps but not so much for your hips.

After training your upper legs, you should proceed to your lower legs, either your calves or dorsi flexors. If you train your calves and your dorsi flexors in the same workout, the order in which you do so really doesn't matter.

So in general, you should start with your hips and literally work down your legs. In other words, the best order of exercise would be hips, upper legs (hamstrings and quadriceps) and lower legs (calves or dorsi flexors).

The Upper Body

Once you've exercised your lower body, you can now direct your attention to your upper body. What's the best order of exercise for training your upper body? Not to be redundant but from a conceptual standpoint, it sounds quite similar to that which has been discussed for your lower body. Multiple-joint movements that are done for your upper body – such as the bench press, seated row and shoulder press – require the use of your arms for assistance. Your arms – your biceps, triceps and forearms – are the weak link in those exercises because they have a smaller amount of muscle mass. So if you fatigue your arms first, you'll weaken an already weak link thereby limiting the workload placed on the muscles of your torso. As a result, it's usually best to train your upper back before your biceps; your biceps before your forearms; and your chest and/ or shoulders before your triceps.

What would happen if you did train your triceps immediately prior to your chest and/or shoulders or your biceps immediately prior to your upper back? In other words, what if you did the tricep extension and then the bench press or the bicep curl and then the seated row? This sequence of exercises would be very effective in fatiguing your arms but not so much for the major muscles of your torso.

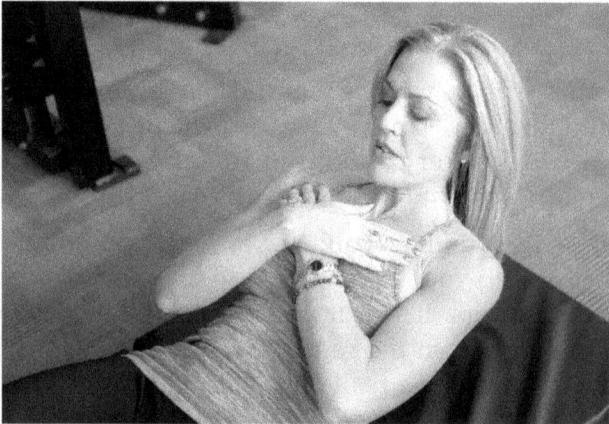

Exercise your abdominals at the end of a workout, not at the beginning. (Photo provided by Luke Carlson.)

You have at least two options for the order in which you train your chest, upper back and shoulders. One way is to do all of the exercises for a given muscle – your chest, for example – and then proceed to the next muscle. Another way is to alternate an exercise that involves a pushing motion (or action) with an exercise that involves a pulling motion. (To avoid confusion, it's important to note that muscles *always* pull when they contract; however, muscular contractions produce motion that can be described as either a push or a pull.) Your chest, anterior portion of your shoulders and triceps are used in pushing motions (and can be referred to as "pushing" muscles); your upper back, posterior portion of your shoulders, biceps and forearms are used in pulling motions (and can be referred to as "pulling" muscles). In a push-pull application, you might do the following sequence for your torso: bench press (push), seated row (pull), incline press (push), underhand lat pulldown (pull), front raise (push), bent-over raise (pull), tricep extension (push) and bicep curl (pull).

Performing all of the exercises for a given muscle before moving to another muscle produces a large amount of fatigue since the muscle being exercised gets little relief (assuming, of course, that the time taken between exercises/sets is minimal); alternating exercises in a push-pull fashion allows one muscle to recover while another muscle is being trained. (You're encouraged to experiment with these two applications and vary them based on your personal preferences and performance objectives.)

So in general, you should start with your chest, upper back and shoulders and literally work down your arms. In other words, the best order of exercise would be torso (chest, upper back and shoulders) and upper arms (biceps and triceps). If you include an exercise for your lower arms (forearms) in your workout, it's best to do it after you complete your upper-arm exercises.

The Mid-Section

Many people begin their workouts by training their mid-section (their abdominals and lower back). But early fatigue of the mid-section isn't advisable.

During intense exercise/activity, your abdominals are involved in forced expiration. Therefore, fatiguing your abdominals early in your workout would detract from your performance in other exercises that involve larger, more powerful muscles.

In one crossover study, 12 subjects ran as far as possible in 12 minutes on an outdoor track on two separate occasions: one time after fatiguing their abdominals and the other time without. To produce fatigue, the subjects inhaled freely through their nose and exhaled through a mouthpiece that offered resistance to breathing. (A previous study found that this type of resistive breathing elicits abdominal fatigue.) In 12 minutes, the subjects ran about 2,872 meters when their abdominals were fatigued and about 2,957 meters when their abdominals weren't. So, prior fatigue of the abdominals resulted in a significant decrease in maximal running distance.

The take-home message is to exercise your abdominals at the *end* of a workout, not at the *beginning*.

The very last muscle that you should train is your lower back. Similar to the abdominals, fatiguing your lower back early in your workout would detract from your performance in other exercises (especially ones that involve the lower back).

So in general, you should end with your mid-section. And the best order of exercise would be abdominals and lower back.

The Neck

As mentioned earlier, individuals who participate in combat sports should train their neck muscles. If you include exercises for your neck in your workout, it makes the most sense to do them at the beginning of your workout or just after you complete your lower-body exercises (prior to beginning your upper-body exercises). This violates the largest-to-smallest rule but at the end of your workout, you will be – and should be – physically and mentally drained. If you wait until this point to train your neck, you'll be less likely to address this all-important area with a desirable level of effort or enthusiasm. Training your neck earlier in your workout when you're less fatigued will yield a more favorable response.

A RECAP

In summary, the best order of exercise in a total-body workout would usually look like this: hips, upper legs (hamstrings and quadriceps), lower legs (calves or dorsi flexors), torso (chest, upper back and shoulders), upper arms (biceps and triceps), abdominals and lower back. If included, exercises for your neck should be done at the beginning of your workout or just after your lower body (prior to the exercises for your torso); exercises for your lower arms (forearms) should be done just after your upper arms.

If you prefer to do a split routine – in which the body is divided or split into parts that are trained over the course of several workouts instead of one total-body workout – the aforementioned order of exercise would still apply. In a workout that targeted your chest, shoulders and triceps, for example, you should still address those body parts from largest to smallest.

9. Frequency of Training

In order for you to achieve optimal increases in strength (and size), your muscles must receive an adequate amount of recovery between your workouts. Intense strength training places large demands on your musculoskeletal system. Compensatory adaptation to these demands occurs during the recovery process.

Believe it or not, your muscles don't get stronger during your workout . . . your muscles get stronger *after* your workout. If the demands are of sufficient magnitude, a muscle is damaged at the cellular level in the form of very small tears. The recovery process is essential in that it permits the damaged muscle the time to repair itself. Think of this as allowing a wound to heal. If you had a scab and picked at it every day, you'd delay the healing process. But if you left it alone, you'd permit the damaged tissue the time to heal. So in a sense, the recovery that follows a workout is a process in which damaged tissue – in this case, muscle tissue – is healed.

There are individual variations in recovery ability; everyone has a different tolerance for exercise. However, a period of at least 48 hours is usually necessary for muscle tissue to recover sufficiently from intense strength training. Keep in mind, too, that intense strength training relies heavily on carbohydrates as the preferred source of energy. When glycogen (carbohydrate) stores are depleted as a result of intense activity, it appears as if about 48 hours are needed to refill those stores.

As such, it's suggested that you do strength training two or three times per week on nonconsecutive days (such as on Monday, Wednesday and Friday). This advice is consistent with the 2011 position stand by the American College of Sports Medicine (ACSM) on the quantity and quality of exercise for healthy adults. (Note that this assumes total-body workouts.)

Sidebar: The process for replenishing glycogen stores is biphasic. In the first phase – assuming that adequate carbohydrates are consumed after an activity – glycogen is resynthesized quickly; glycogen is almost at its pre-activity level within about 24 hours. In the second phase, however, glycogen is resynthesized slowly; glycogen returns to its pre-activity level within about 48 hours (assuming an adequate intake of carbohydrates). In one study, four physical-

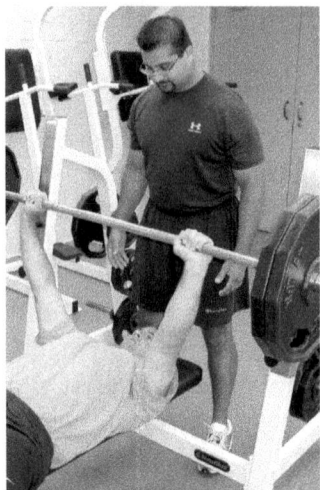

In order for you to achieve optimal increases in strength (and size), your muscles must receive an adequate amount of recovery between workouts (Photo by Peter Silletti.)

education majors were assigned to perform two hours of strenuous activity. Their glycogen reached its pre-activity level 46 hours after the activity; this, despite consuming a carbohydrate-enriched diet – 60% of the calories – during those 46 hours.

An appropriate frequency and volume of strength training can be likened to an appropriate dose of medicine. In order for medicine to improve a condition, it must be taken at specific intervals and in certain amounts. Taking medicine at a greater frequency or in a larger volume than what's needed can have negative effects. Similarly, an overdose of strength training – in which workouts are done too often or have too much volume – can also have negative effects.

Most individuals respond well from three total-body workouts per week. But because of a low tolerance for strength training, others respond more favorably from two total-body workouts per week. In rare circumstances, an individual may respond better from one total-body workout per week. Performing any more than three doses of total-body workouts per week will gradually become counterproductive if the demands placed on your muscles exceed your recovery ability.

Many authorities believe that a muscle begins to lose strength (and size) if it's not adequately stimulated within about 96 hours of a previous workout. Anecdotal reports suggest that it may be more than 96 hours, at least for some individuals. Clearly, however, a loss of strength (and size) will occur after some period of extended inactivity. If you're an athlete, then, it's important for you to continue strength training even while in-season or while competing. However, the workouts should be reduced to twice a week due to the increased level of activity from practices and competitions. One workout should be done as soon as possible following a competition and another not within 48 hours of the next competition. So, an athlete who competes on Tuesdays and Saturdays should do strength training on Wednesdays and Sundays (or Thursdays, providing that it's not within 48 hours of the next competition). From time to time, an athlete may only be able to do strength training once per week because of a particularly heavy schedule such as competing three times in one week or several days in a row.

In general, it appears as if training three days per week is better than training two days per week. But you can still make significant improvements in strength from two weekly workouts. In one study, 117 subjects were randomly assigned to four experimental groups that trained either two or three times per week for either 10 weeks or 18 weeks. (A fifth group acted as a control and didn't train.) The two groups that trained three days per week increased their strength by 21.2% (10 weeks) and 28.4% (18 weeks); the two groups that trained two days per week increased their strength by 13.5% (10 weeks) and 20.9% (18 weeks). So overall, doing two weekly workouts achieved about 80% of the gains in strength as doing three weekly workouts.

How do you know if your muscles have had an adequate amount of recovery? You should see a gradual improvement in the amount of resistance and/or number of repetitions that you're able to do over the course of several weeks. If not, then you're probably not getting enough recovery between your workouts which, again, could be the result of performing too many sets, too many repetitions or too many exercises. Remember, strength training will be effective if it provides an overload, not an overdose.

The Split Routine

A method that has been popularized by bodybuilders and competitive weightlifters is known as the split routine. When using a split routine, the body is split into different parts that are trained on different days.

There are many possibilities for a split routine. One example is to split the muscles such that the hips, legs and mid-section are trained on Monday and Thursday; the chest, shoulders and triceps on Tuesday and Friday; and the upper back, biceps and forearms on Wednesday and Saturday. So in this split routine, each muscle would be trained twice per week during six workouts.

Despite the widespread use of split routines, the method is no more effective than total-body workouts. In one study, 30 female kinesiology students at McMaster University in Canada were assigned to two experimental groups: One group did a split routine consisting of four workouts per week (two for the upper body and two for the lower body) and the other group did two total-body workouts per week. (A third group acted as a control and didn't train.) After 20 weeks of training, it was found that both protocols were equally effective in improving maximum strength, increasing lean-body mass and decreasing body fat.

In another study, 20 men were randomly assigned to two groups: One group did a split routine consisting of three workouts per week that focused on two or three muscle groups per workout; the other group did three total-body workouts per week that addressed all of the muscle groups in each workout. Over the course of a week, both groups performed the same 21 exercises for an identical number of sets and repetitions. After eight weeks of training, there were no significant differences between groups in maximum strength in the bench press and squat as well as muscle thickness of the forearm extensors and thigh. The group that did total-body workouts had a significantly greater increase in muscle thickness of the forearm flexors.

Split routines can be productive as long as they encourage progressive overload and provide

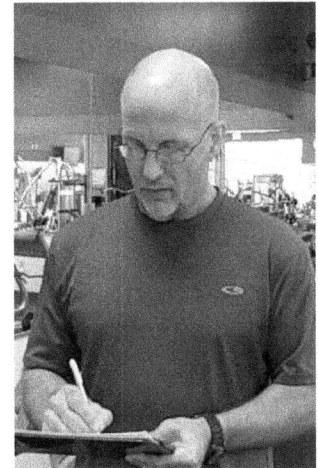

Records are an extremely valuable tool to monitor your progress and make your workouts more productive and more meaningful. (Photo by Patty Durell.)

adequate recovery. It's the latter area in which split routines often fall short. If a split routine is designed correctly, a person won't train the same muscles two days in a row. Recall, however, that about 48 hours are needed for your body to replenish its stockpile of glycogen following intense activity. So if you trained your lower body on Monday with a desirable level of intensity, you exhausted much of your glycogen stores. Even if you train different muscles on Tuesday, your body wouldn't have had the time to return your glycogen stores to its pre-activity level.

Keep in mind, too, that even though you may train part of your body in a workout, you still stress your entire anaerobic pathways (which provide metabolic support for your efforts). Your energy systems don't recover in parts; they recover as a whole. In the aforementioned study that was conducted at McMaster University, the researchers noted that doing fewer workouts per week "would free more days for recovery or other types of training." This is an important consideration for competitive athletes who must invest significant amounts of their time in aerobic, anaerobic and skill training.

If you prefer to use a split routine, make sure that you group your muscles based on their functions and relations with other muscles. For instance, your triceps and shoulders are used to train your chest. So, these muscles should be included in the same workout. Likewise, your biceps and forearms are used to train your upper back. So, these muscles should be included in the same workout.

One final point: From a performance perspective, split routines don't make sense because they're not specific to the muscular involvement in most physical activities. When you use a split routine, you train different muscles on different days. However, a selective use of muscles almost never happens during a physical activity. Rather, you're required to integrate all of your muscles at once. Therefore, it makes little sense for you to prepare for physical activities by training your muscles separately on different days.

10. Record Keeping

Many people believe that they don't need to track their performance because they can remember the resistance that they used and the repetitions that they did. In all likelihood, they've probably been using the same resistance and doing the same repetitions for so long that the information has become firmly entrenched in their long-term memories. In order for you to achieve optimal increases in strength (and size), it's absolutely critical for you to keep written records that are accurate and detailed.

Why? For one thing, records are the history of what you accomplished during each and every exercise of each and every workout. Moreover, records are an extremely valuable tool to monitor your progress and make your workouts more productive and more meaningful. Records can also be used to identify exercises in which you've reached a plateau. In the unfortunate event of an injury, you can also gauge the effectiveness of your rehabilitative training if you have a record of your pre-injury levels of strength.

Regardless of the means that you choose to employ for record keeping, you should be able to track your bodyweight, the date of each workout, the resistance used for each exercise, the number of repetitions performed for each set, the order in which the exercises were completed and any necessary seat adjustments.

Bottom line: Don't underestimate the importance of keeping records as a way to make your strength training more productive and more meaningful.

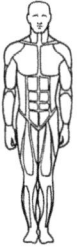

5 Strength Training for Females

Strength training isn't just for males. Many physical, physiological and psychological benefits of strength training have been noted in Chapter 4 but one that's especially important for females is worth mentioning again: an increase in bone mineral density.

Osteoporosis – literally, porous bones – is a condition that's characterized by decreased bone mineral density. According to the National Center for Health Statistics, 2% of American men aged 50 and older have osteoporosis of the hip while 10% of their female counterparts have the same condition. Osteoporosis impacts the quality of life in many ways but perhaps the biggest concern is a greater risk of fractures (mainly to the vertebrae, wrist and hip). Obviously, this could lead to permanent disability. Strength training can increase bone density thereby reducing the risk of osteoporosis (and bone fracture).

DISPELLING MISCONCEPTIONS

It wasn't until the early 1980s or so before it became socially acceptable for females to lift weights. Prior to that time, there were many worries that strength training would produce masculinizing effects.

Gradually, most of these fears have subsided. But even to this day, some concerns continue to linger. The two biggest misconceptions about females who lift weights are that they'll end up losing flexibility and developing large muscles.

Losing Flexibility

When conducted properly, strength training doesn't reduce flexibility. If anything, doing repetitions throughout a full range of motion against a resistance will maintain or even improve flexibility.

Females who have residual fears about becoming less flexible can do a series of stretches both before and after their strength training. As an added measure, they can also stretch the muscles that were involved in an exercise immediately after it's completed. Following the leg extension, for example, an individual can do a stretch for her quadriceps.

Developing Large Muscles

An increase in strength is often accompanied by an increase in size (although the increase in size isn't proportional to the increase in strength). While this is true for both genders, the fact of the matter is that increases in size are much less pronounced in females.

Since the early 1960s, research has shown that most females can achieve an increase in their strength without an increase in their size. In a classic 1974 study that was conducted at the University of California, Davis, Dr. Jack Wilmore – a pioneer in the field of physical education – assigned 47 women and 26 men to do the same training. Both groups did two sets of eight

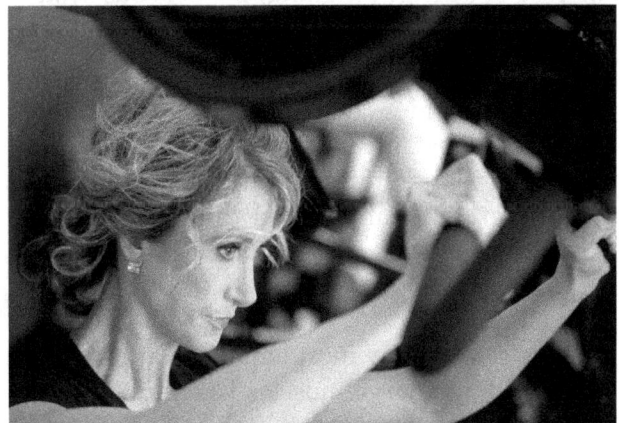

Most females can achieve an increase in their strength without an increase in their size. (Photo provided by Luke Carlson.)

exercises for eight weeks. (This was a 10-week study but initial strength testing wasn't done until after the first two weeks to allow the subjects to learn the proper technique to perform the exercises.) The women significantly improved their strength in the leg press by 29.5% and bench press by 28.6%. Yet, the largest increase in size that was experienced by the women in any one of the 17 areas that were assessed was *less than one-quarter inch*. It's also important to note that the women gained about 2.34 pounds of lean-body mass and lost about 2.38 pounds of fat which, in effect, reduced their percentage of body fat from 24.51 to 22.65%.

More recently is the FAMuSS (Functional Polymorphisms Associated with Human Muscle Size and Strength) Study. In this study, 585 individuals – 243 men and 342 women – did strength training with their non-dominant arm (biceps) for 12 weeks. The cross-sectional area (muscle size) of the biceps increased by 20.4% in men and 17.9% in women. But get this: Isometric strength increased by 22.0% in women and 15.8% in men while dynamic strength increased by 64.1% in women and 39.8% in men.

Sidebar: In general, an increase in strength without an attendant increase in size is thought to be the result of neural adaptation. This is also true of any increase in strength that occurs in the first few weeks of a program. Neural adaptation refers to changes that are made by the nervous system in response to a stimulus. In the case of strength training, the nervous system adapts by becoming more efficient at stimulating (activating) muscle fibers.

It's very evident that females who lift weights can make substantial gains in strength without developing large muscles. From a physiological standpoint, there are at least three reasons why this is true.

Muscle Fiber Type

One reason why most females don't have the potential to get large muscles has to do with the proportion of their fast-twitch (FT) and slow-twitch (ST) fibers. Research has shown that females possess a slightly higher percentage of ST fibers than males. For example, a study that involved 418 subjects reported that females had 51% ST fibers in their vastus lateralis and males had 46%.

As noted in Chapter 3, FT and ST fibers have the potential to increase in size but FT fibers have a much greater potential. Since females have a higher percentage of ST fibers, their potential to increase the size of their muscles is lower.

Testosterone

Another reason why most females don't have the potential to get large muscles pertains to testosterone, a hormone that's typically associated with men but also found in the blood of perfectly normal women. Testosterone prompts muscles to increase in size. Everything else being equal, those who have high levels of testosterone have a greater potential to improve their size than those who have low levels of testosterone. Compared to males, most females possess low levels of this hormone. In fact, the average female has about 5% of the testosterone circulating in her blood as the average male. This small amount of testosterone restricts the degree to which females can increase the size of their muscles.

The small percentage of females who do develop relatively large muscles might have slightly higher levels of testosterone than the average female. In one study, researchers suggested that testosterone may play a role in a female's trainability (the degree to which she responds to strength training). In another study, 10 women participated in a brief but intense strength program. The researchers found a high correlation between their level of testosterone and the size of their muscles.

Body Fat

One more reason why most females can't get large muscles has to do with body fat. Females tend to inherit higher percentages of body fat than males. For example, the average 18- to 22-year-old female has about 22 to 26% body fat, whereas the average male of similar age has about 12 to 16%. A higher percentage of body fat corresponds to a lower percentage of lean-body (or fat-free) mass. This extra body fat tends to soften or mask the effects of strength training.

Females who have very little body fat look more muscular than they actually are because their muscles are more visible. Along these lines, what appears to be an increase in muscle mass from strength training may be the result of a decrease in body fat which makes the same amount of muscle look more noticeable.

Interestingly, the distribution of fat is gender-specific. Even though there are individual differences, males tend to store fat in their abdominal area (aka an android pattern) which produces an apple-shaped look; females tend to store fat in their hips and thighs (aka a gynoid pattern) which produces a pear-shaped look. Moreover, the body type of the average female tends more toward endomorphy (fatness) while the body type of the average male tends more toward ectomorphy (leanness) and mesomorphy (muscularity).

Female Bodybuilders

In case you're wondering about female bodybuilders, they've inherited a greater potential to increase the size of their muscles than the average woman. In other words, female bodybuilders have developed large muscles because of their genetic profile, not simply because they lifted weights. Also, it's well within the realm of possibility that at least some female bodybuilders have used steroids or other performance-enhancing drugs to enhance their muscular development.

Keep in mind, too, that female bodybuilders look much more muscular than normal while posing on stage. When training for a competition, female bodybuilders restrict their caloric consumption – often severely – thereby reducing their body fat and body fluids. Immediately prior to posing on stage, they've also "pumped" their muscles. This engorges their muscles with blood and makes them temporarily bigger, a condition that's known as transient muscular hypertrophy. Finally, the stage lighting as well as their tans and clothing – and even the oil that's rubbed on their bodies – all contribute to making female bodybuilders appear as if they have much larger muscles than they actually do.

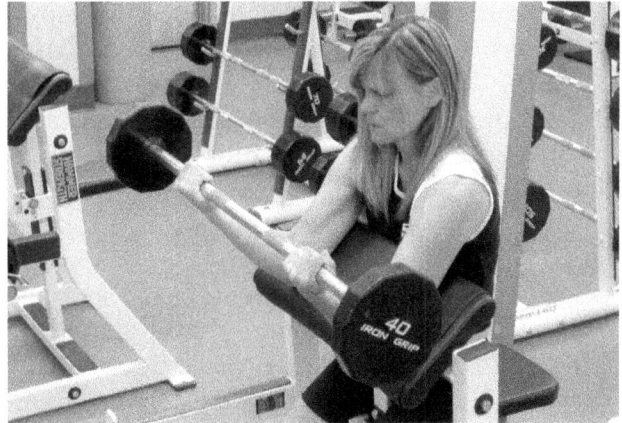

There's no such thing as gender-specific training or gender-specific exercises.

A RECAP

A relatively small number of females have inherited the ingredients that are necessary to attain significant increases in their size. But the overwhelming majority of females can gain considerable strength while experiencing little change in their size. In short, it's physiologically improbable for the average female to develop large muscles that are unsightly or unfeminine.

COMPONENTS OF STRENGTH TRAINING

It must be understood that there's no such thing as gender-specific training (or gender-specific exercises). Even with the use of an electron microscope, it's literally impossible for a scientist to differentiate between the muscle tissue of females and the muscle tissue of males. So in general, females can do the same strength program – and utilize the same exercises – as males.

Females can improve their strength in a manner that's productive, comprehensive, practical, efficient, sustainable and safe by incorporating the 10 components of strength training that are detailed in Chapter 4.

GENDER DIFFERENCES IN STRENGTH

Researchers have investigated gender differences in strength since the early 1900s. This is often done as a measure of absolute strength:

the amount of weight that can be lifted without considering any other factors. But it's also important to examine relative strength: the amount of weight that can be lifted in relation to bodyweight, body composition and muscular size.

Absolute Strength

In terms of absolute strength, the average male tends to be far stronger than the average female. In 1961, a literature review by Dr. Theodor Hettinger found that the absolute total-body strength of females is roughly two thirds (67%) that of males. In 1976, a literature review by Dr. Lloyd Laubach corroborated these results, finding that the absolute total-body strength of females is roughly 63.5% that of males. Since that time, numerous studies have compared the absolute strength levels of males and females and have reported varying degrees of differences. However, research has consistently shown that males tend to be stronger than females in absolute terms.

The differences in absolute strength between males and females vary according to the areas of the body that are being compared. As an example, the review by Dr. Laubach revealed that in comparison to males, the absolute isometric strength of females is about 57 to 86% in the lower body (averaging 71.9%), about 37 to 70% in the mid-section (averaging 63.8%) and about 44 to 79% in the upper body (averaging 59.5%); the absolute dynamic strength of females – lifting, lowering, pulling and pushing – is about 59 to 84% (averaging 68.6%).

The reason why the difference in absolute strength between males and females is less in the lower body than the upper body is probably because both genders have had an equal opportunity to use their lower bodies to a similar degree (such as while standing, walking and running) but not their upper bodies. Another reason that has been cited is that males have wider shoulders than females, giving them a biomechanical advantage in upper-body strength.

Relative Strength

So in absolute terms, males are significantly stronger than females. However, males are significantly larger and heavier than females. In terms of absolute strength, the greater body size of males gives them a decided advantage over females. When assessing gender differences in strength, then, comparisons should be made relative to some measure of size.

As mentioned earlier, the average female has more body fat and less lean-body mass than the average male. And of course, lean-body mass is functional tissue. Let's assign some numbers to this. The average college-aged male who weighs 154 pounds (lb) with 14% body fat has 21.56 pounds of body fat and 132.44 pounds of lean-body mass [154 lb x 14% = 21.56 lb; 154 lb - 21.56 lb = 132.44 lb]. On the other hand, the average college-aged female who weighs 126 pounds with 24% body fat has 30.24 pounds of body fat and 95.76 pounds of lean-body mass [126 lb x 24% = 30.24 lb; 126 lb - 30.24 lb = 95.76 lb]. So in this illustration, the average college-aged male has 22.2% more bodyweight [154 lb versus 126 lb] and 38.3% more lean-body mass [132.44 lb versus 95.76 lb] than the average college-aged female.

In short, the average male has more bodyweight and more lean-body mass – this is to say, more functional tissue – than the average female. Clearly, then, strength must be expressed relative to bodyweight and/or body composition in order to make valid comparisons of males and females.

Strength Relative to Bodyweight and Body Composition

When the disparities in bodyweight and body composition are taken into consideration, the differences in strength between males and females are less substantial. In the study by Dr. Wilmore that was noted earlier, when expressed relative to bodyweight, the leg strength of females was nearly identical to that of males. And when expressed relative to lean-body mass, the leg strength of females was actually slightly higher than males. (In this study, the upper-body strength of men was significantly greater than women regardless of how the values were compared.) Another study reported that the upper-body strength of females averaged 60 to 70% of males relative to bodyweight and 80 to 90% of males relative to lean-body mass. In a study involving 55 women and 48 men, the researchers concluded that gender differences in strength are a function of lean-body mass and body composition. So, it's quite clear that making comparisons relative to body composition basically eliminates any gender difference in strength.

With respect to gender differences in strength relative to bodyweight, it's also interesting to examine highly experienced athletes. This can be done easily by looking at the performances of elite powerlifters. Their accomplishments are a measure of strength – essentially one-repetition maximums (the maximum weight that they can lift one time) – and they compete in weight classes. Of course, the calculations aren't totally precise since someone who "makes weight" in the 60-kilogram class, for example, will likely weigh more than this during the actual competition. Nevertheless, it's still a convenient way to obtain a rough estimate of gender differences in strength relative to bodyweight.

In powerlifting, males and females compete in three different lifts: the squat, bench press and deadlift. The upcoming data were gleaned from the world records of men and women that were officially recognized by the International Powerlifting Federation (IPF) as of June 2011 in seven mutual weight classes: 52.0, 56.0, 60.0, 67.5, 75.0, 82.5 and 90.0 kilograms. (The IPF has since changed the weight classes such that none are the same for men and women.) Relative to bodyweight, performances by females in the squat, bench press and deadlift ranged from 68 to 77% (averaging 72.8%), 64 to 75% (averaging 71.2%) and 70 to 79% (averaging 75.2%) of their male counterparts, respectively. Recall that in the literature review by Dr. Laubach, in comparison to males and without adjusting for bodyweight, the absolute dynamic strength of females – lifting, lowering, pulling and pushing – is about 59 to 84% (averaging 68.6%). So again, the differences

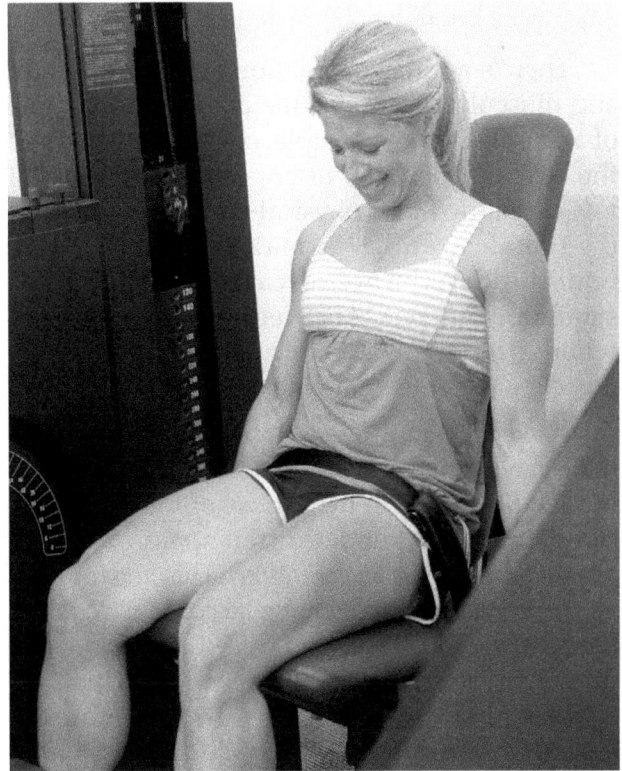

When the disparities in bodyweight and body composition are taken into consideration, the differences in strength between males and females are less substantial. (Photo provided by Luke Carlson.)

in strength between males and females are less significant when bodyweight is considered.

On a related note, something else to ponder is that although the average male is stronger than the average female in terms of absolute strength, many females are much stronger than the average male. According to the IPF, a number of women have lifted more than 3.5 times their bodyweight in the squat and deadlift; at least two women have done the squat with more than four times their bodyweight and one of those women has done the deadlift with more than four times her bodyweight. Also, a number of women have exceeded 2.5 times their bodyweight in the bench press; at least seven women have done the bench press with more than 400 pounds. Needless to say, the vast majority of the male population will never be able to attain such remarkable performances in those three lifts. (Fast fact: At the present time, topping the IPF's list of female powerlifters is Hildeborg Hugdal of Norway with a bench press of 499.4 pounds.)

Strength Relative to Muscular Size

There's a direct correlation between strength and muscular size (here, the cross-sectional area of a muscle). As an example, one study examined the strength per unit of cross-sectional area of muscle tissue of 18 physical-education students (7 females and 11 males) and 5 male bodybuilders. The researchers found no significant differences between males and females when strength was expressed in relation to muscle cross-sectional area.

As such, the differences in strength between males and females appear to be in the *volume* of muscle fibers, not in the *makeup* of muscle fibers. In other words, gender differences in strength are *quantitative*, not *qualitative*. This means that although males usually have larger muscles than females, the force that's produced by equal-sized muscles is the same in both genders. This isn't surprising since muscle tissue of females is essentially the same as the muscle tissue of males.

In short, the ability of a muscle to produce force is independent of gender.

ISSUE: EXERCISE AND PREGNANCY

The fundamental purpose of exercise during pregnancy – including strength training – is to maintain fitness and prepare a woman for labor and delivery. There doesn't appear to be any scientific evidence to suggest that women who exercise during their pregnancy will shorten or ease their labor and delivery. According to the American College of Sports Medicine, however, it's reasonable to expect that exercise will facilitate labor and the recovery from labor.

Potential Benefits

Many other potential benefits are associated with exercising during pregnancy. First of all, women who exercise can better meet the progressive physical demands of pregnancy. By strengthening the muscles of their torso and abdominals, women can compensate for the postural adjustments that typically occur during pregnancy as a result of the forward pull of the growing baby's weight. Women who have stronger muscles can counter fatigue and reduce the severity and frequency of common pregnancy-related discomforts such as low-back pain. In addition, women who do strength training experience minimal biomechanical changes and are better able to maintain their normal activities during pregnancy. Exercising also helps to control the amount of weight that women gain during pregnancy. Finally, improving strength can be good preparation for carrying a baby that may weigh 6 to 10 pounds at birth.

Potential Risks

With regards to a fitness program, the most important consideration for a pregnant woman and her developing fetus is safety. Proper exercise poses little risk to the mother or her fetus. Nonetheless, women who have never participated in a fitness program shouldn't initiate one during their pregnancy. Additionally, women should consult with their physician before starting any fitness program.

Although exercise has little risk during pregnancy, the potential exists for adverse effects to both the mother and the fetus. As such, there are a few areas of concern that must be addressed.

With several precautionary measures for added safety, a pregnant woman can perform the same type of program that's recommended for the general population. If a pregnant woman shows signs of exertional intolerance and/or chronic fatigue, she should reduce her intensity, frequency, volume and/or duration of training. The American College of Obstetricians and Gynecologists advises women to terminate exercise if they experience any of the following conditions: vaginal bleeding; dyspnea (shortness of breath) prior to exercise; dizziness; headache; chest pain; muscle weakness; calf pain or swelling; or decreased fetal movement.

Competing Needs

During exercise, there may be competition for various maternal and fetal physiological needs such as blood flow, oxygen delivery and heat dissipation. The prospect of this biological struggle is greatest during exercise that's performed in the third trimester.

When a person exercises, there's an increased blood flow to the working muscles. In fact, the working muscles may receive 70% or more of the blood flow. During pregnancy, the diversion of oxygen-rich blood to the exercising muscles of the mother leads to a transient reduction in the flow of oxygen-rich blood to the fetus. This threatens the fetus with the possibility of an inadequate supply of blood and oxygen. Exercising with a low to moderate level of intensity for 30 minutes or less doesn't seem to disturb uterine blood flow.

A potential threat to the safety of the developing fetus – especially during the first trimester – is exercise-induced hyperthermia (an increased core temperature). Exercise is associated with a rise in both maternal and fetal core temperatures. The fetus usually maintains a core temperature slightly above that of the mother. In order to dissipate heat, the fetus must depend entirely on the mother's thermo-regulatory abilities. To avoid heat complications, an exercising mother must be adequately hydrated, use a level of intensity that's lower than her pre-pregnancy state and wear light clothing that permits heat loss. In addition, she must be aware of the existing environmental temperature and humidity. Pregnant women must avoid high ambient temperature and humidity during exercise due to potential problems in thermoregulation. During pregnancy, women shouldn't exercise when the ambient temperature is greater than 90 degrees Fahrenheit and the relative humidity exceeds 50%. Finally, workouts shouldn't be more than about 30 minutes in duration so that the fetus isn't exposed to prolonged thermal stress.

Increased Laxity

After contraception, the levels of relaxin increase significantly. Relaxin is a hormone that helps to loosen or, as you might suspect, "relax" the joints and connective tissues. This allows the ribs and pelvic cavity to expand in order to encompass the growing baby and make delivery easier. However, connective tissues soften throughout the entire body and the joints become less stable. The increased laxity of the joints during pregnancy can make women more susceptible to back, hip, knee and ankle injuries. Pregnant women shouldn't overstretch since extreme flexion or extension may be harmful to the joints and connective tissues. (During pregnancy, the aim of flexibility training should be to relieve muscle cramping and alleviate any pain in the low-back area.)

As a countermeasure against the increased laxity of the joints, pregnant women should use slightly higher repetition ranges than suggested for most of the population. Doing higher repetitions requires the use of lighter weights; this, in turn, reduces the orthopedic stress that's placed on their connective tissues (including tendons and ligaments) and joints. Repetition ranges for pregnant women should be about 20 to 25 for the hips, 15 to 20 for the legs and 10 to 15 for the torso.

Exercise Caution

The American College of Obstetricians and Gynecologists recommends that women should avoid exercising in the supine (lying face-up) position after the first trimester. When in this position, the excess weight of the enlarging fetus may obstruct the flow of blood back to the mother's heart.

Also during pregnancy, high-impact activities and movements should be minimized and eventually eliminated. This includes jumping, hopping, bouncing and running. In addition, caution is advised for activities and movements that involve twisting.

Caloric Consumption

The intake of calories must be sufficient to meet the extra energy needs of pregnancy and any exercise that's done. During pregnancy, a woman should consume about 300 calories per day above the amount that's necessary for weight maintenance.

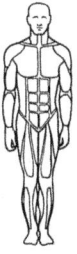

6 Strength Training for Youths

Strength training can be quite beneficial for youths. First and foremost is the fact that it can significantly improve their strength. As youths age, they'll increase their strength from normal growth and maturation. However, these processes may very well be expedited by strength training.

Like all other types of physical training, strength training produces an expenditure of calories that can help to establish a favorable percentage of body fat and improve appearance. Having greater strength can also reduce the frequency and severity of injuries and enhance athletic potential/performance. Moreover, youths can increase their self-confidence and self-esteem during the all-important identity-forming years.

One thing that shouldn't be expected in children and younger adolescents, though, is a noticeable increase in their muscular size. This is because they have low levels of androgens which are growth-promoting hormones. Technically, androgens refer to several hormones in males – the main one is testosterone – but androgens are also present in females. (At younger ages, any improvements in strength are likely due to neural adaptation.)

DISPELLING MISCONCEPTIONS

Two generations ago, the prevailing thought was that youths shouldn't do strength training prior to the development of their secondary sexual characteristics (such as a deeper voice and facial/body hair in boys and breasts and wider hips in girls). These changes usually coincide with the onset of the so-called adolescent growth spurt. It had been believed that doing any strength training prior to this developmental stage would impair or stunt their growth.

Specifically, the worry was that strength training would damage the epiphyseal (or growth) plates which are cartilaginous discs that reside at each end of a long bone (such as the humerus and femur). Injury to the epiphyseal plates can result in pre-mature closure of these structures which could impede the longitudinal growth of a bone.

As a result of this fear, it was recommended that youths should wait until the age of about 13 or 14 before they began strength training. While these concerns were certainly well intended, it turns out that they were unfounded. Attitudes have changed, largely due to a growing body of scientific research that has proven otherwise. Nowadays, participation by youths in strength training has gained much greater acceptance and is endorsed by many organizations, including the American Academy of Pediatrics; the American College of Sports Medicine; the American Orthopaedic Society for Sports Medicine; and the National Strength and Conditioning Association.

When to Begin?

Although there's no clear-cut borderline for determining an appropriate age to begin, research

Research has shown that children as young as 10 can do strength training without risk of injury provided that certain guidelines are followed.

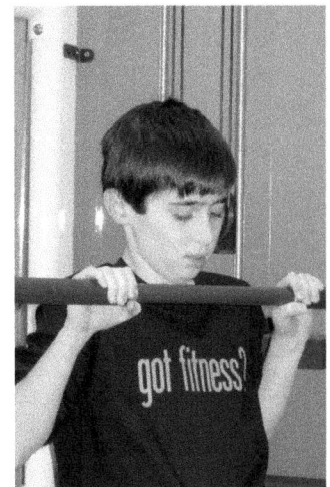

has shown that children as young as 10 can do strength training without risk of injury provided that certain guidelines are followed. Be advised, too, that a youth must be able to stay focused and follow directions before strength training is permitted.

Note: It's helpful to become familiar with several terms that are used frequently in this chapter. Children are boys and girls who haven't developed their secondary sexual characteristics which is about the age of 11 in girls and 13 in boys. Adolescents are girls aged 12 to 18 and boys aged 14 to 18. Youths encompass children and adolescents.

COMPONENTS OF STRENGTH TRAINING

Youths can improve their strength in a manner that's productive, comprehensive, practical, efficient, sustainable and safe by

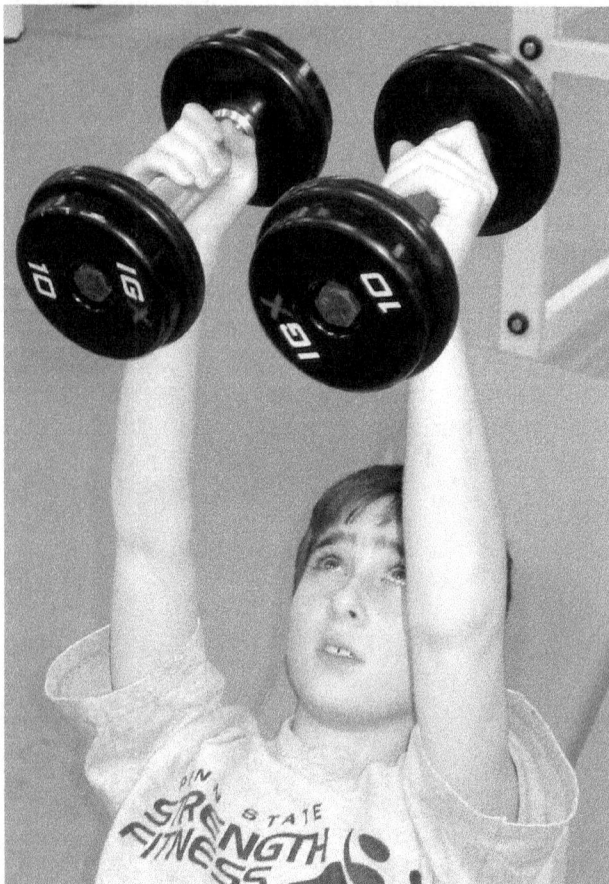

Youths need to perform a higher number of repetitions than most adults.

incorporating these 10 components of strength training:

1. Level of Intensity

A high level of intensity (or effort) is necessary for maximizing the response to strength training. Here, a high level of intensity is characterized by reaching – or at least approaching – the point of muscular fatigue (the point where no additional repetitions can be done with proper technique).

Because of their physical and mental immaturity, however, an appropriate level of intensity for children is to terminate a set a few repetitions short of muscular fatigue or when they feel that they've given a decent effort. As children get older and more mature, they should gradually increase their level of intensity.

2. Progressive Overload

In order for a muscle to get stronger, it must be "asked" to do progressively harder work. To accomplish this, an attempt must be made to increase either the resistance used or the repetitions performed in comparison to a previous workout.

Once the recommended number of repetitions is attained, the progressions in resistance should be made in small increments. Preferably, progressions should be no more than about 5%.

3. Number of Sets

There's no agreement as to how many sets of an exercise should be done by youths. Most of the recommendations, though, are between one and three sets.

Doing one set of each exercise is a productive and an efficient approach to strength training and, for those reasons, is highly recommended. An emphasis should be placed on the *quality* of work that's done in a strength program, not the *quantity* of work.

4. Number of Repetitions

It's generally agreed that youths need to perform a higher number of repetitions than most adults. Doing higher repetitions requires the use of lighter weights; this, in turn, reduces the orthopedic stress that's placed on their bones, connective tissues (including tendons and ligaments) and joints. Repetition ranges for children should be about 20 to 25 for the hips, 15 to 20 for the legs and 10 to 15 for the torso. As they get older and more mature, those repetition ranges can be reduced over time to about 15 to 20 for the hips, 10 to 15 for the legs and 5 to 10 for the torso.

Youths shouldn't try to "max out" or do low-repetition sets. This increases the potential for injury and, therefore, should be discouraged.

5. Proper Technique

To make each exercise safer and more productive, it's important for youths to employ proper technique. The resistance should be raised in a smooth, controlled manner without any explosive or jerking movements. After raising the resistance, there should be a brief pause in the mid-range position. Then, the resistance should be lowered in a smooth, controlled manner. A repetition should be done throughout the greatest possible range of motion that safety allows. Emphasis should be placed on *how well* the weight is lifted, not *how much* weight is lifted.

6. Duration of a Workout

As noted in Chapter 4, more isn't necessarily better when it comes to strength training. The workouts of children should be limited to about 20 to 30 minutes; the workouts of adolescents should be limited to about 30 to 40 minutes.

There's no reason for them to spend much more time than that engaged in strength training. Lengthy workouts can lead to disinterest and dissatisfaction which will decrease adherence to the strength program. Furthermore, lengthy workouts can increase the risk of overuse injuries.

7. Volume of Exercises

Children should perform about nine exercises (one set each) per workout. A workout can consist of one exercise for their hips, hamstrings, quadriceps, calves/dorsi flexors, chest, upper back, shoulders, abdominals and lower back. This lower volume of exercises decreases the potential for overuse injuries and increases the potential

for adherence to the strength program. As they get older and more mature, the volume can be increased to about 14 exercises (one set each) per workout. In this case, a workout can consist of one exercise for their hips, hamstrings, quadriceps, calves/dorsi flexors, biceps, triceps, abdominals and lower back; two exercises (one set each) should be done for their chest, upper back and shoulders. If multiple sets of an exercise are performed, the total number of exercises should be reduced accordingly so as to stay within the aforementioned parameters for the duration and volume of training.

Youths who are involved in combat sports – such as football, judo and wrestling – should also include one or two exercises for their necks; youths who participate in sports or activities that require grip strength – such as baseball, field hockey and tennis – should also include one exercise for their lower arms (forearms).

8. Order of Exercise

A workout should begin with exercises that involve the largest muscles and proceed to those that involve the smallest ones. In general, the order of exercise would be hips, upper legs (hamstrings and quadriceps), lower legs (calves or dorsi flexors), torso (chest, upper back and shoulders), upper arms (biceps and triceps), abdominals and lower back.

If included, exercises for the neck should be done at the beginning of the workout or just after the lower body (prior to exercises for the upper body); exercises for the lower arms should be done after the upper arms.

Incidentally, exercises can be performed with a wide assortment of equipment, including barbells, dumbbells, machines and resistance bands. Youths can also benefit from doing exercises that involve their own bodyweight (such as push-ups, dips, chin-ups, pull-ups and abdominal crunches).

9. Frequency of Training

Care must be taken to ensure that youths get an adequate amount of recovery between workouts. Children should do strength training once or twice per week on nonconsecutive days.

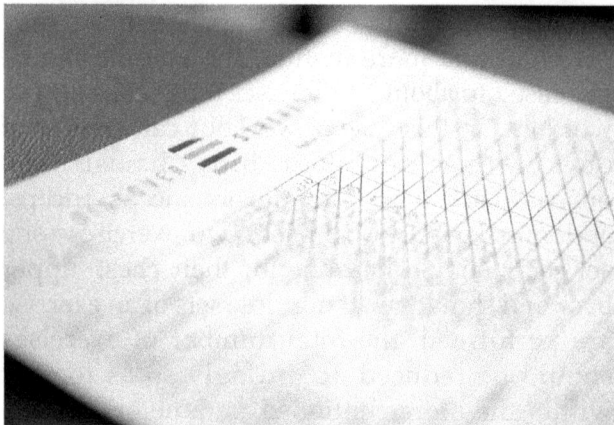

The value of keeping accurate records can't be overemphasized. (Photo provided by Luke Carlson.)

As they get older and more mature, strength training can be increased to two or three times per week on nonconsecutive days. (This assumes total-body workouts.)

10. Records

The value of keeping accurate records can't be overemphasized. A record is a log of what youths have accomplished in their strength program. This is an extremely useful tool to monitor their progress and make their workouts more productive and more meaningful. It can also be used to identify exercises in which they've reached a plateau.

SUPERVISION

It's of utmost importance that youths are monitored closely during their strength training. Competent and qualified individuals should provide adequate instruction in the proper performance of all exercises and direct supervision of all workouts. Simply put, an emphasis must be placed on safety.

ISSUE: PRACTICAL PROGRESSIONS

As mentioned earlier, an important aspect of strength training is progressive overload. It's well worth looking at how this can be incorporated in a practical manner.

Recall that with strength training, progression can be achieved by doing more repetitions or using more resistance in comparison to a previous workout. A practical progression that works well with children (and beginners) is to have them start with a resistance that allows them to easily reach the low end of the repetition range. Then, have them try to do one more repetition every workout or two. When they reach the high end of the repetition range, increase the resistance in their next workout by the smallest amount available and have them aim for the low end of the repetition range.

Example: In today's workout, Ryan did 10 repetitions with 30 pounds in the lat pulldown. In his next five workouts, he lifted the same weight for 11, 12, 13, 14 and 15 repetitions. In his next workout, the weight was increased to 31.25 pounds and he dropped back to 10 repetitions. In his next five workouts with that weight, he did 11, 12, 13, 14 and 15 repetitions. At this point, the weight was increased to 32.5 pounds and the aforementioned cycle repeated (dropping back to 10 repetitions).

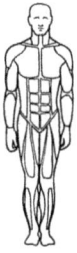

7 Strength Training for Older Adults

A slow but steady increase in life expectancy has resulted in the progressive aging of the American population. In 1990, for example, the median age was 32.9; in 2016, it was 37.9. Even more revealing is that between 1990 and 2016, the number of people aged 55 to 64 increased by 96.8% – nearly doubling from 21.1 million to 41.6 million – which, in 2016, was 12.8% of the US population. And during that same 26-year span, the number of people aged 65 and over increased by 58.2% – from 31.2 million to 49.4 million – which, in 2016, was 15.3% of the US population.

Older adults who do strength training stand to reap numerous rewards. For one thing, strength training can thwart the ravaging effects of osteoporosis. As people age, they have an increased risk of osteoporosis which means that they have a decreased bone mineral density. Although there are individual differences, bone density declines by about 0.5% or more per year after the age of 40. The result of a decrease in bone density is bones that are more porous and more prone to fracture. Also of importance is that with older adults, fractured bones take a longer time to heal. The good news is that strength training can increase bone density which decreases the risk of bone fractures.

With aging comes an increase in body fat; the rate is about 1.5 pounds per year. However, the *amount* of fat might be of less concern than the *distribution* of fat. In general, there are two types of body fat: subcutaneous (located just beneath the surface of the skin) and visceral (located around the major organs of the torso which are collectively referred to as the viscera). Younger adults store about half of their fat as subcutaneous fat and half of their fat as visceral fat; older adults store a higher percentage of their fat as visceral fat. It's well known that visceral fat – which, as noted, surrounds major organs (especially those of the abdomen such as the liver, kidneys, stomach and intestines) – is associated with an increased risk of cardiovascular and metabolic diseases, including diabetes, heart disease and hypertension. Similar to other types of physical training, strength training can produce a loss of body fat (visceral as well as subcutaneous).

Through strength training, older adults can also improve their overall mental health and well-being. This includes a reduced risk of depression and anxiety. In addition, they'll enhance various aspects of their cognitive function such as memory and attention.

Note: There's no clear guideline as to what age defines an older adult. This is partly due to the fact that everyone ages at different rates. The fact of the matter is that chronological age has nothing to do with physiological age. The recommendations that appear in this chapter are intended for those who are 65 and older but could be applicable for individuals who are much younger, depending on their level of fitness and function.

Older adults who do strength training stand to reap numerous rewards. (Photo by Fred Fornicola.)

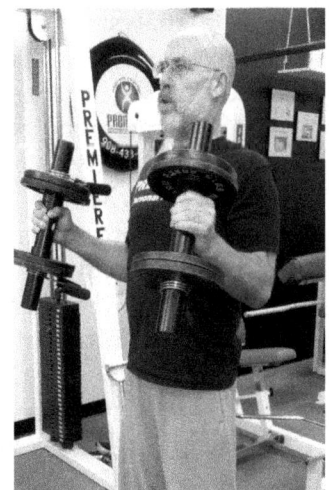

71

DISPELLING MISCONCEPTIONS

Perhaps the biggest misconception about older adults is that because of their advanced age, they'll experience little or no response to strength training in terms of the strength and size of their muscles. However, research tells another story.

Muscular Strength

As people age, they gradually lose muscular strength. In fact, strength usually peaks between the ages of 20 and 30 and then remains relatively stable until the age of about 45. But by the age of 50, strength declines progressively and precipitously with increasing age. Between the ages of 50 and 60, strength drops by about 1.5% per year and 3.0% per year thereafter. The loss of strength may actually be significant enough to hinder daily activities that nearly everyone else takes for granted such as rising from a chair or even walking.

The decline in strength is likely due to a loss of muscle mass. (The term for an age-related loss of muscle mass and strength is sarcopenia.) Indeed, studies show that much of the loss of strength is due to *quantitative* changes in the muscle, not *qualitative* changes. In other words, the muscles of older adults still function basically the same way as when they were younger; it's just that they have less muscle mass. (On a related note, research has found that a selective atrophy of fast-twitch fibers occurs with aging.)

While a loss of strength is inevitable, strength training can slow the rate of decline. A meta-analysis is a scientific way to combine the results of separate studies that examine the same topic. One meta-analysis pooled data from 47 studies that looked at the effects of strength training on older adults. The studies involved a total of 1,079 men and women who ranged in age from 50 to 83. The meta-analysis found that, on average, older adults who did strength training had significant improvements in strength in their lower body (29% in the leg press and 33% in the leg extension) and upper body (24% in the chest press and 25% in the lat pulldown).

Muscular Size

As people age, they gradually lose muscular size. Between the ages of 25 and 55, individuals lose muscle mass at the rate of about one-half pound per year. So, the average 55-year-old has 15 less pounds of muscle than at age 25. The loss of lean-body mass intensifies after the mid-50s.

Early studies that investigated the effects of strength training in older adults found marked gains in muscular strength but little evidence of any gains in muscular size. Because of the absence of significant hypertrophy, researchers speculated that the increases in strength achieved by older adults were due to neural adaptation. But in 1988, researchers at Tufts University in Boston reported significant increases in muscular strength *and* size. In this landmark study, 12 men (aged 60 to 72) did three sets of eight repetitions on the leg extension and leg curl, using one limb at a time. Each repetition took six to nine seconds to complete. They trained three times per week for 12 weeks. The subjects increased the strength of their right quadriceps by 116.7%, their left quadriceps by 107.4%, their right hamstrings by 226.7% and their left hamstrings by 226.7%. This was accompanied by an increase in the cross-sectional area of their right quadriceps by 11.9% and their left quadriceps by 9.3%.

And get this: Gains in muscular size can be made by older adults *even into their 90s*. In one study, 10 men and women (aged 86 to 96) did three sets of eight repetitions on the leg extension, using one limb at a time. Each repetition took six to nine seconds to complete. They trained three times per week for eight weeks. The nine subjects who completed the study increased the strength of their right quadriceps by 174% and their left quadriceps by 180%. (One subject stopped after four weeks due to a previous injury.) Also, seven subjects who had data for both pre- and post-testing increased the muscle area of the total mid-thigh (the quadriceps, hamstrings and adductors) in their non-dominant leg by 9%. Of no small importance is that at the end of the study, two subjects no longer needed canes for assistance in walking.

More recently, a meta-analysis pooled data from 49 studies that looked at the effects of strength training on older adults. The studies involved a total of 1,328 men and women who ranged in age from 50 to 83. The meta-analysis found that, on average, older adults who did strength training 2.8 times per week for 20.5 weeks increased their lean-body mass by about 2.4 pounds. This might seem small but remember that after the age of 25, people lose about one-half pound of lean-body mass per year.

COMPONENTS OF STRENGTH TRAINING

Older adults can improve their strength in a manner that's productive, comprehensive, practical, efficient, sustainable and safe by incorporating these 10 components of strength training:

1. Level of Intensity

A high level of intensity (or effort) is necessary for maximizing the response to strength training. Here, a high level of intensity is characterized by reaching – or at least approaching – the point of muscular fatigue (the point where no additional repetitions can be done with proper technique).

Some older adults might not tolerate training to muscular fatigue, however. Those who aren't comfortable with this level of intensity can terminate a set a few repetitions short of muscular fatigue or when they feel that they've given a decent effort. As they become more accustomed to strength training, they should gradually increase their level of intensity.

2. Progressive Overload

In order for a muscle to get stronger, an attempt must be made to increase either the resistance used or the repetitions performed in comparison to a previous workout.

Once the recommended number of repetitions is attained, the progressions in resistance should be made in small increments. Preferably, progressions should be no more than about 5%.

3. Number of Sets

There's no agreement as to how many sets of an exercise should be done by older adults. Most of the recommendations, though, are between one and three sets.

Doing one set of each exercise is a productive and an efficient approach to strength training and, for those reasons, is highly recommended. An emphasis should be placed on the *quality* of work that's done in a strength program, not the *quantity* of work.

4. Number of Repetitions

Older adults should perform a higher number of repetitions than their younger counterparts. Doing higher repetitions requires the use of lighter weights; this, in turn, reduces the orthopedic stress that's placed on their bones, connective tissues and joints. Repetition ranges for older adults should be about 20 to 25 for the hips, 15 to 20 for the legs and 10 to 15 for the torso.

5. Proper Technique

To make each exercise safer and more productive, older adults must use proper technique. The resistance should be raised in a smooth, controlled manner without any explosive or jerking movements. After raising the resistance, there should be a brief pause in the mid-range position. Then, the resistance should be lowered in a smooth, controlled manner. A repetition should be done throughout the greatest possible range of motion that safety allows.

Older adults who suffer from arthritis should use a range of motion that's pain-free. Note that their pain-free range could change from one day to the next.

6. Duration of a Workout

More isn't necessarily better when it comes to strength training. The workouts of older adults should be limited to about 30 to 40 minutes. If more recovery is needed, the workouts should be limited to about 20 to 30 minutes.

Lengthy workouts can lead to disinterest and dissatisfaction which will decrease adherence to the strength program. Furthermore, lengthy workouts can increase the risk of overuse injuries and joint pain.

7. Volume of Exercises

Older adults can accomplish a total-body workout with 14 exercises or less. The focal point for the majority of these exercises should be their major muscles: their hips, legs and torso. A workout can consist of one exercise (one set each) for their hips, hamstrings, quadriceps, calves/dorsi flexors, biceps, triceps, abdominals and lower back; two exercises (one set each) should be done for their chest, upper back and shoulders.

If more recovery is needed, older adults can perform about nine exercises (one set each) per workout. In this case, a workout can consist of one exercise (one set each) for their hips, hamstrings, quadriceps, calves/dorsi flexors, chest, upper back, shoulders, abdominals and lower back. This lower volume of exercises decreases the potential for overuse injuries and increases the potential for adherence to the strength program.

8. Order of Exercise

A workout should begin with exercises that involve the largest muscles and proceed to those that involve the smallest ones. In general, the order of exercise would be hips, upper legs (hamstrings and quadriceps), lower legs (calves or dorsi flexors), torso (chest, upper back and shoulders), upper arms (biceps and triceps), abdominals and lower back.

9. Frequency of Training

Care must be taken to ensure that older adults get an adequate amount of recovery between workouts. Older adults should do strength training two or three times per week on nonconsecutive days. If more recovery is needed, the frequency should be reduced to once or twice per week on nonconsecutive days. (This assumes total-body workouts.)

10. Records

It's important for older adults to keep accurate records of what they've accomplished in their strength program. It's an extremely useful tool to monitor progress and make their workouts more productive and more meaningful. Records can also be used to identify exercises in which a plateau has been reached. In the event of an injury, the effectiveness of rehabilitative training

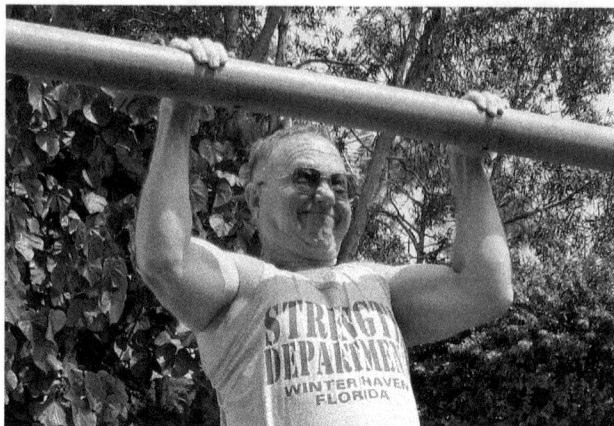

By engaging in a strength program on a regular basis, older adults will be able to slow down the weight gain that's associated with aging. (Photo by Margaret Bryan.)

can be gauged if there's a record of their pre-injury levels of strength.

ISSUE: WEIGHT GAIN WITH AGING

It has been noted that between the ages of 25 and 55, people lose about one-half pound of muscle mass per year. And as people age, they also gain body fat at a rate of about 1.5 pounds per year. So the net gain in weight is one pound per year but it's really a two-pound change in body composition.

Suppose that at the age of 25, a man weighed 154 pounds and his body fat was 14%. This means that he had 21.56 pounds of body fat and 132.44 pounds of lean-body mass. And now, 30 years later at the age of 55, his weight has increased by 30 pounds – one pound per year – to 184 pounds. But it's really a 60-pound swing in body composition as his body fat has increased by 45 pounds (to 66.56 pounds) and his lean-body mass has decreased by 15 pounds (to 117.44 pounds). So over the span of 30 years, his body fat has more than doubled, rising from 14 to 36.17%.

As people get older, it's natural for them to lose muscle mass and gain body fat. But by engaging in a strength program on a regular basis, they'll be able to slow down the weight gain that's associated with aging.

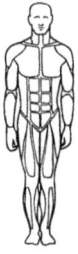

8 Free-Weight Exercises

Most fitness centers have at least some free weights (namely, barbells and dumbbells). And with good reason since free weights are perhaps the most popular pieces of equipment for strength training.

MAJOR MOMENTS IN HISTORY

The chronicle of free-weight exercises contains many evolutionary events and inventions of considerable significance. Let's see how these historic moments have led to our present-day barbells and dumbbells.

Barbells

In the early 1830s, Hippolyte Triat – a professional strongman from France – performed feats of strength in front of audiences that had paid to see his shows; later, he operated several "fashionable" gymnasiums in Europe. An etching from 1854 of his gymnasium in Paris – at the time one of the largest in the world with more than 9,000 square feet of space that included balconies for spectators – shows "pupils" exercising together in what resembled a modern group-fitness class. On the walls were numerous spherical-ended bars. The existence of these "bars with spheres" has led researchers to believe that Trait invented the so-called globe barbell.

Be that as it may, the first actual use of the term barbell didn't appear until almost two decades later. In 1870, a book that was authored by Madame (Lucie) Brenner – who operated a gymnasium in London – described a "bar-bell" that was 4.5 feet in length with wooden spheres on each end.

These and other early barbells were of "fixed" weight; the barbells had solid globes (spheres) at each end that were constructed of wood or iron, meaning that the resistance couldn't be made heavier or lighter. In effect, a different barbell was needed for a different weight. Among other things, this made it extremely difficult to employ progressive overload.

Later barbells had hollow globes that could be filled with lead shot or sand. Although this made it possible to adjust the resistance, the process wasn't necessarily convenient; in all likelihood, it took some time – and patience – to load both globes with an equal amount of fill.

An advancement in the design of adjustable barbells occurred in the United States in 1889. That year, Samuel Stockburger of Canton, Ohio, filed a patent application for an "exercising bar" that was four to six feet in length with the gripping area made of "spring material, preferably of hickory or ash wood." The bar had removable weights which he referred to as "metal disks." Stockburger's concept was a step in the right direction but being made of wood, the bar couldn't be loaded with too much weight.

In 1902, Alan Calvert of Philadelphia filed a patent application for his version of an adjustable "bar-bell." Later that year, Calvert founded the Milo Bar-Bell Company – named after the legendary Milo of Croton – which is considered

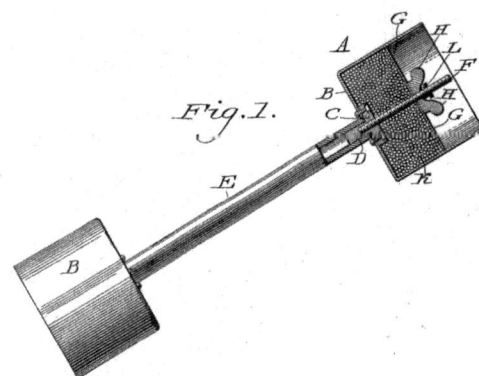

A patent drawing for Alan Calvert's adjustable "bar-bell." (Image from Calvert, 1902.)

75

to be the first company to manufacture and sell adjustable barbells in the United States. Instead of having hollow spheres, the ends of his barbell had hollow, canister-like chambers. (Think of the chambers as large cans.) Resistance was added to the barbell by pouring "a mass of pellets, particles or small pieces of weighting material, preferably shot" through an opening of each chamber. The contents of each chamber were then compacted by turning a wing nut which tightened what essentially was a lid. For the first time in this country, a barbell was commercially available in which the resistance could be adjusted – though still not very quickly – which effectively ended the need to have a different barbell for a different weight. (The original model was advertised as being adjustable from 20 to 200 pounds.) By 1909, his company was selling plate-loading barbells. Largely because of Calvert, the American public was given access to equipment for strength training that for the most part had only been available to professional strongmen. Equally important was that individuals now had the means to overload their muscles with progressively greater demands. (Fast fact: The Milo Bar-Bell Company went bankrupt in 1935 and was acquired by Bob Hoffman for $4,000; Hoffman founded the York Barbell Company in 1938.)

Dumbbells

A dumbbell is essentially a shorter version of a barbell that's intended for use with one hand. In the historical timeline of free-weight exercises, the dumbbell actually predates the barbell by about two millennia.

The fact of the matter is that people have been using dumbbells – or dumbbell-like objects – to improve their might and muscle since ancient times. In the sixth century BC or earlier – that's at least 2,500 years ago – Greek athletes employed hand-held weights known as halteres (the singular of which is halter). The oblong-shaped halteres were fitted to the hands and usually weighed anywhere from about 3.3 to 5.5 pounds (though some exceeded 10 pounds). Athletes used the halteres to propel themselves farther during the standing long jump. There's some debate as to exactly how this was done but it's

suspected that prior to takeoff, the athletes positioned the halteres behind their bodies. At takeoff, they swung the halteres forward and then prior to landing, they swung the halteres backward. Around the same period of time, individuals used halteres to develop their strength, doing exercises that resembled the lunge, shoulder press and some type of back extension. Accordingly, halteres have the honor of being the first dumbbells. (Fast fact: Researchers calculated that when using halteres that weighed between about 4.4 to 9.8 pounds, performance in the standing long jump improved by 5 to 7%.)

In past cultures, strength was a necessity . . . and not just for men. In the early 1900s, a Roman mosaic that dates back to the fourth century was discovered in Sicily. The artwork depicts 10 women, one of whom is engaging in some type of physical activity with a pair of hand-held weights that bears a striking resemblance to modern-day dumbbells.

Exactly when the term dumbbell was first coined is a matter of dispute. Some make the case for Joseph Addison who wrote in 1711 that he exercised for "an hour every morning upon a dumb bell that is placed in a corner of [his] room." Others believe that the dumbbell didn't get its name until the middle of the 18th century in Merrie Olde England when a church handbell – minus the clappers – was secured to each end of a short handle. At the time, anyone who couldn't speak was referred to as dumb. Some researchers suspect that because the clapper-less handbell made no sound, it was christened a dumb bell.

Regardless, use of the term dumbbell became much more common by the 1770s. As it turns out, Benjamin Franklin – one of our founding fathers and the gentleman whose face adorns a C-note – was a big proponent of exercising with dumbbells. In August 1772, while living in London, he penned a letter to his son William – then the governor of New Jersey when it was a British colony – in which he described the "dumb bell" as an exercise that was "compendious" (or comprehensive). Clearly, Ben Franklin was no dumbbell. (Fast fact: In 1766, Governor Franklin issued a charter to establish Queens College in the town of New Brunswick which would become Rutgers University.)

Similar to the barbells of the 1850s, the dumbbells of that era were of "fixed" weight with solid globes at each end that couldn't be made heavier or lighter, meaning that a different dumbbell was needed for a different weight. In 1859, Dr. George Barker Windship – a physician from Boston who was a renowned practitioner of strength training – made a dumbbell with hollow globes that were secured to the ends of an iron handle. The resistance could be adjusted by filling the globes with lead shot. That same year, Dr. Windship began giving lectures on health in which he also extolled the virtues of strength training. After the lectures, Dr. Windship – who had been dubbed the American Samson by *The Times* of London – performed feats of strength for those in attendance who paid to hear his lecture and see his performance; his first "successful" lecture/demonstration in June 1859 cost 25 cents or about $7.13 in 2018 money. (Nine days earlier, during his first attempt at a lecture/demonstration, he succumbed to stage fright and fainted.)

In 1860, Daniel Savage – another Bostonian – filed a patent application for his "graduated dumb-bells" which contained interlocking pieces or "shells" that were nested inside the globes. The resistance could be adjusted by adding or removing one or more of the internal pieces while preserving the spherical shape of the globes. In 1865, Dr. Windship filed a patent application for his "graduated dumb-bells" that could be adjusted from eight to 101 pounds in 0.5-pound increments by adding or removing metal disks or plates. That same year, David Butler – yet another Bostonian – also filed a patent for his adjustable "dumb-bells" which were quite similar to those of Savage.

These days, most fitness centers offer solid dumbbells of "fixed" weight. Adjustable dumbbells are still employed but on a limited basis, mostly in residential settings where having multiple pairs of dumbbells isn't practical or affordable. The general operation of the modern adjustable dumbbell harkens back to the adjustable dumbbell that was invented by Dr. Windship in 1865.

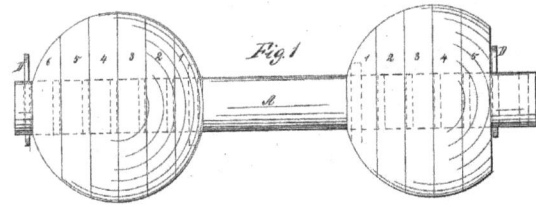

A patent drawing for Dr. George Windship's "graduated dumb-bells." (Image from Windship, 1865.)

MAJOR COMPANIES

The major companies that sell barbells, plates and dumbbells currently include Intek Strength; Iron Grip® Barbell Company; Ivanko® Barbell Company; Troy® Barbell and Fitness; and York® Barbell.

ADVANTAGES OF FREE WEIGHTS

In comparison to machines, free weights offer the following advantages:

1. Free weights are generally less costly than machines.

In trying to furnish a fitness center with a limited or tight budget, the most important consideration in choosing equipment may very well be the price. It could easily cost $40,000 for a complete "line" of state-of-the-art selectorized equipment (10 to 12 machines). And larger fitness centers require far more than one line of machines. A considerable amount of free weights could be purchased for much less of an investment.

Plate-loaded machines tend to be less expensive than selectorized machines. Not to be overlooked, however, is a hidden cost: A few thousand pounds or more of barbell plates may need to be purchased to serve as the resistance.

2. Free weights give you more variety per dollar.

Most machines that are geared toward commercial use are designed to perform only one or two functions. An abdominal machine, for example, can only be used to train the abdominals. On the other hand, a bar and several hundred pounds of plates can allow you to perform exercises for just about every major muscle in your body.

3. Free weights can accommodate everyone regardless of their size from the tallest individual to the shortest.

When it comes to free weights, it's safe to say that one size fits all. Those who are at an extreme in terms of skeletal height and/or limb length may not be able to fit properly on some machines. This could make it difficult – or outright impossible – for some individuals to include certain machines in their strength program.

4. Having to balance free weights requires a greater involvement of synergistic muscles.

The degree to which this is considered as an advantage is debatable, though, since the significance of using synergistic muscles remains unclear. (A muscle is said to act as a synergist if it's used to prevent an undesired movement of a joint.)

ADVANTAGES OF DUMBBELLS

In this discussion, mention must be made of some benefits that are specific to dumbbells. In comparison to machines, dumbbells offer the following advantages:

1. Dumbbells can provide variety to your workout.

Remember, every exercise that can be performed with a barbell can also be performed with dumbbells. This means that every barbell exercise has a dumbbell counterpart that can be used as an alternative exercise.

2. With dumbbells, you have unrestricted freedom to change the position of your hands to best suit your natural biomechanics and level of comfort.

For instance, you can do a bicep curl with dumbbells using a traditional grip (palms facing up), a parallel grip (palms facing each other), a reverse grip (palms facing down) or even a grip that's somewhere in between.

3. Dumbbells force your limbs to work independently.

Most people are often stronger – and more flexible – on one side of their body than the other. Usually, this isn't a significant difference. But when there's a significant difference in the strength between limbs, the use of dumbbells is highly recommended. This is an important consideration for rehabilitative training, too. In this case, an individual may need to work one limb at a time while using a lighter weight for the injured limb. It should be noted that many machines have independent movement arms which also allow you to work your limbs in an independent fashion.

THE EXERCISES

This chapter describes and illustrates the safest and most productive exercises that can be performed with free weights and your bodyweight. Included in the discussions of each exercise are the muscle(s) strengthened (if two or more muscles are involved, the first one listed is the prime mover), suggested repetitions (the time that the targeted muscles should be loaded is shown in parentheses), start/finish position, performance description and training tips for making the exercise safer and more productive.

These 36 exercises are described in this chapter: deadlift, ball squat, lunge, step-up, seated calf raise, standing calf raise, dorsi flexion, bench press, incline press, decline press, dip, bent-arm fly, bench row, bent-over row, chin-up, pull-up, pullover, shoulder press, lateral raise, front raise, bent-over raise, internal rotation, external rotation, upright row, shoulder shrug, scapulae adduction, bicep curl, tricep extension, wrist flexion, wrist extension, finger flexion, abdominal crunch, knee-up, side bend, back extension and stiff-leg deadlift.

DEADLIFT

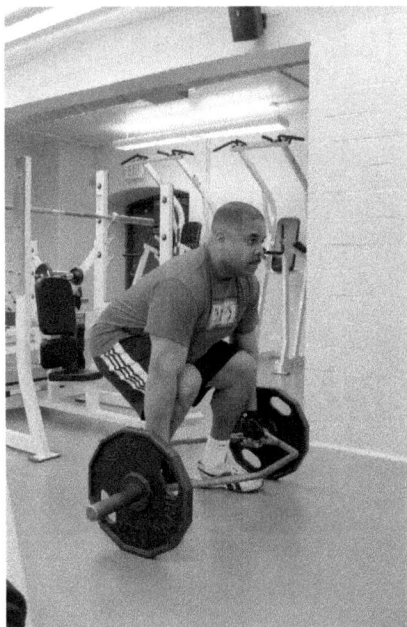

Start/Finish Position

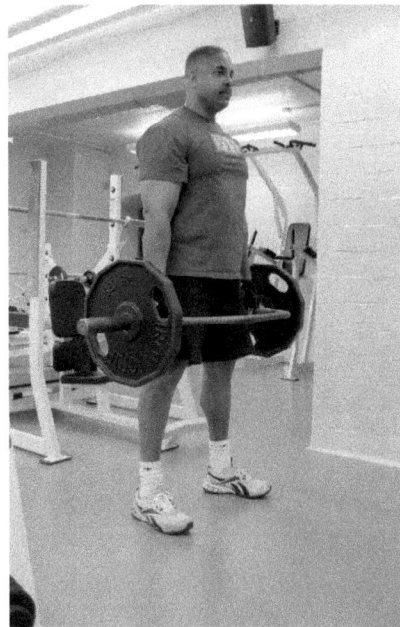

Mid-Range Position

Muscles Strengthened: gluteus maximus, hamstrings, quadriceps, erector spinae and forearms

Suggested Repetitions: 15 to 20 (or 90 to 120 seconds)

Start/Finish Position: Step inside the opening of a trap bar and spread your feet slightly wider than shoulder-width apart. Reach down and grasp the bar on the outside of your legs with a parallel grip (your palms facing each other). Lower your hips until your upper legs are almost parallel to the floor. Flatten your back and look up slightly. Place most of your bodyweight on your heels. Straighten yor arms.

Performance Description: Stand upright by straightening your legs and torso. Pause briefly in this mid-range position (your legs and torso straight) and then lower the bar under control to the start/finish position (your legs and torso bent).

Training Tips:

- Avoid raising your hips too early. This negates their effectiveness and causes you to do the exercise almost entirely with your lower back. Ideally, your hips, legs and lower back should work together. However, your hips and legs should do most of the work.

- Exert force through your heels, not the balls of your feet.

- Avoid "locking" or "snapping" your knees in the mid-range position. Also, avoid hyperextending your torso (leaning backward excessively) in the mid-range position.

- Keep your arms straight, head up and back flat.

- Refrain from bouncing the weight off the floor between repetitions.

- You can also perform this exercise with a barbell and dumbbells. When doing this exercise with a barbell, use an alternating grip (your dominant palm facing forward and non-dominant palm facing backward); when doing this exercise with dumbbells, use a parallel grip and keep the weights at your sides.

- Use wrist straps if you have difficulty in maintaining your grip on the bar.

- This exercise may be contraindicated if you have low-back pain, hyperextended elbows or an exceptionally long torso and/or legs.

BALL SQUAT

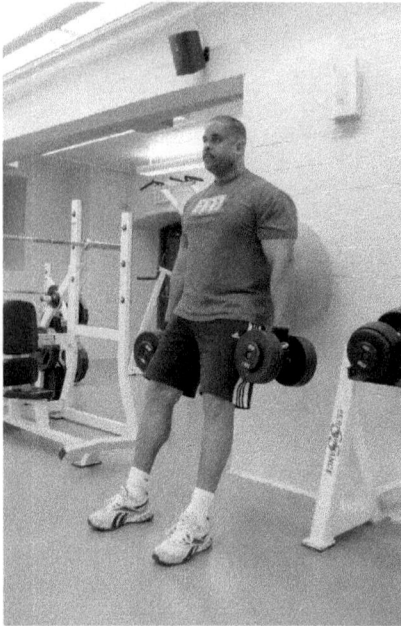

Start/Finish Position

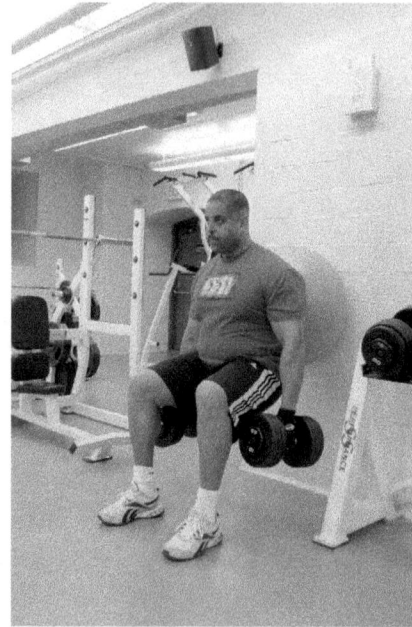

Mid-Range Position

Muscles Strengthened: gluteus maximus, hamstrings, quadriceps and forearms

Suggested Repetitions: 15 to 20 (or 90 to 120 seconds)

Start/Finish Position: Grasp a dumbbell with each hand. Stand with your back toward a wall and have a spotter or training partner place a stability ball between your lower back and the wall. Position your feet so that your upper legs will be parallel to the floor and lower legs will be perpendicular to the floor in the mid-range position. Spread your feet slightly wider than shoulder-width apart and point them straight ahead. Keep your legs almost completely straight. Place most of your bodyweight on your heels. Straighten your arms and point your palms toward each other.

Performance Description: Lower your body under control to the mid-range position (your upper legs parallel to the floor). Without bouncing, return to the start/finish position (your legs almost completely straight).

Training Tips:

- Exert force through your heels, not the balls of your feet.
- Avoid "locking" or "snapping" your knees in the start/finish position.
- If you can't do 15 repetitions, perform this exercise without the dumbbells.
- Use wrist straps if you have difficulty in maintaining your grip on the dumbbells.

LUNGE

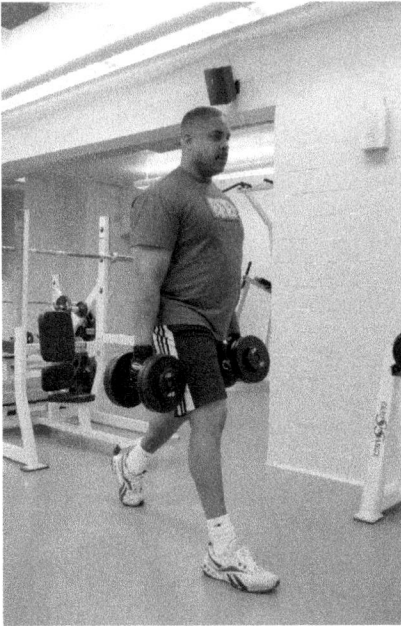

Start/Finish Position

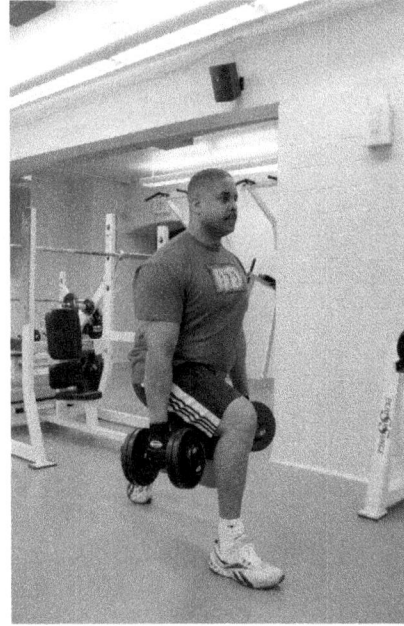

Mid-Range Position

Muscles Strengthened: gluteus maximus, hamstrings, quadriceps and forearms

Suggested Repetitions: 15 to 20 (or 90 to 120 seconds)

Start/Finish Position: Grasp a dumbbell with each hand. Step forward with your right foot and position your right lower leg so that it's perpendicular to the floor. Elevate your left heel off the floor. Point your feet straight ahead. Keep your torso erect and your right leg almost completely straight. Place most of your bodyweight on your right heel. Straighten your arms and point your palms toward each other.

Performance Description: Lower your body under control to the mid-range position (your right upper leg parallel to the floor). Without bouncing, return to the start/finish position (your right leg almost completely straight). Repeat the exercise for the other side of your body (with your left foot forward).

Training Tips:

- Exert force through your heel, not the ball of your foot.
- Avoid "locking" or "snapping" your knee in the start/finish position.
- If you can't do 15 repetitions, perform this exercise without the dumbbells.
- Use wrist straps if you have difficulty in maintaining your grip on the dumbbells.

STEP-UP

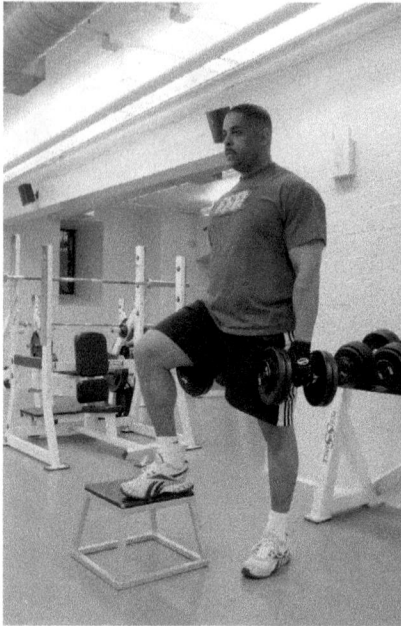

Start/Finish Position

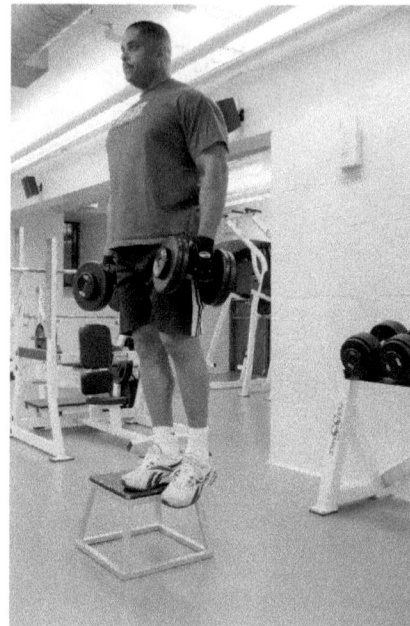

Mid-Range Position

Muscles Strengthened: gluteus maximus, hamstrings, quadriceps and forearms

Suggested Repetitions: 15 to 20 (or 90 to 120 seconds)

Start/Finish Position: Grasp a dumbbell with each hand. Place your right foot on a step that's about 18 to 24 inches high (or something similar that's stable). Position your right lower leg so that it's perpendicular to the floor. Straighten your left leg. Point your feet straight ahead. Place most of your bodyweight on your right heel. Straighten your arms and point your palms toward each other.

Performance Description: Step up with your right leg until it's almost completely straight. Pause briefly in this mid-range position (your right leg almost completely straight) and then lower your body under control to the start/finish position (your right leg bent). Repeat the exercise for the other side of your body.

Training Tips:

- Avoid using your non-exercising leg to assist your exercising leg.
- Exert force through your heel, not the ball of your foot.
- Avoid "locking" or "snapping" your knee in the mid-range position.
- If you can't do 15 repetitions, perform this exercise without the dumbbells.
- Use wrist straps if you have difficulty in maintaining your grip on the dumbbells.

SEATED CALF RAISE

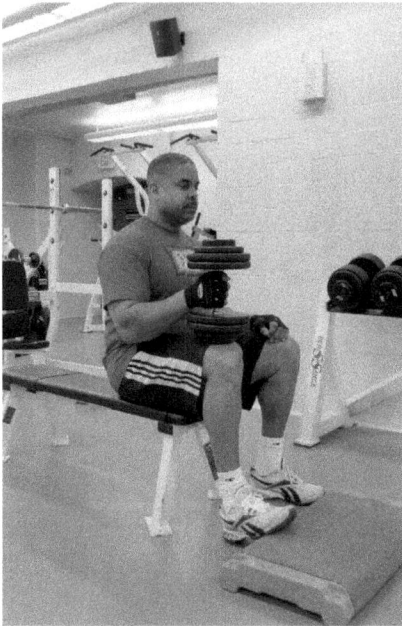

Start/Finish Position

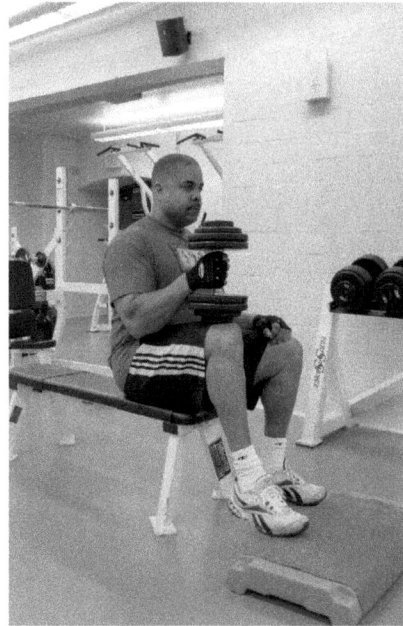

Mid-Range Position

Muscle Strengthened: soleus

Suggested Repetitions: 10 to 15 (or 60 to 90 seconds)

Start/Finish Position: Grasp a dumbbell with your right hand. Sit down near the end of a utility bench (or stool). Place the ball of your right foot on the edge of a step (or something similar that's stable) and lower your heel. Position the dumbbell on the top of your right upper leg near your knee and hold it in place.

Performance Description: Rise up onto your toes as high as possible. Pause briefly in this mid-range position (your ankle straight) and then lower your leg under control to the start/finish position (your heel near the floor). Repeat the exercise for the other side of your body.

Training Tips:

- Use a step or something similar that's at least several inches high to obtain an adequate stretch.
- Avoid this exercise if you have shin splints.

STANDING CALF RAISE

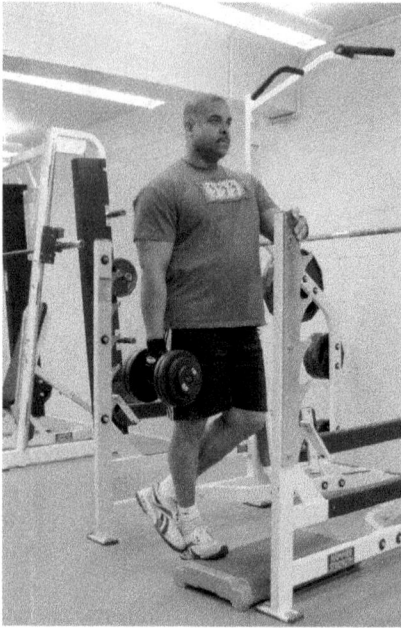

Start/Finish Position

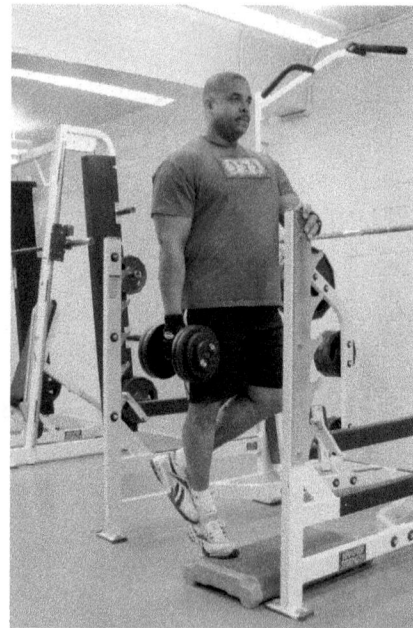

Mid-Range Position

Muscle Strengthened: gastrocnemius

Suggested Repetitions: 10 to 15 (or 60 to 90 seconds)

Start/Finish Position: Grasp a dumbbell with your right hand. Place the ball of your right foot on the edge of a step (or something similar that's stable and offers a place to hold with your left hand to maintain your balance) and lower your heel. Keep your torso erect and straighten your right leg but don't "lock" your knee. Cross your left ankle behind your right ankle.

Performance Description: Rise up onto your toes as high as possible. Pause briefly in this mid-range position (your ankle straight) and then lower your body under control to the start/finish position (your heel near the floor). Repeat the exercise for the other side of your body (with the dumbbell in your left hand).

Training Tips:

• Use a step or something similar that's at least several inches high to obtain an adequate stretch.

• Avoid using your hips and legs. Movement should only occur at your ankle joint.

• Refrain from doing this exercise with a weight placed on your shoulders. This compresses the spinal column.

• If you can't do 10 repetitions, perform this exercise without the dumbbells.

• Use wrist straps if you have difficulty in maintaining your grip on the dumbbell.

• Avoid this exercise if you have shin splints.

DORSI FLEXION

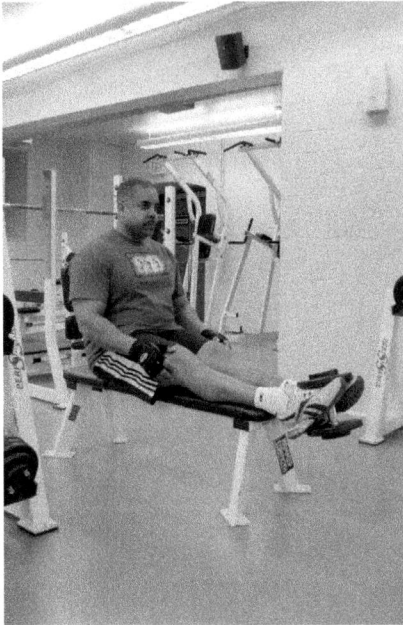

Start/Finish Position

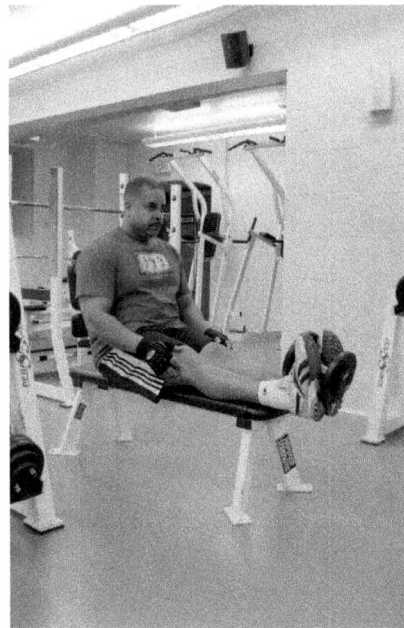

Mid-Range Position

Muscles Strengthened: dorsi flexors

Suggested Repetitions: 10 to 15 (or 60 to 90 seconds)

Start/Finish Position: Grasp a dumbbell with your preferred hand. Sit down near the end of a utility bench and place the dumbbell between your feet. Slide your hips back so that your legs lie across the length of the back pad. Position your heels slightly over the end of the bench and point your toes away from your body.

Performance Description: Keeping your legs flat on the back pad, raise the dumbbell as high as possible. Pause briefly in this mid-range position (your ankles bent) and then lower the dumbbell under control to the start/finish position (your ankles straight).

Training Tips:

- Avoid moving your torso forward and backward. Movement should only occur at your ankle joint.
- This exercise may be contraindicated if you have shin splints.

BENCH PRESS

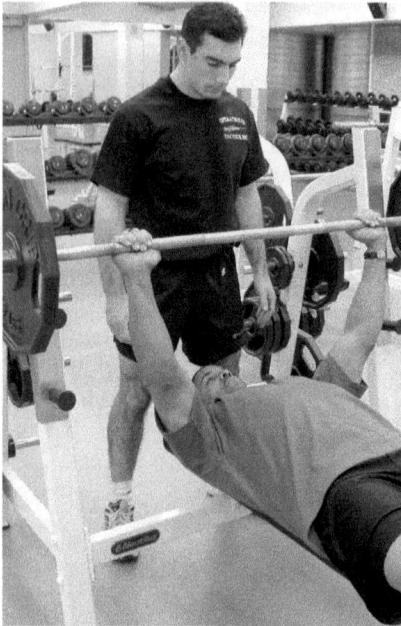
Start/Finish Position

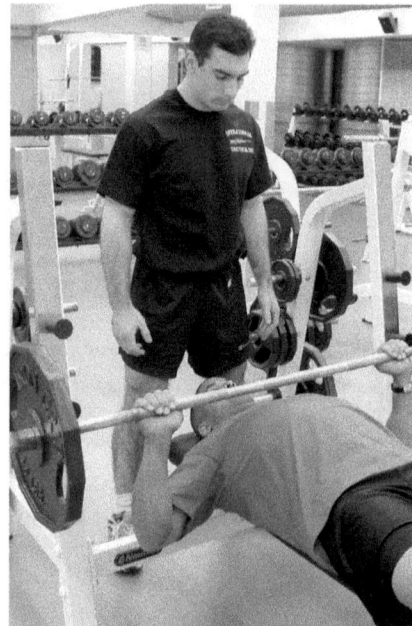
Mid-Range Position

Muscles Strengthened: chest, anterior deltoid and triceps

Suggested Repetitions: 5 to 10 (or 30 to 60 seconds)

Start/Finish Position: Lie down on an Olympic supine (flat) bench and place your feet flat on the floor. Grasp a barbell and spread your hands slightly wider than shoulder-width apart. Lift the bar out of the "gun rack" or have a spotter give you assistance. Keep your arms almost completely straight (without "locking" your elbows).

Performance Description: Lower the bar under control to the mid-range position (the bar touching the middle part of your chest). Without bouncing the bar off your chest, push it up to the start/finish position (your arms almost completely straight).

Training Tips:

- Perform this exercise with a spotter.
- Avoid using an excessively wide grip. This reduces your range of motion.
- Keep your hips on the bench.
- If you have low-back pain, place your feet flat on the end of the bench or a stool. This reduces the stress in your low-back region.
- Avoid "locking" or "snapping" your elbows in the start/finish position.
- You can also perform this exercise with dumbbells.
- This exercise may be contraindicated if you have shoulder-impingement syndrome.

INCLINE PRESS

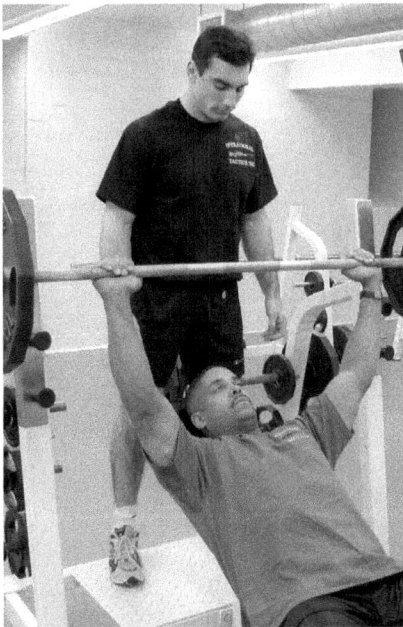

Start/Finish Position

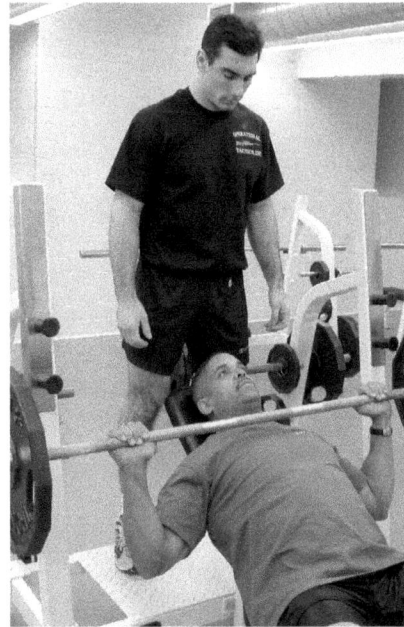

Mid-Range Position

Muscles Strengthened: chest (upper portion), anterior deltoid and triceps

Suggested Repetitions: 5 to 10 (or 30 to 60 seconds)

Start/Finish Position: Sit down on an Olympic incline bench and place your feet flat on the floor (or on the footplate if one is provided). Grasp a barbell and spread your hands slightly wider than shoulder-width apart. Lift the bar out of the "gun rack" or have a spotter give you assistance. Keep your arms almost completely straight (without "locking" your elbows).

Performance Description: Lower the bar under control to the mid-range position (the bar touching the upper part of your chest near your collarbones). Without bouncing the bar off your chest, push it up to the start/finish position (your arms almost completely straight).

Training Tips:

- · Perform this exercise with a spotter.
- Avoid using an excessively wide grip. This reduces your range of motion.
- Keep your hips on the seat pad.
- Avoid "locking" or "snapping" your elbows in the start/finish position.
- You can also perform this exercise with dumbbells.
- This exercise may be contraindicated if you have shoulder-impingement syndrome.

DECLINE PRESS

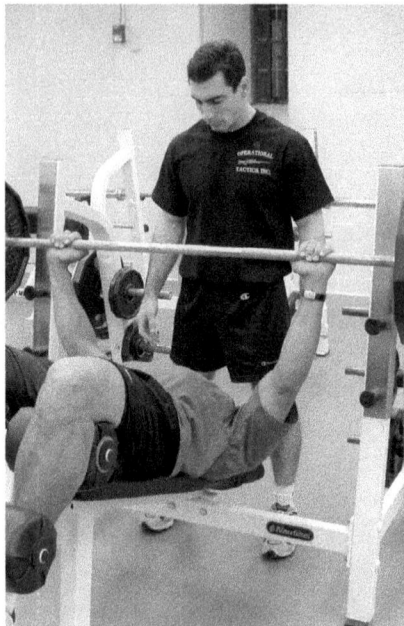

Start/Finish Position

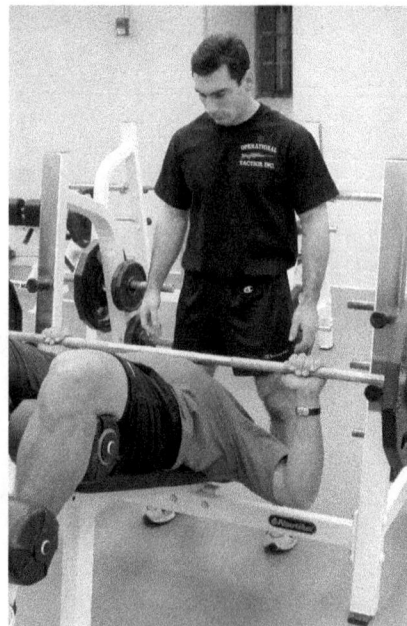

Mid-Range Position

Muscles Strengthened: chest (lower portion), anterior deltoid and triceps

Suggested Repetitions: 5 to 10 (or 30 to 60 seconds)

Start/Finish Position: Lie down on an Olympic decline bench and place your legs over the roller pads and against the shin pads. Grasp a barbell and spread your hands slightly wider than shoulder-width apart. Lift the bar out of the "gun rack" or have a spotter give you assistance. Keep your arms almost completely straight (without "locking" your elbows).

Performance Description: Lower the bar under control to the mid-range position (the bar touching the lower part of your chest near the tip of your breastbone). Without bouncing the bar off your chest, push it up to the start/finish position (your arms almost completely straight).

Training Tips:

- Perform this exercise with a spotter.
- Avoid using an excessively wide grip. This reduces your range of motion.
- Keep your hips on the bench.
- Avoid "locking" or "snapping" your elbows in the start/finish position.
- You can also perform this exercise with dumbbells.
- This exercise may be contraindicated if you have shoulder-impingement syndrome.

DIP

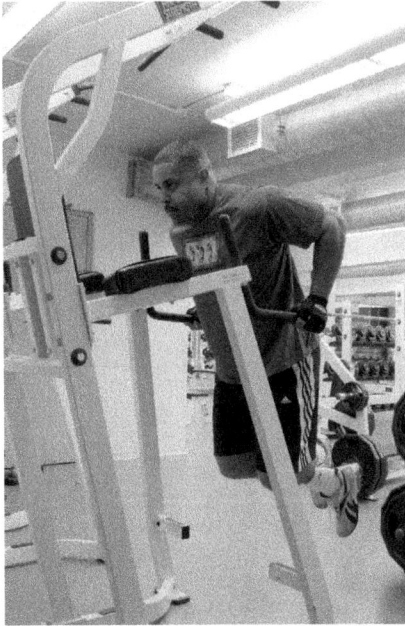

Start/Finish Position

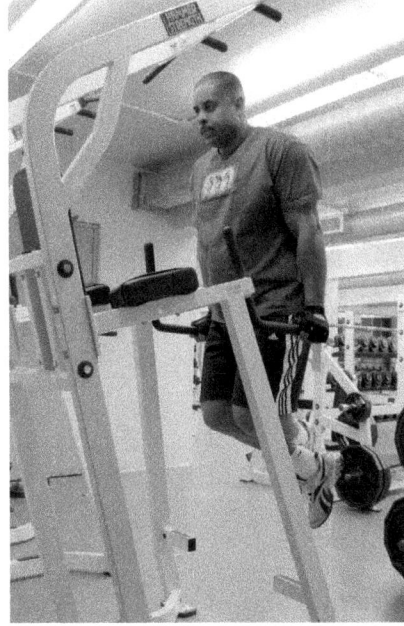

Mid-Range Position

Muscles Strengthened: chest (lower portion), anterior deltoid and triceps

Suggested Repetitions: 5 to 10 (or 30 to 60 seconds)

Start/Finish Position: Grasp the dip bars (or handles) with a parallel grip (your palms facing each other). Bend your arms so that your upper arms are roughly parallel to the floor. Lift your feet off the floor, bend your knees and cross your ankles.

Performance Description: Push your body up until your arms are almost completely straight (without "locking" your elbows). Pause briefly in this mid-range position (your arms almost completely straight) and then lower your body under control to the start/finish position (your arms bent).

Training Tips:

- Avoid swinging your body back and forth. Movement should only occur at your shoulder and elbow joints.

- Avoid "locking" or "snapping" your elbows in the mid-range position.

- If you can do 10 repetitions or more using your bodyweight, increase the workload by attaching additional weight to your waist, performing the exercise with a slower speed of movement or having a spotter apply manual resistance to your waist.

- After reaching muscular fatigue, you can overload your muscles further by stepping up to the mid-range position and lowering your body under control to the start/finish position for 3 to 5 negative-only repetitions.

- This exercise may be contraindicated if you have shoulder-impingement syndrome.

BENT-ARM FLY

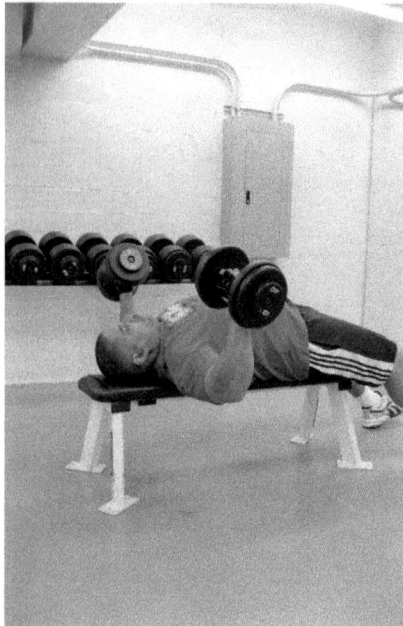

Start/Finish Position

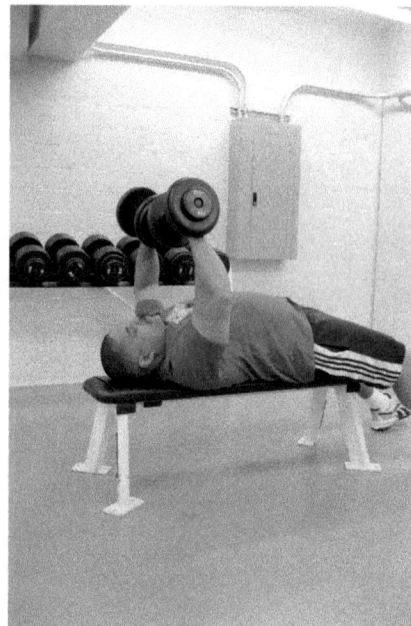

Mid-Range Position

Muscles Strengthened: chest and anterior deltoid

Suggested Repetitions: 5 to 10 (or 30 to 60 seconds)

Start/Finish Position: Grasp a dumbbell with each hand. Lie down on a utility bench and place your feet flat on the floor. Position the dumbbells near your shoulders so that they're even with your chest. Bend your arms so that the angle between your upper and lower arms is about 90 degrees. Point your palms toward your legs.

Performance Description: Keeping the same angle between your upper and lower arms, bring the dumbbells together directly over your chest. Pause briefly in this mid-range position (the dumbbells directly over your chest) and then lower the dumbbells under control to the start/finish position (the dumbbells near your shoulders).

Training Tips:

- This exercise is also referred to as a chest fly and a pec fly.
- Avoid straightening your arms as you raise the dumbbells. This changes the exercise from a bent-arm fly into a bench press. (When raising the dumbbells, imagine that you're hugging a tree.)
- Keep your hips on the bench.
- If you have low-back pain, place your feet on the end of the bench or a stool. This reduces the stress in your low-back region.
- This exercise may be contraindicated if you have shoulder-impingement syndrome.

BENCH ROW

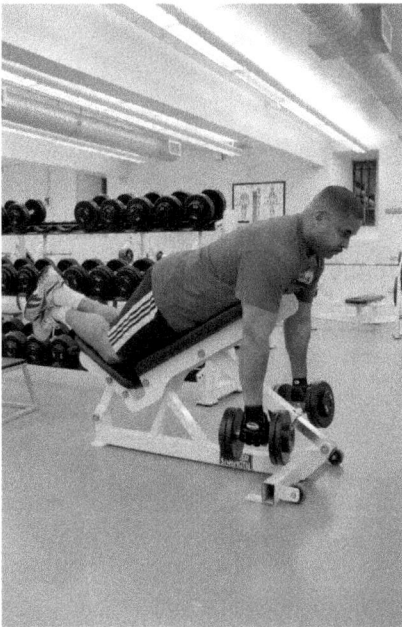

Start/Finish Position

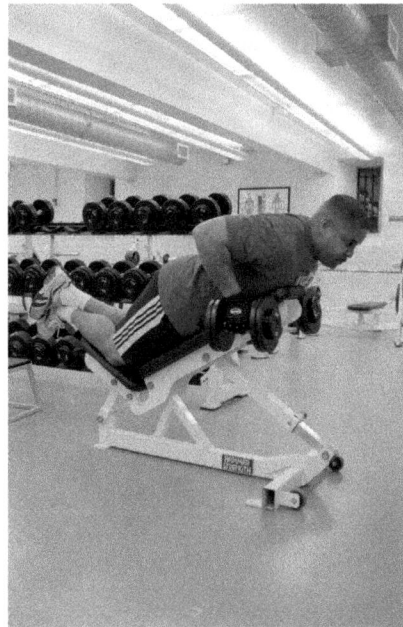

Mid-Range Position

Muscles Strengthened: upper back, biceps and forearms

Suggested Repetitions: 5 to 10 (or 30 to 60 seconds)

Start/Finish Position: Grasp a dumbbell with each hand. Kneel on the seat pad of an adjustable incline bench. Lie forward against the bench and position the dumbbells directly below your torso. Straighten your arms with your palms facing each other.

Performance Description: Pull the dumbbells up to your shoulders. Pause briefly in this mid-range position (your arms bent) and then lower the dumbbells under control to the start/finish position (your arms completely straight).

Training Tips:

- Do this exercise with one limb at a time if you have a shoulder or an arm injury, a gross difference in the strength between your limbs or desire a training variation.

- You can also perform this exercise with your upper arms positioned away from your torso. Doing this involves less of your upper back and more of your posterior deltoid, trapezius and rhomboids. In this case, your upper arms would be perpendicular to your torso in the mid-range position and your palms would be facing backward.

- Use wrist straps if you have difficulty in maintaining your grip on the dumbbells.

- This exercise may be contraindicated if you have hyperextended elbows.

BENT-OVER ROW

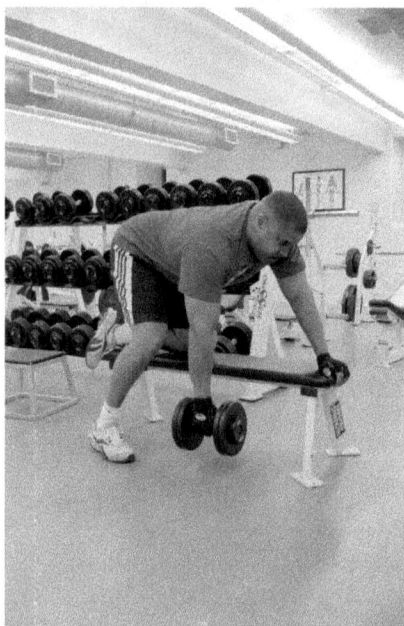

Start/Finish Position

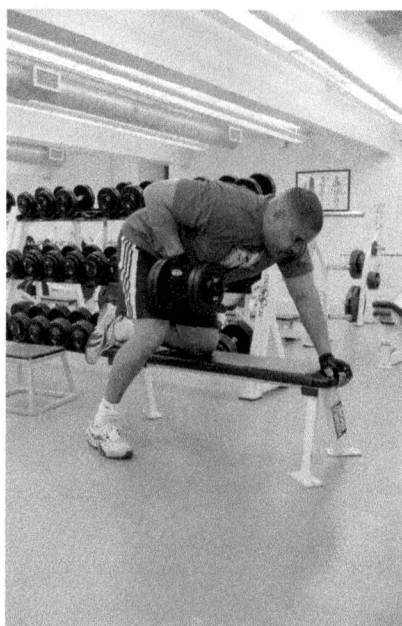

Mid-Range Position

Muscles Strengthened: upper back, biceps and forearms

Suggested Repetitions: 5 to 10 (or 30 to 60 seconds)

Start/Finish Position: Grasp a dumbbell with your right hand. Place your left hand and left knee on a utility bench and position your right foot on the floor at a comfortable distance from the bench. Straighten your right arm with your palm facing the bench.

Performance Description: Pull the dumbbell up to your right shoulder. Pause briefly in this mid-range position (your arm bent) and then lower the dumbbell under control to the start/finish position (your arm completely straight). Repeat the exercise for the other side of your body (with your right hand and right knee on the bench).

Training Tips:

- Avoid using your legs and rotating your torso. Movement should only occur at your shoulder and elbow joints.

- You can also perform this exercise with your upper arm positioned away from your torso. Doing this involves less of your upper back and more of your posterior deltoid, trapezius and rhomboids. In this case, your upper arm would be perpendicular to your torso and your palm would be facing backward in the mid-range position.

- Use wrist straps if you have difficulty in maintaining your grip on the dumbbell.

- This exercise may be contraindicated if you have a hyperextended elbow.

CHIN-UP

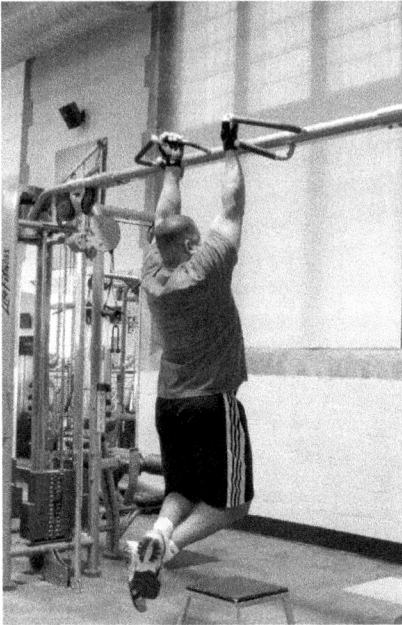

Start/Finish Position

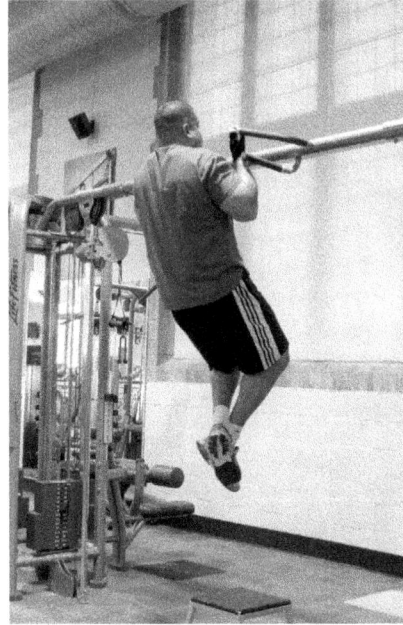

Mid-Range Position

Muscles Strengthened: upper back, biceps and forearms

Suggested Repetitions: 5 to 10 (or 30 to 60 seconds)

Start/Finish Position: Reach up, grasp a chin-up/pull-up bar (or handles) with your palms facing toward you and spread your hands approximately shoulder-width apart. Bring your body to a "dead hang" and cross your ankles.

Performance Description: Pull your body up so that your upper chest touches the bar and draw your elbows backward. Pause briefly in this mid-range position (your arms bent) and then lower your body under control to the start/finish position (your arms completely straight).

Training Tips:

- Avoid swinging your body forward and backward. Movement should only occur at your shoulder and elbow joints.

- If you can't do 5 repetitions using your bodyweight, you can exercise the same muscles in a similar fashion by performing the underhand lat pulldown (as described in Chapter 9).

- If you can do 10 repetitions or more using your bodyweight, increase the workload by attaching additional weight to your waist, performing the exercise with a slower speed of movement or having a spotter apply manual resistance to your waist.

- After reaching muscular fatigue, you can overload your muscles further by stepping up to the mid-range position and lowering your body under control to the start/finish position for 3 to 5 negative-only repetitions.

- Use wrist straps if you have difficulty in maintaining your grip on the bar.

- This exercise may be contraindicated if you have hyperextended elbows.

PULL-UP

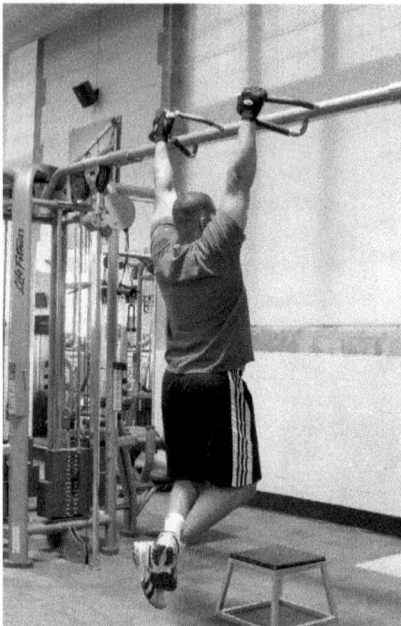

Start/Finish Position

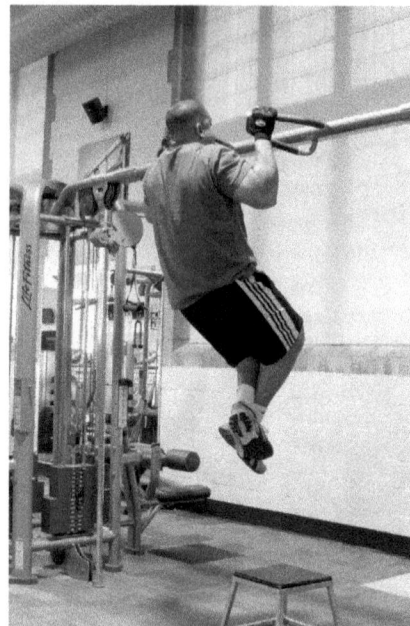

Mid-Range Position

Muscles Strengthened: upper back, biceps and forearms

Suggested Repetitions: 5 to 10 (or 30 to 60 seconds)

Start/Finish Position: Reach up, grasp a chin-up/pull-up bar (or handles) with your palms facing away from you and spread your hands several inches wider than shoulder-width apart. Bring your body to a "dead hang" and cross your ankles.

Performance Description: Pull your body up so that your upper chest touches the bar and draw your elbows backward. Pause briefly in this mid-range position (your arms bent) and then lower your body under control to the start/finish position (your arms straight).

Training Tips:

- Avoid swinging your body forward and backward. Movement should only occur at your shoulder and elbow joints.

- Avoid using an excessively wide grip. This reduces your range of motion.

- If you can't do 5 repetitions using your body-weight, you can exercise the same muscles in a similar fashion by performing the overhand lat pulldown (as described in Chapter 9).

- If you can do 10 repetitions or more using your bodyweight, increase the workload by attaching additional weight to your waist, performing the exercise with a slower speed of movement or having a spotter apply manual resistance to your waist.

- After reaching muscular fatigue, you can overload your muscles further by stepping up to the mid-range position and lowering your body under control to the start/finish position for 3 to 5 negative-only repetitions.

- Performing pull-ups with an overhand grip (your palms facing away from you) isn't as biomechanically efficient as performing chin-ups with an underhand grip (your palms facing toward you). But this exercise is still quite productive with an overhand grip.

- Use wrist straps if you have difficulty in maintaining your grip on the bar.

- You can also perform this exercise with the bar positioned behind your head/neck. However, this may be contraindicated if you have shoulder-impingement syndrome. This exercise may also be contraindicated if you have hyperextended elbows.

PULLOVER

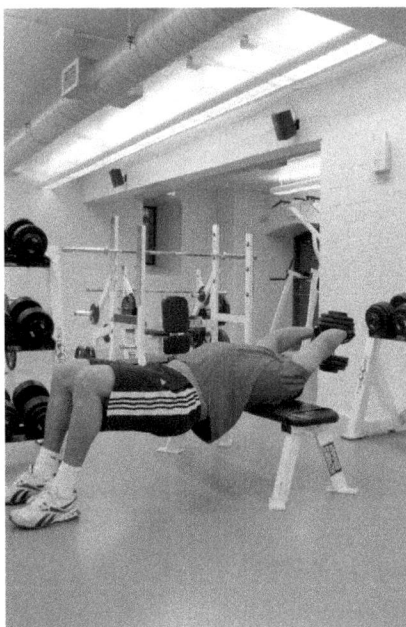

Start/Finish Position

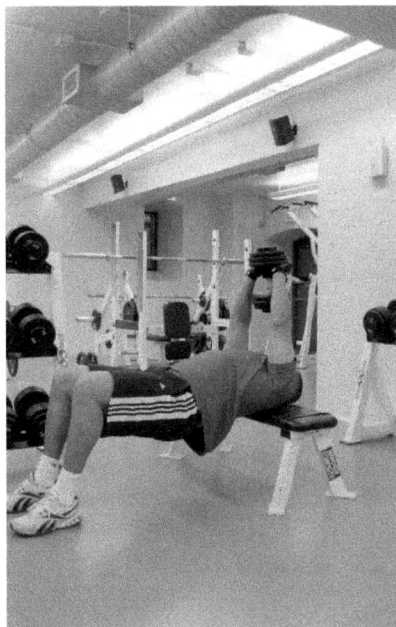

Mid-Range Position

Muscle Strengthened: upper back

Suggested Repetitions: 5 to 10 (or 30 to 60 seconds)

Start/Finish Position: Grasp a dumbbell with both hands. Lie on a utility bench so that your torso is perpendicular to the length of the bench and place your feet flat on the floor. Hold the dumbbell by placing your palms against the innermost plate (not the handle). Position your elbows near or slightly past your head and keep your arms almost completely straight. (A spotter can assist you in positioning a heavy dumbbell.)

Performance Description: Keeping your arms almost completely straight, pull the dumbbell directly over your head. Pause briefly in this mid-range position (the dumbbell directly over your head) and then lower the dumbbell under control to the start/finish position (your elbows near or slightly past your head).

Training Tips:

- You can also perform this exercise with a barbell and an EZ curl bar (spreading your hands about 4 to 6 inches apart).

- This exercise may be contraindicated if you have shoulder-impingement syndrome or low-back pain.

SHOULDER PRESS

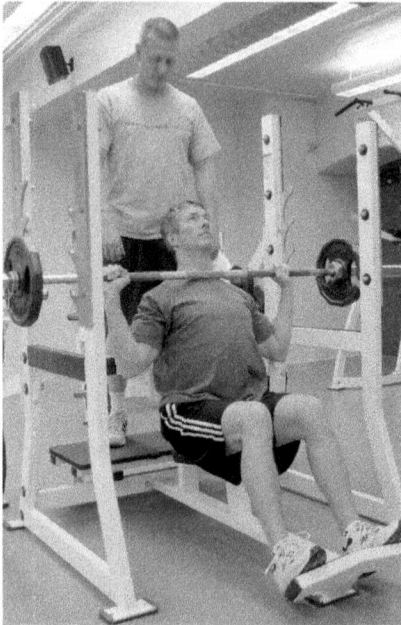

Start/Finish Position

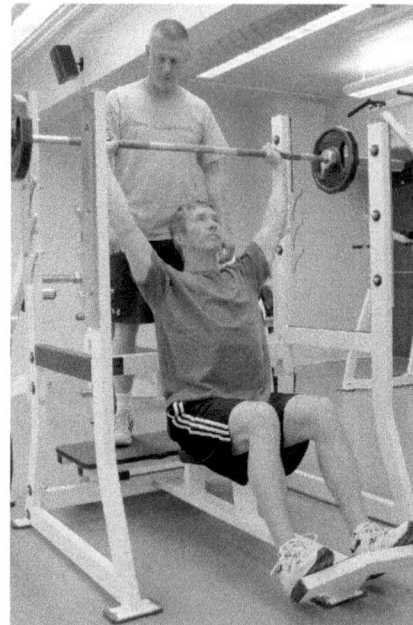

Mid-Range Position

Muscles Strengthened: anterior deltoid and triceps

Suggested Repetitions: 5 to 10 (or 30 to 60 seconds)

Start/Finish Position: Sit down on an Olympic military bench and place your feet flat on the floor (or on the footplate if one is provided). Grasp a barbell and spread your hands slightly wider than shoulder-width apart. Lift the bar out of the "gun rack" or have a spotter give you assistance. Place the bar on the upper part of your chest near your collarbones. (If the bench doesn't have a rack, two spotters can place the bar in the same position.)

Performance Description: Push the bar up until your arms are almost completely straight (without "locking" your elbows). Pause briefly in this mid-range position (your arms almost completely straight) and then lower the bar under control to the start/finish position (your arms bent).

Training Tips:

- This exercise is also referred to as an overhead press, a seated press and a military press.
- Perform this exercise with a spotter.
- Avoid using an excessively wide grip. This reduces your range of motion.
- Keep your hips on the seat pad and your feet flat on the floor.
- Avoid "locking" or "snapping" your elbows in the mid-range position.
- You can also perform this exercise with dumbbells.
- You can also perform this exercise with the bar positioned behind your head/neck. However, this may be contraindicated if you have shoulder-impingement syndrome. This exercise may also be contraindicated if you have low-back pain.

.

LATERAL RAISE

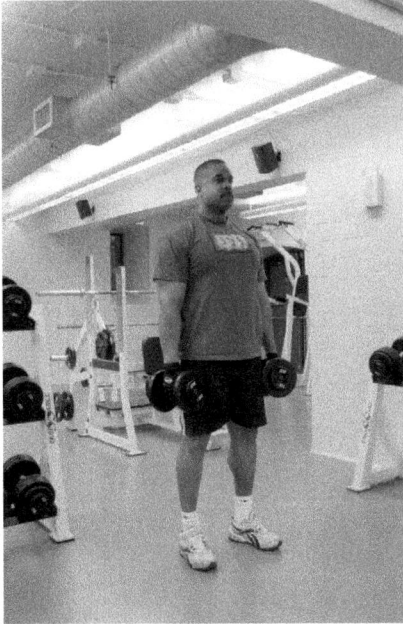

Start/Finish Position

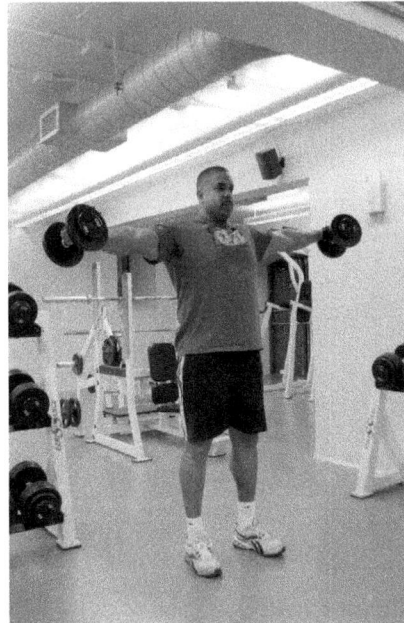

Mid-Range Position

Muscles Strengthened: middle deltoid and trapezius (upper and lower portions)

Suggested Repetitions: 5 to 10 (or 30 to 60 seconds)

Start/Finish Position: Grasp a dumbbell with each hand. Position the dumbbells against the sides of your upper legs with your palms facing each other. Straighten your arms and spread your feet about shoulder-width apart.

Performance Description: Keeping your arms fairly straight, raise the dumbbells sideways until your arms are parallel to the floor. Pause briefly in this mid-range position (your arms parallel to the floor) and then lower the dumbbells under control to the start/finish position (your arms at your sides).

Training Tips:

- Avoid using your legs and moving your torso forward and backward. Movement should only occur at your shoulder joints.

- Raise your arms only to the point at which they're parallel to the floor.

- Your palms should be facing the floor in the mid-range position.

- Do this exercise with one limb at a time if you have a shoulder or an arm injury, a gross difference in the strength between your limbs or desire a training variation.

97

FRONT RAISE

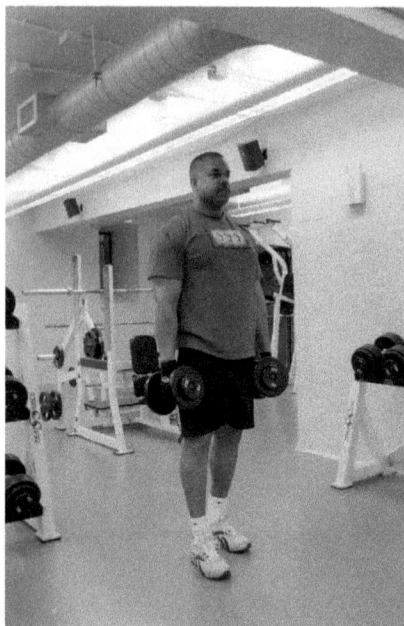

Start/Finish Position

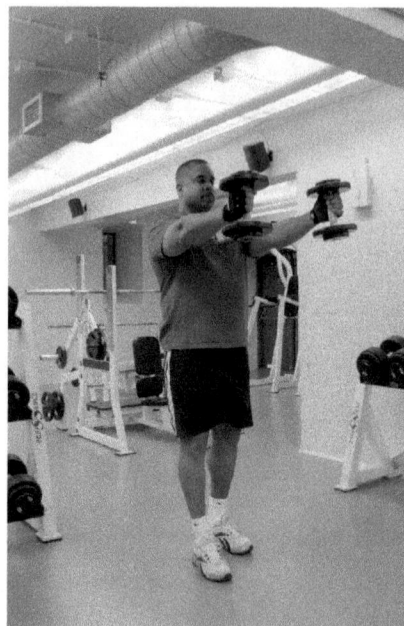

Mid-Range Position

Muscle Strengthened: anterior deltoid

Suggested Repetitions: 5 to 10 (or 30 to 60 seconds)

Start/Finish Position: Grasp a dumbbell with each hand. Position the dumbbells against the sides of your upper legs with your palms facing each other. Straighten your arms and spread your feet a comfortable distance apart with one foot slightly in front of the other.

Performance Description: Keeping your arms fairly straight, raise the dumbbells forward until your arms are parallel to the floor. Pause briefly in this mid-range position (your arms parallel to the floor) and then lower the dumbbells under control to the start/finish position (your arms at your sides).

Training Tips:

- Avoid using your legs and moving your torso forward and backward. Movement should only occur at your shoulder joints.

- Raise your arms only to the point at which they're parallel to the floor.

- Your palms should be facing each other in the mid-range position.

- Do this exercise with one limb at a time if you have a shoulder or an arm injury, a gross difference in the strength between your limbs or desire a training variation.

BENT-OVER RAISE

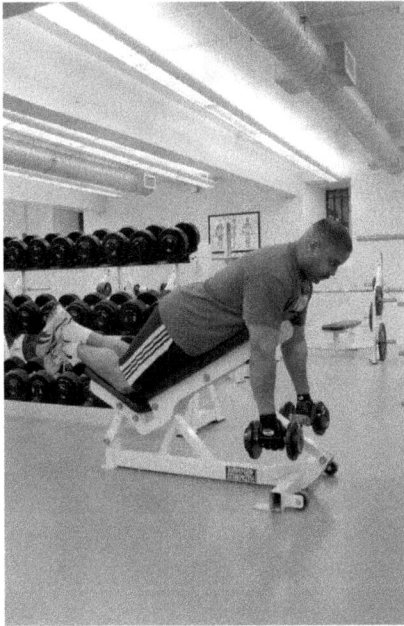

Start/Finish Position

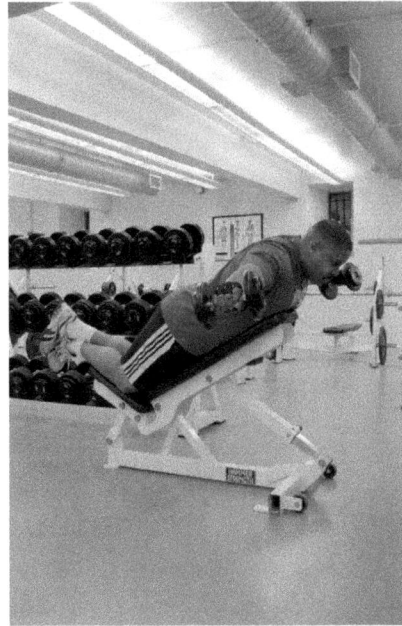

Mid-Range Position

Muscles Strengthened: posterior deltoid, trapezius (middle and lower portions) and rhomboids

Suggested Repetitions: 5 to 10 (or 30 to 60 seconds)

Start/Finish Position: Grasp a dumbbell with each hand. Kneel on the seat pad of an adjustable incline bench. Lie forward against the bench and position the dumbbells directly below your torso. Straighten your arms and point your palms toward each other.

Performance Description: Keeping your arms fairly straight, raise the dumbbells sideways until your arms are parallel to the floor. Pause briefly in this mid-range position (your arms parallel to the floor) and then lower the dumbbells under control to the start/finish position (your hands near the floor).

Training Tips:

- This exercise is also referred to as a posterior raise.
- Raise your arms only to the point at which they're parallel to the floor.
- Your palms should be facing the floor and your upper arms should be perpendicular to your torso in the mid-range position.

INTERNAL ROTATION

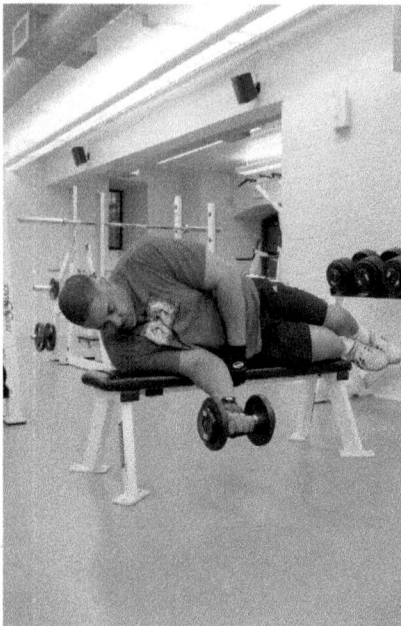

Start/Finish Position

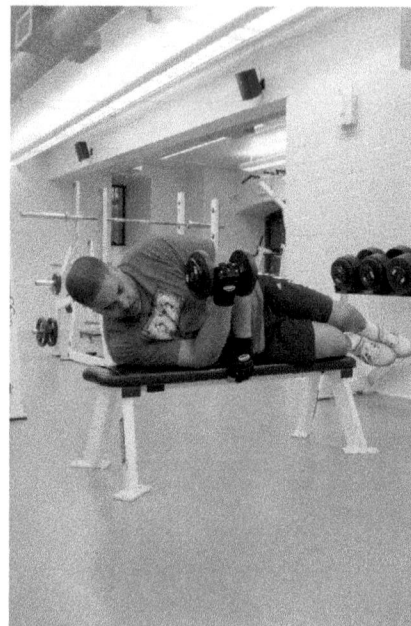

Mid-Range Position

Muscles Strengthened: internal rotators

Suggested Repetitions: 8 to 10 (or 50 to 60 seconds)

Start/Finish Position: Grasp a dumbbell with your right hand. Lie down on a utility bench on your right side and draw your knees toward your torso. Position your right elbow just in front of your torso and bend your right arm so that the angle between your upper and lower arms is about 90 degrees. Point your right palm upward.

Performance Description: Keeping the same angle between your upper and lower arms, pull the dumbbell to your left shoulder. Pause briefly in this mid-range position (your hand near your mid-section) and then lower the dumbbell under control to the start/finish position (your hand away from your mid-section). Repeat the exercise for the other side of your body (with your left side on the bench).

Training Tips:

- Avoid rotating your torso. Movement should only occur at your shoulder joint.

- Refrain from lying directly on your upper arm.

- This exercise can also be done with a resistance band. The band should be secured to an object that won't move such as a machine. While standing, grasp the free handle of the band and pull it horizontally toward your body in the fashion described above.

- Do this exercise on a bench (instead of the floor) to obtain a greater range of motion and permit a better stretch.

EXTERNAL ROTATION

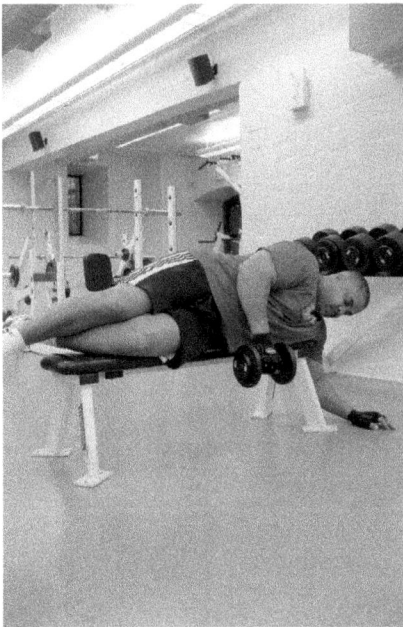

Start/Finish Position

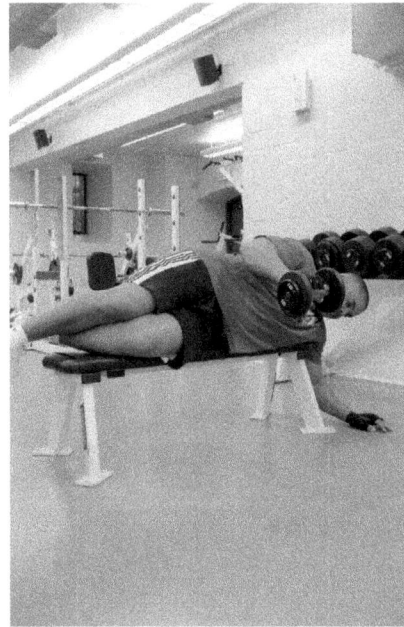

Mid-Range Position

Muscles Strengthened: external rotators

Suggested Repetitions: 8 to 10 (or 50 to 60 seconds)

Start/Finish Position: Grasp a dumbbell with your right hand. Lie down on a utility bench on your left side and draw your knees toward your torso. Position your left arm just in front of your torso and lean back slightly. Keep your right elbow against your side and bend your right arm so that the angle between your upper and lower arms is about 90 degrees. Point your right palm downward.

Performance Description: Keeping the same angle between your upper and lower arms, raise the dumbbell as high as possible. Pause briefly in this mid-range position (your hand away from your mid-section) and then lower the dumbbell under control to the start/finish position (your hand near your mid-section). Repeat the exercise for the other side of your body (with your right side on the bench).

Training Tips:

- Avoid rotating your torso. Movement should only occur at your shoulder joint.
- This exercise can also be done with a resistance band. The band should be secured to an object that won't move such as a machine. While standing, grasp the free handle of the band and pull it horizontally away from your body in the fashion described above.
- Do this exercise on a bench (instead of the floor) to obtain a greater range of motion and permit a better stretch.

UPRIGHT ROW

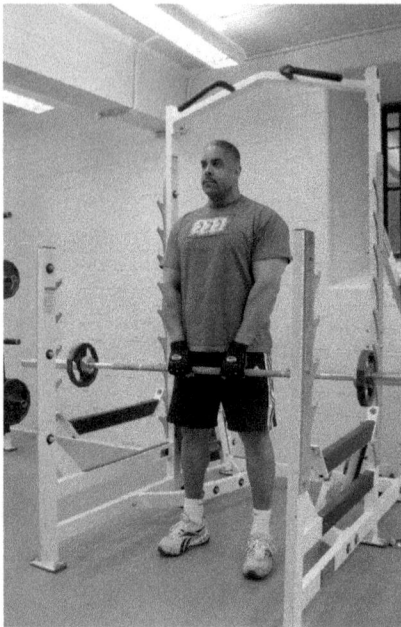

Start/Finish Position

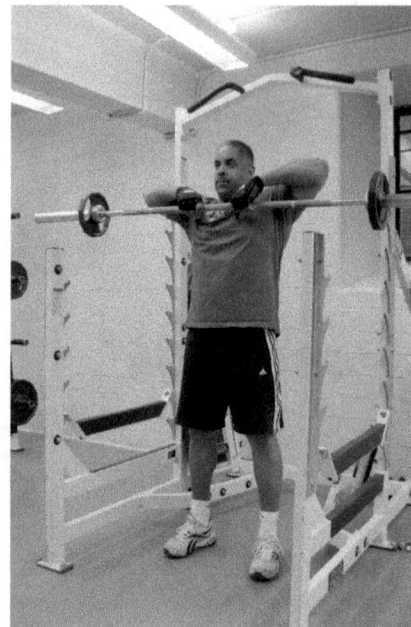

Mid-Range Position

Muscles Strengthened: trapezius (upper and lower portions), biceps and forearms

Suggested Repetitions: 5 to 10 (or 30 to 60 seconds)

Start/Finish Position: Grasp a barbell with your hands spread about 8 to 10 inches apart with your palms facing toward you. Straighten your arms and spread your feet approximately shoulder-width apart.

Performance Description: Pull the bar up until your upper arms are parallel to the floor. (Your elbows should be slightly higher than your hands in this position.) Pause briefly in this mid-range position (your arms bent) and then lower the bar under control to the start/finish position (your arms completely straight).

Training Tips:

- Avoid using your legs and moving your torso forward and backward. Movement should only occur at your shoulder and elbow joints.

- You can also perform this exercise with dumbbells. In this case, grasp the dumbbells with your palms facing toward you and hold them in front of your body about 8 to 10 inches apart.

- Keep the bar close to your body.

- Use wrist straps if you have difficulty in maintaining your grip on the bar.

- This exercise may be contraindicated if you have shoulder-impingement syndrome. This exercise may also be contraindicated if you have hyperextended elbows or low-back pain.

SHOULDER SHRUG

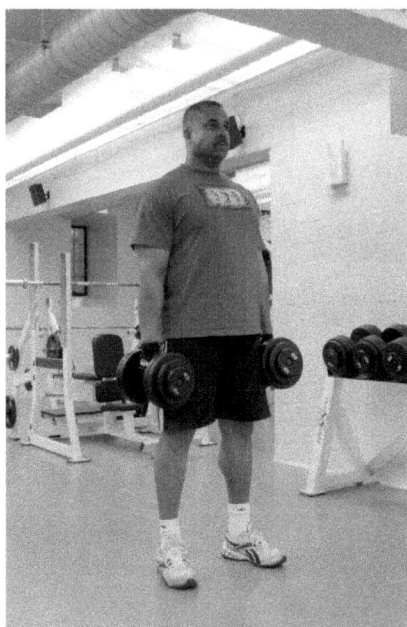

Start/Finish Position

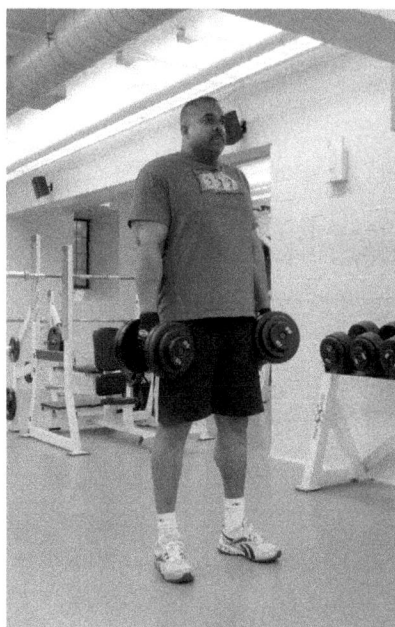

Mid-Range Position

Muscles Strengthened: trapezius (upper and lower portions) and forearms

Suggested Repetitions: 8 to 10 (or 50 to 60 seconds)

Start/Finish Position: Grasp a dumbbell with each hand. Position the dumbbells against the sides of your upper legs with your palms facing each other. Straighten your arms and spread your feet about shoulder-width apart.

Performance Description: Keeping your arms and legs fairly straight, pull the dumbbells up as high as possible (with the intent of trying to touch your shoulders to your ears as if to say, "I don't know"). Pause briefly in this mid-range position (your shoulders near your ears) and then lower the dumbbells under control to the start/finish position (your shoulders away from your ears).

Training Tips:

- Avoid "rolling" your shoulders in the mid-range position.

- Avoid using your legs and moving your torso forward and backward. Movement should only occur at your shoulder joints.

- You can also perform this exercise with a barbell and trap bar. When doing this exercise with a barbell, grasp the bar with both hands approximately shoulder-width apart with your palms facing toward you; when doing this exercise with a trap bar, use a parallel grip.

- Do this exercise with one limb at a time if you have a shoulder or an arm injury, a gross difference in the strength between your limbs or desire a training variation.

- Use wrist straps if you have difficulty in maintaining your grip on the dumbbells.

- This exercise may be contraindicated if you have hyperextended elbows or low-back pain.

SCAPULAE ADDUCTION

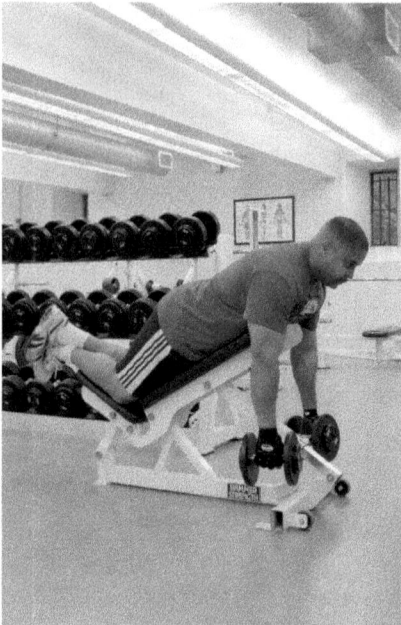

Start/Finish Position

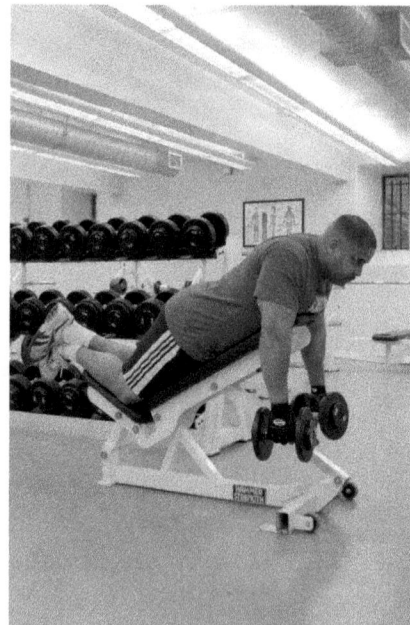

Mid-Range Position

Muscles Strengthened: trapezius (middle and lower portions), rhomboids and forearms

Suggested Repetitions: 8 to 10 (or 50 to 60 seconds)

Start/Finish Position: Grasp a dumbbell with each hand. Kneel on the seat pad of an adjustable incline bench. Lie forward against the bench and position the dumbbells directly below your torso. Straighten your arms with your palms facing each other.

Performance Description: Keeping your arms fairly straight, pull the dumbbells up as high as possible (with the intent of trying to "pinch" your shoulder blades together). Pause briefly in this mid-range position (your shoulder blades together) and then lower the dumbbells under control to the start/finish position (your shoulder blades apart).

Training Tips:

- Do this exercise with one limb at a time if you have a shoulder or an arm injury, a gross difference in the strength between your limbs or desire a training variation.

- Use wrist straps if you have difficulty in maintaining your grip on the dumbbells.

- This exercise may be contraindicated if you have hyperextended elbows.

BICEP CURL

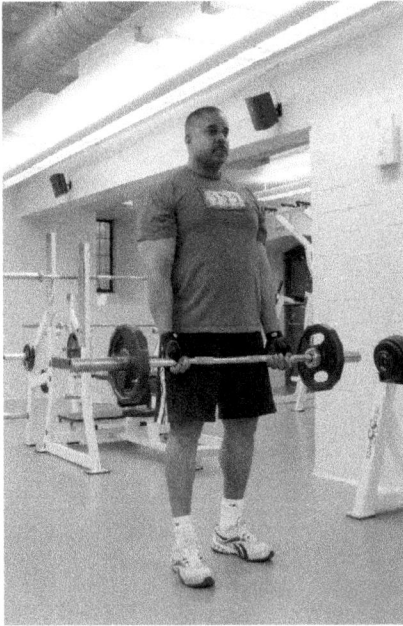

Start/Finish Position

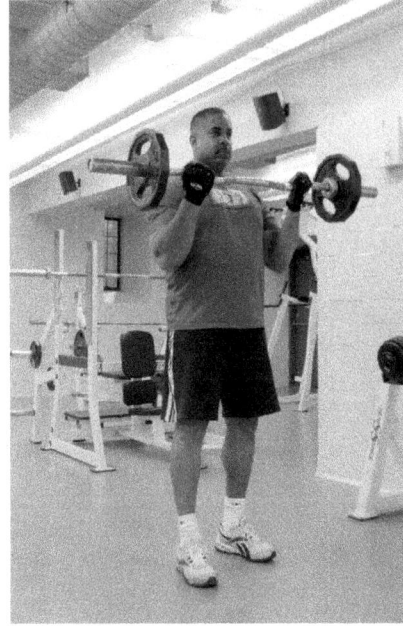

Mid-Range Position

Muscles Strengthened: biceps and forearms

Suggested Repetitions: 5 to 10 (or 30 to 60 seconds)

Start/Finish Position: Grasp an EZ curl barbell with your hands spaced slightly wider than shoulder-width apart and your palms facing away from you. Straighten your arms and spread your feet a comfortable distance apart with one foot slightly in front of the other.

Performance Description: Pull the bar below your chin. Pause briefly in this mid-range position (your arms bent) and then lower the bar under control to the start/finish position (your arms completely straight).

Training Tips:

- Keep your elbows against the sides of your torso.

- Avoid using your legs and moving your torso forward and backward. Movement should only occur at your elbow joints.

- You can also perform this exercise with a barbell and dumbbells. When doing this exercise with dumbbells, use a parallel grip (your palms facing each other) in the start/finish position. As you raise the dumbbells, gradually supinate (turn) your hands so that they're facing toward your shoulders in the mid-range position. Reverse this action when you return the dumbbells to the start/finish position.

- Do this exercise with one limb at a time if you have a shoulder or an arm injury, a gross difference in the strength between your limbs or desire a training variation.

- This exercise may be contraindicated if you have hyperextended elbows.

TRICEP EXTENSION

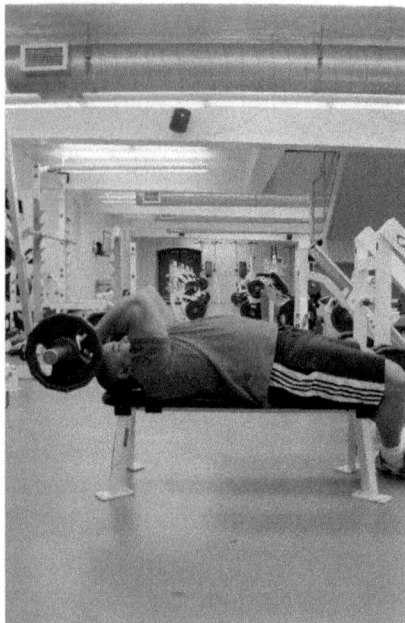

Start/Finish Position

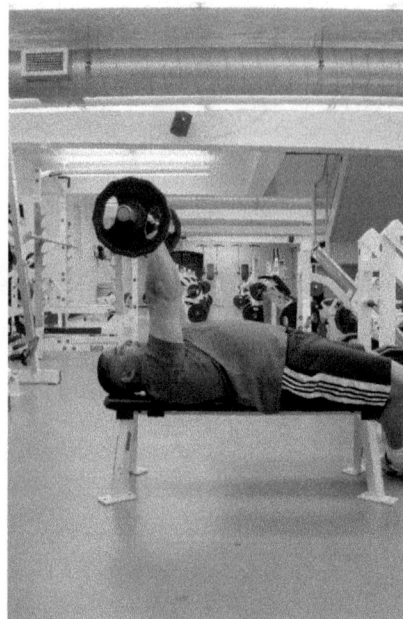

Mid-Range Position

Muscle Strengthened: triceps

Suggested Repetitions: 5 to 10 (or 30 to 60 seconds)

Start/Finish Position: Grasp an EZ curl bar with your hands spread about 4 to 6 inches apart with your palms facing toward you. Lie down on a utility bench and place your feet flat on the floor. Position your upper arms so that they're perpendicular to the floor and point your elbows toward your knees. Lower the bar until it's near your forehead.

Performance Description: Push the bar up until your arms are almost completely straight. Pause briefly in this mid-range position (your arms almost completely straight) and then lower the bar under control to the start/finish position (your arms bent).

Training Tips:

- Keep your upper arms perpendicular to the floor and your elbows pointed toward your knees.

- Keep your hips on the bench.

- If you have low-back pain, place your feet on the end of the bench or a stool. This reduces the stress in your low-back region.

- You can also perform this exercise while sitting or standing. In both cases, keep your upper arms perpendicular to the floor and raise and lower the bar behind your head.

- You can also perform this exercise with a barbell and dumbbells.

- Do this exercise with one limb at a time if you have a shoulder or an arm injury, a gross difference in the strength between your limbs or desire a training variation.

- This exercise may be contraindicated if you have shoulder-impingement syndrome.

WRIST FLEXION

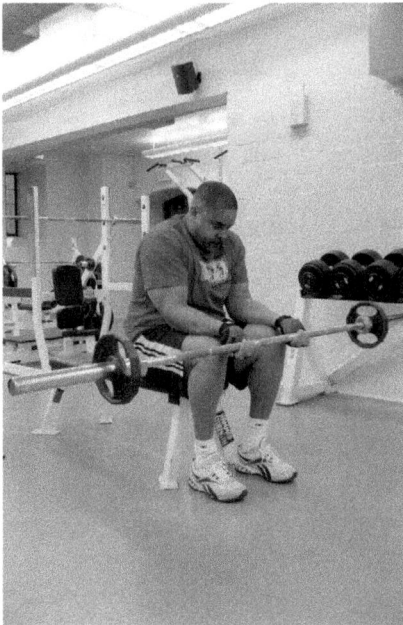

Start/Finish Position

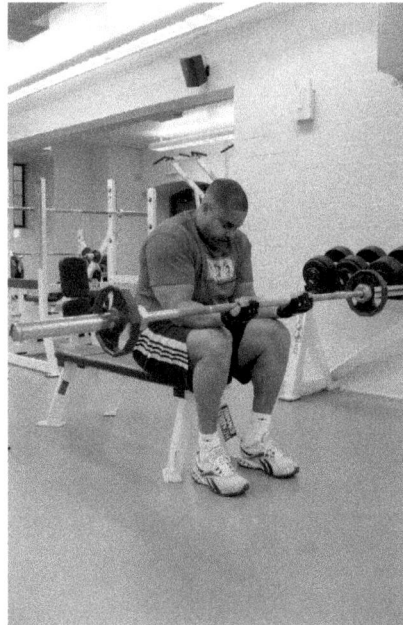

Mid-Range Position

Muscles Strengthened: wrist flexors

Suggested Repetitions: 8 to 10 (or 50 to 60 seconds)

Start/Finish Position: Grasp a barbell with your hands spread about 4 to 6 inches apart and your palms facing up. Position your thumbs underneath the bar alongside your fingers. Sit down near the end of a utility bench and place the back of your forearms on your upper legs so that your wrists are over your kneecaps. Lean forward slightly so that the angle between your upper and lower arms is about 90 degrees or less.

Performance Description: Pull the bar up as high as possible. Pause briefly in this mid-range position (your wrists bent) and then lower the bar under control to the start/finish position (your wrists extended).

Training Tips:

- Keep your forearms on your upper legs.
- Do this exercise with your thumbs underneath the bar. This increases your range of motion.
- Avoid using your legs and moving your torso forward and backward. Movement should only occur at your wrist joints.
- Do this exercise with one limb at a time if you have an arm injury, a gross difference in the strength between your limbs or desire a training variation.
- You can also perform this exercise with dumbbells.

WRIST EXTENSION

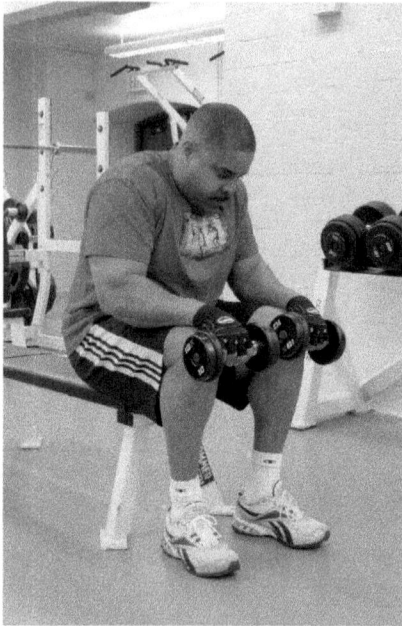

Start/Finish Position

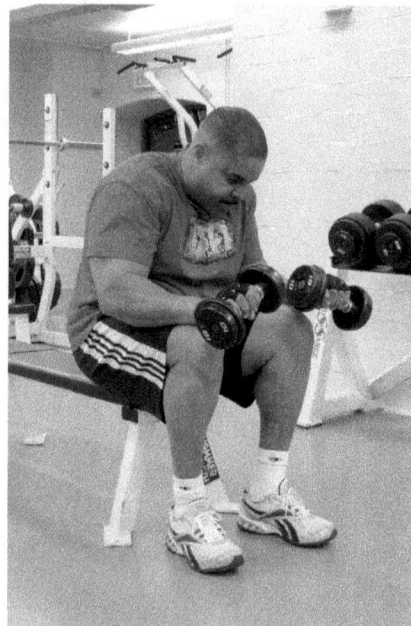

Mid-Range Position

Muscles Strengthened: wrist extensors

Suggested Repetitions: 8 to 10 (or 50 to 60 seconds)

Start/Finish Position: Grasp a dumbbell with each hand. Sit down near the end of a utility bench and place the front of your forearms on your upper legs so that your wrists are over your kneecaps and your palms are facing down. Lean forward slightly so that the angle between your upper and lower arms is about 90 degrees or less.

Performance Description: Pull the dumbbells up as high as possible. Pause briefly in this mid-range position (your wrists extended) and then lower the dumbbells under control to the start/finish position (your wrists bent).

Training Tips:

- Keep your forearms on your upper legs.
- Avoid using your legs and moving your torso forward and backward. Movement should only occur at your wrist joints.
- Do this exercise with dumbbells rather than a barbell. This makes it more comfortable on your wrist joints.
- Do this exercise with one limb at a time if you have an arm injury, a gross difference in the strength between your limbs or desire a training variation.

FINGER FLEXION

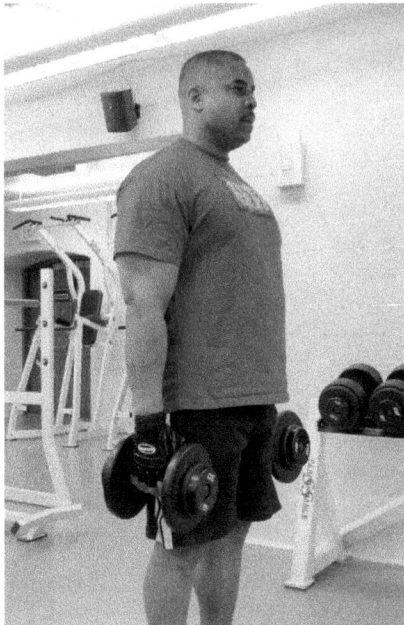
Start/Finish Position

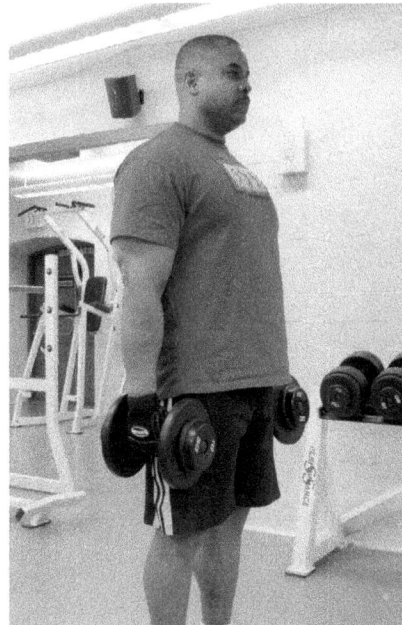
Mid-Range Position

Muscles Strengthened: finger flexors

Suggested Repetitions: 8 to 10 (or 50 to 60 seconds)

Start/Finish Position: Grasp a dumbbell with each hand. Position the dumbbells against the sides of your upper legs with your palms facing each other. Straighten your arms and spread your feet about shoulder-width apart. Allow the dumbbells to roll down your hands to your fingertips.

Performance Description: Keeping your arms fairly straight, pull the dumbbells up to your thumbs. Pause briefly in this mid-range position (your fingers flexed) and then lower the dumbbells under control to the start/finish position (your fingers extended).

Training Tips:

- Avoid using your legs and arms. Movement should only occur at your finger joints.
- Squeeze the dumbbells as hard as possible in the mid-range position.
- Lower the dumbbells all the way down to your fingertips.
- You can also perform this exercise with a barbell (keeping the bar in front of your legs and grasping it with either your palms facing toward you or away from you).
- Do this exercise with one limb at a time if you have an arm injury, a gross difference in the strength between your limbs or desire a training variation.

ABDOMINAL CRUNCH

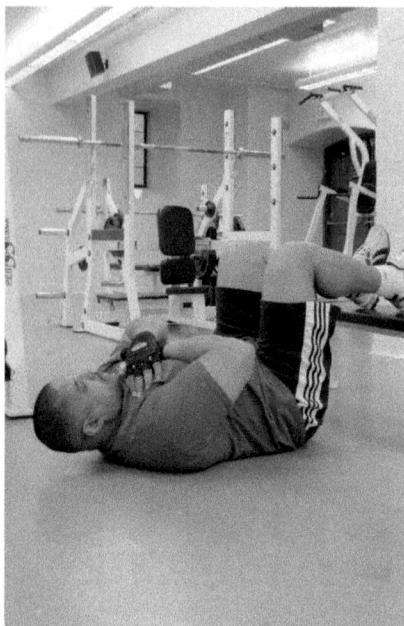

Start/Finish Position

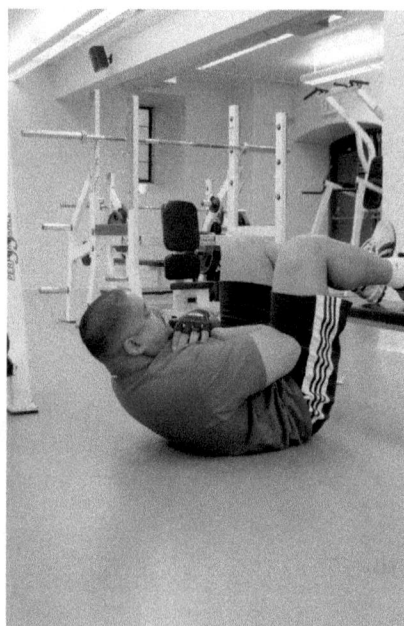

Mid-Range Position

Muscle Strengthened: rectus abdominis

Suggested Repetitions: 8 to 10 (or 50 to 60 seconds)

Start/Finish Position: Lie down on the floor and place the back of your lower legs on a utility bench (or stool). Position your upper legs so that they're perpendicular to the floor and the angle between your upper and lower legs is about 90 degrees. Fold your arms across your chest and bring your head toward your chest so that the upper portion of your shoulder blades doesn't touch the floor.

Performance Description: Pull your torso as close to your upper legs as possible. Pause briefly in this mid-range position (your torso bent) and then lower your torso under control to the start/finish position (your torso straight).

Training Tips:

- Avoid touching the floor with your shoulder blades. This removes the load from your abdominals.

- Avoid snapping your head forward. Movement should only occur at your hip joint and mid-section.

- If you can do 10 repetitions or more using your bodyweight, increase the workload by holding additional weight against your chest, performing the exercise with a slower speed of movement or having a spotter apply manual resistance to your shoulders.

- After reaching muscular fatigue, you can overload your muscles further by grasping the backs of your upper legs, pulling your torso to the mid-range position and lowering your torso under control to the start/finish position for 3 to 5 negative-only repetitions.

- This exercise may be contraindicated if you have low-back pain.

KNEE-UP

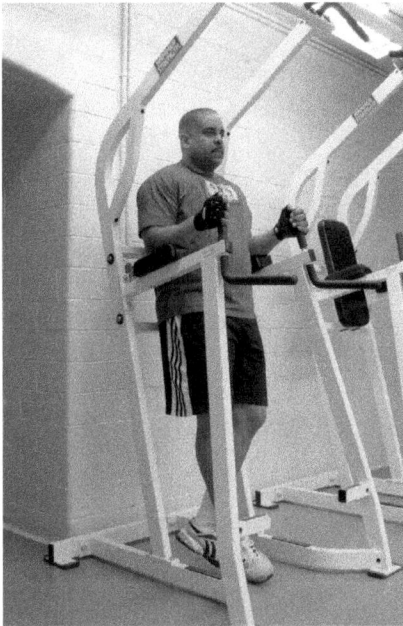

Start/Finish Position

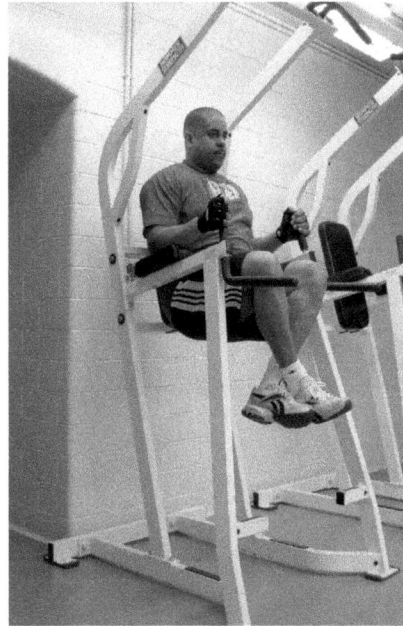

Mid-Range Position

Muscles Strengthened: iliopsoas and rectus abdominis (lower portion)

Suggested Repetitions: 8 to 10 (or 50 to 60 seconds)

Start/Finish Position: Place your lower arms on the forearm pads. Grasp the handles. Straighten your legs and cross your ankles.

Performance Description: Pull your knees up as close to your chest as possible. Pause briefly in this mid-range position (your knees near your chest) and then lower your legs under control to the start/finish position (your legs hanging down).

Training Tips:

- Avoid swinging your body forward and backward. Movement should only occur at your hip and knee joints.

- If you can do 10 repetitions or more using your bodyweight, increase the workload by performing the exercise with a slower speed of movement or having a spotter apply manual resistance to your upper legs.

SIDE BEND

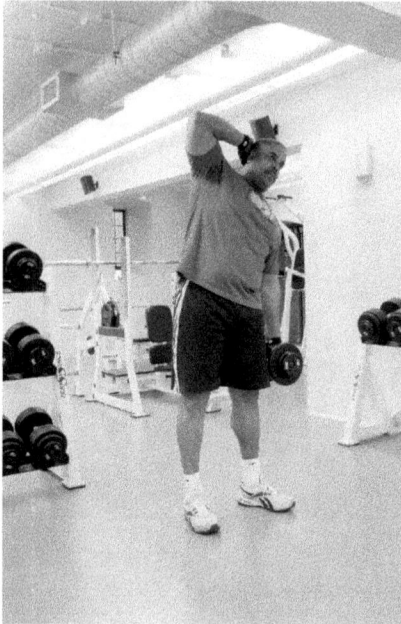

Start/Finish Position

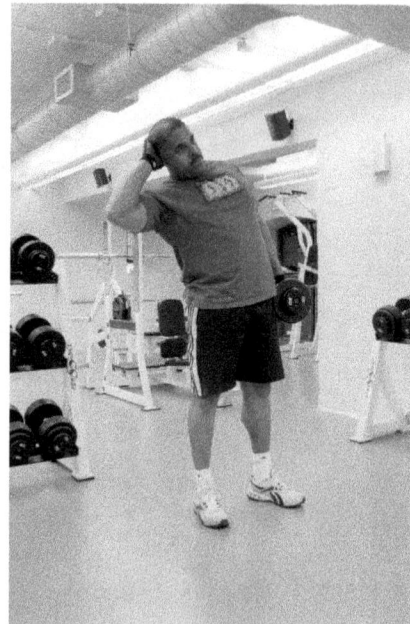

Mid-Range Position

Muscles Strengthened: obliques, erector spinae and forearms

Suggested Repetitions: 8 to 10 (or 50 to 60 seconds)

Start/Finish Position: Grasp a dumbbell with your left hand. Position the dumbbell against the side of your upper leg with your palm facing your leg. Spread your feet about shoulder-width apart. Place your right palm against the right side of your head. Keep your hips in the same position and bend your torso to the left as far as possible.

Performance Description: Without moving your hips, bring your torso to the right as far as possible. Pause briefly in this mid-range position (your torso bent to the right) and then lower the dumbbell under control to the start/finish position (your torso bent to the left). Repeat the exercise for the other side of your body.

Training Tips:

- Avoid moving your hips. Movement should only occur at your mid-section.
- Refrain from bending forward at the waist.
- Keep your feet flat on the floor.
- Use wrist straps if you have difficulty in maintaining your grip on the dumbbell.
- This exercise may be contraindicated if you have low-back pain.

BACK EXTENSION

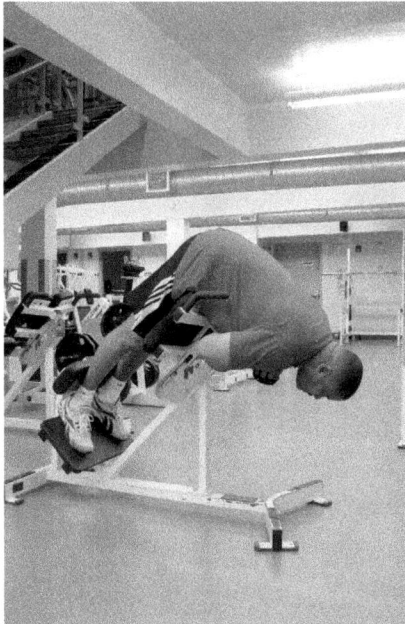

Start/Finish Position

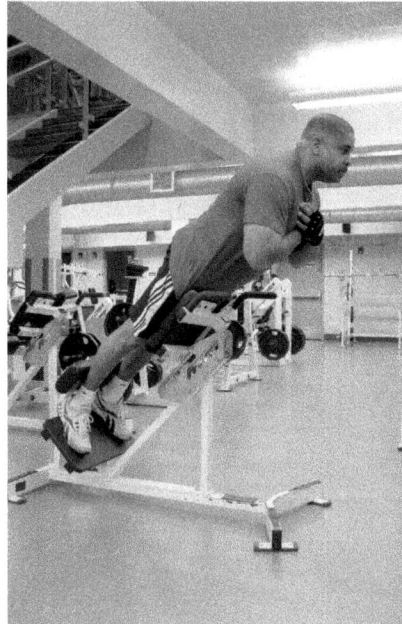

Mid-Range Position

Muscles Strengthened: erector spinae, gluteus maximus and hamstrings

Suggested Repetitions: 10 to 15 (or 60 to 90 seconds)

Start/Finish Position: Place your feet flat on the footboard and the back of your lower legs against the leg pads. Position your pelvis against the hip pads so that your navel is above the edges. Allow your torso to hang down and fold your arms across your chest.

Performance Description: Raise your torso until it's aligned with your upper legs. Pause briefly in this mid-range position (your torso straight) and then lower your torso under control to the start/finish position (your torso bent).

Training Tips:

- Avoid hyperextending your torso (leaning backward excessively) in the mid-range position.
- Avoid snapping your head backward. Movement should only occur at your hip joint and mid-section.
- If you can do 15 repetitions or more using your bodyweight, increase the workload by holding additional weight against your chest, performing the exercise with a slower speed of movement or having a spotter apply manual resistance to your upper back.
- This exercise may be contraindicated if you have low-back pain.

STIFF-LEG DEADLIFT

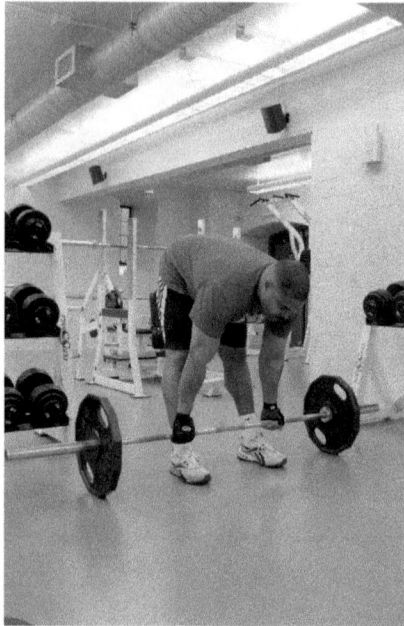

Start/Finish Position

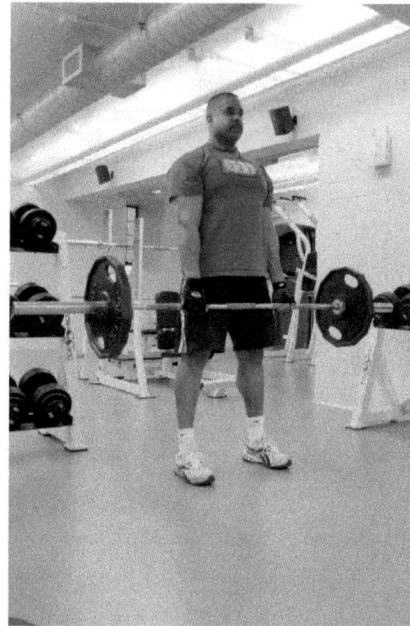

Mid-Range Position

Muscles Strengthened: erector spinae, gluteus maximus, hamstrings and forearms

Suggested Repetitions: 10 to 15 (or 60 to 90 seconds)

Start/Finish Position: Spread your feet slightly narrower than shoulder-width apart. Reach down and grasp a bar on the inside of your legs with an alternating grip (your dominant palm facing forward and non-dominant palm facing backward). Straighten your legs but don't "lock" your knees. Place most of your bodyweight on your heels. Straighten your arms.

Performance Description: Stand upright by straightening your torso. Pause briefly in this mid-range position (your torso straight) and then lower the bar under control to the start/finish position (your torso bent).

Training Tips:

- Keep your arms and legs straight as you perform this exercise. Unlike the deadlift, your lower back should do most of the work.
- Exert force through your heels, not the balls of your feet.
- Avoid "locking" or "snapping" your knees in the mid-range position. Also, avoid hyperextending your torso (leaning backward excessively) in the mid-range position.
- Refrain from bouncing the weight off the floor between repetitions.
- You can also perform this exercise with dumbbells.
- Use wrist straps if you have difficulty in maintaining your grip on the bar.
- This exercise may be contraindicated if you have low-back pain, hyperextended elbows or an exceptionally long torso and/or legs.

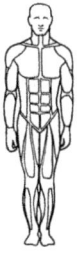

9 Machine Exercises

The two most popular types of machines are selectorized and plate-loaded. With a selectorized machine, the resistance can be adjusted – or selected – by inserting a selector pin or key into a weight stack of flat, rectangular-shaped plates that travel up and down a pair of steel guide rods; with a plate-loaded machine, the resistance can be adjusted by adding barbell plates to or removing barbell plates from "horns" that are attached to its movement arms.

MAJOR MOMENTS IN HISTORY

The machines that reside in fitness centers have a rich history that overflows with many evolutionary events and inventions of considerable significance. Let's see how these historic moments have led to our present-day machines.

The Polymachinon

In 1829, Captain James (nee Giacomo) Chiosso – an Italian inventor and later a professor of gymnastics at University College in London – created what's thought by many to be the first exercise machine. Over the course of many years, Captain Chiosso revised his original machine at least four times in order to correct what he thought were deficiencies in its form and function. Although its inner workings were concealed within a tall, wooden, box-like structure, the final version – referred to as the Gymnastic and Calisthenic Polymachinon – greatly resembled a modern-day multi-station, cable-column machine; for all intents and purposes, it was a functional trainer of yesteryear.

As many as 10 individuals could use the machine at a time and perform a wide assortment of exercises that addressed all of the major muscles, including the neck flexion, neck extension, squat, hip abduction, hip adduction, leg curl, leg extension, chest press, lat pulldown and back extension. The resistance could be adjusted by adding plates to or removing plates from rods that were housed within numerous compartments that corresponded to different stations around the column. The Polymachinon never really gained much acceptance as an exercise machine, probably because of its close ties to gymnastics.

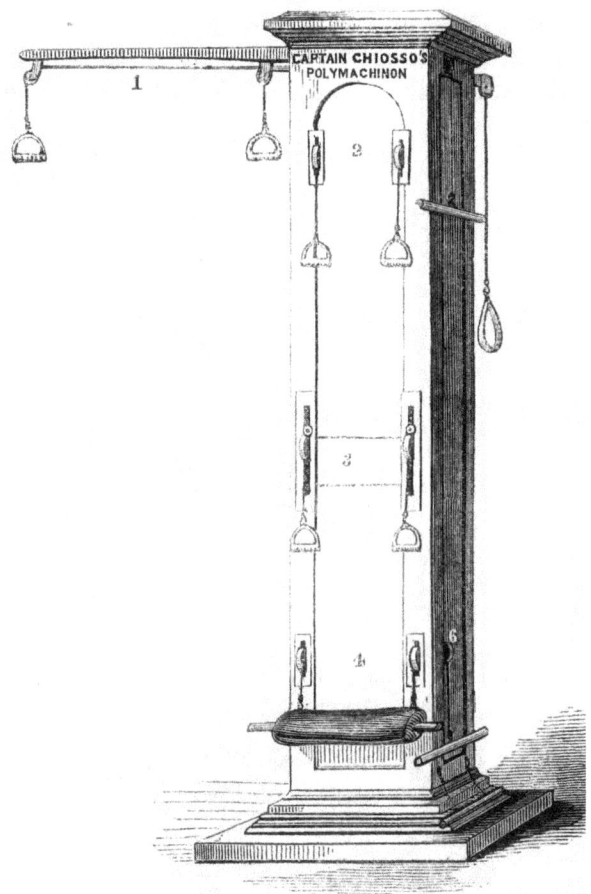

The polymachinon – created in 1829 by Captain James Chiosso – is thought by many to be the first exercise machine. (Image from Chiosso, 1855.)

The Health-Lift Machines

From the late 1860s to the late 1870s, an enormously popular exercise was the health-lift. Essentially, the health-lift is a partial deadlift. Whereas in performing a traditional deadlift, the weight is lifted from the floor level, in performing a partial deadlift, the weight is lifted from the mid-thigh level. This abbreviated range of motion allowed individuals to lift very heavy weights, a practice that was in vogue at the time. In addition, the health-lift was viewed by many in the medical community as a miraculous exercise that could be used to treat or "cure" virtually any ailment that was imaginable, ranging from diseases to deformities.

A number of individuals – many of whom were physicians – have been regarded as or have professed to inventing a mechanized version of the health-lift, including Dr. David Butler, Dr. Frank Reilly and Dr. George Barker Windship. As to who was the first person to do so is debatable. Some claims don't have much merit.

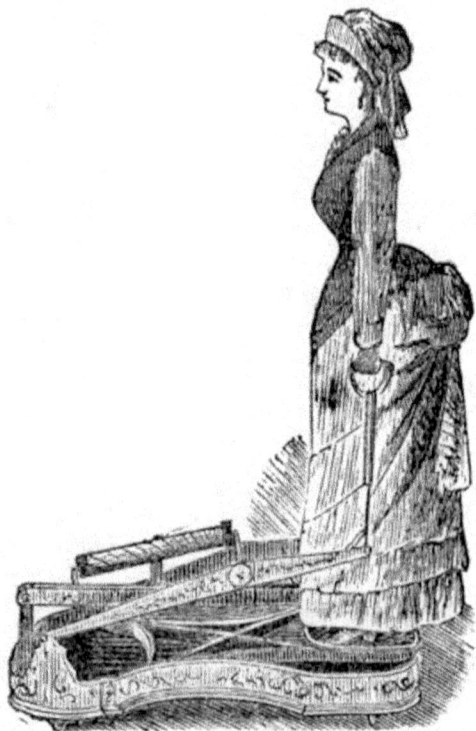

The Reactionary Lifter – a mechanized version of the health-lift – was invented by Reverend Charles Mann in or around 1870. (Image from Health-Lift Company, 1876.)

For example, Dr. Windship's "machine" hardly qualifies as such . . . unless standing on a wooden platform over a hole in the ground and using a rope and handle to lift a barrel of rocks and sand that was in the hole fits your definition of a machine.

By 1868, Dr. Butler – who promoted a system of training called "The Lifting Cure" – had created a plate-loaded health-lift machine. Up to that point in time, all of the health-lift machines used plates as resistance. But that changed in 1870 when Reverend Charles Mann of Orange, New Jersey, filed a patent application for a health-lift machine that he referred to as the Reactionary Lifter. The resistance on this machine could be adjusted "instantly" from 20 to 1,200 pounds through "a combination of levers and a movable fulcrum"; no external source of resistance was required.

In using the Reactionary Lifter, a person stood on a platform between two levers with handles. The person reached down and grasped the handles with a parallel grip (the palms facing each other). To do the exercise, the person simply stood upright by straightening the legs and torso. The action is quite similar to that of grasping the levers of a wheelbarrow and standing upright.

Reverend Mann sold his machine through the Reactionary Lifter Company of Newark, New Jersey. However, the rights to manufacture and sell the machine were soon purchased by the Health-Lift Company of New York City. Its cost was $100 in 1876 or about $2,224 in 2018 money.

The Reactionary Lifter was billed as "the only scientific system of physical training" and required "minimum time for maximum results" (specifically, 10 minutes a day). It was, arguably, one of the most hyped products in history, said to relieve constipation, diarrhea, dyspepsia, morning sickness during pregnancy, rheumatism, sciatica and even "restores displaced organs to their natural position." Testimonials for the machine came from physicians, clergymen, "eminent lawyers," "prominent individuals," musicians and vocalists and athletes. One of the most interesting endorsements came from P. T. Barnum – yes, *that*

P. T. Barnum – who stated that the Reactionary Lifter "afforded great relief" for his "dizzy turns, numbness in wrist and spine [and] headache" when medical treatment wasn't effective.

Fascination with the health-lift was very brief, only lasting about a decade. It's thought that the premature death of Dr. Windship in 1876 at the age of 42 – perhaps the most famous advocate of the health-lift – was a major factor in the demise of the exercise.

"Apparatus for Physical Culture"

As noted earlier, it may have been a stretch to associate Dr. Windship with inventing a mechanized health-lift. But in 1873, he filed a patent application for an "Apparatus for Physical Culture" which was a true multi-exercise machine.

Included among the exercises that could be done on the machine were the leg press (which he called "foot-shoving"), chest press ("hand-shoving"), lat pulldown ("down-pulling") and row. The machine also had a horizontal bar that could be employed for the chin-up/pull-up. (In an early application of record keeping, Dr. Windship's instructions for using the machine made note of an "exercise card" on which an individual "marks on it the weight lifted and the number of times lifted.")

Medico-Mechanische Therapie

In 1865, around the time that the health-lift mania began to take root in America, Dr. Gustav Zander – a Swedish physician – founded a medical institute in Stockholm. The facility contained more than two dozen machines that he had invented. His "medico-mechanische therapie" – loosely translated as medical-mechanical therapy – was originally intended as a way to treat physical ailments but was later promoted as a way to exercise.

When first introduced, Dr. Zander's "mechanical method" of treatment and exercise was met with sharp criticism. At the time, a "manual method" of treatment and exercise was the standard approach. This was based on the teachings of Per Henrik Ling, a fellow-countryman who advocated "free exercises" that

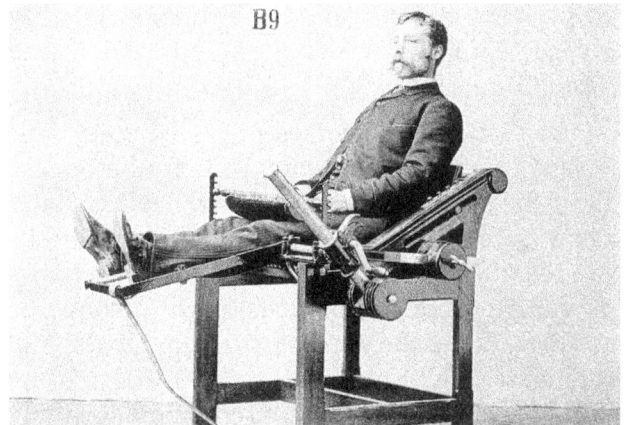

This seated leg curl was invented by Dr. Gustav Zander more than a century ago yet is incredibly similar to modern machines in terms of both design and function. (Image from Levertin, 1893.)

were done "without apparatus." (More on that point in Chapter 10.)

Over time, Dr. Zander's methods and machines gained greater acceptance and his medical institutes began to spread across Europe and elsewhere. In 1911, at the peak of its popularity, 202 institutes bore his name. All but 14 of these were located in European countries but a handful or so were established in America. The first institute in this country to offer a complete "line" of his machines opened in New York City in 1890, on East 59th Street near the edge of Central Park. In addition to the medical setting, Dr. Zander's machines appeared in gymnasiums as well as spas and resorts such as the famous Greenbrier® Resort in West Virginia. In fact, the RMS *Titanic* – the "unsinkable" British ocean liner that sunk in less than three hours after colliding with an iceberg in 1912 – offered a gymnasium to its first-class passengers that included stationary cycles, rowers and several of Dr. Zander's machines.

To say that Dr. Zander was more than a century ahead of his time is no exaggeration. Many of his machines were incredibly similar to modern machines in terms of both design and function. He was the first person to create a series of single-station machines that addressed all of the major muscles. Among his machines – of which there were eventually about 30 for "active movements" – were the seated leg curl, lat pulldown, bicep curl and torso rotation; he even invented a machine for wrist supination and pronation.

Dr. Zander's machines provided adjustable resistance by changing the position of a weight along the movement arm (or lever). His machines also provided variable resistance throughout the range of motion by the way in which the movement arm changed its angle during the performance of the exercise, a design feature that was incredibly advanced for the 1860s; it's the same basic concept that's used in modern-day plate-loaded machines. In ranges of motion where an individual had a biomechanical advantage and could produce more force, the movement arm was closer to horizontal and the machine offered more resistance; in ranges of motion where an individual had a biomechanical disadvantage and could produce less force, the movement arm was closer to vertical and the machine offered less resistance. In effect, where an individual had more leverage, the machine gave less leverage and where an individual had less leverage, the machine gave more leverage. The end result was greater muscular effort throughout the range of motion.

His machines all but disappeared by the early 1930s. Most researchers attribute this to the global impact of World War I and the subsequent Great Depression.

Sidebar: Gymnasiums of that era were much different from gymnasiums of this era. During the mid- to late-1800s, gymnasiums placed a heavy emphasis on gymnastics; so when you "hit the gym," you "did gymnastics." In those days, even the term gymnastics had a much different meaning. Back then, gymnastics referred to activities that were done for treatment (medical gymnastics) or exercise (educational gymnastics) and were mainly calisthenic-type movements. And a gymnast referred to a therapist or teacher/instructor.

Pulley-Weight "Appliances"

In 1879, Dr. Dudley Sargent – a physician, inventor and pioneer in physical education who pushed for its nationwide acceptance – was appointed the director of the Hemenway

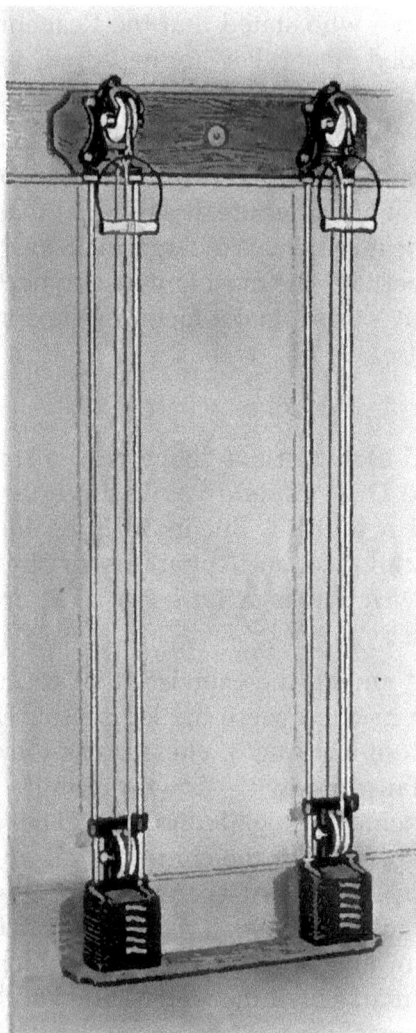

This wall-mounted, pulley-weight "appliance" was invented by Dr. Dudley Sargent in or around the late 1870s. (Image from Narragansett Machine Company, 1905.)

Gymnasium at Harvard University. He remained in that position for the next 40 years, until retiring in 1919. During the first five years of his employment, Dr. Sargent was also an assistant professor of physical training.

His arrival at Harvard coincided with that of the newly built Hemenway Gymnasium, a construction project that cost $110 thousand or about $2.62 million in 2018 money. At the time, the sticker price of Hemenway made it the most expensive college gymnasium in the country.

When Hemenway opened its doors in January 1880, the inventory of equipment included 80 pieces of Dr. Sargent's pulley-weight "appliances" and other machines as well as horizontal bars, parallel bars, pommel horses, rings, climbing ropes, ladders and "dumb-bells." Prior to arriving in Cambridge, Dr. Sargent had tinkered with pulley-weight machines but Harvard gave him the opportunity to let his imagination run wild.

In its simplest form, his pulley machine consisted of a single weight stack, two guide rods, a rope/cord, a pulley and a handle. A variation of this employed two weight stacks with high pulleys that swiveled so that the two handles could be used in combination and in different directions, making it act a lot like a functional trainer of today. Most of these machines were wall-mounted units. Dr. Sargent also invented pulley-based equipment for specific body parts, including the following machines: chest (by some accounts, his most popular machine), dip, "abdominal chair," wrist roller, finger flexion and neck.

The system that was advocated by Dr. Sargent departed from traditional practices in two ways. Although Dr. Sargent's background and experience included gymnastics – at age 18, he even performed acrobatic stunts with a traveling circus – his system placed a heavy emphasis on exercise with machine-based equipment, not gymnastic-based equipment. Also, his system was geared toward individual activity, not group activity.

Dr. Sargent's equipment – along with his training system and method for tests and measurements – soon spread to hundreds of high schools, colleges, YMCAs and other institutions across the United States. In fact, the popularity of his pulley machines was so great that a strong case can be made for this being the point in history when exercise broke away from its gymnastic-based roots and began to take on the appearance of training as is now performed.

The legacy of Dr. Sargent lives on in other ways. In 1881, he founded the Sargent School for Physical Education which became part of Boston University in 1929. It's now known as the Boston University College of Health and Rehabilitation Sciences: Sargent College. (Fast

fact: In 1921, Dr. Sargent developed the Sargent Jump Test; today, it's simply referred to as the vertical jump.)

The Universal® Gym

In 1957, the Universal® Gym Company developed the first multi-station selectorized machine. Invented by Harold Zinkin – who was a "regular" at Muscle Beach in Santa Monica, California, and finished second in the 1945 Mr. America bodybuilding contest – the Universal® Gym was a revolutionary machine with multiple weight stacks that were strategically positioned around what amounted to a large, metal cube-like frame.

The company manufactured different models of the Universal® Gym with names that hark back to the days of ancient Rome and Greece, including the Centurion, Gladiator, Maximus and Spartan. Standard features varied but the Centurion – perhaps the most well-known model – had five weight stacks. Three were used for the leg press, bench press and shoulder press; and two were attached to high and low pulleys which allowed the underhand/overhand lat pulldown and tricep extension (on the high pulley) and the bicep curl, upright row and seated row (on the low pulley). Also available on the Centurion were an adjustable abdominal board for the sit-up/crunch, handles for the dip and chin-up/pull-up and stations for the hip flexion and back extension. The models could be customized to some extent. For instance, the adjustable abdominal board could be swapped for the vertical chest (pec fly) or leg extension/leg curl.

The Universal® Gym was a device of sheer brilliance. This was demonstrated in both design and function.

Its design was amazingly simple. The guts of the Centurion, for example, consisted of five weight stacks, 10 guide rods (two per weight stack), two cables and three movement arms. Moreover, all of the parts were exposed – meaning that none were hidden from view – which made a Universal® Gym extremely easy to maintain. Despite its simplicity, the machine was incredibly durable. And a Universal® Gym didn't take up too much real estate, either; its basic footprint was about 14 feet by 16 feet or about 224 square feet.

Its function was exceedingly effective. The machine allowed for multiple exercises (or stations) that could accommodate multiple users at one time. (A "fully loaded" version of the Centurion had enough stations for 10 users.) The compact arrangement of a Universal® Gym – and the fact that the resistance could be adjusted quickly and easily – made it ideal for circuit training which was all the rage in the United States throughout much of the 1960s and 1970s.

In 1974, the company introduced Dynamic Variable Resistance (DVR) on its Centurion model. DVR was created by Dr. Gideon Ariel – who earned his doctoral degree in exercise science from the University of Massachusetts – and employed on the three weight stacks that were used for pressing movements: the leg press, bench press and shoulder press. At the top of each weight stack was a "sleeve mechanism" with a roller that was positioned above the movement arm. As an exercise was performed, the roller slid back and forth along the movement arm thereby changing the length of the resistance arm (defined as the distance from the axis of rotation – or fulcrum – to the point where the resistance is applied). In ranges of motion where an individual had a biomechanical advantage and could produce more force, the sleeve moved away from the axis of rotation which made the resistance arm longer and the machine offered more resistance; in ranges of motion where an individual had a biomechanical disadvantage and could produce less force, the sleeve moved closer to the axis of rotation which made the resistance arm shorter and the machine offered less resistance. In effect, where an individual had more leverage, the machine gave less leverage and where an individual had less leverage, the machine gave more leverage. The end result was greater muscular effort throughout the range of motion. (Fast fact: Dr. Ariel graduated from the famed Wingate Institute in Netanya, Israel; he competed for Israel in the 1960 Rome Olympics in the shot put and the 1964 Tokyo Olympics in the discus.)

The Universal® Gym proved to be immensely popular for several decades, especially in high schools, colleges and YMCAs; it was said that at one point, more than 5,000 machines were sold *per year*. According to a 1975 company brochure, the US Military Academy in West Point, New York, had 13 multi-station machines alone; Princeton University had six. Its use was so widespread that Universal® became a generic term for any multi-station machine in the same vein that Band-Aid® became a generic term for any adhesive bandage and Kleenex® became a generic term for any tissue. By the early 1990s, sales of Universal® machines had peaked. The company went into bankruptcy in 1996 and never again held the same lofty status in the industry.

Nautilus® Machines

A company that transformed the fitness landscape with its chain-driven machines was Nautilus® Sports/Medical Industries which was founded by Arthur Jones. Legend has it that Jones built the first Nautilus® machine in 1948 – a prototype pullover that used barbell plates for resistance – on a front porch in Tulsa, Oklahoma. But it wasn't until November 1970 – after 27 different versions of the pullover machine were built and tested – that Nautilus® actually sold and delivered a machine to a customer (said to be Dana Brigham who was an attorney in Miami). As you may have guessed, the machine was a plate-loaded pullover. (Technically, the first "customer" was Lloyd "Red" Lerille – winner of the 1960 Mr. America bodybuilding contest and owner of a health club in Lafayette, Louisiana – who paid cash for a Nautilus® machine in August 1970. However, that machine was a prototype.)

The establishment of Nautilus® couldn't have come at a more opportune time for Jones. The early 1970s marked the embryonic stage of the so-called fitness boom, a major moment in history when aerobic training and strength training went mainstream. Almost overnight, it suddenly became fashionable to exercise. And Nautilus® filled that niche. Without a doubt, Nautilus® helped to energize the fitness boom.

Hundreds of fitness centers sprouted up across the United States and Canada with Nautilus® machines as the main or lone attraction. Amazingly, Jones allowed business owners to include Nautilus® in the names of their fitness centers without requiring them to pay him any franchise fees or royalties. Its use was so extensive and trendy that instead of saying "I work out," people often bragged, "I do Nautilus®."

At the heart of a Nautilus® machine was a spiral-shaped pulley known as a cam. Gary Jones – Arthur's son – is credited with designing the Nautilus® cam . . . at the age of 17. As an exercise was performed, the asymmetrical cam rotated around its axis thereby changing the length of the resistance arm (aka effective radius). In ranges of motion where an individual had a biomechanical advantage and could produce more force, the effective radius of the cam was larger and the machine offered more resistance; in ranges of motion where an individual had a biomechanical disadvantage and could produce less force, the effective radius of the cam was smaller and the machine offered less resistance. In effect, where an individual had more leverage, the machine gave less leverage and where an individual had less leverage, the machine gave more leverage. The end result was greater muscular effort throughout the range of motion. (Fast fact: Nautilus® derives its name from the spiral shape of the cam which bears a close likeness to the spiral shape of a chambered nautilus shell.)

Nautilus® mainly produced single-station machines but also offered at least five "double" machines: The compound leg (leg extension and leg press); double chest (arm cross and decline press); pullover/torso arm; behind neck/torso arm; and double shoulder (lateral raise and overhead press). As the name suggests, a double machine consisted of two exercises: a single-joint movement (aka a simple or primary movement) and a multiple-joint movement (aka a compound or secondary movement).

The design of these double machines was based on the Pre-Exhaustion Principle, a training tactic that was popularized by Jones in the early 1970s. The idea was to perform a single-joint movement to "pre-exhaust" (or pre-fatigue) the major muscle that you're trying to work. This was followed quickly by a multiple-joint movement to gain assistance from other surrounding muscles to work the pre-exhausted muscle to a much greater degree of fatigue. In using the double-chest machine, for example, you'd do the single-joint movement (the arm cross; essentially a pec fly) to pre-exhaust your chest and anterior deltoid. As soon as possible following the completion of that exercise, you'd do the multiple-joint movement (the decline press) which will employ your triceps to assist your pre-exhausted chest and anterior deltoid to produce a level of fatigue that would normally be impossible. Even though the Nautilus® double machines have gone the way of the dinosaur and the phone book, the Pre-Exhaustion Principle can still be done with free weights, machines and manual resistance.

Around 1985, Nautilus® began to manufacture and sell a complete line of plate-loaded machines that were then referred to as leverage machines. At the time, the machines had chrome-plated frames and, as the name implies, required the use of barbell plates as resistance. Gary Jones is also credited with designing the Nautilus® leverage machines. Interestingly, these leverage machines employed the same basic concept to vary the resistance as Dr. Zander's machines.

In 1986, Arthur Jones – whose arrogant, abrasive and cantankerous personality was as legendary as his contributions to the fitness industry — sold the company to a Texas oilman named Travis Ward. Jones, in turn, quickly founded MedX® Corporation, a company that specialized in medical-testing and -training devices but also produced high-quality selectorized machines and, for a few years in the early 2000s, plate-loaded machines (known as the Avenger line).

The Nautilus® brand was never really the same after the 1986 sale. In fact, the company filed for bankruptcy in 1990. Nautilus® is still in existence but since 2011, has focused on the residential (home) market.

Hammer Strength® Machines

The Nautilus® leverage machines were actually the forerunners of the Hammer Strength® machines that were introduced in 1989. The company – formed by a trio of business partners that included Gary Jones – enjoyed immediate success and continues to manufacture the premiere plate-loaded machines in the world. (Fast fact: Nautilus® acquired Universal Gym in 2006 but soon thereafter discontinued the brand; Brunswick Corporation – the parent company of Life Fitness® – acquired Hammer Strength® in 1997 and Cybex® in 2016, continuing to sell products under both names.)

MAJOR COMPANIES

The major companies that sell selectorized and/or plate-loaded machines currently include Cybex®; Hammer Strength®; Life Fitness®; Pendulum™; Precor®; and Technogym®.

ADVANTAGES OF MACHINES

In comparison to free weights, machines offer the following advantages:

1. Machines allow you to perform some exercises that can't be done with free weights.

This includes hip abduction, hip adduction, leg curl, leg extension and lat pulldown as well as those for the neck. These machine exercises and others have a valuable role in a comprehensive strength program.

2. Most machines provide variable resistance.

As an exercise is performed, the biomechanical leverage of your skeletal system changes which makes the movement feel easier in some positions and harder in others. (Plotting these changes on a graph reveals what's known as a strength curve.)

A properly designed machine automatically varies the resistance to match the changes in your biomechanical leverage. In positions in which you have superior leverage (and superior strength), the machine creates a mechanical disadvantage and offers more resistance; in positions in which you have inferior leverage (and inferior strength), the machine creates a mechanical advantage and offers less resistance. The end result is greater muscular effort throughout the range of motion (ROM).

During a typical free-weight exercise, there's adequate resistance for your muscles in their weakest positions but not enough in their strongest positions. Because of this, the amount of resistance that you can use is limited to that which you can handle in your position of least leverage. There are, however, a few free-weight exercises that provide somewhat adequate resistance throughout most of the ROM including wrist flexion/extension, shoulder shrug and calf raise.

3. Most machines don't require you to balance the weight.

Not having to balance the weight means that it will be easier for you to concentrate on the proper performance of the exercise. Some individuals – particularly those who have very little experience in strength training – might worry more about balancing the weight effectively than about performing the exercise properly. Furthermore, you're likely to spend excessive energy in balancing the weight. Because synergistic muscles aren't involved when the weight is balanced, machines can also work the targeted muscles to a greater degree.

4. Workouts are usually more time-efficient when machines are employed.

Some individuals don't have an abundance of free time to spend in the fitness center. The resistance on selectorized machines can be set by moving a pin to select a weight rather than by fiddling around changing plates. Of course, plates must be changed when using plate-loaded machines.

5. In general, machines can provide direct resistance over a greater ROM compared to a similar free-weight exercise.

For example, a machine pullover can offer direct resistance over as much as 270 degrees

ROM around your shoulder joint. In contrast, a barbell or dumbbell pullover can offer direct resistance over about 100 degrees ROM around your shoulder joint. Therefore, a pullover done with a machine is much more efficient than a pullover done with free weights because the targeted muscles are loaded over a greater ROM. This holds true for just about all machine exercises compared to their free-weight counterparts.

6. Machines are more practical than free weights during rehabilitative training.

Suppose that you injured your left knee. Many exercises with free weights would be quite difficult or uncomfortable – if not impossible – to perform. However, you could still train your entire torso, your right leg and possibly even both hips if you have access to machines. Actually, you could exercise on most machines with very little discomfort even if your arm or leg was immobilized in a cast. For instance, if your wrist was casted such that you were unable to grasp a barbell or dumbbell, you could still perform many upper-body exercises with machines, including the pec fly, pullover and lateral raise.

7. Machines allow you to train alone in a relatively safe manner.

Any barbell exercise that involves lifting a weight overhead – such as a bench press, incline press or shoulder press – should only be done under the watchful eye of a competent spotter. Doing so reduces the potential for an unexpected mishap such as getting trapped under a weighted bar. With machines, you can't get pinned by a weight in a precarious position. It should be noted that with dumbbells, you can't "get stuck" either since you can simply lower the weights to the floor.

THE EXERCISES

This chapter describes and illustrates the safest and most productive exercises that can be performed with machines. (Generic descriptions are given in this chapter that can be applied to equipment from different manufacturers.) Included in the discussions of each exercise are the muscle(s) involved (if two or more muscles are involved, the first one listed is the prime mover), suggested repetitions (the time that the targeted muscles should be loaded is shown in parentheses), start/finish position, performance description and training tips for making the exercise safer and more productive.

These 36 exercises are described in this chapter: leg press, hip extension, hip flexion, hip abduction, hip adduction, prone leg curl, seated leg curl, leg extension, seated calf raise, calf extension, dorsi flexion, chest press, seated dip, pec fly, seated row, underhand lat pulldown, overhand lat pulldown, pullover, shoulder press, lateral raise, rear deltoid, internal rotation, external rotation, upright row, scapulae adduction, bicep curl, tricep extension, wrist flexion, wrist extension, abdominal crunch, side bend, torso rotation, back extension, neck flexion, neck extension and neck lateral flexion.

LEG PRESS

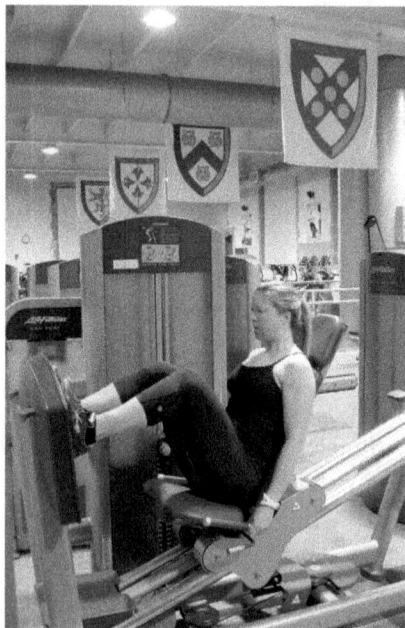

Start/Finish Position

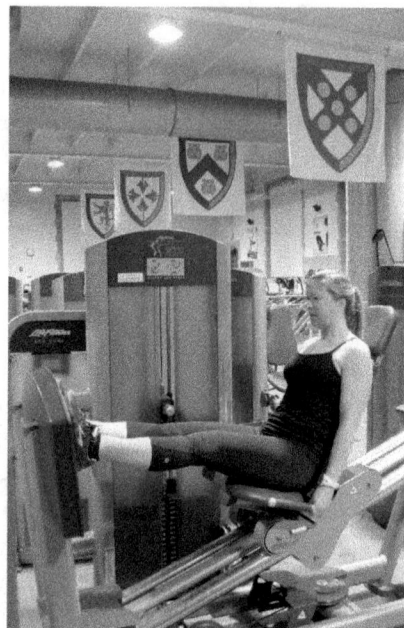

Mid-Range Position

Muscles Strengthened: gluteus maximus, hamstrings and quadriceps

Suggested Repetitions: 15 to 20 (or 90 to 120 seconds)

Start/Finish Position: Adjust the seat carriage so that the angle between your upper and lower legs will be about 90 degrees. Sit down and place your feet on the footplate so that they're slightly wider than shoulder-width apart. Position your lower legs so that they're parallel to the floor. Grasp the handles that are located on the sides of the seat pad.

Performance Description: Push the footplate forward until your legs are almost completely straight (without "locking" your knees). Pause briefly in this mid-range position (your legs almost completely straight) and then lower the weight under control to the start/finish position (your legs bent).

Training Tips:

• The angle of the back pad can be adjusted on some machines. As the back pad is positioned less upright, there's more emphasis on the gluteus maximus (your buttocks). Also note that when the back pad is less upright, the seat must be moved closer to the footplate to maintain the same range of motion as when the back pad is more upright.

• Exert force through your heels, not the balls of your feet.

• Avoid "locking" or "snapping" your knees in the mid-range position.

• You can also perform this exercise with a plate-loaded machine.

• Do this exercise with one limb at a time if you have a hip, leg, knee or ankle injury, a gross difference in the strength between your limbs or desire a training variation.

HIP EXTENSION

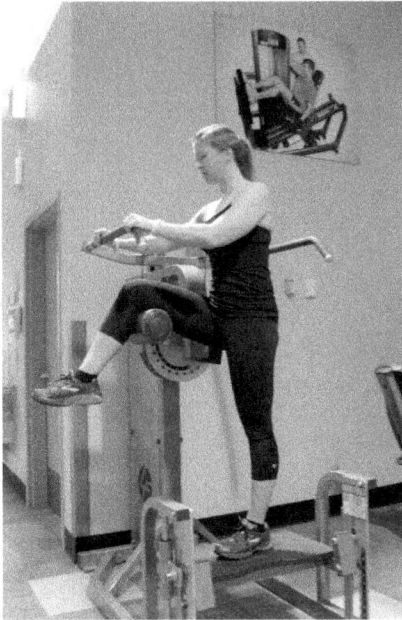

Start/Finish Position

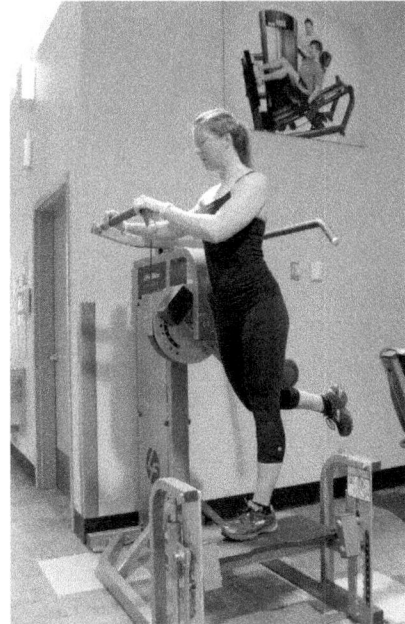

Mid-Range Position

Muscles Strengthened: gluteus maximus and hamstrings

Suggested Repetitions: 15 to 20 (or 90 to 120 seconds)

Start/Finish Position: Adjust the platform so that your hip will be aligned with the axis of rotation. Adjust the movement arm to accommodate your level of flexibility. Place your right upper leg on top of the roller pad. Keep your torso erect and straighten your left leg. Grasp the bar with both hands.

Performance Description: Drive your leg backward while gradually straightening it. Pause briefly in this mid-range position (your leg completely straight) and then lower the weight under control to the start/finish position (your leg bent). Repeat the exercise for the other side of your body.

Training Tips:

- Avoid moving your torso forward and backward. Movement should only occur at your hip and knee joints.

- Attempt to raise the weight as high as possible in the mid-range position to ensure that you're obtaining a maximum contraction of the target muscles.

HIP FLEXION

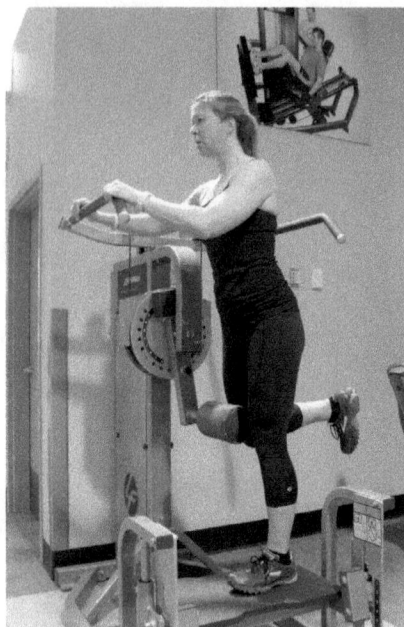

Start/Finish Position

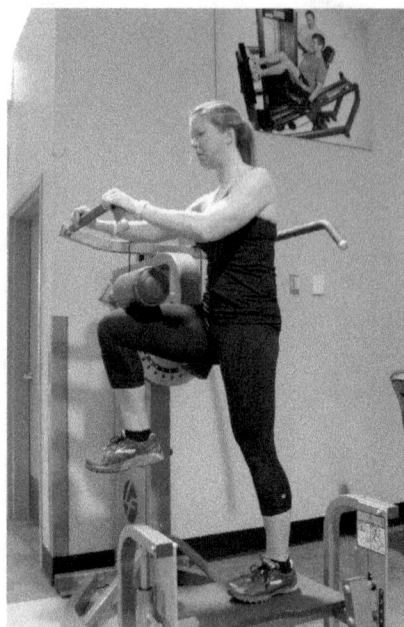

Mid-Range Position

Muscle Strengthened: iliopsoas

Suggested Repetitions: 15 to 20 (or 90 to 120 seconds)

Start/Finish Position: Adjust the platform so that your hip will be aligned with the axis of rotation. Adjust the movement arm to accommodate your level of flexibility. Place your right upper leg behind the roller pad. Keep your torso erect and straighten your left leg. Grasp the bar with both hands.

Performance Description: Bring your knee toward your chest while gradually bending your leg. Pause briefly in this mid-range position (your knee near your chest) and then lower the weight under control to the start/ finish position (your leg hanging down). Repeat the exercise for the other side of your body.

Training Tips:

- Avoid moving your torso forward and backward. Movement should only occur at your hip and knee joints.

- Attempt to raise the weight as high as possible in the mid-range position to ensure that you're obtaining a maximum contraction of the target muscles.

HIP ABDUCTION

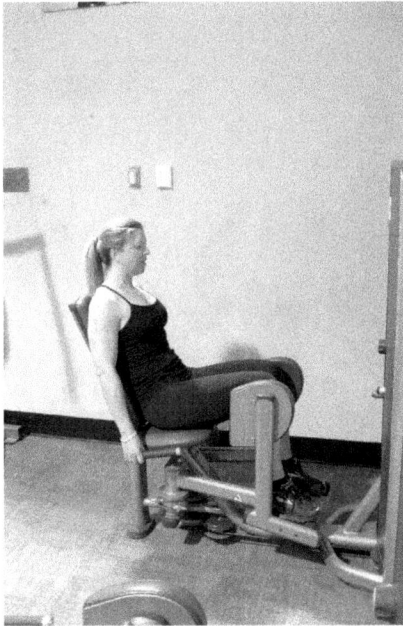

Start/Finish Position

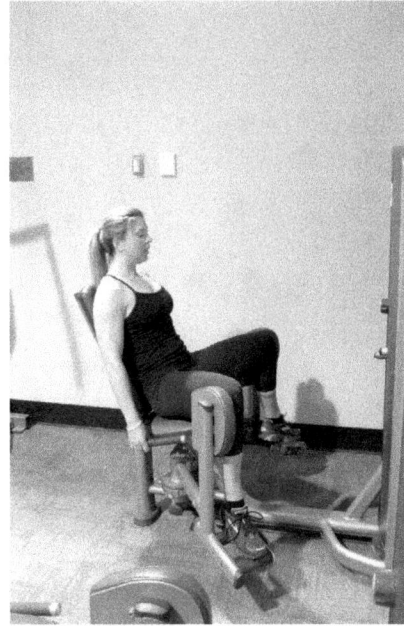

Mid-Range Position

Muscles Strengthened: gluteus medius and gluteus minimus

Suggested Repetitions: 10 to 15 (or 60 to 90 seconds)

Start/Finish Position: Sit down, place your legs on the thigh pads and position your feet on the foot pegs. Grasp the handles that are located on the sides of the seat pad.

Performance Description: Spread your legs apart as far as possible. Pause briefly in this mid-range position (your legs apart) and then lower the weight under control to the start/finish position (your legs together).

Training Tips:

- The angle of the back pad can be adjusted on some machines. In this case, adjust the back pad so that it's as upright as possible.

- Attempt to raise the weight as high as possible in the mid-range position to ensure that you're obtaining a maximum contraction of the target muscles.

- You can also perform this exercise with a plate-loaded machine.

HIP ADDUCTION

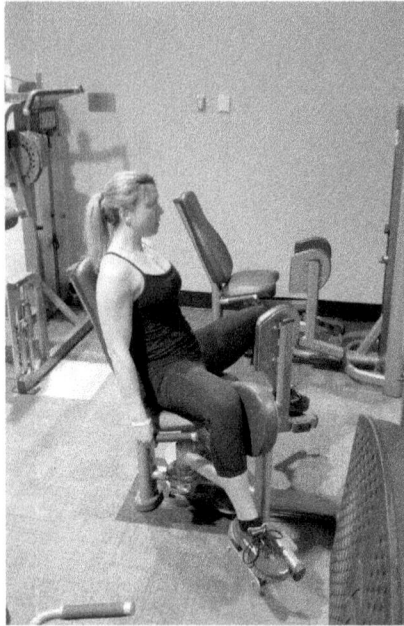

Start/Finish Position

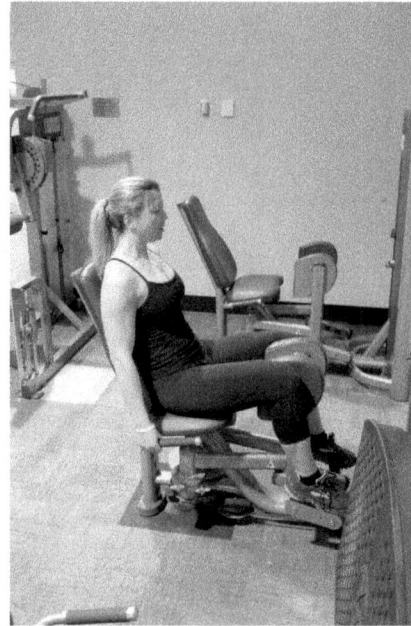

Mid-Range Position

Muscles Strengthened: hip adductors

Suggested Repetitions: 10 to 15 (or 60 to 90 seconds)

Start/Finish Position: Adjust the movement arms to accommodate your level of flexibility. Sit down, place your legs on the thigh pads and position your feet on the foot pegs. Grasp the handles that are located on the sides of the seat pad.

Performance Description: Bring your legs as close together as possible. Pause briefly in this mid-range position (your legs together) and then lower the weight under control to the start/finish position (your legs apart).

Training Tips:

- The angle of the back pad can be adjusted on some machines. In this case, adjust the back pad so that it's as upright as possible.

- Attempt to raise the weight as high as possible in the mid-range position to ensure that you're obtaining a maximum contraction of the target muscles.

- You can also perform this exercise with a plate-loaded machine.

PRONE LEG CURL

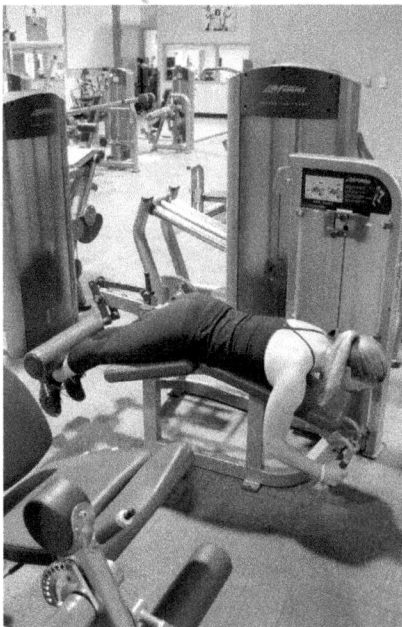

Start/Finish Position

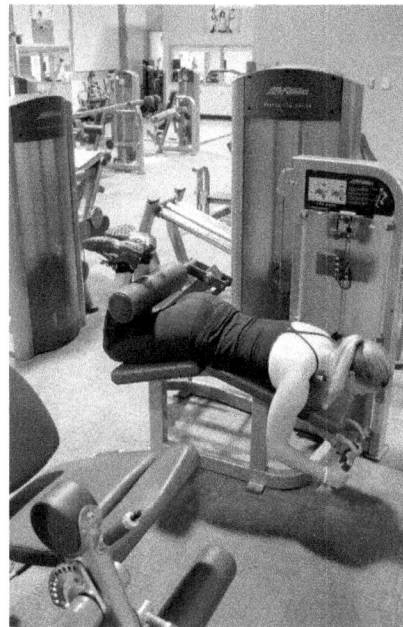

Mid-Range Position

Muscles Strengthened: hamstrings

Suggested Repetitions: 10 to 15 (or 60 to 90 seconds)

Start/Finish Position: Adjust the roller pad so that it will be just above your heels. Adjust the movement arm to accommodate your level of flexibility. Lie face down and place your lower legs underneath the roller pad. Position the tops of your kneecaps just over the edge of the thigh pad. (By doing this, your knees will be aligned with the axis of rotation.) Grasp the handles that are located in front of the chest pad.

Performance Description: Pull your heels as close to your hips as possible. Pause briefly in this mid-range position (your heels near your hips) and then lower the weight under control to the start/finish position (your legs completely straight).

Training Tips:

- Avoid raising your torso. Movement should only occur at your knee joints.
- The angle between your upper and lower legs should be about 90 degrees or less in the mid-range position.
- Attempt to raise the weight as high as possible in the mid-range position to ensure that you're obtaining a maximum contraction of the target muscles.
- You can also perform this exercise with a plate-loaded machine.
- Do this exercise with one limb at a time if you have a leg, knee or ankle injury, a gross difference in the strength between your limbs or desire a training variation.
- This exercise may be contraindicated if you have hyperextended knees or low-back pain.

SEATED LEG CURL

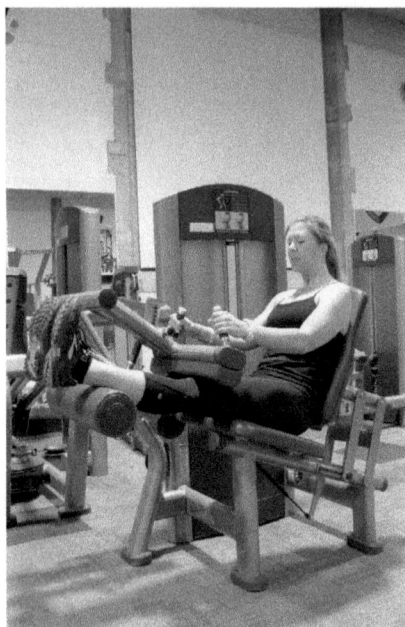

Start/Finish Position

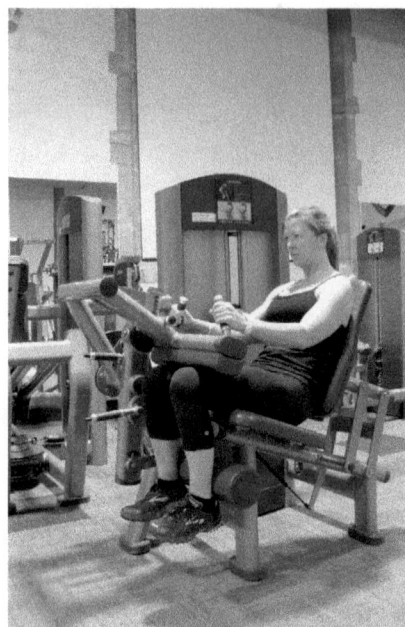

Mid-Range Position

Muscles Strengthened: hamstrings

Suggested Repetitions: 10 to 15 (or 60 to 90 seconds)

Start/Finish Position: Adjust the back pad so that your knees will be aligned with the axis of rotation. Adjust the roller pad so that that it will be just above your heels. Adjust the movement arm to accommodate your level of flexibility. Sit down and place your lower legs on top of the roller pad. Lower the thigh pad so that it presses against your upper legs. Grasp the handles that are located above the thigh pad (or on the sides of the seat pad).

Performance Description: Pull your heels as close to your hips as possible. Pause briefly in this mid-range position (your heels near your hips) and then lower the weight under control to the start/finish position (your legs completely straight). Raise the thigh pad when you finish performing the exercise.

Training Tips:

• Performing this exercise in the seated position produces less stress in the low-back region than performing it in the prone position.

• Avoid moving your torso forward and backward. Movement should only occur at your knee joints.

• The angle between your upper and lower legs should be about 90 degrees or less in the mid-range position.

• Attempt to raise the weight as high as possible in the mid-range position to ensure that you're obtaining a maximum contraction of the target muscles.

• You can also perform this exercise with a plate-loaded machine.

• Do this exercise with one limb at a time if you have a leg, knee or ankle injury, a gross difference in the strength between your limbs or desire a training variation.

• This exercise may be contraindicated if you have hyperextended knees.

LEG EXTENSION

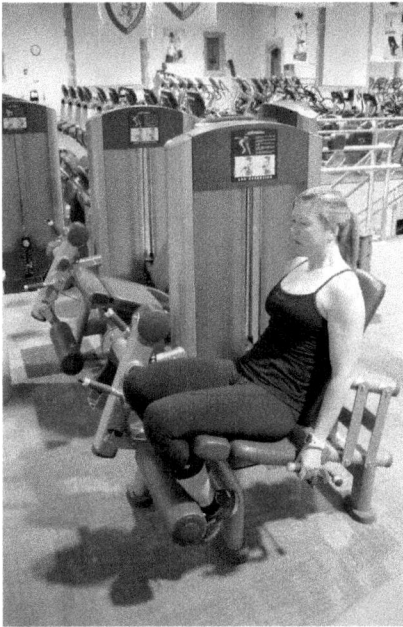

Start/Finish Position

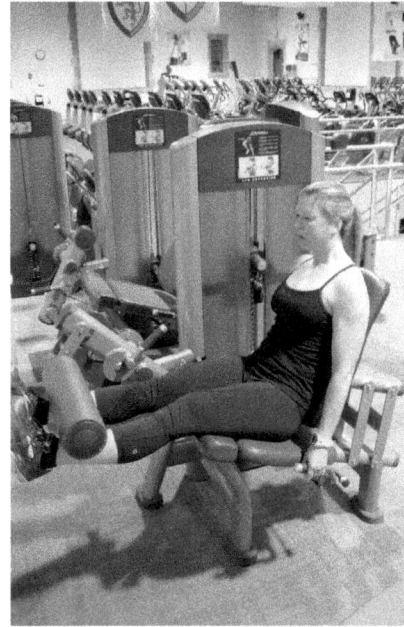

Mid-Range Position

Muscles Strengthened: quadriceps

Suggested Repetitions: 10 to 15 (or 60 to 90 seconds)

Start/Finish Position: Adjust the back pad so that your knees will be aligned with the axis of rotation. Adjust the roller pad so that it will be just above your instep. Adjust the movement arm to accommodate your level of flexibility. Sit down and place your lower legs behind the roller pad. Fasten the waist belt (if one is provided). Grasp the handles that are located on the sides of the seat pad.

Performance Description: Straighten your legs as completely as possible. Pause briefly in this mid-range position (your legs completely straight) and then lower the weight under control to the start/finish position (your legs bent).

Training Tips:

- Avoid moving your torso forward and backward. Movement should only occur at your knee joints.
- Attempt to raise the weight as high as possible in the mid-range position to ensure that you're obtaining a maximum contraction of the target muscles.
- You can also perform this exercise with a plate-loaded machine.
- Do this exercise with one limb at a time if you have a leg, knee or ankle injury, a gross difference in the strength between your limbs or desire a training variation.

131

SEATED CALF RAISE

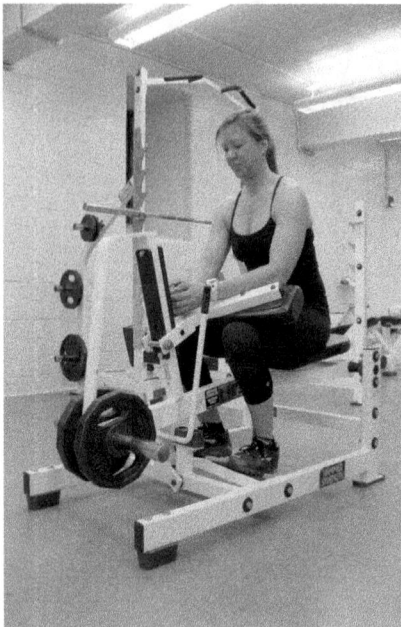

Start/Finish Position

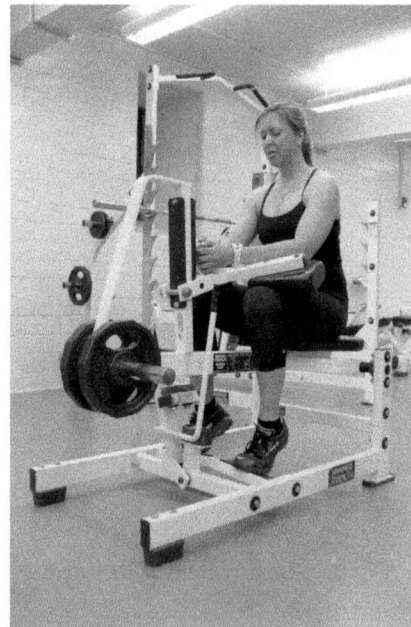

Mid-Range Position

Muscle Strengthened: soleus

Suggested Repetitions: 10 to 15 (or 60 to 90 seconds)

Start/Finish Position: Sit down, place the balls of your feet on the edge of the footplate and lower your heels. Lower the thigh pads so that they press against your upper legs. Rise up onto your toes slightly and push the lever arm to the left. (This frees the movement arm so that you have a full range of motion.) Grasp the handle (or hold onto the sides of the seat pad) and lower your heels.

Performance Description: Rise up onto your toes as high as possible. Pause briefly in this mid-range position (your ankles straight) and then lower the weight under control to the start/finish position (your heels near the floor). Rise up onto your toes slightly and push the lever arm to the right when you finish performing the exercise. (This holds the movement arm in place so that you can exit the machine.)

Training Tips:

- Avoid using your arms and moving your torso forward and backward. Movement should only occur at your ankle joints.

- Attempt to raise the weight as high as possible in the mid-range position to ensure that you're obtaining a maximum contraction of the target muscles.

- Do this exercise with one limb at a time if you have a leg, knee or ankle injury, a gross difference in the strength between your limbs or desire a training variation.

- Avoid this exercise if you have shin splints.

CALF EXTENSION

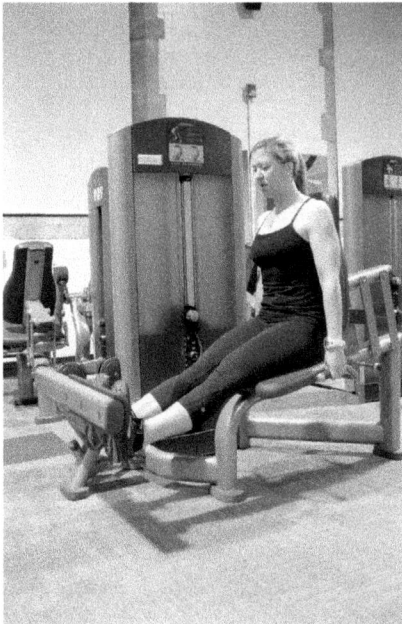

Start/Finish Position

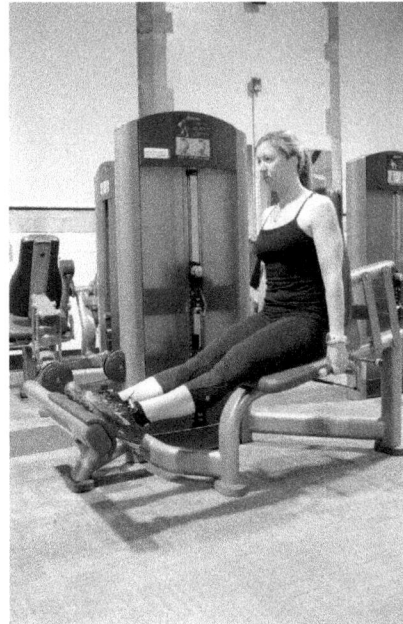

Mid-Range Position

Muscle Strengthened: gastrocnemius

Suggested Repetitions: 10 to 15 (or 60 to 90 seconds)

Start/Finish Position: Adjust the back pad to accommodate the length of your legs. Sit down, place the balls of your feet on the edge of the footplate and lower your heels. Straighten your legs but don't "lock" your knees. Grasp the handles that are located on the sides of the seat pad.

Performance Description: Extend your ankles as far as possible. Pause briefly in this mid-range position (your ankles straight) and then lower the weight under control to the start/finish position (your ankles bent).

Training Tips:

• Avoid using your hips and legs. Movement should only occur at your ankle joints.

• Attempt to raise the weight as high as possible in the mid-range position to ensure that you're obtaining a maximum contraction of the target muscles.

• Do this exercise with one limb at a time if you have a leg, knee or ankle injury, a gross difference in the strength between your limbs or desire a training variation.

• Avoid this exercise if you have shin splints.

DORSI FLEXION

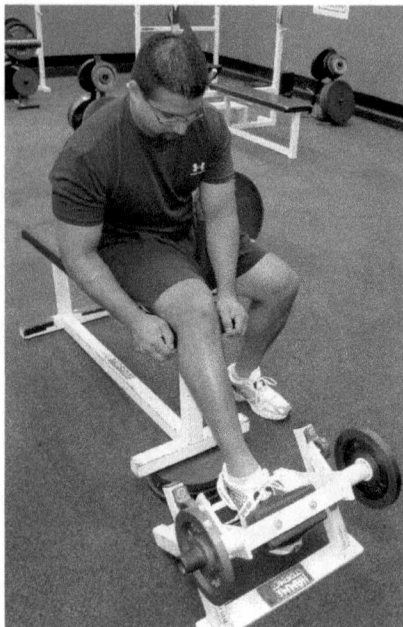

Start/Finish Position

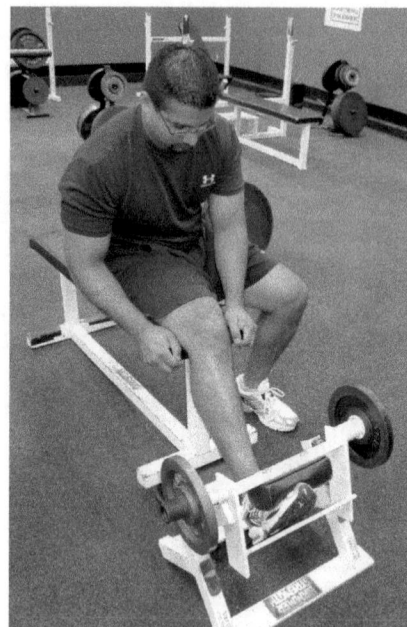

Mid-Range Position

Muscles Strengthened: dorsi flexors

Suggested Repetitions: 10 to 15 (or 60 to 90 seconds)

Start/Finish Position: Sit down near the end of a utility bench (or a stool). Place the back of your right knee against the end of the pad. Position your right foot on the footplate so that the ankle pad is against your instep. Grasp the sides of the bench.

Performance Description: Keeping your leg flat on the bench, pull your right foot up as high as possible. Pause briefly in this mid-range position (your ankle bent) and then lower the weight under control to the start/ finish position (your ankle straight). Repeat the exercise for the other side of your body.

Training Tips:

• Avoid moving your torso forward and backward. Movement should only occur at your ankle joint.

• Attempt to raise the weight as high as possible in the mid-range position to ensure that you're obtaining a maximum contraction of the target muscles.

• This exercise may be contraindicated if you have shin splints.

CHEST PRESS

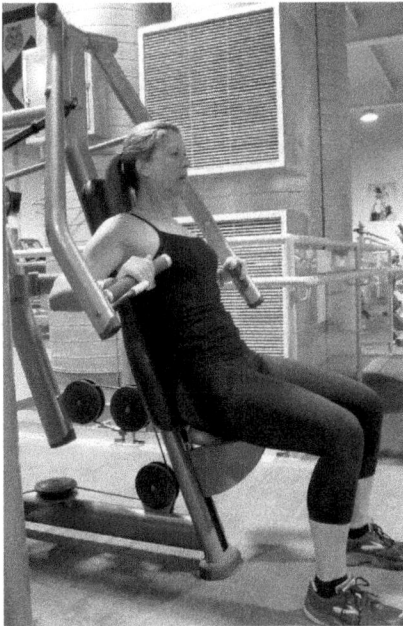

Start/Finish Position

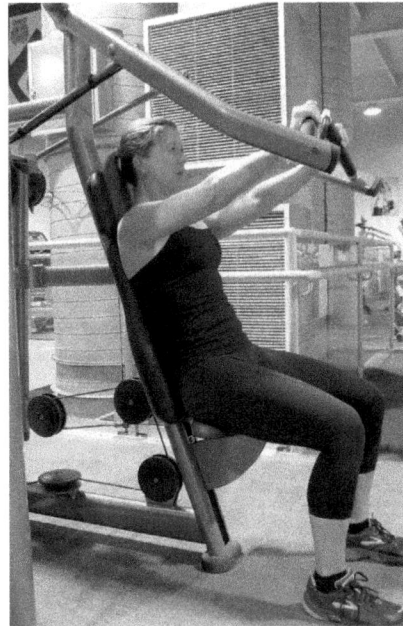

Mid-Range Position

Muscles Strengthened: chest, anterior deltoid and triceps

Suggested Repetitions: 5 to 10 (or 30 to 60 seconds)

Start/Finish Position: Adjust the seat pad so that your hands will be just below your shoulders in the start/finish position. Adjust the movement arms to accommodate your level of flexibility. Sit down and place your feet flat on the floor. Grasp the handles with a narrow grip.

Performance Description: Push the handles forward until your arms are almost completely straight (without "locking" your elbows). Pause briefly in this mid-range position (your arms almost completely straight) and then lower the weight under control to the start/finish position (your hands near your shoulders).

Training Tips:

- The back pad can be adjusted on some machines. Moving it forward increases the range of motion and allows a greater stretch.

- Multiple grips are available on some machines. A parallel grip reduces the stress in your shoulder joints.

- Keep your hips on the seat pad and your torso against the back pad. Movement should only occur at your shoulder and elbow joints.

- Avoid "locking" or "snapping" your elbows in the mid-range position.

- You can also perform this exercise with a plate-loaded machine.

- Do this exercise with one limb at a time if you have a shoulder or an arm injury, a gross difference in the strength between your limbs or desire a training variation.

- This exercise may be contraindicated if you have shoulder-impingement syndrome.

SEATED DIP

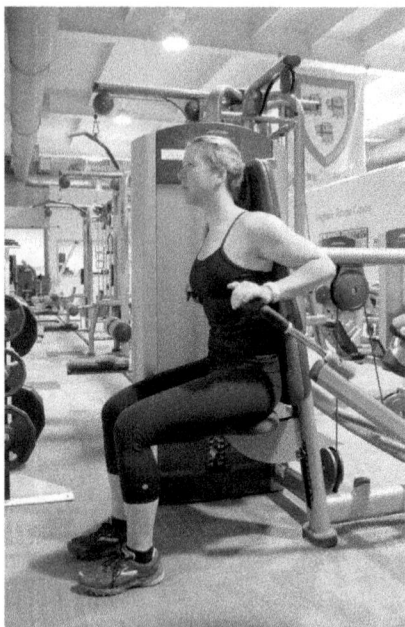

Start/Finish Position

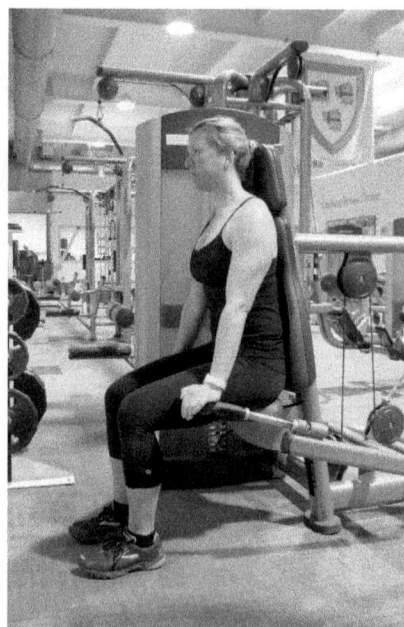

Mid-Range Position

Muscles Strengthened: chest (lower portion), anterior deltoid and triceps

Suggested Repetitions: 5 to 10 (or 30 to 60 seconds)

Start/Finish Position: Adjust the seat pad so that your hands will be just below your shoulders in the start/ finish position. Adjust the movement arms to accommodate the width of your shoulders. Sit down and place your feet flat on the floor. Grasp the handles.

Performance Description: Push the handles down until your arms are almost completely straight (without "locking" your elbows). Pause briefly in this mid-range position (your arms almost completely straight) and then lower the weight under control to the start/finish position (your arms bent).

Training Tips:

- Keep your hips on the seat pad and your torso against the back pad. Movement should only occur at your shoulder and elbow joints.

- Avoid "locking" or "snapping" your elbows in the mid-range position.

- You can also perform this exercise with a plate-loaded machine.

- Do this exercise with one limb at a time if you have a shoulder or an arm injury, a gross difference in the strength between your limbs or desire a training variation.

- This exercise may be contraindicated if you have shoulder-impingement syndrome.

PEC FLY

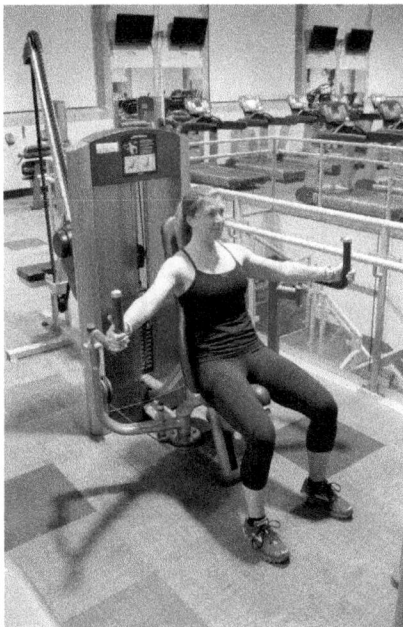

Start/Finish Position

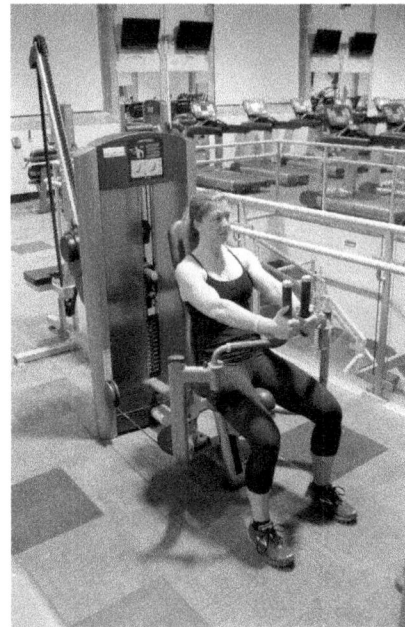

Mid-Range Position

Muscles Strengthened: chest and anterior deltoid

Suggested Repetitions: 5 to 10 (or 30 to 60 seconds)

Start/Finish Position: Adjust the seat pad so that your elbows will be slightly lower than your shoulders in the start/finish position. Adjust the movement arms to accommodate your level of flexibility. Sit down and place your feet flat on the floor. Grasp the handles with a parallel grip (your palms facing each other).

Performance Description: Keeping your arms fairly straight, bring the handles as close together as possible. Pause briefly in this mid-range position (your hands together) and then lower the weight under control to the start/finish position (your hands apart).

Training Tips:

- This exercise is also referred to as a chest fly.

- Keep your hips on the seat pad and your torso against the back pad. Movement should only occur at your shoulder joints.

- You can also perform this exercise with a plate-loaded machine.

- Do this exercise with one limb at a time if you have a shoulder or an arm injury, a gross difference in the strength between your limbs or desire a training variation.

- This exercise may be contraindicated if you have shoulder-impingement syndrome.

SEATED ROW

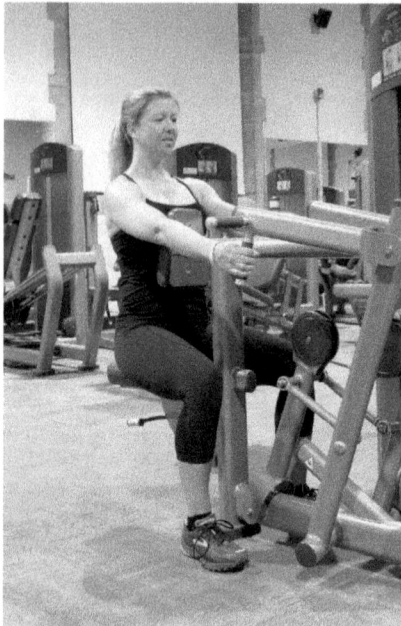

Start/Finish Position

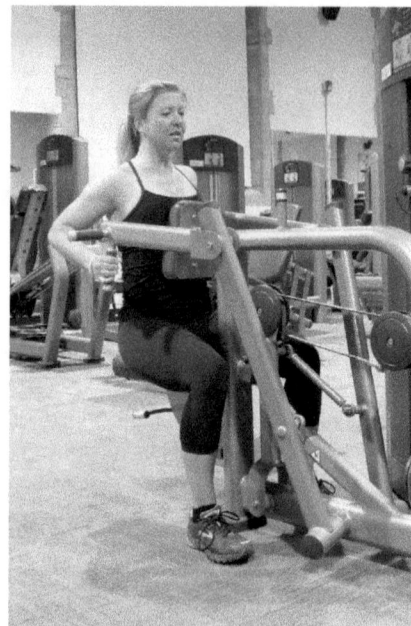

Mid-Range Position

Muscles Strengthened: upper back, biceps and forearms

Suggested Repetitions: 5 to 10 (or 30 to 60 seconds)

Start/Finish Position: Adjust the chest pad so that your arms will be completely straight in the start/finish position. Adjust the seat pad so that your hands will be just below your shoulders in the mid-range position. Sit down, lean forward against the chest pad and place your feet flat on the floor (or on the footplate if one is provided). Grasp the handles with a parallel grip (your palms facing each other).

Performance Description: Pull the handles just below your shoulders. Pause briefly in this mid-range position (your arms bent) and then lower the weight under control to the start/finish position (your arms completely straight).

Training Tips:

- You can also perform this exercise with your upper arms positioned away from your torso using an overhand grip. Doing this involves less of your upper back and more of your posterior deltoid, trapezius and rhomboids. In this case, your upper arm would be perpendicular to your torso and your palms would be facing down in the mid-range position.

- Avoid moving your torso forward and backward. Movement should only occur at your shoulder and elbow joints.

- Attempt to raise the weight as high as possible in the mid-range position to ensure that you're obtaining a maximum contraction of the target muscles.

- You can also perform this exercise with a plate-loaded machine.

- Do this exercise with one limb at a time if you have a shoulder or an arm injury, a gross difference in the strength between your limbs or desire a training variation.

- Use wrist straps if you have difficulty in maintaining your grip on the handles.

- This exercise may be contraindicated if you have hyperextended elbows.

UNDERHAND LAT PULLDOWN

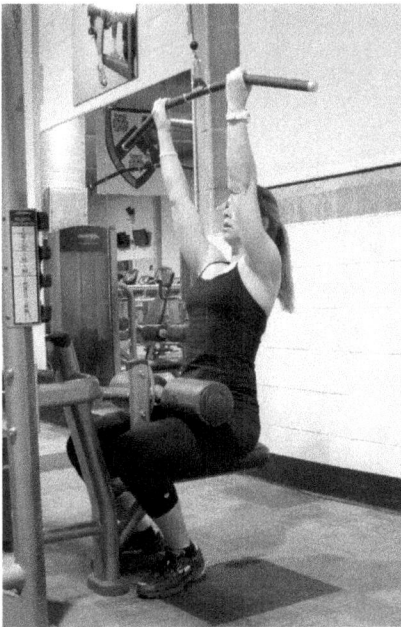

Start/Finish Position

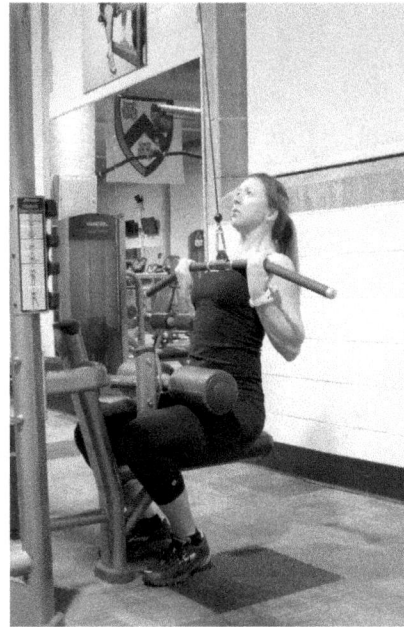

Mid-Range Position

Muscles Strengthened: upper back, biceps and forearms

Suggested Repetitions: 5 to 10 (or 30 to 60 seconds)

Start/Finish Position: Reach up, grasp a bar with your palms facing toward you and spread your hands approximately shoulder-width apart. Sit down, position your upper legs under the roller pads and place your feet flat on the floor. Lean back slightly.

Performance Description: Pull the bar down to your upper chest and draw your elbows backward. Pause briefly in this mid-range position (your arms bent) and then lower the weight under control to the start/finish position (your arms completely straight).

Training Tips:

- Avoid moving your torso forward and backward. Movement should only occur at your shoulder and elbow joints.

- Attempt to raise the weight as high as possible in the mid-range position to ensure that you're obtaining a maximum contraction of the target muscles.

- You can also perform this exercise with a plate-loaded machine.

- Do this exercise with one limb at a time (with a handle instead of a bar) if you have a shoulder or an arm injury, a gross difference in the strength between your limbs or desire a training variation.

- Use wrist straps if you have difficulty in maintaining your grip on the bar.

- This exercise may be contraindicated if you have hyperextended elbows.

OVERHAND LAT PULLDOWN

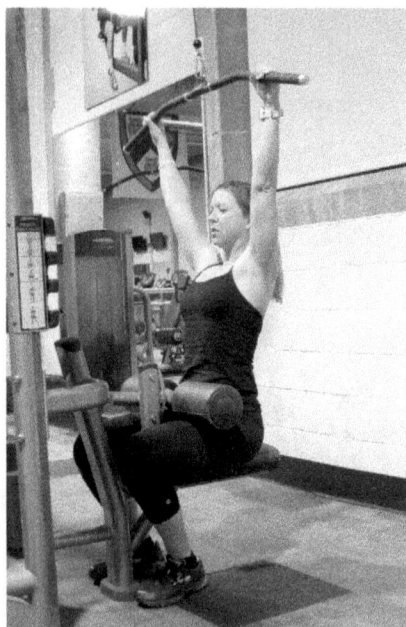

Start/Finish Position

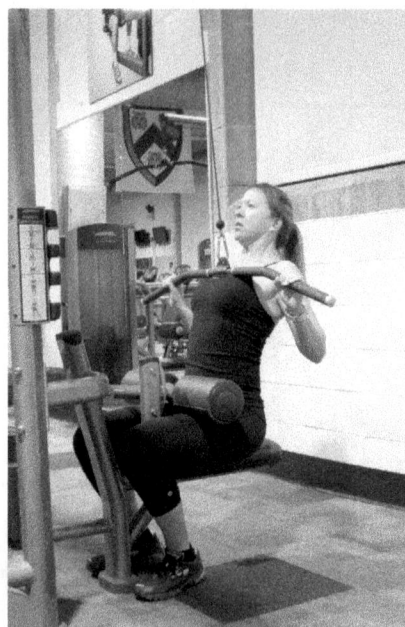

Mid-Range Position

Muscles Strengthened: upper back, biceps and forearms

Suggested Repetitions: 5 to 10 (or 30 to 60 seconds)

Start/Finish Position: Reach up, grasp a bar with your palms facing away from you and space your hands several inches wider than shoulder-width apart. Sit down, position your upper legs under the roller pads and place your feet flat on the floor. Lean back slightly.

Performance Description: Pull the bar down to your upper chest and draw your elbows backward. Pause briefly in this mid-range position (your arms bent) and then lower the weight under control to the start/finish position (your arms completely straight).

Training Tips:

- Avoid moving your torso forward and backward. Movement should only occur at your shoulder and elbow joints.

- Avoid using an excessively wide grip. This reduces your range of motion.

- Attempt to raise the weight as high as possible in the mid-range position to ensure that you're obtaining a maximum contraction of the target muscles.

- You can also perform this exercise with a plate-loaded machine.

- Do this exercise with one limb at a time (with a handle instead of a bar) if you have a shoulder or an arm injury, a gross difference in the strength between your limbs or desire a training variation.

- Performing a lat pulldown with an overhand grip (your palms facing away from you) isn't as biomechanically efficient as performing a lat pulldown with an underhand grip (your palms facing toward you). But this exercise is still quite productive when done with an overhand grip.

- Use wrist straps if you have difficulty in maintaining your grip on the bar.

- You can also perform this exercise with the bar positioned behind your head/neck. However, this may be contraindicated if you have shoulder-impingement syndrome. This exercise may also be contraindicated if you have hyperextended elbows.

PULLOVER

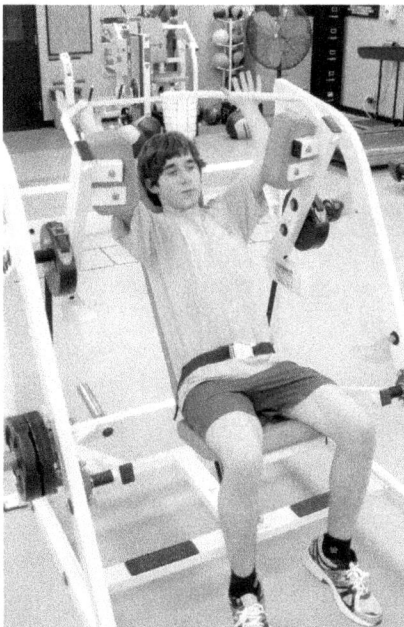

Start/Finish Position

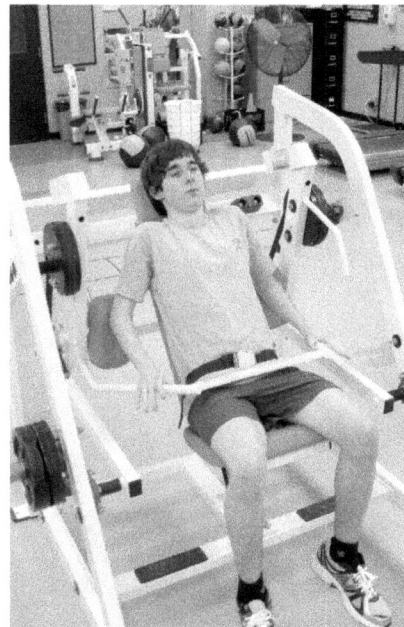

Mid-Range Position

Muscle Strengthened: upper back

Suggested Repetitions: 5 to 10 (or 30 to 60 seconds)

Start/Finish Position: Adjust the seat pad so that the side part of your shoulders will be aligned with the axis of rotation in the start/finish position. Sit down and place your feet flat on the floor. Fasten the waist belt (if one is provided). Position the back of your upper arms on the elbow pads. Place your palms on the bar and open your hands (extend your fingers).

Performance Description: Pull the bar down to your mid-section. Pause briefly in this mid-range position (the bar against your mid-section) and then lower the weight under control to the start/finish position (your elbows near or slightly past your head).

Training Tips:

- Avoid moving your torso forward and backward. Movement should only occur at your shoulder joints.

- Exert force against the elbow pads with your upper arms, not your hands. This isolates your upper back.

- If you're unable to keep your upper arms against the elbow pads, you can grasp the bar with an underhand grip and pull with your hands instead of your upper arms. This doesn't allow you to isolate your upper back but it will make the exercise more comfortable for you to perform.

- Attempt to raise the weight as high as possible in the mid-range position to ensure that you're obtaining a maximum contraction of the target muscles.

- You can also perform this exercise with a selectorized machine.

- Do this exercise with one limb at a time if you have a shoulder or an arm injury, a gross difference in the strength between your limbs or desire a training variation.

- This exercise may be contraindicated if you have shoulder-impingement syndrome.

SHOULDER PRESS

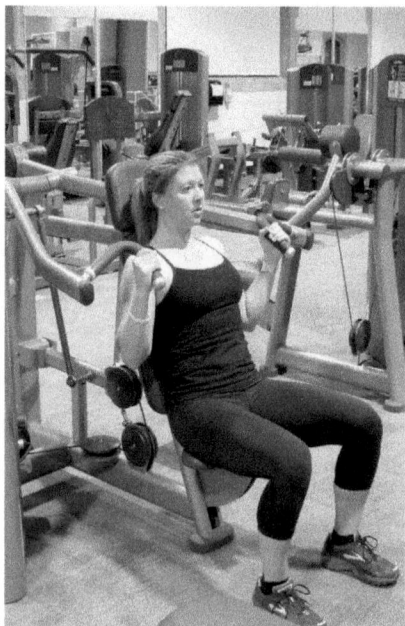

Start/Finish Position

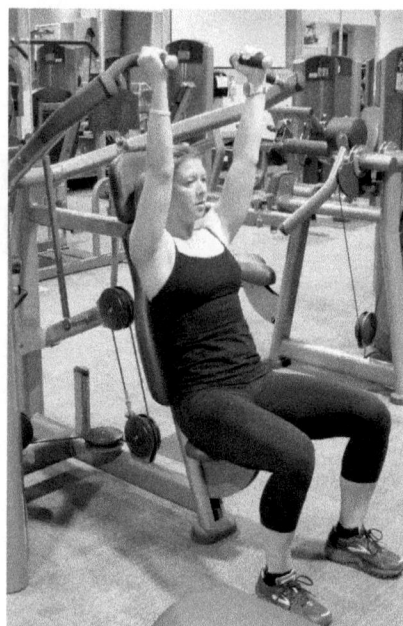

Mid-Range Position

Muscles Strengthened: anterior deltoid and triceps

Suggested Repetitions: 5 to 10 (or 30 to 60 seconds)

Start/Finish Position: Adjust the seat pad so that your hands will be near your shoulders in the start/finish position. Sit down and place your feet flat on the floor. Reach up and grasp the handles with a parallel grip (your palms facing each other).

Performance Description: Push the handles up until your arms are almost completely straight (without "locking" your elbows). Pause briefly in this mid-range position (your arms almost completely straight) and then lower the weight under control to the start/finish position (your arms bent).

Training Tips:

- This exercise is also referred to as an overhead press, a seated press and a military press.
- Multiple grips are available on some machines. A parallel grip reduces the stress in your shoulder joints.
- Keep your hips on the seat pad and your feet flat on the floor.
- Avoid "locking" or "snapping" your elbows in the mid-range position.
- You can also perform this exercise with a plate-loaded machine.
- Do this exercise with one limb at a time if you have a shoulder or an arm injury, a gross difference in the strength between your limbs or desire a training variation.
- This exercise may be contraindicated if you have shoulder-impingement syndrome or low-back pain.

LATERAL RAISE

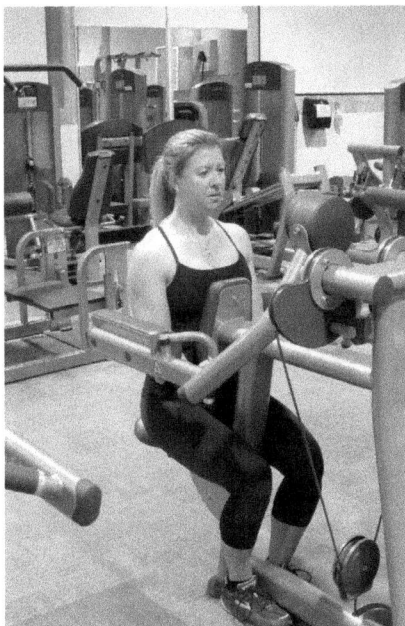

Start/Finish Position

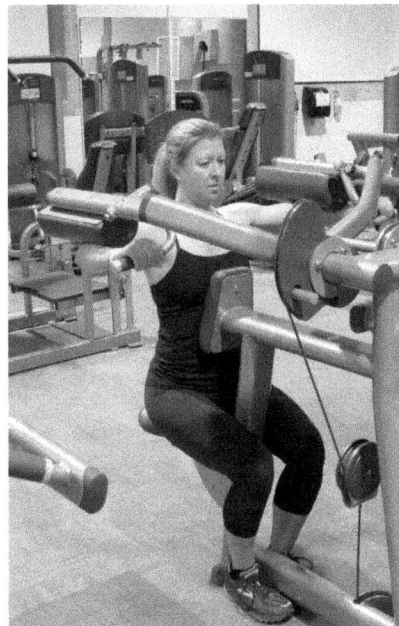

Mid-Range Position

Muscles Strengthened: middle deltoid and trapezius (upper and lower portions)

Suggested Repetitions: 5 to 10 (or 30 to 60 seconds)

Start/Finish Position: Adjust the seat pad so that the front part of your shoulders will be aligned with the axis of rotation in the start/finish position. Sit down and place your feet flat on the floor. Position your upper arms against the forearm pads. Grasp the handles with a parallel grip (your palms facing each other).

Performance Description: Raise your arms sideways until they're parallel to the floor. Pause briefly in this mid-range position (your arms parallel to the floor) and then lower the weight under control to the start/finish position (your arms at your sides).

Training Tips:

• Keep your hips on the seat pad and your feet flat on the floor. Movement should only occur at your shoulder joints.

• Raise your arms only to the point where they're parallel to the floor.

• Your palms should be facing the floor in the mid-range position.

• You can also perform this exercise with a plate-loaded machine.

• Do this exercise with one limb at a time if you have a shoulder or an arm injury, a gross difference in the strength between your limbs or desire a training variation.

REAR DELTOID

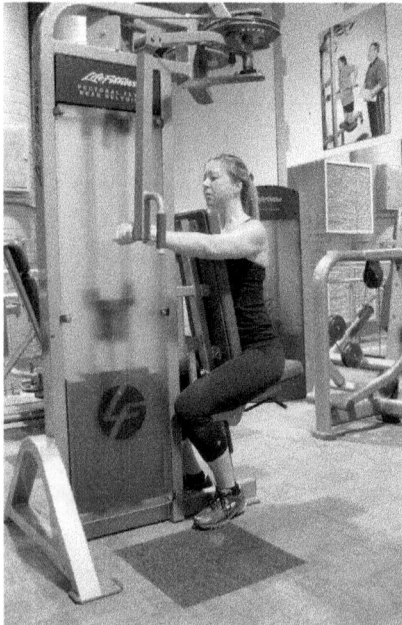

Start/Finish Position

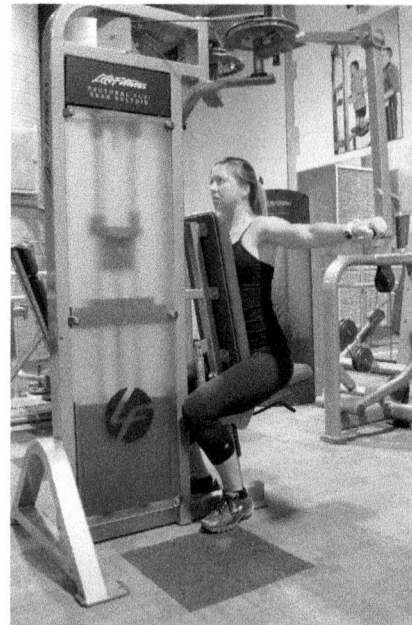

Mid-Range Position

Muscles Strengthened: posterior deltoid, trapezius (middle and lower portions) and rhomboids

Suggested Repetitions: 5 to 10 (or 30 to 60 seconds)

Start/Finish Position: Adjust the seat pad so that your elbows will be slightly lower than your shoulders in the start/finish position. Adjust the movement arms to accommodate your level of flexibility. Sit down and place your feet flat on the floor. Grasp the handles.

Performance Description: Keeping your arms fairly straight, pull the handles back as far as possible. Pause briefly in this mid-range position (your hands apart) and then lower the weight under control to the start/finish position (your hands together).

Training Tips:

- Avoid moving your torso forward and backward. Movement should only occur at your shoulder joints.

- Attempt to raise the weight as high as possible in the mid-range position to ensure that you're obtaining a maximum contraction of the target muscles.

- You can also perform this exercise with a plate-loaded machine.

- Do this exercise with one limb at a time if you have a shoulder or an arm injury, a gross difference in the strength between your limbs or desire a training variation.

INTERNAL ROTATION

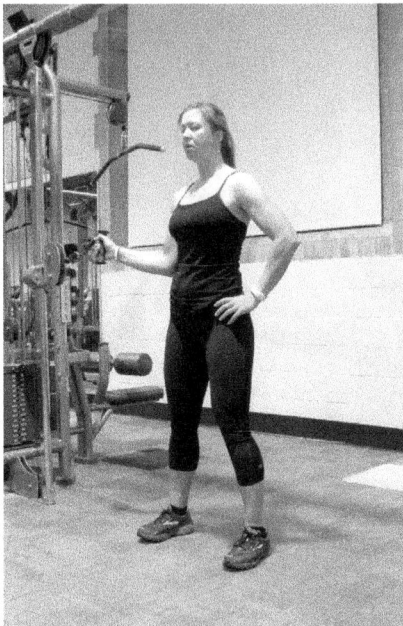

Start/Finish Position

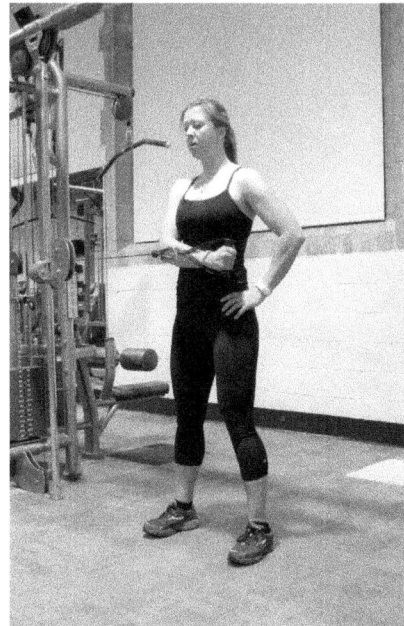

Mid-Range Position

Muscles Strengthened: internal rotators

Suggested Repetitions: 8 to 10 (or 50 to 60 seconds)

Start/Finish Position: Adjust the pulley so that it's even with your right elbow. Grasp a handle with your right hand. Position your body so that your right side faces the pulley. Place your left hand on your left hip and spread your feet about shoulder-width apart. Place your right elbow against the right side of your torso and bend your right arm so that the angle between your upper and lower arms is about 90 degrees. (By doing this, your right lower arm will be parallel to the floor.) Position the handle away from your mid-section.

Performance Description: Keeping the same angle between your upper and lower arms, pull the handle to your mid-section. Pause briefly in this mid-range position (your hand near your mid-section) and then lower the weight under control to the start/finish position (your hand away from your mid-section). Repeat the exercise for the other side of your body.

Training Tips:

- Keep your elbow against the side of your torso and your lower arm parallel to the floor.
- Avoid rotating your torso. Movement should only occur at your shoulder joint.
- You can also perform this exercise with a plate-loaded machine.

145

EXTERNAL ROTATION

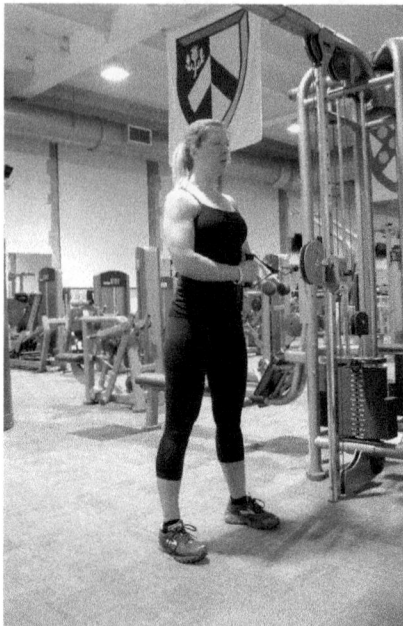

Start/Finish Position

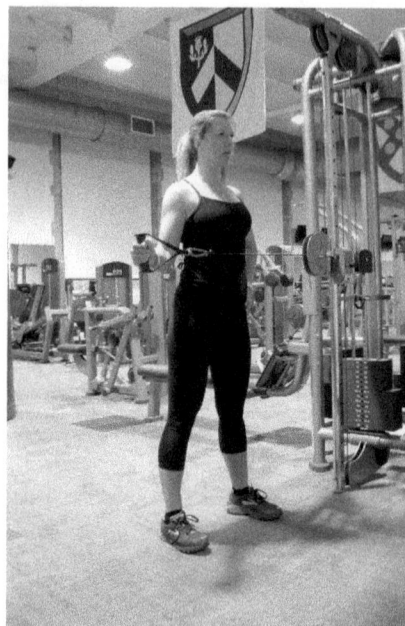

Mid-Range Position

Muscles Strengthened: external rotators

Suggested Repetitions: 8 to 10 (or 50 to 60 seconds)

Start/Finish Position: Adjust the pulley so that it's even with your right elbow. Grasp a handle with your right hand. Position your body so that your left side faces the pulley. Place your left hand on your left hip and spread your feet about shoulder-width apart. Place your right elbow against the right side of your torso and bend your right arm so that the angle between your upper and lower arms is about 90 degrees. (By doing this, your right lower arm will be parallel to the floor.) Position the handle near your mid-section.

Performance Description: Keeping the same angle between your upper and lower arms, pull the handle away from your mid-section. Pause briefly in this mid-range position (your hand away from your mid-section) and then lower the weight under control to the start/finish position (your hand near your mid-section). Repeat the exercise for the other side of your body.

Training Tips:

- Keep your elbow against the side of your torso and your lower arm parallel to the floor.

- Avoid rotating your torso. Movement should only occur at your shoulder joint.

- You can also perform this exercise with a plate-loaded machine.

UPRIGHT ROW

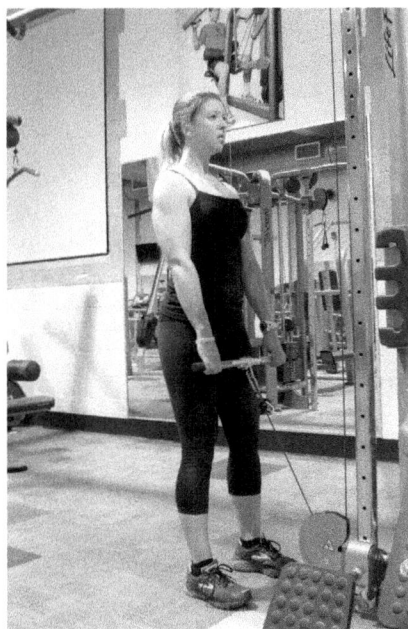

Start/Finish Position

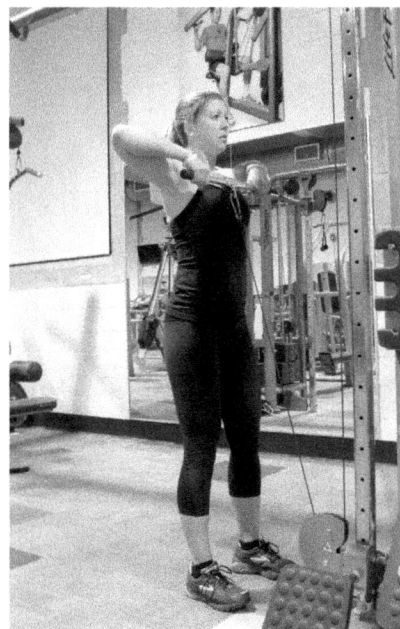

Mid-Range Position

Muscles Strengthened: trapezius (upper and lower portions), biceps and forearms

Suggested Repetitions: 5 to 10 (or 30 to 60 seconds)

Start/Finish Position: Adjust the pulley so that it's near the floor. Grasp a bar with your hands spaced about 8 to 10 inches apart and your palms facing you. Straighten your arms and spread your feet approximately shoulder-width apart.

Performance Description: Pull the bar up until your upper arms are parallel to the floor. (Your elbows should be slightly higher than your hands in this position.) Pause briefly in this mid-range position (your arms bent) and then lower the bar under control to the start/finish position (your arms completely straight).

Training Tips:

- Avoid using your legs and moving your torso forward and backward. Movement should only occur at your shoulder and elbow joints.
- Keep the bar close to your body.
- You can also perform this exercise with a plate-loaded machine.
- Do this exercise with one limb at a time (with a handle instead of a bar) if you have a shoulder or an arm injury, a gross difference in the strength between your limbs or desire a training variation.
- Use wrist straps if you have difficulty in maintaining your grip on the bar.
- This exercise may be contraindicated if you have shoulder-impingement syndrome. This exercise may also be contraindicated if you have hyperextended elbows or low-back pain.

SCAPULAE ADDUCTION

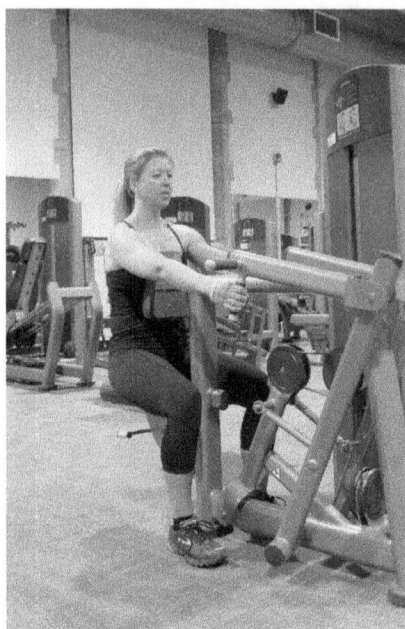

Start/Finish Position   *Mid-Range Position*

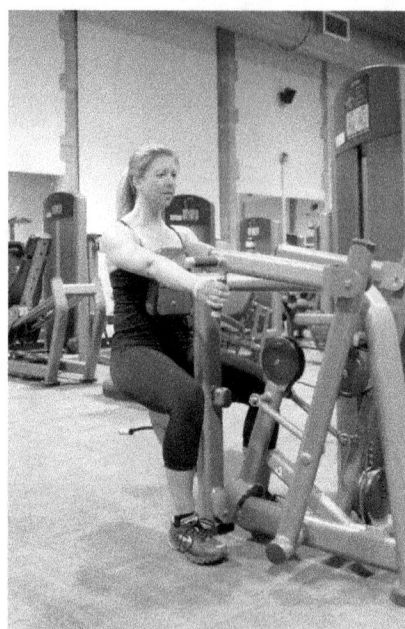

Muscles Strengthened: trapezius (middle and lower portions), rhomboids and forearms

Suggested Repetitions: 8 to 10 (or 50 to 60 seconds)

Start/Finish Position: Adjust the chest pad so that your arms will be completely straight in the start/finish position. Adjust the seat pad so that your arms will be parallel to the floor in the start/finish position. Sit down, lean forward against the chest pad and place your feet flat on the floor (or on the footplate if one is provided). Grasp the handles with a parallel grip (your palms facing each other).

Performance Description: Keeping your arms fairly straight, pull the handles back as far as possible (with the intent of trying to "pinch" your shoulder blades together). Pause briefly in this mid-range position (your shoulder blades together) and then lower the weight under control to the start/finish position (your shoulder blades apart).

Training Tips:

- Avoid moving your torso forward and backward. Movement should only occur at your shoulder and elbow joints.
- Attempt to raise the weight as high as possible in the mid-range position to ensure that you're obtaining a maximum contraction of the target muscles.
- You can also perform this exercise with a plate-loaded machine.
- Do this exercise with one limb at a time if you have a shoulder or an arm injury, a gross difference in the strength between your limbs or desire a training variation.
- Use wrist straps if you have difficulty in maintaining your grip on the handles.
- This exercise may be contraindicated if you have hyperextended elbows.

BICEP CURL

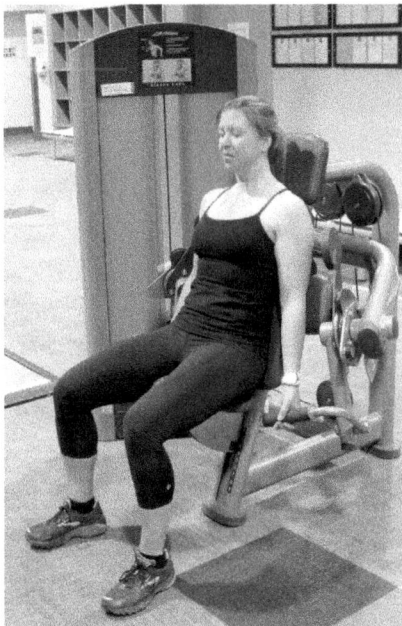

Start/Finish Position

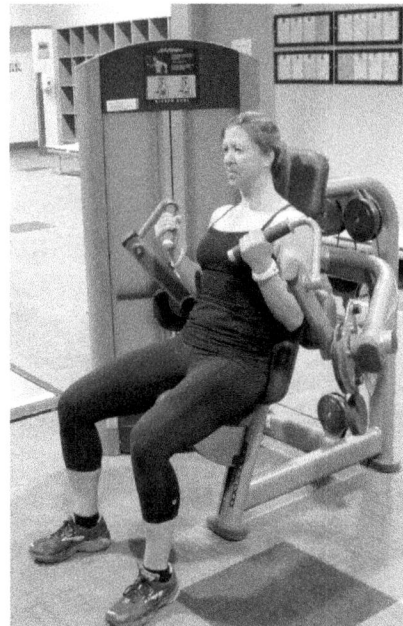

Mid-Range Position

Muscles Strengthened: biceps and forearms

Suggested Repetitions: 5 to 10 (or 30 to 60 seconds)

Start/Finish Position: Adjust the seat pad so that your elbows will be aligned with the axis of rotation in the start/finish position. Sit down and place your feet flat on the floor. Position your upper arms against the arm pads. Grasp the handles with your palms facing forward.

Performance Description: Pull the handles up to your shoulders. Pause briefly in this mid-range position (your arms bent) and then lower the weight under control to the start/finish position (your arms completely straight).

Training Tips:

- Avoid using your legs and moving your torso forward and backward. Movement should only occur at your elbow joints.

- Keep your upper arms against the arm pads.

- Attempt to raise the weight as high as possible in the mid-range position to ensure that you're obtaining a maximum contraction of the target muscles.

- You can also perform this exercise with a cable column and plate-loaded machine.

- Do this exercise with one limb at a time if you have a shoulder or an arm injury, a gross difference in the strength between your limbs or desire a training variation.

- This exercise may be contraindicated if you have hyperextended elbows.

TRICEP EXTENSION

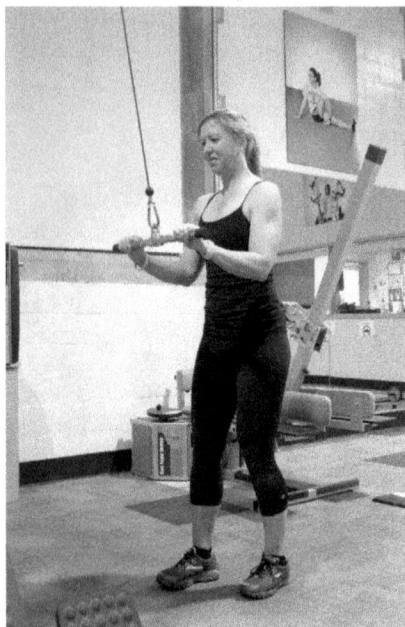

Start/Finish Position

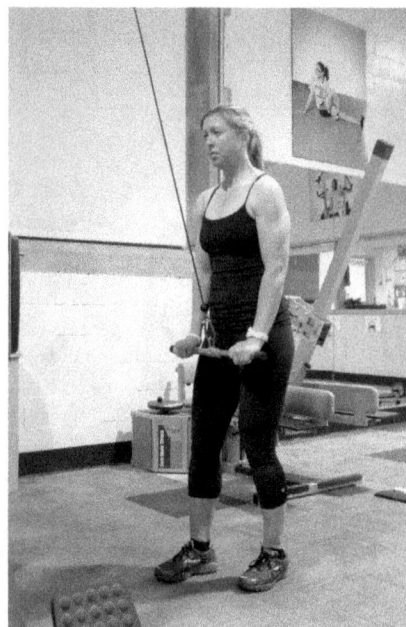

Mid-Range Position

Muscle Strengthened: triceps

Suggested Repetitions: 5 to 10 (or 30 to 60 seconds)

Start/Finish Position: Reach up and grasp a bar with your hands spaced about 4 to 6 inches apart and your palms facing downward. Pull the bar down and position your elbows against the sides of your torso. Spread your feet a comfortable distance apart with one foot slightly in front of the other.

Performance Description: Push the bar down until your arms are completely straight. Pause briefly in this mid-range position (your arms completely straight) and then lower the weight under control to the start/finish position (your arms bent).

Training Tips:

- Keep your elbows against the sides of your torso.
- You can also perform this exercise with a selectorized machine.
- Do this exercise with one limb at a time (with a handle instead of a bar) if you have a shoulder or an arm injury, a gross difference in the strength between your limbs or desire a training variation.

WRIST FLEXION

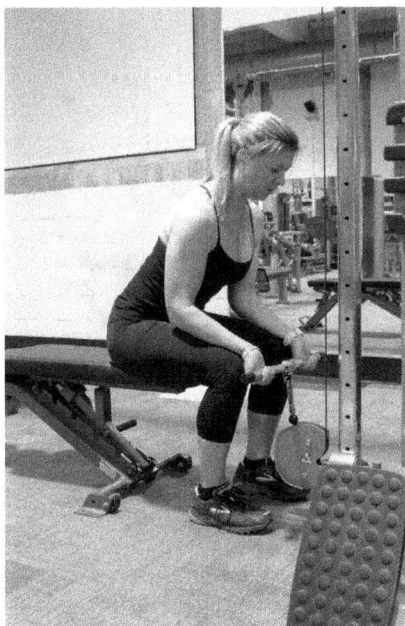

Start/Finish Position

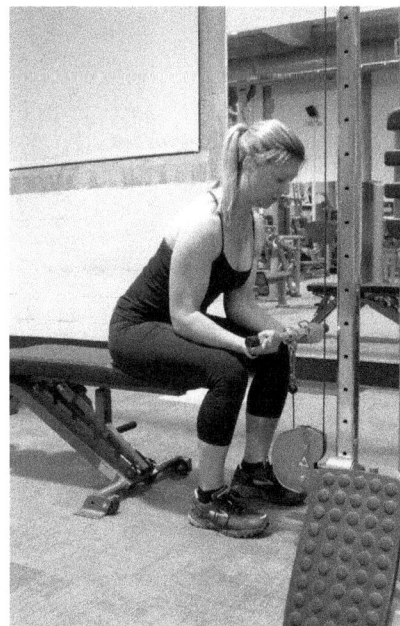

Mid-Range Position

Muscles Strengthened: wrist flexors

Suggested Repetitions: 8 to 10 (or 50 to 60 seconds)

Start/Finish Position: Adjust the pulley so that it's near the floor. Reach down and grasp a bar with your hands spread about 4 to 6 inches apart and your palms facing up. Position your thumbs underneath the bar alongside your fingers. Sit down near the end of a utility bench and place the back of your forearms on your upper legs so that your wrists are over your kneecaps. Lean forward slightly so that the angle between your upper and lower arms is about 90 degrees or less.

Performance Description: Pull the bar up as high as possible. Pause briefly in this mid-range position (your wrists bent) and then lower the weight under control to the start/finish position (your wrists extended).

Training Tips:

- Keep your forearms on your upper legs.

- Do this exercise with your thumbs underneath the bar. This increases your range of motion.

- Avoid using your legs and moving your torso forward and backward. Movement should only occur at your wrist joints.

- Attempt to raise the weight as high as possible in the mid-range position to ensure that you're obtaining a maximum contraction of the target muscles.

- Do this exercise with one limb at a time (with a handle instead of a bar) if you have a shoulder or an arm injury, a gross difference in the strength between your limbs or desire a training variation.

WRIST EXTENSION

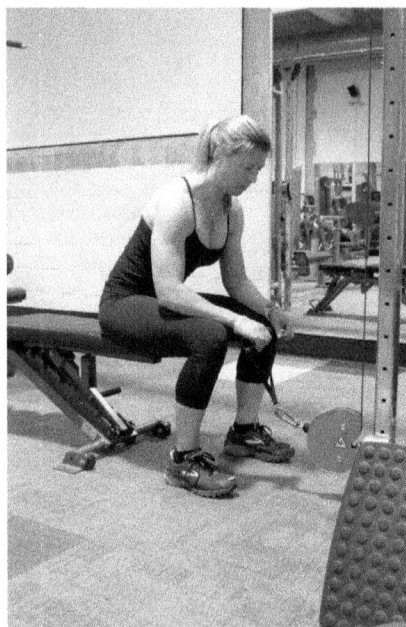

Start/Finish Position

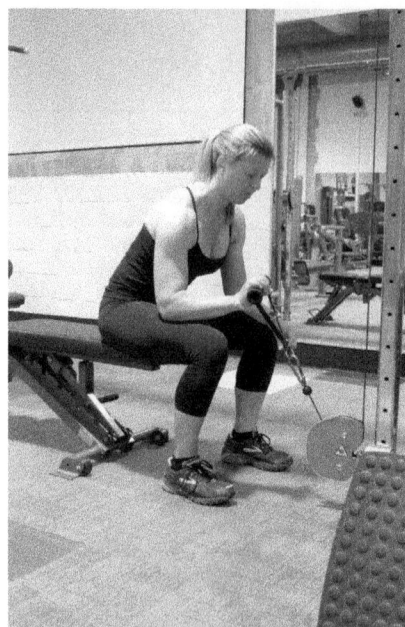

Mid-Range Position

Muscle Strengthened: wrist extensors

Suggested Repetitions: 8 to 10 (or 50 to 60 seconds)

Start/Finish Position: Adjust the pulley so that it's near the floor. Reach down and grasp a handle with your right hand. Sit down near the end of a utility bench and place the front of your right forearm on your right upper leg so that your wrist is over your kneecap and your palm is facing down. Lean forward slightly so that the angle between your upper and lower arms is about 90 degrees or less.

Performance Description: Pull the handle up as high as possible. Pause briefly in this mid-range position (your wrist extended) and then lower the weight under control to the start/finish position (your wrist bent). Repeat the exercise for the other side of your body.

Training Tips:

- Keep your forearm on your upper leg.

- Avoid using your leg and moving your torso forward and backward. Movement should only occur at your wrist joint.

- Attempt to raise the weight as high as possible in the mid-range position to ensure that you're obtaining a maximum contraction of the target muscles.

- Do this exercise with a handle rather than a bar. This makes it more comfortable on your wrist joint.

ABDOMINAL CRUNCH

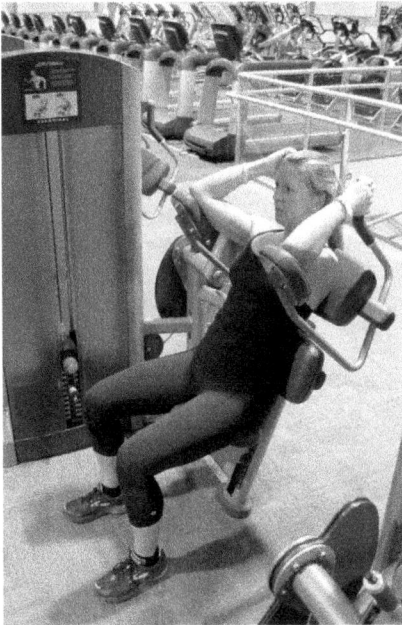

Start/Finish Position

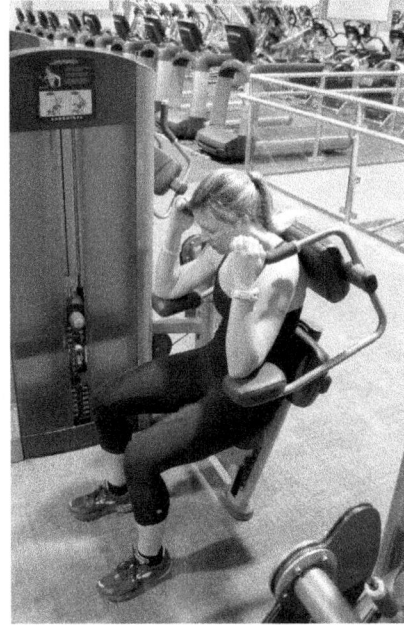

Mid-Range Position

Muscle Strengthened: rectus abdominis

Suggested Repetitions: 8 to 10 (or 50 to 60 seconds)

Start/Finish Position: Adjust the seat pad so that your navel ("belly button") will be aligned with the axis of rotation in the start/finish position. Sit down and place your feet flat on the floor. Position the back of your upper arms on the elbow pads. Place your palms on the handles and open your hands (extend your fingers).

Performance Description: Pull your torso as close to your upper legs as possible. Pause briefly in this mid-range position (your torso bent) and then lower the weight under control to the start/finish position (your torso straight).

Training Tips:

- Avoid snapping your head forward. Movement should only occur at your hip joint and mid-section.

- Exert force against the elbow pads with your upper arms, not your hands. This isolates your abdominals.

- If you're unable to keep your upper arms against the elbow pads, you can grasp the handles with a parallel grip (your palms facing each other) and pull with your hands instead of your upper arms. This doesn't allow you to isolate your abdominals but it will make the exercise more comfortable for you to perform.

- Attempt to raise the weight as high as possible in the mid-range position to ensure that you're obtaining a maximum contraction of the target muscles.

- You can also perform this exercise with a plate-loaded machine.

- This exercise may be contraindicated if you have low-back pain or shoulder-impingement syndrome.

SIDE BEND

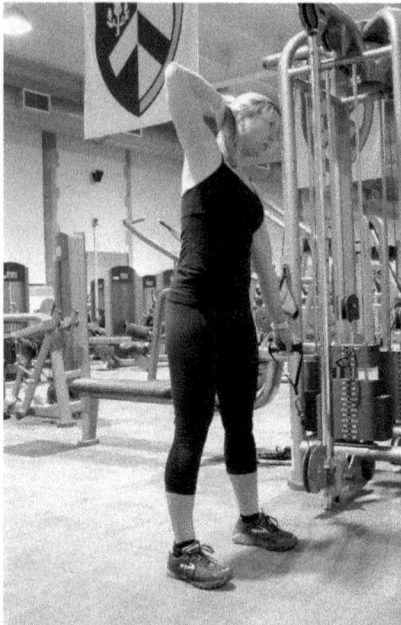

Start/Finish Position

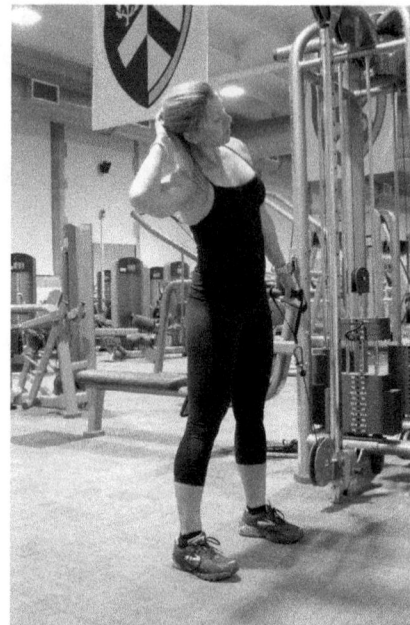

Mid-Range Position

Muscles Strengthened: obliques, erector spinae and forearms

Suggested Repetitions: 8 to 10 (or 50 to 60 seconds)

Start/Finish Position: Adjust the pulley so that it's near the floor. Reach down and grasp a handle with your left hand. Position your body so that your left side faces the pulley. Position the handle near the side of your upper leg with your palm facing your leg. Spread your feet about shoulder-width apart. Place your right palm against the right side of your head. Keep your hips in the same position and bend your torso to the left as far as possible.

Performance Description: Without moving your hips, bring your torso to the right as far as possible. Pause briefly in this mid-range position (your torso bent to the right) and then lower the weight under control to the start/finish position (your torso bent to the left). Repeat the exercise for the other side of your body.

Training Tips:

- Avoid moving your hips. Movement should only occur at your mid-section.
- Refrain from bending forward at the waist.
- Keep your feet flat on the floor.
- Attempt to raise the weight as high as possible in the mid-range position to ensure that you're obtaining a maximum contraction of the target muscles.
- Use wrist straps if you have difficulty in maintaining your grip on the handle.
- This exercise may be contraindicated if you have low-back pain.

TORSO ROTATION

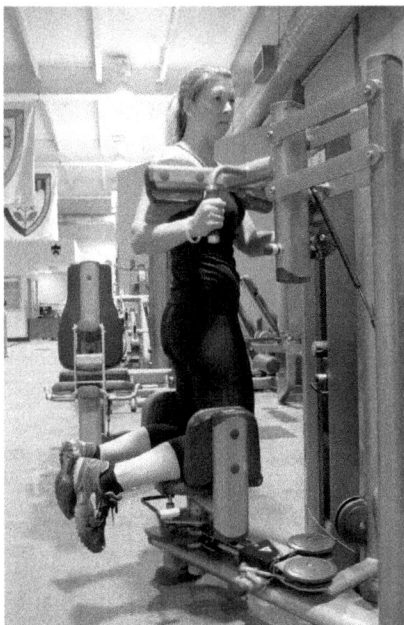

Start/Finish Position

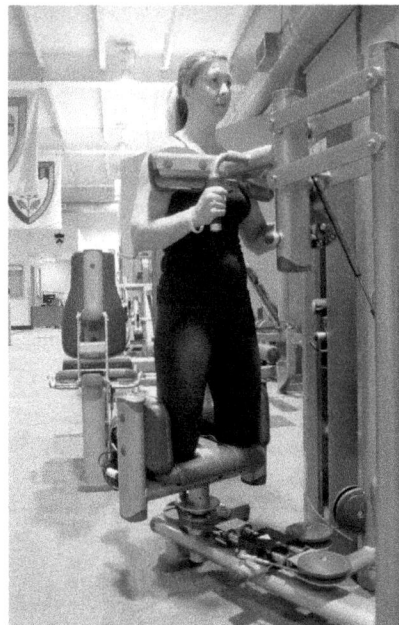

Mid-Range Position

Muscles Strengthened: obliques and erector spinae

Suggested Repetitions: 8 to 10 (or 50 to 60 seconds)

Start/Finish Position: Adjust the chest pads so that they will be centered on your chest in the start/finish position. Adjust the movement arm clockwise to accommodate your level of flexibility. Kneel down on the knee pad and position the side part of your thighs against the thigh pads. Grasp the handles with a parallel grip (your palms facing each other).

Performance Description: Rotate your torso to the right as far as possible. Pause briefly in this mid-range position (your torso rotated to the right) and then lower the weight under control to the start/finish position (your torso rotated to the left). Repeat the exercise for the other side of your body (adjusting the movement arm counterclockwise to accommodate your level of flexibility).

Training Tips:

- Attempt to raise the weight as high as possible in the mid-range position to ensure that you're obtaining a maximum contraction of the target muscles.

- This exercise may be contraindicated if you have low-back pain.

155

BACK EXTENSION

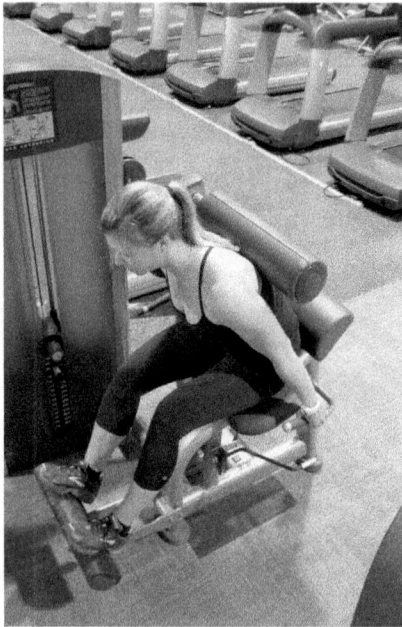

Start/Finish Position

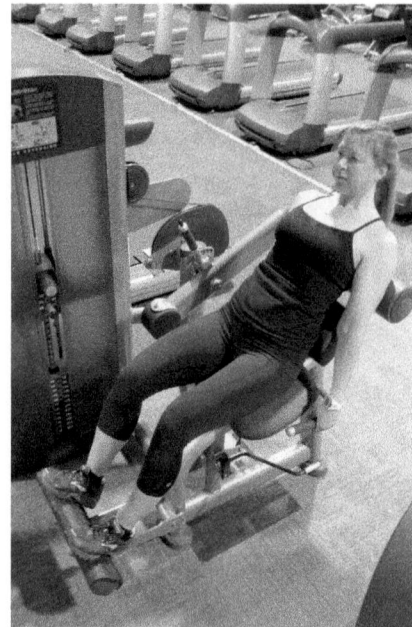

Mid-Range Position

Muscles Strengthened: erector spinae, gluteus maximus and hamstrings

Suggested Repetitions: 10 to 15 (or 60 to 90 seconds)

Start/Finish Position: Adjust the movement arm to accommodate your level of flexibility. Adjust the footplate so that your legs will be almost completely straight in the start/finish position. Sit down and place your feet flat on the footplate. Position your upper back against the roller pad. Grasp the handles that are located on the sides of the seat pad.

Performance Description: Extend your torso backward until it's aligned with your upper legs. Pause briefly in this mid-range position (your torso straight) and then lower the weight under control to the start/finish position (your torso bent).

Training Tips:

- Avoid snapping your head backward. Movement should only occur at your hip joint and mid-section.

- Keep your hips on the seat pad and your feet flat on the footplate.

- This exercise may be contraindicated if you have low-back pain.

NECK FLEXION

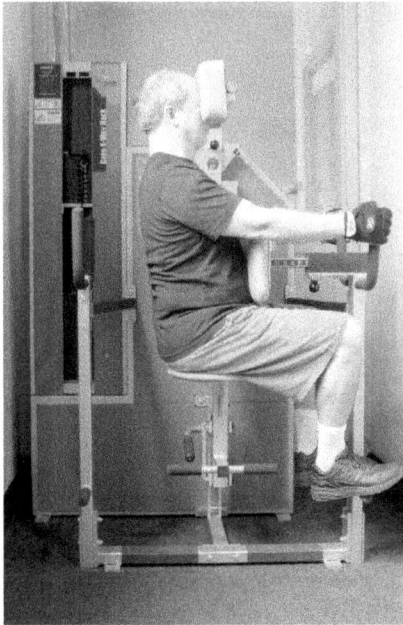

Start/Finish Position

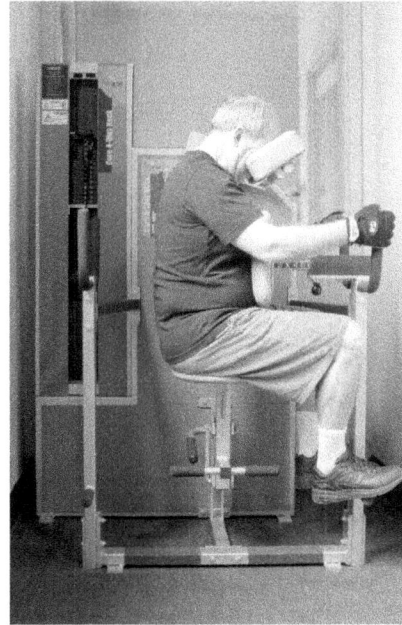

Mid-Range Position

Muscle Strengthened: sternocleidomastoideus

Suggested Repetitions: 8 to 10 (or 50 to 60 seconds)

Start/Finish Position: Adjust the seat pad so that your laryngeal prominence ("Adam's apple") will be aligned with the axis of rotation in the start/finish position. Adjust the torso pad so that your torso will be even with the axis of rotation in the start/finish position. Adjust the movement arm so that your head will be perpendicular to the floor in the start/finish position. Sit down, position the front part of your head against the head pad and place your feet flat on the floor (or on the foot pedal if one is provided). Grasp the handles with a parallel grip (your palms facing each other).

Performance Description: Pull your head as close to your chest as possible. Pause briefly in this mid-range position (your chin near your chest) and then lower the weight under control to the start/finish position (your head perpendicular to the floor).

Training Tips:

• Avoid moving your head backward beyond the point at which it's perpendicular to the floor.

• Avoid moving your torso forward and backward. Movement should only occur at your neck.

• Keep your hips on the seat pad and your feet flat on the floor.

• Attempt to raise the weight as high as possible in the mid-range position to ensure that you're obtaining a maximum contraction of the target muscles.

• You can also perform this exercise with a plate-loaded machine.

NECK EXTENSION

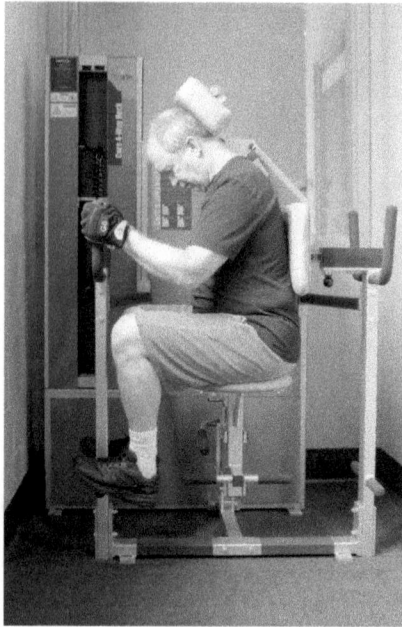

Start/Finish Position

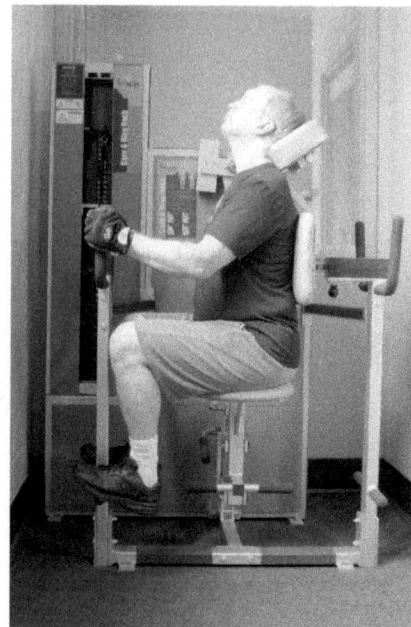

Mid-Range Position

Muscles Strengthened: neck extensors and trapezius (upper portion)

Suggested Repetitions: 8 to 10 (or 50 to 60 seconds)

Start/Finish Position: Adjust the seat pad so that your laryngeal prominence ("Adam's apple") will be aligned with the axis of rotation in the start/finish position. Adjust the torso pad so that your torso will be even with the axis of rotation in the start/finish position. Adjust the movement arm to accommodate your level of flexibility. Sit down, position the back part of your head against the head pad and place your feet flat on the floor (or on the foot pedal if one is provided). Grasp the handles with a parallel grip (your palms facing each other). Position your chin near your chest.

Performance Description: Extend your head backward as far as possible. Pause briefly in this mid-range position (your neck extended) and then lower the weight under control to the start/finish position (your chin near your chest).

Training Tips:

- Avoid moving your torso forward and backward. Movement should only occur at your neck.

- Keep your hips on the seat pad and your feet flat on the floor.

- Attempt to raise the weight as high as possible in the mid-range position to ensure that you're obtaining a maximum contraction of the target muscles.

- You can also perform this exercise with a plate-loaded machine.

NECK LATERAL FLEXION

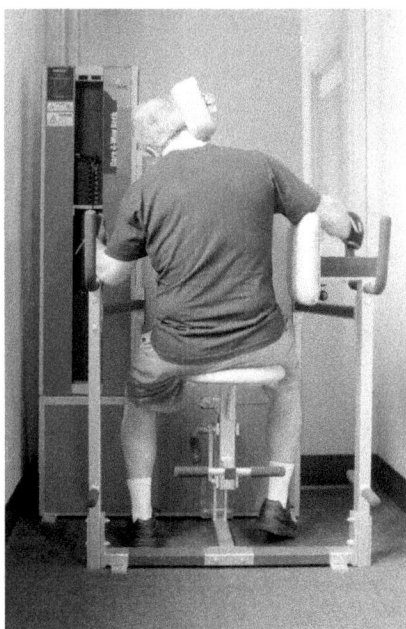

Start/Finish Position

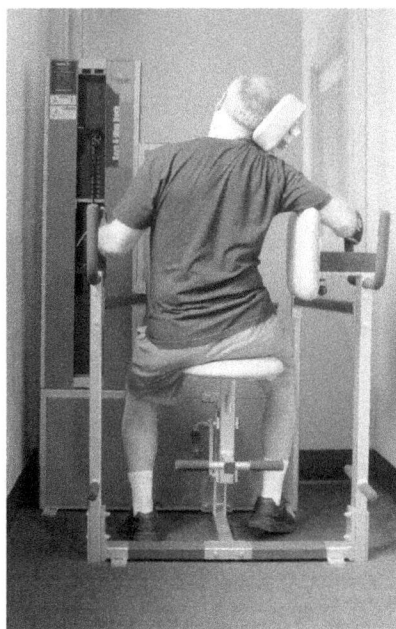

Mid-Range Position

Muscle Strengthened: sternocleidomastoideus

Suggested Repetitions: 8 to 10 (or 50 to 60 seconds)

Start/Finish Position: Adjust the seat pad so that your laryngeal prominence ("Adam's apple") will be aligned with the axis of rotation in the start/finish position. Adjust the torso pad so that it doesn't restrict your range of motion. Adjust the movement arm to accommodate your level of flexibility. Sit down, position the right side of your head against the head pad and place your feet flat on the floor (or on the foot pedal if one is provided). Grasp the handles with a parallel grip (your palms facing each other). Position your head so that it's near your left shoulder.

Performance Description: Pull your head to your right shoulder. Pause briefly in this mid-range position (your head near your right shoulder) and then lower the weight under control to the start/finish position (your head near your left shoulder). Repeat the exercise for the other side of your body.

Training Tips:

• Avoid moving your torso. Movement should only occur at your neck.

• Keep your hips on the seat pad and your feet flat on the floor.

• Attempt to raise the weight as high as possible in the mid-range position to ensure that you're obtaining a maximum contraction of the target muscles.

• You can also perform this exercise with a plate-loaded machine.

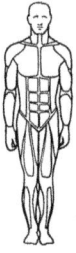

10 Manual-Resistance Exercises

Manual resistance (aka partner resistance) has been referred to as a productive alternative for improving strength with little or no equipment. It's an extremely effective way of strength training in which one individual supplies the resistance for another individual.

MAJOR MOMENTS IN HISTORY

It may be surprising to learn that the concept of manual resistance has actually been around for more than 200 years. The origin of these exercises can be traced back to the Swedish system of gymnastics which was developed by Per Henrik Ling – a Swedish physical educator and innovator – in the early 1800s. His "free exercises" – basically calisthenics – were done "without apparatus" in a setting that bore resemblance to a modern group-fitness class albeit much more regimented. Led by a "teacher," the "pupils" stood in formation and were expected to do the exercises in unison – almost literally by the numbers – with a motion and precision that were akin to military drill. In fact, many of the "commands" were lifted straight from the vernacular of the armed forces, including "fall in," "attention," "at ease" and "right face." Ling – known as the father of Swedish gymnastics – alluded to manual resistance when he wrote: "Resistance may consist of gravity, the opposing force of antagonizing muscles, or that which is exerted by another person." Partner-resistance exercises were referred to by Ling as "combined active movements," "exercises with single assistance" and "exercises with support." Guidelines for the "supporter" – the spotter – included this directive: "Resistance is to be given steadily, and in proportion to the power of the person resisted; there must be no violence, and the resistance must not be so strong as to stop the movement of a limb altogether."

In the United States, Dr. Diocletian (Dio) Lewis – a physician and pioneer in physical education – alluded to manual resistance around the early 1860s. In the August 1862 issue of *The Atlantic Monthly*, Dr. Lewis authored an article that described several exercises in which an individual pulled one or two wooden gymnastic rings that were held by another person who offered resistance. He wrote: "In most exercises there must be some resistance. How much better that this should be another human being, rather than a pole, ladder, or bar!" And that same year, he authored a book called *The New Gymnastics for Men, Women, and Children* which included descriptions and

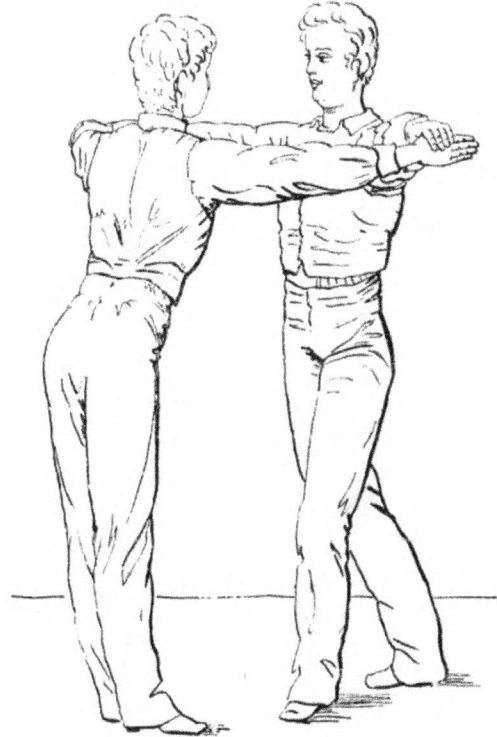

Per Henrik Ling promoted this partner-resistance exercise and others more than 200 years ago. (Image from Ling, PH, and H Ling, 1893.)

161

drawings of numerous partner-resistance exercises which he called "mutual-help exercises." (Fast fact: In 1863, Dr. Lewis founded the Boston Normal Institute for Physical Education, a college that was devoted to training teachers.)

A revival of manual resistance occurred during the late 1970s when the exercises were refined and galvanized by Dan Riley who was then the strength coach at Penn State. In 1979, he gave a presentation at the second annual National Strength Coaches Association convention in Chicago where most of the nearly 300 people in attendance were exposed to manual resistance for the very first time. And Coach Riley's 1982 book, *Maximum Muscular Fitness: Strength Training without Equipment*, was dedicated exclusively to this form of exercise. His early efforts brought manual resistance mainstream and are largely responsible for its continued popularity among strength coaches at the scholastic, collegiate and professional levels as well as personal trainers and physical therapists.

Self-Resistance Exercise

A novel iteration of manual-resistance exercise – self-resistance exercise – was promoted nearly a century ago. The backstory of self-resistance exercise is exceedingly important in the annals of strength training.

In February 1904, 11-year-old Angelo Siciliano and his mother, Francesca Fiorelli, immigrated to the United States from Italy, entering the country through historic Ellis Island. Siciliano would achieve epic fame as Charles Atlas, a name that has become as synonymous with fitness as any other with the possible exception of Jack LaLanne. In 1921, Atlas won the title of "World's Most Handsome Man." The competition was actually a photo contest in which the entrants submitted their pictures and measurements to *Physical Culture* magazine. For his, ahem, efforts, Atlas was given the choice of two prizes: a "satisfactory contract for motion picture work" – said to be the next *Tarzan* movie – or $1,000. He took the dough (about $13,847 in 2018 money). In 1922, Atlas won the title of "America's Most Perfectly Developed Man" which, over time, somehow expanded into the

"World's Most Perfectly Developed Man." At any rate, the title was bestowed on him by virtue of beating 774 other men in a bona fide physique contest that was held in the second Madison Square Garden (located in Manhattan on the site of the present New York Life Building). For winning the contest, Atlas was awarded $1,000. He also received a diploma. Yes, a *diploma* (bearing the name Charles Siciliano Atlas).

Atlas claimed that he developed his award-winning physique without the use of equipment (although it seems as if he "supplemented" his training with barbells and dumbbells). In 1923, he established a business that sold his system of training through the mail. A major selling point was that the system didn't require any equipment; it involved a variety of bodyweight, isometric and self-resistance exercises. But things didn't go as planned and his company went bankrupt by the late 1920s. With the help of Charles Roman – a veritable genius in marketing and advertising – Atlas rebooted the company in 1929. Their partnership spawned a highly lucrative mail-order business that was one of the most successful, influential and memorable in history. And not just in regards to the fitness industry; in regards to *any* industry. Their early success was truly remarkable, given the Stock Market Crash of 1929 and subsequent Great Depression.

In addition to exercises, the 12-lesson course – which Roman named Dynamic Tension® – included advice on nutrition and personal grooming (such as hair/skin care and bathing). Atlas passed away in 1972 but his legacy lives on. The company – known as Charles Atlas, Ltd. – continues to do business more than 90 years after it was first established. In fact, you can still purchase his original course – in English or Spanish – for the current price of $49.95. (Fast fact: In 1936, a bitter feud between Atlas and Bob Hoffman – the founder of the York Barbell Company who famously referred to Dynamic Tension® as Dynamic Hooey – landed in front of the Federal Trade Commission with Hoffman having claimed that Atlas used barbells and dumbbells to build his physique; the commission ruled in favor of Atlas.)

Sidebar: Advertisements for Dynamic Tension® – many of which had the look of a comic strip – targeted male insecurities and anxieties. In one classic advertisement, a man named Joe (or Mac) has a confrontation on a beach with "a big bully" who threatens to "smash [his] face" if he wasn't "so skinny [he] might dry up and blow away." To make matters worse, Joe's female companion – who witnessed the one-sided exchange – tells him that he's a "little boy." Frustrated, Joe sends away for Dynamic-Tension®, follows the course and quickly improves his strength and physique. He returns to the beach and punches the bully in the face – for no apparent reason other than the bully was in the vicinity – saying, "Here's something that I owe you!" This prompts his female companion to tell Joe "You are a real man after all." Another woman who's sunbathing nearby with a male companion remarks "Gosh! What a build." Text over Joe's head proclaims him "HERO OF THE BEACH." This marketing strategy was wildly successful; when Roman passed away in 1999, it was estimated that the company had produced $60 million in sales since 1929.

ADVANTAGES AND DISADVANTAGES

Manual resistance has many advantages. First of all, little or no equipment is required. Because of this, the exercises can be done just about anywhere without having to go to a fitness center. In addition, there's little or no expense. This is an important consideration for those with a limited or tight budget. Manual resistance is also a way of training large numbers of individuals in an extremely time-efficient fashion. This makes manual resistance well-suited for groups of athletes after practice and certain group-fitness classes. (Regardless of the size of the group, one half are the lifters while the other half are the spotters.)

Manual resistance has several disadvantages. The major drawback is that the resistance can't be quantified thereby making it impossible to monitor progress. Another disadvantage of manual resistance is that it requires a competent spotter.

GENERAL TECHNIQUE

In order for manual resistance to be productive, the exercises must be performed with proper technique. The following are general guidelines for the lifter and spotter:

The Lifter

As in lifting any weight, the lifter should perform the repetitions in a smooth, controlled manner without any explosive or jerking movements and throughout the greatest possible range of motion (ROM) that safety allows. The resistance (as applied by the spotter) should be raised in at least one to two seconds and lowered in at least three to four seconds.

The lifter should reach – or at least approach – the point of muscular fatigue within about 10 to 15 repetitions for the lower body and 5 to 10 repetitions for the torso. (Muscular fatigue should occur within about 8 to 10 repetitions for torso exercises that have an abbreviated ROM.) It should be noted that these ranges are based on six-second repetitions.

As an alternative to counting repetitions, the exercises can be performed for a prescribed amount of time. In this case, the lifter should reach muscular fatigue within about 60 to 90 seconds for the lower body and about 30 to 60 seconds for the torso. (Muscular fatigue should occur within about 50 to 60 seconds for torso exercises that have an abbreviated ROM.)

Also, the lifter must keep the muscles loaded throughout the entire exercise. Finally, the lifter must communicate to the spotter whether the resistance is too little or too much.

The Spotter

As an exercise is performed, the biomechanical leverage of your skeletal system changes which makes the movement feel easier in some positions and harder in others. Because of this, the spotter must vary the resistance throughout the lifter's entire ROM in an attempt to match the changes in biomechanical leverage. In positions in which the lifter has superior leverage (and superior strength), the spotter offers more resistance; in positions in which the lifter has inferior leverage (and inferior strength), the spotter offers less resistance. The end result is greater muscular effort throughout the range of motion. And since eccentric strength is greater than concentric strength (in the same exercise), the spotter must apply more resistance when the lifter performs the negative phase of each repetition.

The spotter must also regulate the resistance in accordance with the lifter's momentary level of strength. This means that the spotter must furnish less resistance as the lifter fatigues during each repetition. In addition, the spotter must control the speed with which the lifter performs the repetitions. Lastly, the spotter should provide the lifter with feedback on technique and motivate the lifter with words of encouragement.

THE EXERCISES

This chapter describes and illustrates the safest and most productive exercises that can be performed with manual resistance. Included in the discussions of each exercise are the muscle(s) strengthened (if two or more muscles are involved, the first muscle listed is the prime mover), suggested repetitions (the time that the targeted muscles should be loaded is shown in parentheses), start/finish position, performance description and training tips for making the exercise safer and more productive. (Note: In the accompanying photographs, the lifter is wearing the darker shirt.)

These 24 exercises are described in this chapter: hip abduction, hip adduction, prone leg curl, seated leg curl, leg extension, dorsi flexion, push-up, bent-arm fly, bent-over row, seated row, lat pulldown, shoulder press, lateral raise, front raise, bent-over raise, internal rotation, external rotation, bicep curl, tricep extension, wrist pronation, wrist supination, abdominal crunch, neck flexion and neck extension.

HIP ABDUCTION

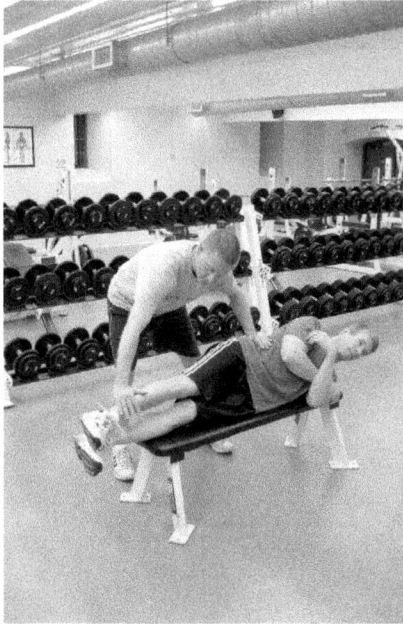

Start/Finish Position

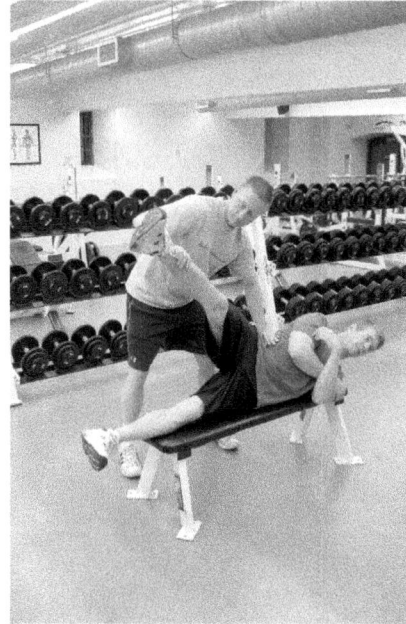

Mid-Range Position

Muscles Strengthened: gluteus medius and gluteus minimus

Suggested Repetitions: 10 to 15 (or 60 to 90 seconds)

Start/Finish Position: Lie down on a utility bench (or the floor) on the left side of your body and straighten your legs. Point your right toes toward your right knee. The spotter should stand or kneel behind you and apply resistance against your right ankle.

Performance Description: Raise your right leg as high as possible as the spotter provides resistance evenly throughout the full range of motion. Pause briefly in this mid-range position (your legs apart) and then resist as the spotter pushes your leg back to the start/finish position (your legs together). Repeat the exercise for the other side of your body (with your right side on the bench).

Training Tips:

- The spotter should apply resistance above your knee if you suffer from a hyperextended knee or other joint pain.

- Refrain from bending forward at the waist.

- Attempt to raise your leg as high as possible in the mid-range position to ensure that you're obtaining a maximum contraction of the target muscles.

- After reaching muscular fatigue, you can overload your muscles further by having the spotter lift your leg to the mid-range position and then push it back to the start/finish position as you resist for 3 to 5 negative-only repetitions.

HIP ADDUCTION

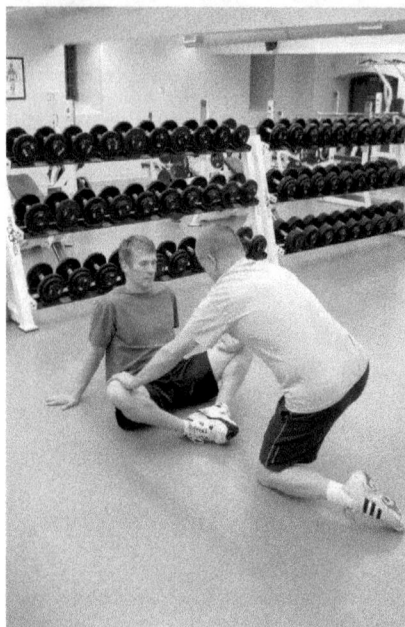

Start/Finish Position

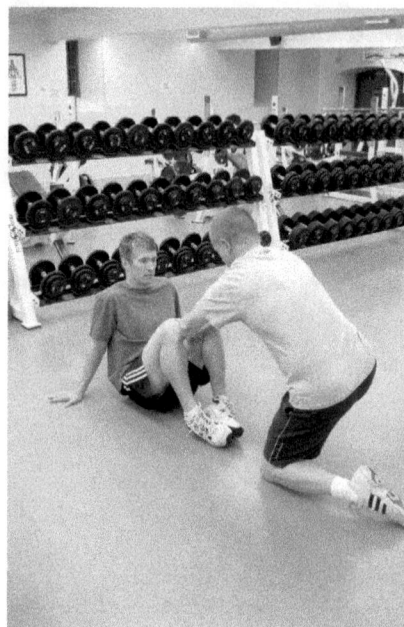

Mid-Range Position

Muscles Strengthened: hip adductors

Suggested Repetitions: 10 to 15 (or 60 to 90 seconds)

Start/Finish Position: Sit down on the floor, bend your legs and place the soles of your feet together. Position your feet close to your hips and spread your knees apart. Place your hands alongside your hips and lean back slightly. The spotter should kneel in front of you and apply resistance against the inside of your knees.

Performance Description: Bring your knees as close together as possible as the spotter provides resistance evenly throughout the full range of motion. Pause briefly in this mid-range position (your knees together) and then resist as the spotter pushes your legs back to the start/finish position (your knees apart).

Training Tips:

- Attempt to bring your knees as close together as possible in the mid-range position to ensure that you're obtaining a maximum contraction of the target muscles.

- After reaching muscular fatigue, you can overload your muscles further by having the spotter lift your legs to the mid-range position and then push them back to the start/finish position as you resist for 3 to 5 negative-only repetitions.

PRONE LEG CURL

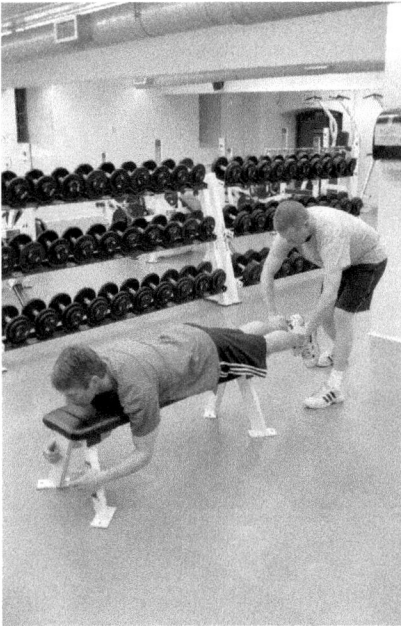

Start/Finish Position

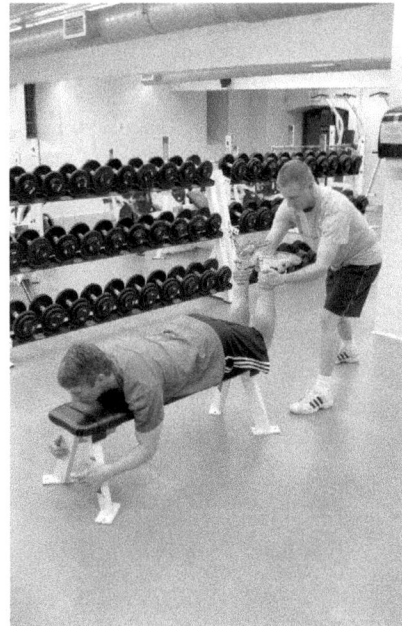

Mid-Range Position

Muscles Strengthened: hamstrings

Suggested Repetitions: 10 to 15 (or 60 to 90 seconds)

Start/Finish Position: Lie face down on a utility bench (or the floor) and straighten your legs. Position the tops of your kneecaps just over the edge the back pad. Grasp the front edge of the bench. The spotter should stand or kneel behind you and apply resistance against your heels.

Performance Description: Pull your heels as close to your hips as possible as the spotter provides resistance evenly throughout the full range of motion. Pause briefly in this mid-range position (your heels near your hips) and then resist as the spotter pulls your heels back to the start/finish position (your legs completely straight).

Training Tips:

- Avoid raising your torso. Movement should only occur at your knee joints.

- The angle between your upper and lower legs should be about 90 degrees or less in the mid-range position.

- Attempt to bring your heels as close to your hips as possible in the mid-range position to ensure that you're obtaining a maximum contraction of the target muscles.

- Do this exercise with one limb at a time if you have a leg, knee or ankle injury, a gross difference in the strength between your limbs or desire a training variation.

- After reaching muscular fatigue, you can overload your muscles further by having the spotter lift your lower legs to the mid-range position and then pull them back to the start/finish position as you resist for 3 to 5 negative-only repetitions.

- This exercise may be contraindicated if you have hyperextended knees or low-back pain.

167

SEATED LEG CURL

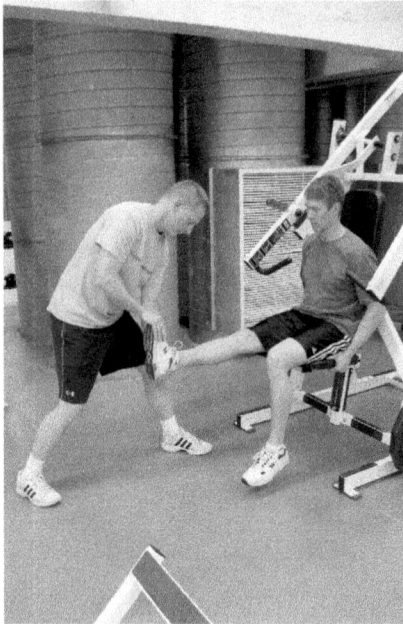

Start/Finish Position

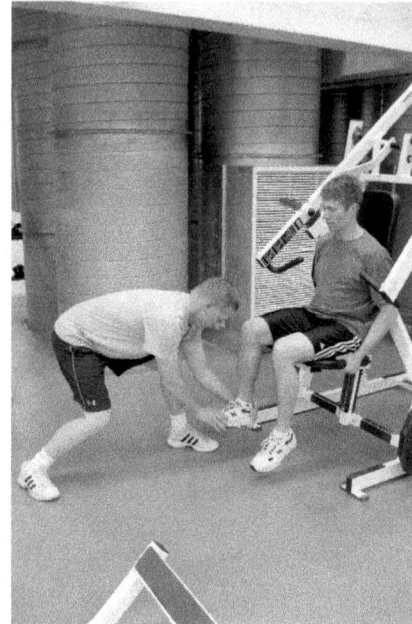

Mid-Range Position

Muscles Strengthened: hamstrings

Suggested Repetitions: 10 to 15 (or 60 to 90 seconds)

Start/Finish Position: Sit down on a machine (or table or chair) that's high enough so that your feet don't touch the floor and straighten your right leg. Grasp the sides of the seat pad. The spotter should stand or kneel in front of you and apply resistance against your right heel.

Performance Description: Pull your heel as close to your hip as possible as the spotter provides resistance evenly throughout the full range of motion. Pause briefly in this mid-range position (your heel near your hip) and then resist as the spotter pulls your heel back to the start/finish position (your leg completely straight). Repeat the exercise for the other side of your body.

Training Tips:

- Performing this exercise in the seated position produces less stress in the low-back region than performing it in the prone position.

- Avoid moving your torso forward and backward. Movement should only occur at your knee joint.

- The angle between your upper and lower leg should be about 90 degrees or less in the mid-range position.

- Attempt to bring your heel as close to your hip as possible in the mid-range position to ensure that you're obtaining a maximum contraction of the target muscles.

- After reaching muscular fatigue, you can overload your muscles further by having the spotter bring your lower leg to the mid-range position and then pull it back to the start/finish position as you resist for 3 to 5 negative-only repetitions.

- This exercise may be contraindicated if you have hyperextended knees.

LEG EXTENSION

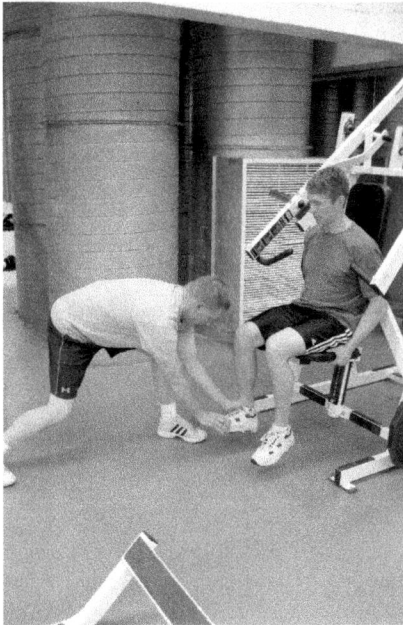

Start/Finish Position

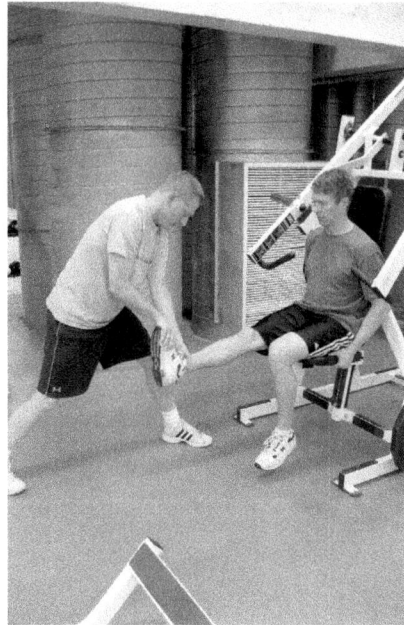

Mid-Range Position

Muscles Strengthened: quadriceps

Suggested Repetitions: 10 to 15 (or 60 to 90 seconds)

Start/Finish Position: Sit down on a machine (or table or chair) that's high enough so that your feet don't touch the floor and bend your right leg. Grasp the sides of the seat pad. The spotter should stand or kneel in front of you and apply resistance against your right instep.

Performance Description: Straighten your right leg as completely as possible as the spotter provides resistance evenly throughout the full range of motion. Pause briefly in this mid-range position (your leg completely straight) and then resist as the spotter pushes your ankle back to the start/finish position (your leg bent). Repeat the exercise for the other side of your body.

Training Tips:

• Avoid moving your torso forward and backward. Movement should only occur at your knee joint.

• Attempt to straighten your leg as high as possible in the mid-range position to ensure that you're obtaining a maximum contraction of the target muscles.

• After reaching muscular fatigue, you can overload your muscles further by having the spotter lift your lower leg to the mid-range position and then push it back to the start/finish position as you resist for 3 to 5 negative-only repetitions.

DORSI FLEXION

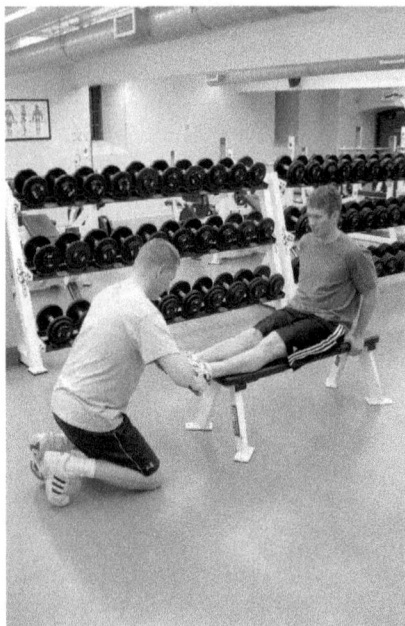

Start/Finish Position

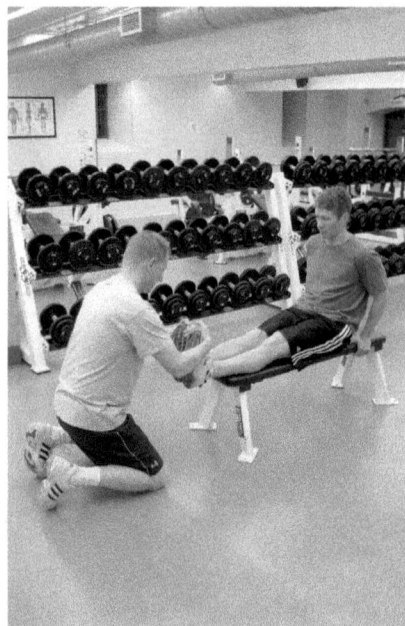

Mid-Range Position

Muscles Strengthened: dorsi flexors

Suggested Repetitions: 10 to 15 (or 60 to 90 seconds)

Start/Finish Position: Sit down on a utility bench. Place your legs across the length of it. Position your heels over the end of the back pad and point your toes away from your body. Grasp the sides of the bench. The spotter should stand or kneel in front of you and apply resistance against your insteps.

Performance Description: Keeping your legs flat on the bench, pull your feet up as high as possible as the spotter provides resistance evenly throughout the full range of motion. Pause briefly in this mid-range position (your ankles bent) and then resist as the spotter pulls your feet back to the start/finish position (your ankles straight).

Training Tips:

- Avoid moving your torso forward and backward. Movement should only occur at your ankle joints.

- Attempt to raise your feet as high as possible in the mid-range position to ensure that you're obtaining a maximum contraction of the target muscles.

- Do this exercise with one limb at a time if you have a leg, knee or ankle injury, a gross difference in the strength between your limbs or desire a training variation.

- After reaching muscular fatigue, you can overload your muscles further by having the spotter bring your feet to the mid-range position and then pull them back to the start/finish position as you resist for 3 to 5 negative-only repetitions.

- This exercise may be contraindicated if you have shin splints.

PUSH-UP

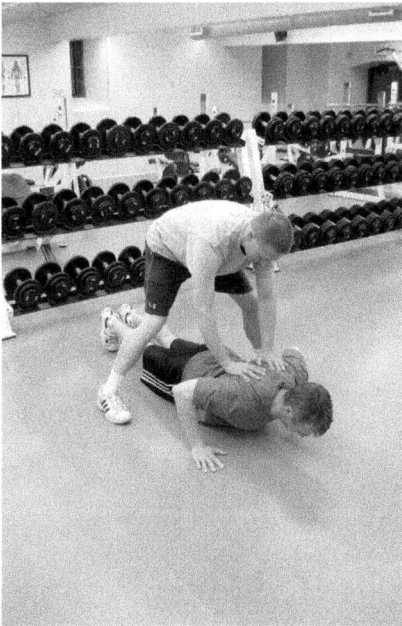

Start/Finish Position

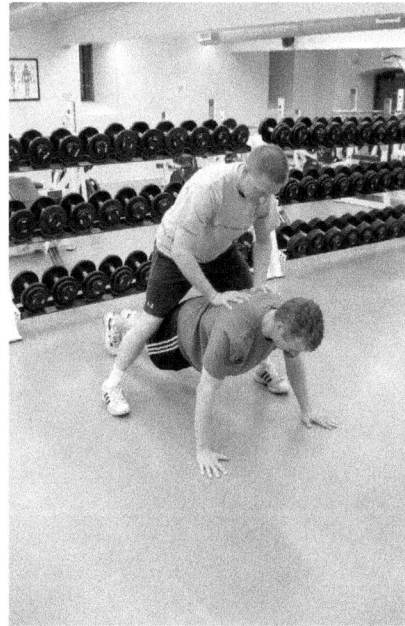

Mid-Range Position

Muscles Strengthened: chest, anterior deltoid and triceps

Suggested Repetitions: 5 to 10 (or 30 to 60 seconds)

Start/Finish Position: Lie face down on the floor, straighten your legs and curl your toes under your feet. Place your palms on the floor and spread your hands slightly wider than shoulder-width apart. The spotter should straddle your torso and apply resistance against your upper back.

Performance Description: Push your body up until your arms are almost completely straight (without "locking" your elbows) as the spotter provides resistance evenly throughout the full range of motion. Pause briefly in this mid-range position (your arms almost completely straight) and then resist as the spotter pushes you back to the start/finish position (your arms bent).

Training Tips:

- Avoid using an excessively wide hand position. This reduces your range of motion.
- Avoid arching your lower back. Your torso should remain aligned with your lower body.
- Avoid "locking" or "snapping" your elbows in the mid-range position.
- If you can't do 5 repetitions using your bodyweight, you can increase your biomechanical leverage by performing this exercise in the kneeling position.
- After reaching muscular fatigue, you can overload your muscles further by having the spotter lift your body to the mid-range position and then push it back to the start/finish position as you resist for 3 to 5 negative-only repetitions.
- This exercise may be contraindicated if you have shoulder-impingement syndrome.

BENT-ARM FLY

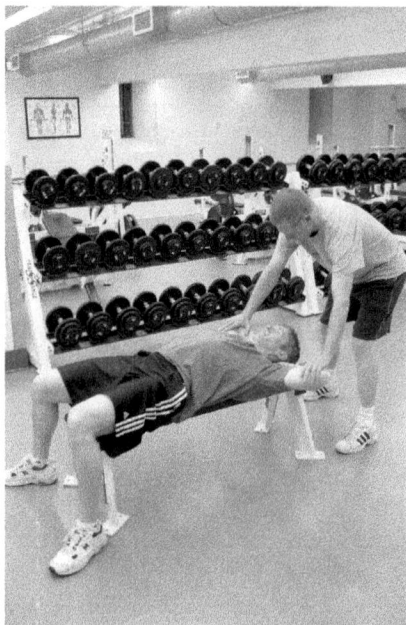

Start/Finish Position

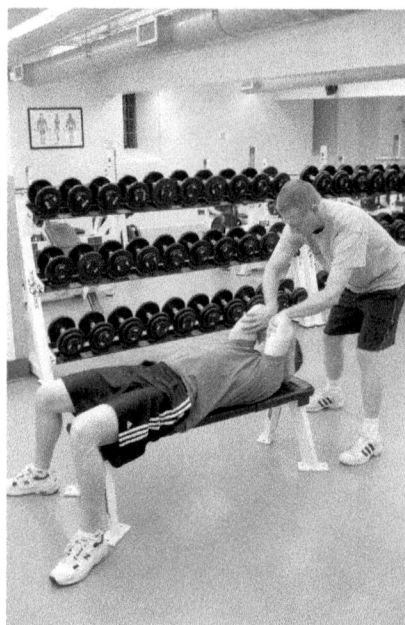

Mid-Range Position

Muscles Strengthened: chest and anterior deltoid

Suggested Repetitions: 5 to 10 (or 30 to 60 seconds)

Start/Finish Position: Lie down on a utility bench (or the floor) and interlock your fingers behind your head. Place your feet flat on the floor. The spotter should stand or kneel behind your head and apply resistance against the inside of your elbows.

Performance Description: Keeping your head against the back pad, bring your elbows as close together as possible as the spotter provides resistance evenly throughout the full range of motion. Pause briefly in this mid-range position (your elbows together) and then resist as the spotter pushes your arms back to the start/finish position (your elbows apart).

Training Tips:

- Keep your head, hips and torso against the back pad and your feet flat on the floor. Movement should only occur at your shoulder joints.

- If you have low-back pain, place your feet flat on the end of the bench or a stool. This reduces the stress in your low-back region.

- Do this exercise with one limb at a time if you have a shoulder or an arm injury, a gross difference in the strength between your limbs or desire a training variation.

- After reaching muscular fatigue, you can overload your muscles further by having the spotter lift your arms to the mid-range position and then push them back to the start/finish position as you resist for 3 to 5 negative-only repetitions.

- This exercise may be contraindicated if you have shoulder-impingement syndrome.

BENT-OVER ROW

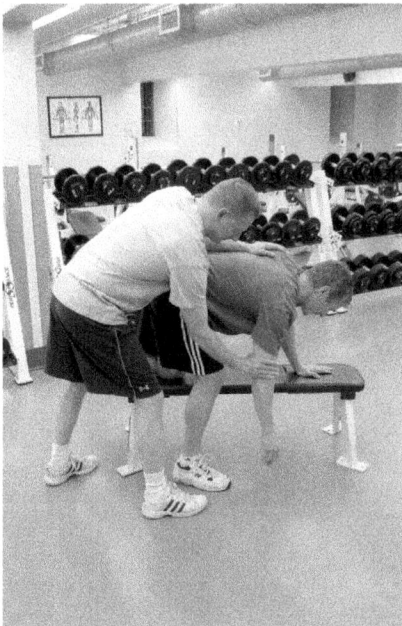

Start/Finish Position

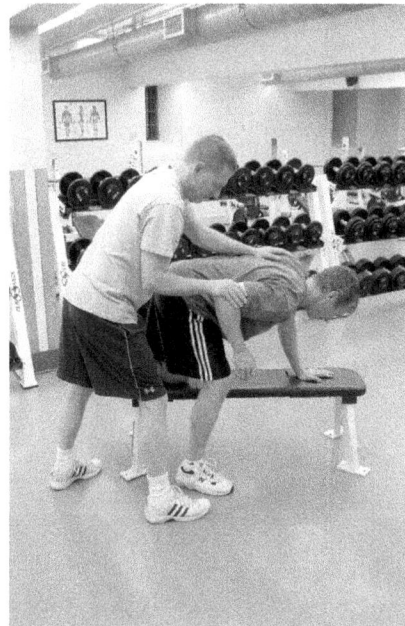

Mid-Range Position

Muscle Strengthened: upper back

Suggested Repetitions: 5 to 10 (or 30 to 60 seconds)

Start/Finish Position: Place your left hand and left knee on a utility bench and position your right foot on the floor a comfortable distance from the bench. Position your right arm so that it's perpendicular to the floor and open your right hand (extend your fingers). Straighten your right arm and point your palm toward the bench. The spotter should stand along the right side of your torso and apply resistance against the back of your right upper arm near your elbow.

Performance Description: Pull your elbow up as high as possible as the spotter provides resistance evenly throughout the full range of motion. Pause briefly in this mid-range position (your arm bent) and then resist as the spotter pushes your arm back to the start/finish position (your arm completely straight). Repeat the exercise for the other side of your body (with your right hand and right knee on the bench).

Training Tips:

• Keep your hand open (your fingers extended).

• Avoid using your legs and rotating your torso. Movement should only occur at your shoulder and elbow joints.

• You can also perform this exercise with your upper arm positioned away from your torso. Doing this involves less of your upper back and more of your posterior deltoid, trapezius and rhomboids. In this case, your upper arm would be perpendicular to your torso and your palm would be facing backward in the mid-range position.

• This exercise is a multiple-joint movement when performed with dumbbells but a single-joint movement when performed with manual resistance because the resistance is applied above your elbow, not to your hand.

• After reaching muscular fatigue, you can overload your muscles further by having the spotter lift your arm to the mid-range position and then push it back to the start/finish position as you resist for 3 to 5 negative-only repetitions.

SEATED ROW

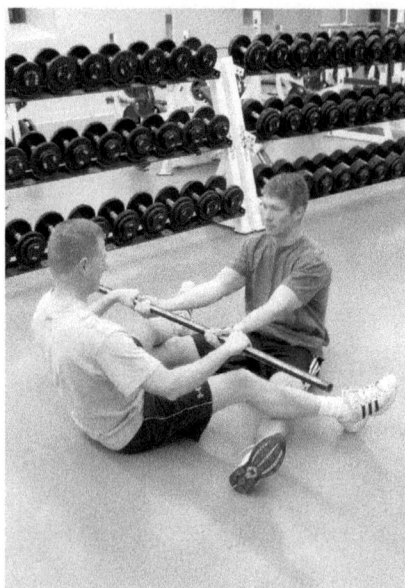

Start/Finish Position

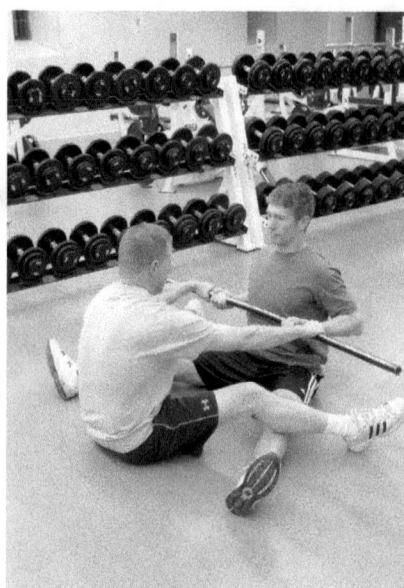

Mid-Range Position

Muscles Strengthened: upper back, biceps and forearms

Suggested Repetitions: 5 to 10 (or 30 to 60 seconds)

Start/Finish Position: Sit down on the floor, straighten your legs and spread them apart. Grasp a long stick (or similar object) with your palms facing up and space your hands approximately shoulder-width apart. Straighten your arms and lean back slightly. The spotter should sit down on the floor between your legs and grasp the stick on the outside of your grip with palms facing down.

Performance Description: Pull the stick to your mid-section as the spotter provides resistance evenly throughout the full range of motion. Pause briefly in this mid-range position (your arms bent) and then resist as the spotter pulls your arms back to the start/finish position (your arms completely straight).

Training Tips:

- The spotter should provide resistance by bending forward and backward at the waist to involve the larger, more powerful muscles of the lower back.

- You can also perform this exercise with your upper arms positioned away from your torso using an overhand grip. Doing this involves less of your upper back and more of your posterior deltoid, trapezius and rhomboids. In this case, your upper arm would be perpendicular to your torso and your palms would be facing down in the mid-range position.

- Avoid using an excessively wide grip. This reduces your range of motion.

- Avoid moving your torso forward and backward. Movement should only occur at your shoulder and elbow joints.

- Do this exercise with one limb at a time if you have a shoulder or an arm injury, a gross difference in the strength between your limbs or desire a training variation.

- Use wrist straps if you have difficulty in maintaining your grip on the stick.

- After reaching muscular fatigue, you can overload your muscles further by having the spotter bring the stick to the mid-range position and then pull it back to the start/finish position as you resist for 3 to 5 negative-only repetitions.

- This exercise may be contraindicated if you have hyperextended elbows.

174

LAT PULLDOWN

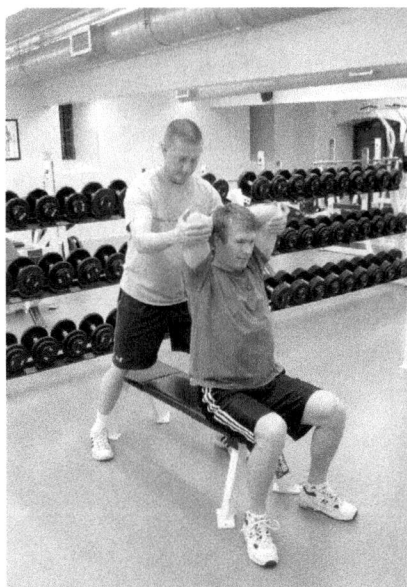

Start/Finish Position

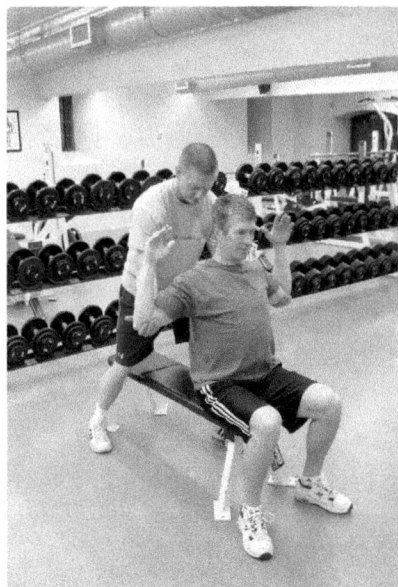

Mid-Range Position

Muscle Strengthened: upper back

Suggested Repetitions: 5 to 10 (or 30 to 60 seconds)

Start/Finish Position: Sit down on a utility bench (or stool or chair) and place your upper arms near the sides of your head. Cross your lower arms above your head and open your hands (extend your fingers). The spotter should stand behind you and apply resistance against the back of your upper arms near your elbows.

Performance Description: Keeping your upper arms aligned with your torso, pull your elbows down to your sides as the spotter provides resistance evenly throughout the full range of motion. Pause briefly in this mid-range position (your upper arms near the sides of your body) and then resist as the spotter pulls your arms back to the start/finish position (your upper arms near the sides of your head).

Training Tips:

- Keep your hands open (your fingers extended).

- Avoid moving your hands in front of your face. Your hands should remain out of your sight.

- This exercise is a multiple-joint movement when performed with a machine but it becomes a single-joint movement when using manual resistance because the load is applied above your elbows, not to your hands.

- Do this exercise with one limb at a time if you have a shoulder or an arm injury, a gross difference in the strength between your limbs or desire a training variation.

- After reaching muscular fatigue, you can overload your muscles further by having the spotter bring your arms to the mid-range position and then pull them back to the start/finish position as you resist for 3 to 5 negative-only repetitions.

- This exercise may be contraindicated if you have shoulder-impingement syndrome.

SHOULDER PRESS

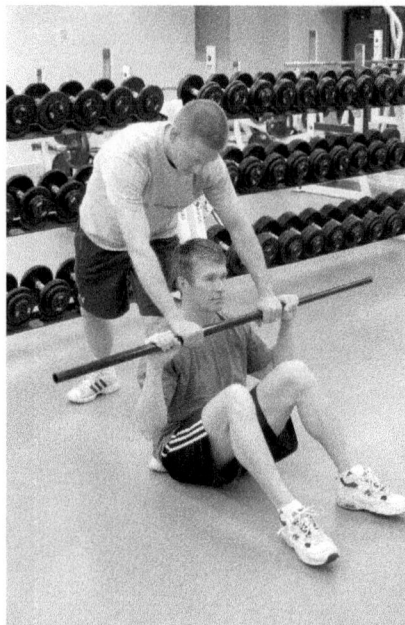

Start/Finish Position

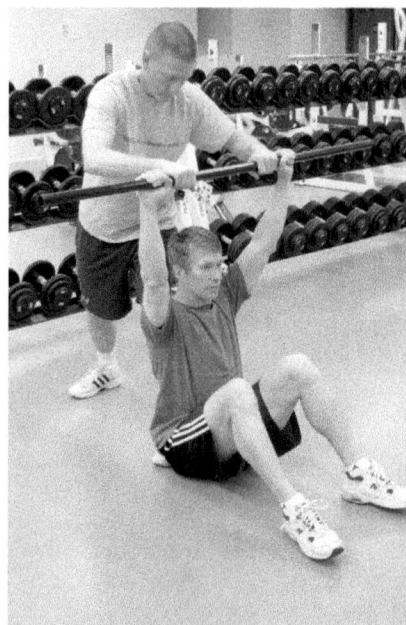

Mid-Range Position

Muscles Strengthened: anterior deltoid and triceps

Suggested Repetitions: 5 to 10 (or 30 to 60 seconds)

Start/Finish Position: Sit down on the floor, bend your legs and place your feet flat on the floor. Grasp a long stick (or similar object) and spread your hands slightly wider than shoulder-width apart. Place the stick on the upper part of your chest near your collarbones. The spotter should stand behind you, place one leg behind your torso for you to lean against and grasp the stick on the inside of your grip with palms facing down.

Performance Description: Push the stick up until your arms are almost completely straight (without "locking" your elbows) as the spotter provides resistance evenly throughout the full range of motion. Pause briefly in this mid-range position (your arms almost completely straight) and then resist as the spotter pushes the stick back to the start/finish position (your arms bent).

Training Tips:

- Avoid using an excessively wide grip. This reduces your range of motion.

- Avoid "locking" or "snapping" your elbows in the mid-range position.

- Do this exercise with one limb at a time if you have a shoulder or an arm injury, a gross difference in the strength between your limbs or desire a training variation.

- After reaching muscular fatigue, you can overload your muscles further by having the spotter lift the stick to the mid-range position and then push it back to the start/finish position as you resist for 3 to 5 negative-only repetitions.

- You can also perform this exercise with the stick positioned behind your head/neck. However, this may be contraindicated if you have shoulder-impingement syndrome. This exercise may also be contraindicated if you have low-back pain.

LATERAL RAISE

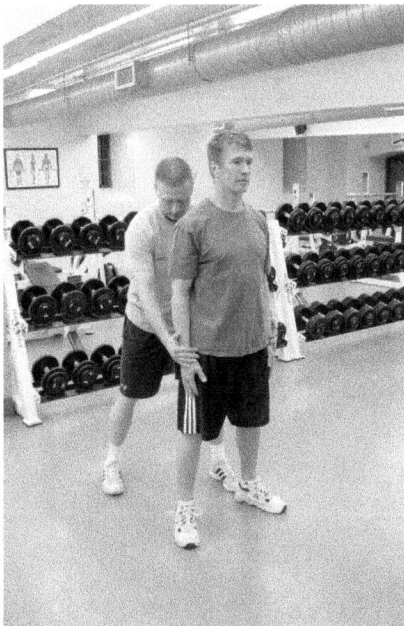

Start/Finish Position

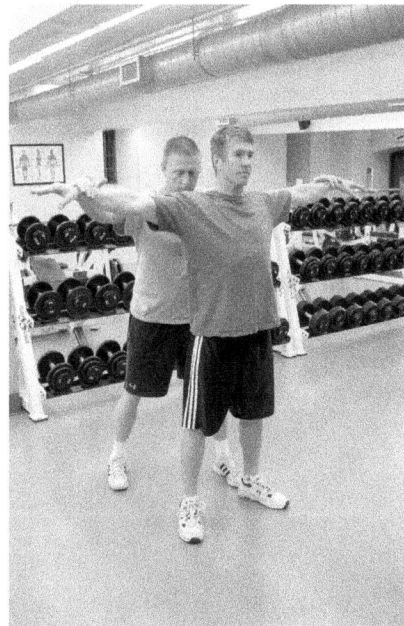

Mid-Range Position

Muscles Strengthened: middle deltoid and trapezius (upper and lower portions)

Suggested Repetitions: 5 to 10 (or 30 to 60 seconds)

Start/Finish Position: Position your hands against the sides of your upper legs with your palms facing each other and open your hands (extend your fingers). Straighten your arms and spread your feet about shoulder-width apart. The spotter should stand behind you and apply resistance near your wrists.

Performance Description: Keeping your arms fairly straight, raise them sideways until they're parallel to the floor as the spotter provides resistance evenly throughout the full range of motion. Pause briefly in this mid-range position (your arms parallel to the floor) and then resist as the spotter pushes your arms back to the start/finish position (your arms at your sides).

Training Tips:

- The spotter should apply resistance above your elbows if you suffer from a hyperextended elbow or other joint pain.
- Keep your hands open (your fingers extended).
- Avoid using your legs and moving your torso forward and backward. Movement should only occur at your shoulder joints.
- Raise your arms only to the point at which they're parallel to the floor.
- Your palms should be facing the floor in the mid-range position.
- Do this exercise with one limb at a time if you have a shoulder or an arm injury, a gross difference in the strength between your limbs or desire a training variation.
- After reaching muscular fatigue, you can overload your muscles further by having the spotter lift your arms to the mid-range position and then push them back to the start/finish position as you resist for 3 to 5 negative-only repetitions.

FRONT RAISE

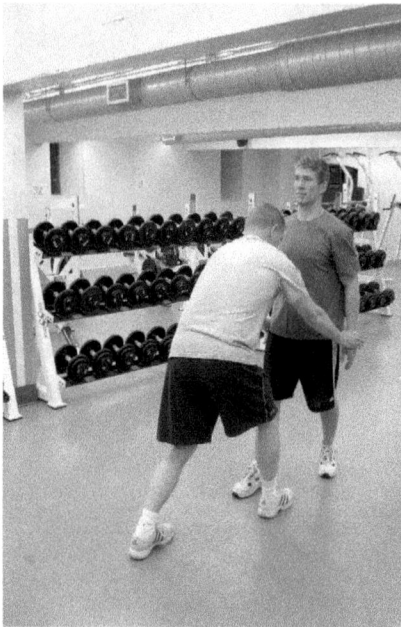

Start/Finish Position

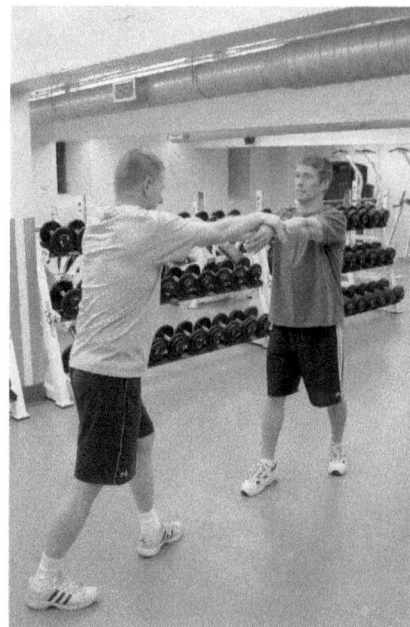

Mid-Range Position

Muscle Strengthened: anterior deltoid

Suggested Repetitions: 5 to 10 (or 30 to 60 seconds)

Start/Finish Position: Position your hands slightly past your hips with your palms facing each other and open your hands (extend your fingers). Straighten your arms and spread your feet a comfortable distance apart with one foot slightly in front of the other. The spotter should stand in front of you, place one foot to the inside of your forward foot and apply resistance against your wrists.

Performance Description: Keeping your arms fairly straight, raise them forward until they're parallel to the floor as the spotter applies resistance evenly throughout the full range of motion. Pause briefly in this mid-range position (your arms parallel to the floor) and then resist as the spotter pushes your arms back to the start/finish position (your arms past your hips).

Training Tips:

- The spotter should apply resistance above your elbows if you suffer from a hyperextended elbow or other joint pain.

- The spotter's front foot should slide backward as you raise your arms up to the mid-range position and forward as you lower your arms to the start/finish position.

- Keep your hands open (your fingers extended).

- Avoid using your legs and moving your torso forward and backward. Movement should only occur at your shoulder joints.

- Raise your arms only to the point at which they're parallel to the floor.

- Your palms should be facing each other in the mid-range position.

- Do this exercise with one limb at a time if you have a shoulder or an arm injury, a gross difference in the strength between your limbs or desire a training variation.

- After reaching muscular fatigue, you can overload your muscles further by having the spotter lift your arms to the mid-range position and then push them back to the start/finish position as you resist for 3 to 5 negative-only repetitions.

BENT-OVER RAISE

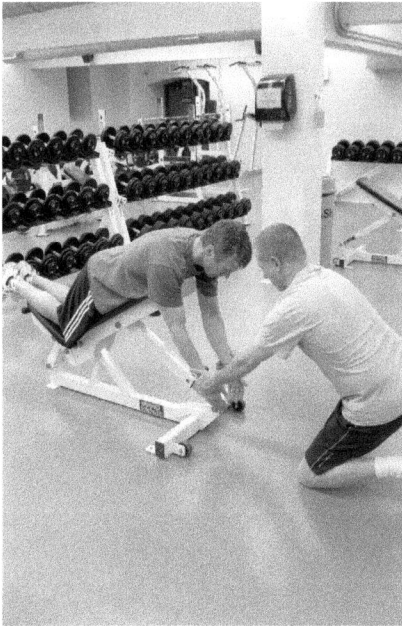

Start/Finish Position

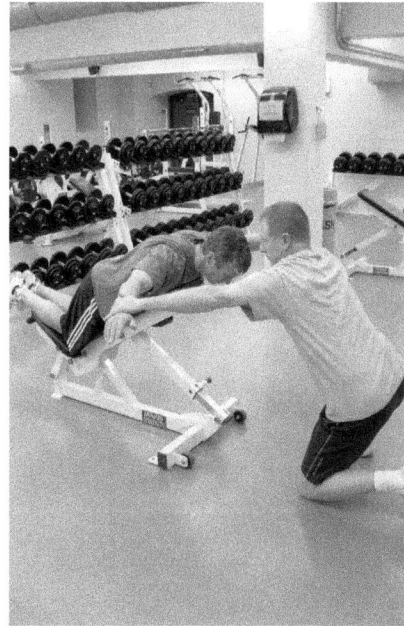

Mid-Range Position

Muscles Strengthened: posterior deltoid, trapezius (middle and lower portions) and rhomboids

Suggested Repetitions: 5 to 10 (or 30 to 60 seconds)

Start/Finish Position: Kneel on the seat pad of an adjustable incline bench. Lie forward against the bench, position your arms so that they're perpendicular to your torso and open your hands (extend your fingers). Straighten your arms and point your palms toward each other. The spotter should stand or kneel in front of you and apply resistance against your wrists.

Performance Description: Keeping your arms fairly straight, raise your arms sideways until they're parallel to the floor as the spotter applies resistance evenly throughout the full range of motion. Pause briefly in this mid-range position (your arms parallel to the floor) and then resist as the spotter pushes your arms back to the start/finish position (your arms hanging down).

Training Tips:

- The spotter should apply resistance above your elbows if you suffer from a hyperextended elbow or other joint pain.

- Keep your hands open (your fingers extended).

- Raise your arms only to the point at which they're parallel to the floor.

- Your palms should be facing the floor and your upper arms should be perpendicular to your torso in the mid-range position.

- Do this exercise with one limb at a time if you have a shoulder or an arm injury, a gross difference in the strength between your limbs or desire a training variation.

- After reaching muscular fatigue, you can overload your muscles further by having the spotter lift your arms to the mid-range position and then push them back to the start/finish position as you resist for 3 to 5 negative-only repetitions.

INTERNAL ROTATION

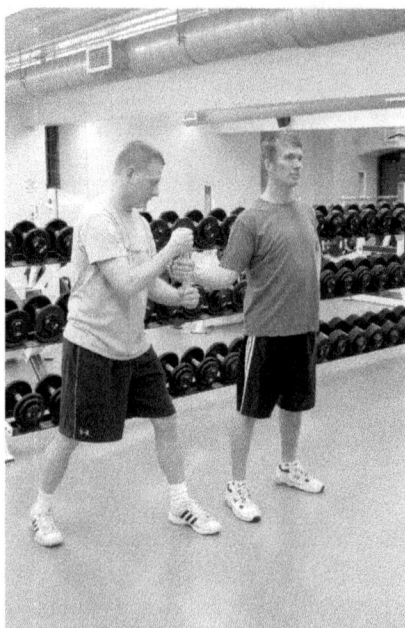

Start/Finish Position

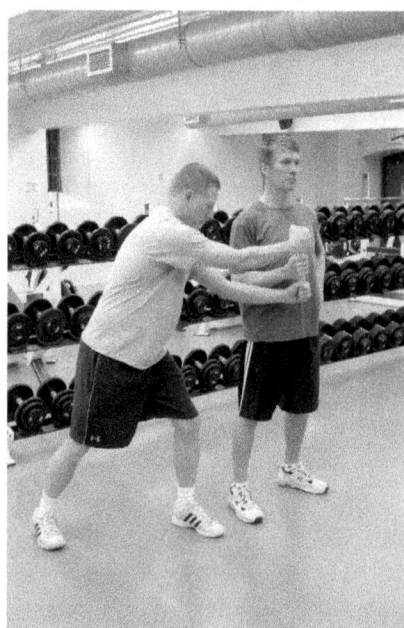

Mid-Range Position

Muscles Strengthened: internal rotators

Suggested Repetitions: 8 to 10 (or 50 to 60 seconds)

Start/Finish Position: Grasp a small stick (or similar object) with your right hand. Place your left hand on your left hip and spread your feet about shoulder-width apart. Place your right elbow against the right side of your torso and bend your right arm so that the angle between your upper and lower arms is about 90 degrees. (By doing this, your right lower arm will be approximately parallel to the floor.) Position the stick away from your mid-section. The spotter should stand alongside you and grasp the stick above and below your right hand.

Performance Description: Keeping the same angle between your upper and lower arms, pull the stick to your mid-section as the spotter applies resistance evenly throughout the full range of motion. Pause briefly in this mid-range position (your hand near your mid-section) and then resist as the spotter pulls the stick back to the start/finish position (your hand away from your mid-section). Repeat the exercise for the other side of your body.

Training Tips:

- Keep your elbow against the side of your torso and your lower arm parallel to the floor.
- Avoid rotating your torso. Movement should only occur at your shoulder joint.
- After reaching muscular fatigue, you can overload your muscles further by having the spotter bring the stick to the mid-range position and then pull it back to the start/finish position as you resist for 3 to 5 negative-only repetitions.

EXTERNAL ROTATION

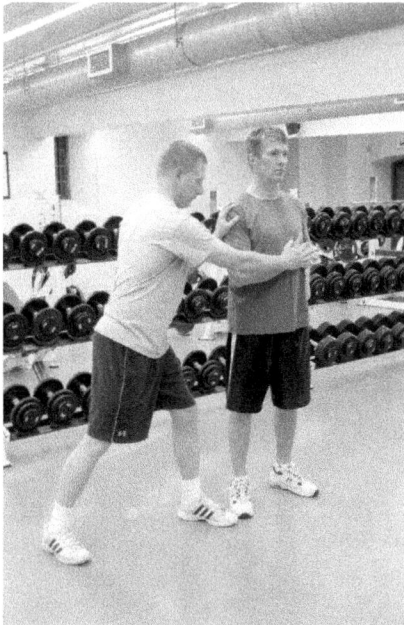

Start/Finish Position

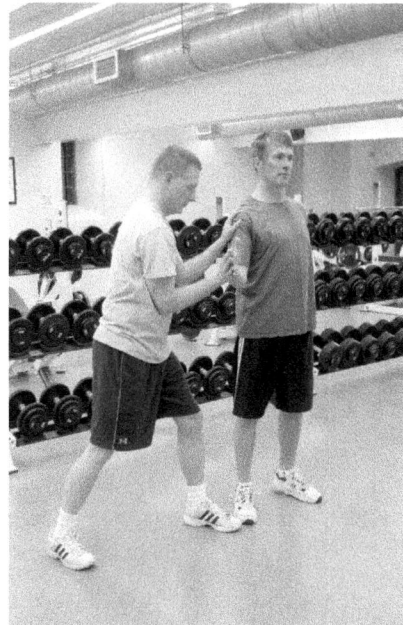

Mid-Range Position

Muscles Strengthened: external rotators

Suggested Repetitions: 8 to 10 (or 50 to 60 seconds)

Start/Finish Position: Place your left hand on your left hip and spread your feet about shoulder-width apart. Place your right elbow against the right side of your torso and bend your right arm so that the angle between your upper and lower arms is about 90 degrees. (By doing this, your right lower arm will be approximately parallel to the floor.) Position your right palm near your mid-section and open your hand (extend your fingers). The spotter should stand alongside you and apply resistance against your right wrist.

Performance Description: Keeping the same angle between your upper and lower arms, push your hand away from your mid-section as the spotter applies resistance evenly throughout the full range of motion. Pause briefly in this mid-range position (your hand away from your mid-section) and then resist as the spotter pushes your hand back to the start/finish position (your hand near your mid-section). Repeat the exercise for the other side of your body.

Training Tips:

- Keep your hand open (your fingers extended).

- Keep your elbow against the side of your torso and your lower arm parallel to the floor.

- Avoid rotating your torso. Movement should only occur at your shoulder joint.

- After reaching muscular fatigue, you can overload your muscles further by having the spotter bring your hand to the mid-range position and then push it back to the start/finish position as you resist for 3 to 5 negative-only repetitions.

BICEP CURL

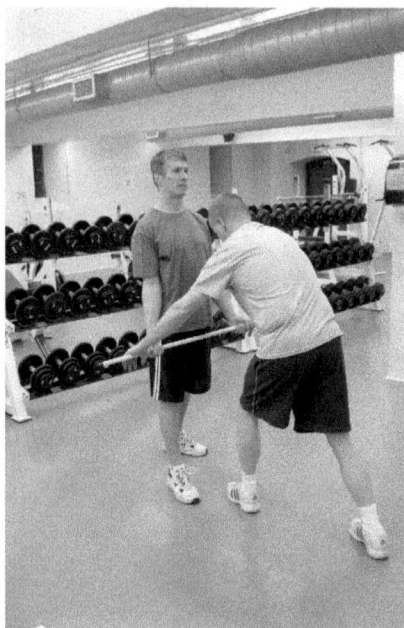

Start/Finish Position

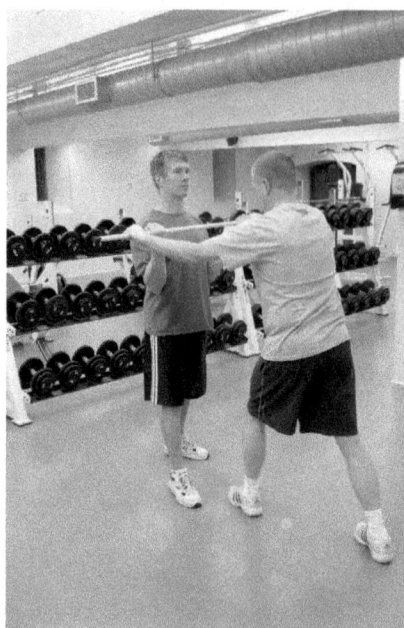

Mid-Range Position

Muscles Strengthened: biceps and forearms

Suggested Repetitions: 5 to 10 (or 30 to 60 seconds)

Start/Finish Position: Grasp a long stick (or similar object) with your hands spaced slightly wider than shoulder-width apart and your palms facing away from you. Spread your feet a comfortable distance apart with one foot slightly in front of the other. Straighten your arms. The spotter should stand in front of you and grasp the stick on the outside of your grip with palms facing down.

Performance Description: Pull the stick below your chin as the spotter applies resistance evenly throughout the full range of motion. Pause briefly in this mid-range position (your arms bent) and then resist as the spotter pulls the stick back to the start/finish position (your arms completely straight).

Training Tips:

- Keep your elbows against the sides of your torso.

- Avoid using your legs and moving your torso forward and backward. Movement should only occur at your elbow joints.

- Do this exercise with one limb at a time if you have a shoulder or an arm injury, a gross difference in the strength between your limbs or desire a training variation.

- After reaching muscular fatigue, you can overload your muscles further by having the spotter lift the stick to the mid-range position and then pull it back to the start/finish position as you resist for 3 to 5 negative-only repetitions.

- This exercise may be contraindicated if you have hyperextended elbows.

TRICEP EXTENSION

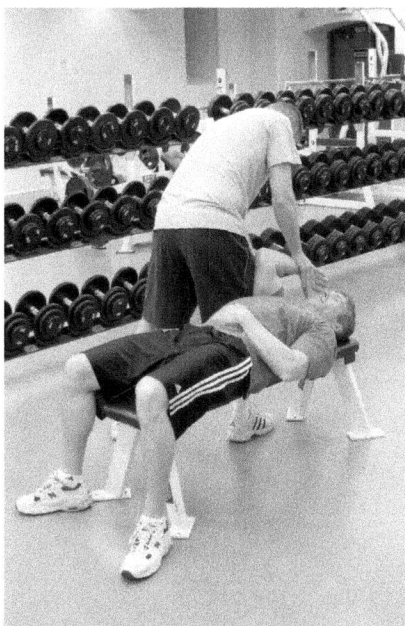

Start/Finish Position

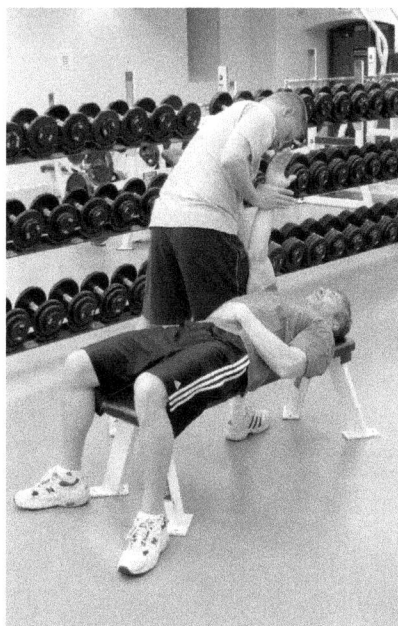

Mid-Range Position

Muscle Strengthened: triceps

Suggested Repetitions: 5 to 10 (or 30 to 60 seconds)

Start/Finish Position: Lie down on a utility bench and place your feet flat on the floor. Position the back of your right upper arm against the spotter's right thigh so that it's perpendicular to the floor and point your right elbow toward your right knee. Place your right hand near the right side of your head with your palm facing your ear and open your hand (extend your fingers). The spotter should apply resistance against your right wrist.

Performance Description: Push your hand up until your arm is almost completely straight as the spotter applies resistance evenly throughout the full range of motion. Pause briefly in this mid-range position (your arm almost completely straight) and then resist as the spotter pushes your lower arm back to the start/finish position (your arm bent). Repeat the exercise for the other side of your body.

Training Tips:

- Keep your hand open (your fingers extended).
- Keep your upper arm perpendicular to the floor and your elbow pointed toward your knee.
- Keep your hips on the bench.
- If you have low-back pain, place your feet on the end of the bench or a stool. This reduces the stress in your low-back region.
- You can also perform this exercise while sitting or standing. In both cases, keep your upper arm perpendicular to the floor and raise and lower your arm behind your head.
- After reaching muscular fatigue, you can overload your muscles further by having the spotter lift your hand to the mid-range position and then push it back to the start/finish position as you resist for 3 to 5 negative-only repetitions.

WRIST PRONATION

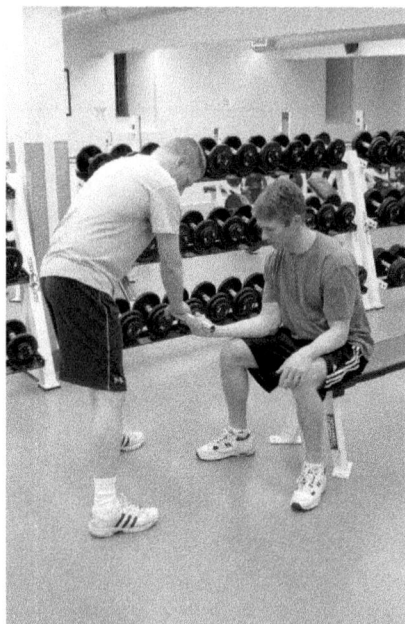

Start/Finish Position

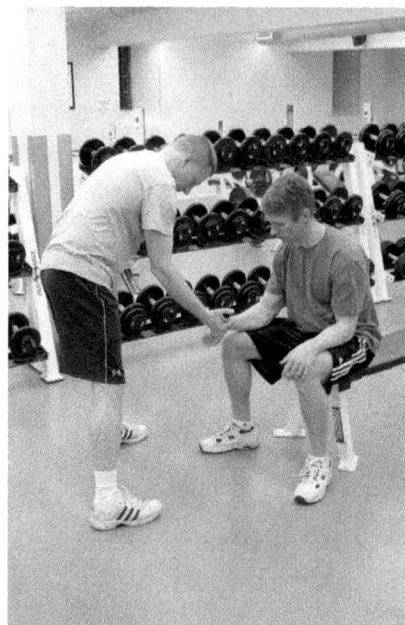

Mid-Range Position

Muscles Strengthened: wrist pronators

Suggested Repetitions: 8 to 10 (or 50 to 60 seconds)

Start/Finish Position: Grasp the end of a small stick (or similar object) with your right hand. Sit down near the end of a utility bench and place the back of your right forearm on your right upper leg so that your wrist is over your kneecap and your palm is facing up. Lean forward slightly so that the angle between your upper and lower arms is about 90 degrees or less. The spotter should stand or kneel in front of you and grasp the other end of the stick.

Performance Description: Turn your hand downward as the spotter applies resistance evenly throughout the full range of motion. Pause briefly in this mid-range position (your palm down) and then resist as the spotter pushes the stick back to the start/finish position (your palm up). Repeat the exercise for the other side of your body.

Training Tips:

- Keep your forearm on your upper leg.
- Avoid using your leg and moving your torso forward and backward. Movement should only occur at your wrist joint.
- After reaching muscular fatigue, you can overload your muscles further by having the spotter bring the stick to the mid-range position and then push it back to the start/finish position as you resist for 3 to 5 negative-only repetitions.

WRIST SUPINATION

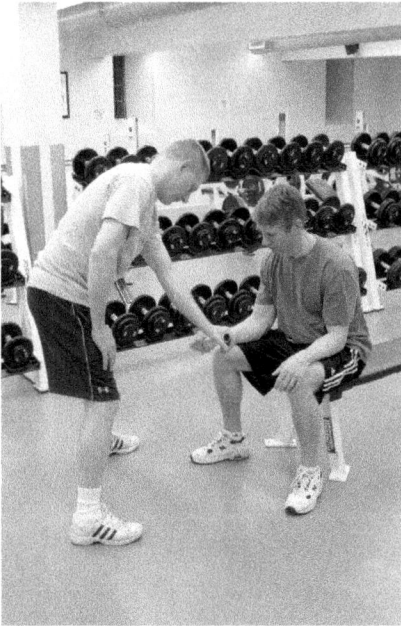

Start/Finish Position

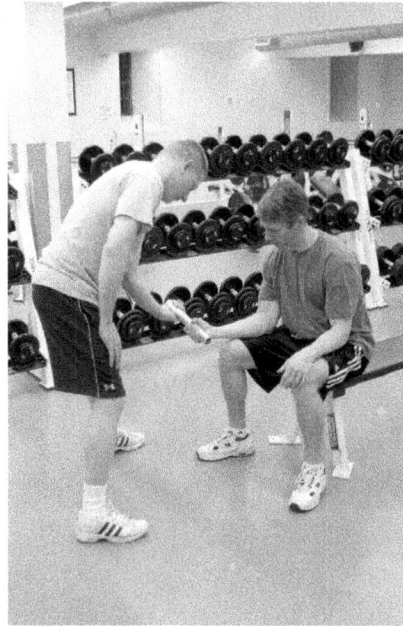

Mid-Range Position

Muscles Strengthened: wrist supinators

Suggested Repetitions: 8 to 10 (or 50 to 60 seconds)

Start/Finish Position: Grasp the end of a small stick (or similar object) with your right hand. Sit down near the end of a utility bench and place the front of your right forearm on your right upper leg so that your wrist is over your kneecap and your palm is facing down. Lean forward slightly so that the angle between your upper and lower arms is about 90 degrees or less. The spotter should stand or kneel in front of you and grasp the other end of the stick.

Performance Description: Turn your hand upward as the spotter applies resistance evenly throughout the full range of motion. Pause briefly in this mid-range position (your palm up) and then resist as the spotter pulls the stick back to the start/finish position (your palm down). Repeat the exercise for the other side of your body.

Training Tips:

- Keep your forearm on your upper leg.

- Avoid using your leg and moving your torso forward and backward. Movement should only occur at your wrist joint.

- After reaching muscular fatigue, you can overload your muscles further by having the spotter bring the stick to the mid-range position and then pull it back to the start/finish position as you resist for 3 to 5 negative-only repetitions.

185

ABDOMINAL CRUNCH

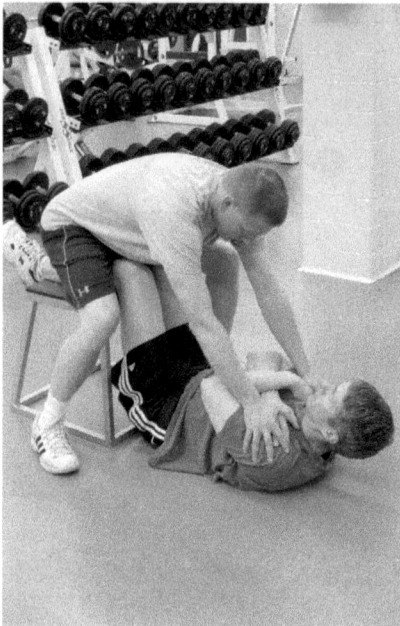

Start/Finish Position

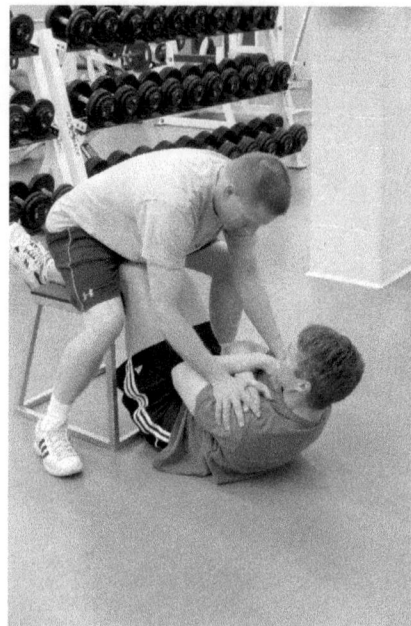

Mid-Range Position

Muscle Strengthened: rectus abdominis

Suggested Repetitions: 8 to 10 (or 50 to 60 seconds)

Start/Finish Position: Lie down on the floor and place the back of your lower legs on a utility bench (or stool). Position your upper legs so that they're perpendicular to the floor and the angle between your upper and lower legs is about 90 degrees. Fold your arms across your chest and bring your head toward your chest so that the upper portion of your shoulder blades doesn't touch the floor. The spotter should sit on your lower legs and apply resistance against the front part of your shoulders.

Performance Description: Pull your torso as close to your upper legs as possible as the spotter applies resistance evenly throughout the full range of motion. Pause briefly in this mid-range position (your torso bent) and then resist as the spotter pushes your torso back to the start/finish position (your torso straight).

Training Tips:

- Avoid touching the floor with your shoulder blades. This removes the load from your abdominals.

- Avoid snapping your head forward. Movement should only occur at your hip joint and mid-section.

- After reaching muscular fatigue, you can overload your muscles further by having the spotter lift your torso to the mid-range position and then push it back to the start/finish position as you resist for 3 to 5 negative-only repetitions.

- This exercise may be contraindicated if you have low-back pain.

NECK FLEXION

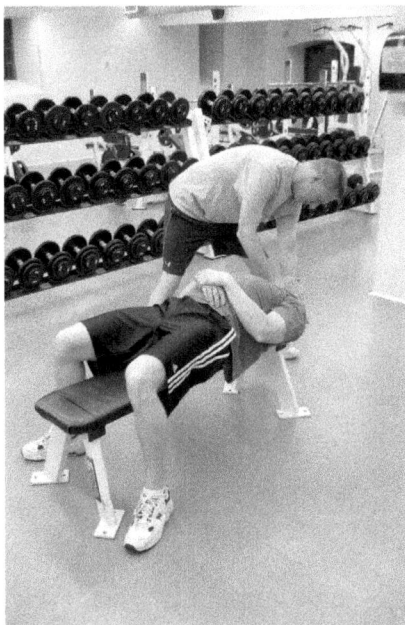

Start/Finish Position

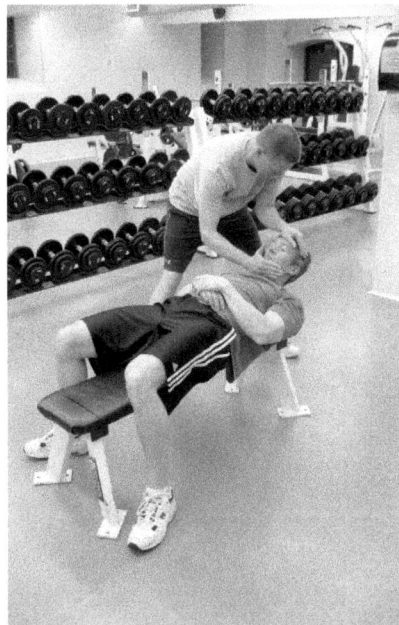

Mid-Range Position

Muscle Strengthened: sternocleidomastoideus

Suggested Repetitions: 8 to 10 (or 50 to 60 seconds)

Start/Finish Position: Lie down on a utility bench and place your feet flat on the floor. Position your head over the end of the back pad. Place your hands on your mid-section. The spotter should stand or kneel alongside your head and apply resistance against your chin with one hand and your forehead with the other.

Performance Description: Pull your head as close to your chest as possible as the spotter applies resistance evenly throughout the full range of motion. Pause briefly in this mid-range position (your chin near your chest) and then resist as the spotter pushes your head back to the start/finish position (your head hanging down).

Training Tips:

- The resistance must be applied carefully since the cervical spine is involved.
- Keep your hips and torso on the bench.
- If you have low-back pain, place your feet flat on the end of the bench or a stool. This reduces the stress in your low-back region.
- You can also perform this exercise while sitting on the floor. In this case, the spotter would sit or kneel behind you and apply resistance against your chin with one hand and your forehead with the other.
- After reaching muscular fatigue, you can overload your muscles further by having the spotter lift your head to the mid-range position and then push it back to the start/finish position as you resist for 3 to 5 negative-only repetitions.

NECK EXTENSION

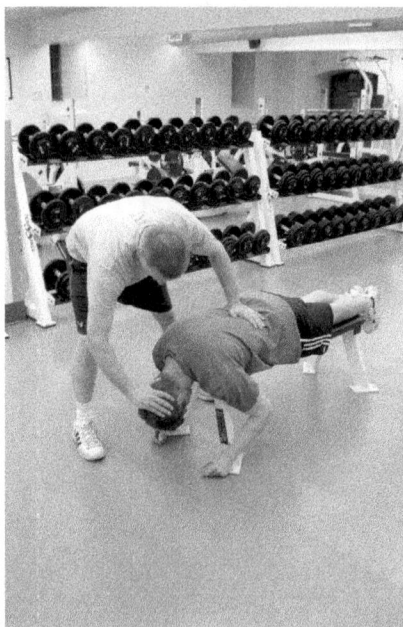

Start/Finish Position

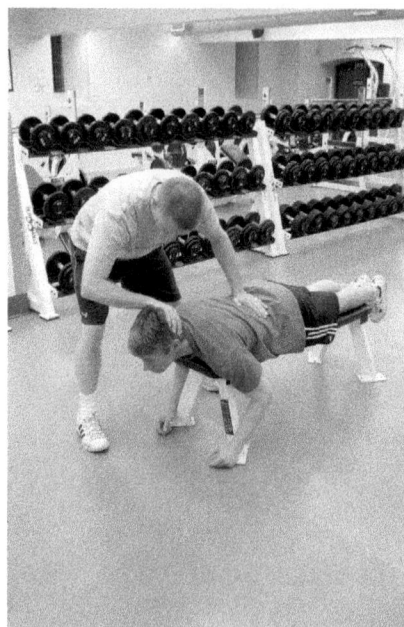

Mid-Range Position

Muscles Strengthened: neck extensors and trapezius (upper portion)

Suggested Repetitions: 8 to 10 (or 50 to 60 seconds)

Start/Finish Position: Lie face down on a utility bench and place your hands on the floor. Position your legs across the length of the back pad and your head over the end of the back pad with your chin near your chest. The spotter should stand or kneel alongside your head and apply resistance against the back of your head with one hand and your back with the other.

Performance Description: Extend your head backward as far as possible as the spotter applies resistance evenly throughout the full range of motion. Pause briefly in this mid-range position (your neck extended) and then resist as the spotter pushes your head back to the start/finish position (your chin near your chest).

Training Tips:

• The resistance must be applied carefully since the cervical spine is involved.

• Keep your torso on the bench.

• You can also perform the exercise while on your hands and knees.

• After reaching muscular fatigue, you can overload your muscles further by having the spotter lift your head to the mid-range position and then push it back to the start/finish position as you resist for 3 to 5 negative-only repetitions.

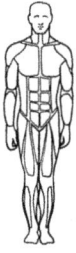

11 Designing and Varying the Strength Program

Your strength program can be designed and varied in countless ways, incorporating a wide assortment of exercises and equipment. But designing and varying the strength program involves much more than merely doing specific exercises and/or using certain equipment.

PROGRAM DESIGN

A number of elements go into program design. What follows are some things that must be considered.

The Training Week

An important aspect of program design is planning the training week. Here are several options for scheduling total-body workouts:

- Do three workouts per week on any nonconsecutive days such as Monday/Wednesday/Friday; Monday/Wednesday/Saturday; Tuesday/Thursday/Sunday; or some other combination.

- Do two workouts per week on any nonconsecutive days such as Monday/Thursday; Monday/Friday; Tuesday/Friday; Tuesday/Saturday; or some other combination. Note that the two workouts should be scheduled so that the time between them is roughly the same. If the two workouts for the week are on Monday and Thursday, for example, then an individual would have 72 hours between Monday and Thursday and 96 hours between Thursday and Monday. This is more favorable than if the two workouts for the week are on Monday and Wednesday. Here, an individual would have 48 hours between Monday and Wednesday and 120 hours between Wednesday and Monday.

- Do one workout every third day such as Monday, Thursday, Sunday, Wednesday, Saturday, Tuesday, Friday and so on. In a three-week period, then, an individual will get seven workouts: One week in which three workouts are done and two weeks in which two workouts are done.

Workouts can be performed three times per week, two times per week, every third day or with whatever scheme is most appropriate for each individual based on age, maturation, personal preferences, social situations and academic and athletic/recreational obligations. Keep in mind that all of these factors will change over time. As a result, it's not always practical to employ a rigid schedule or regular pattern of days to do strength training. The idea, though, is to implement the schedule that best meets your needs and maintains your enthusiasm while giving your body sufficient time to recover from previous workouts so as to avoid overtraining.

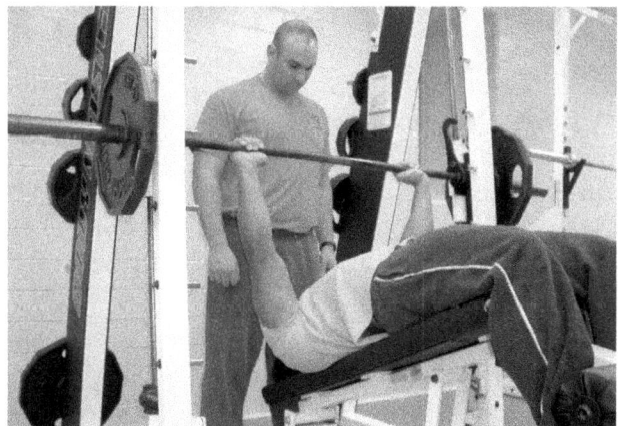

Implement the schedule that best meets your needs and maintains your enthusiasm while giving your body sufficient time to recover from previous workouts.

189

Sets and Repetitions

Two components of strength training are sets and repetitions. As noted in Chapter 4, the number of sets that are needed to increase muscular strength (and size) are debatable; and the number of repetitions that are needed to increase strength (and size) are variable. A wide assortment of "set-rep schemes" can be employed but the most common recommendation is in the range of one to three sets and 5 to 20 repetitions.

From a practical – and historical – perspective of sets and repetitions, it's interesting to revisit the contribution of Dr. Thomas DeLorme. It was mentioned in Chapter 4 that in 1944, as a physician in the US Army, Dr. DeLorme developed a protocol of "heavy resistance exercise" that he used to strengthen the muscles of soldiers who were wounded and/or injured during World War II. The protocol was 7 to 10 sets of 10 repetitions per exercise.

After the war ended, Dr. DeLorme left the Army. In 1948, while working at the Massachusetts General Hospital in Boston, he and Dr. Arthur Watkins rebooted the original protocol, scaling it back to three sets of 10 repetitions and referring to it as "progressive resistance exercise." (Fast fact: DeLorme has enjoyed a great deal of fame – among other things being dubbed the father of progressive resistance exercise – while Watkins has remained largely unknown.)

The sets that are done in the DeLorme-Watkins Protocol are based on a 10-repetition maximum (10-RM; the maximum weight that can be lifted 10 times). The first set is done with 50% of a 10-RM and the second set is done with 75% of a 10-RM. After these two "warm-up sets," the "work set" is done with 100% of a 10-RM.

For example, suppose that the most weight that you can lift for 10 repetitions is 200 pounds or 10 x 200. In this case, you'd do a set of 10 x 100 followed by a set of 10 x 150 then a set of 10 x 200.

In 1951, Dr. Andrew Zinovieff – a physician at the United Oxford Hospitals in England – developed a variation of the DeLorme-Watkins Protocol with a radical twist. Zinovieff felt that the protocol as outlined by DeLorme and Watkins produced so much fatigue that other than "in exceptional cases," it would be very difficult to perform a work set with 100% of a 10-RM after doing warm-up sets with 50% of a 10-RM and 75% of a 10-RM.

Like the DeLorme-Watkins Protocol, the three sets in the Zinovieff Protocol are based on a 10-RM. Unlike the DeLorme-Watkins Protocol – and here's the twist – the three sets are done in the reverse order. With the Zinovieff Protocol, the first set is done with 100% of a 10-RM. After this work set, the second set is done with 75% of a 10-RM and the third set is done with 50% of a 10-RM.

For example, suppose that the most weight that you can lift for 10 repetitions is 10 x 200. In this case, you'd do a set of 10 x 200 followed by a set of 10 x 150 then a set of 10 x 100.

As you can see, the Zinovieff Protocol is literally the exact opposite of the DeLorme-Watkins Protocol. The basic idea is to use as much weight as possible during the first set and then systematically reduce the weight in the sets that follow to offset the fatigue that was created during the previous efforts.

When the two protocols go toe-to-toe, which one is the winner? In one study, 50 subjects were randomly assigned to perform the leg extension using either the DeLorme-Watkins Protocol or the Zinovieff Protocol three times per week for nine weeks. The study found that both protocols produced roughly the same improvements in strength. In another study, 32 subjects were randomly assigned to perform the half squat – a partial squat – using either the DeLorme-Watkins Protocol or the Zinovieff Protocol two times per week for four weeks. This study found the same results as the other one: There was no significant difference between the two protocols.

So why the history lesson? Well, the DeLorme-Watkins Protocol – or reasonable facsimiles of the protocol – remains fairly popular more than 70 years after it was first introduced. In fact, "three sets of 10" has probably been prescribed and performed more than any other single protocol in history.

In addition, certain elements of the DeLorme-Watkins Protocol are found in other protocols, most notably those that are done in a traditional "pyramid" style. At the base of the pyramid, the first set is done with a relatively light weight for high repetitions. In ascending the pyramid, each subsequent set is done with an increased amount of weight and a decreased number of repetitions. At the top of the pyramid, the last set is done with a relatively heavy weight for low repetitions. This type of system is sometimes referred to as an ascending pyramid or pyramiding up.

An example of an ascending pyramid is 10 x 135, 8 x 185, 6 x 205 and 4 x 215.

But let's not forget about Zinovieff. Essentially, his protocol is a reverse of the ascending pyramid – think of an upside-down pyramid – and certain elements of it are found in some protocols. At the top of the pyramid, the first set is done with a relatively heavy weight – the most weight that can be handled – for a designated number of repetitions (which can range anywhere from 5 to as many as 20, depending on the exercise). In descending the pyramid, each subsequent set is done with a decreased amount of weight and number of repetitions. At the bottom of the pyramid, the last set is done with a relatively light weight for low repetitions. Usually, all sets are done to the point of muscular fatigue. This type of system is sometimes referred to as a descending pyramid or pyramiding down.

An example of a descending pyramid is 10 x 205, 8 x 165, 6 x 135 and 4 x 115.

A popular application of this system is to use a minimal amount of recovery between sets thereby making it a very time-efficient method of training. When done in this manner, it's known as drop sets, strip sets, breakdowns or burnouts.

Volume of Exercises

Recall from Chapter 4 that most people can perform a total-body workout using no more than about 14 exercises. In this case, you should do one exercise for your hips, hamstrings, quadriceps, calves/dorsi flexors, biceps, triceps,

abdominals and lower back. Since your shoulder joint permits freedom of movement at a variety of angles, you should perform two exercises for your chest, upper back and shoulders.

If you participate in a combat sport – such as football, rugby, boxing, judo and wrestling – your workout should include an additional two to four exercises for your neck to strengthen and protect your cervical area against catastrophic injury. If you participate in sports or activities that require grip strength – such as baseball, golf and tennis – you should include one exercise for your lower arms (forearms).

There's nothing inherently wrong with doing additional exercises in order to emphasize a particular muscle. But if your level of strength begins to plateau in one or more exercises, it's probably because you're overtraining: You're unable to recover from the volume of your training.

Also keep in mind that placing too much emphasis on one muscle may eventually produce abnormal development and/or create an imbalance of strength between two muscles which can predispose you to injury. For instance, too much emphasis on your chest may lead to a round-shouldered appearance; too much emphasis on your quadriceps may lead to problems with your hamstrings.

Agonists and Antagonists

At this point, it's necessary to define two terms: agonist and antagonist. An agonist is a muscle that causes movement; an antagonist is a muscle that opposes movement of the agonist. As an example, consider your biceps and triceps. Your biceps on the front of your upper arm bend (or flex) your elbow and your triceps on the back of your upper arm straighten (or extend) your elbow. When one of these muscles acts as an agonist, the other acts as an antagonist. (Note: An agonist is also referred to as a prime mover.)

In general, your muscles are arranged in pairs that have opposing positions and functions. In addition to the biceps-triceps partnership, other agonist/antagonist pairings include your hip abductors and hip adductors; hamstrings and quadriceps; calves and dorsi flexors; chest and upper back; anterior deltoid and posterior deltoid; internal rotators and external rotators; wrist flexors and wrist extensors; and abdominals and lower back.

It's important to provide agonist/antagonist muscles with an equal – or nearly equal – amount of stimulus. In doing so, you'll ensure that you're not overemphasizing one muscle or underemphasizing another; this, in turn, will reduce your risk of producing abnormal development or creating an imbalance of strength between two muscles.

One study investigated shoulder-impingement (SIS) among men who did strength training on a regular basis. Among the 55 individuals were 24 with SIS and 31 without SIS. The researchers looked at several characteristics of the shoulder, including a comparison of the strength between a pair of agonist/antagonist muscles: the internal rotators and external rotators. In the group with SIS, the strength of their external rotators was 49.3% of their internal rotators; in the group without SIS, the strength of their external rotators was 65.2% of their internal rotators. It's normal for the internal rotators to be stronger than the external rotators but in this study, those with SIS had a significantly greater difference in strength than those without SIS. It's thought that an imbalance in the strength of the internal and external rotators contributes to SIS. Unfortunately, in most strength programs, the internal rotators get overtrained and the external rotators get overlooked.

The point is that you should perform approximately the same volume of training – roughly the same number of exercises, sets and repetitions – for pairs of agonist/antagonist muscles. In short, don't emphasize a particular muscle without also addressing its antagonistic counterpart with a similar volume of training.

Types of Movements

Essentially, there are two types of movements: single joint and multiple joint. A single-joint movement (aka a simple or primary movement) involves action of one joint. A good example is a pullover in which the upper arm

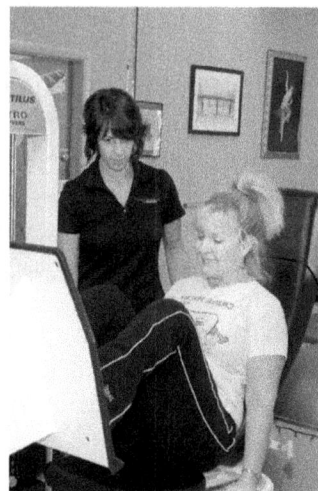

The main advantage of a multiple-joint movement is that it engages a relatively large amount of muscle mass in one exercise. (Photo by Pilar Martinez.)

moves about the shoulder joint. The main advantage of a single-joint movement is that it usually provides muscle isolation.

A multiple-joint movement (aka a compound or secondary movement) involves action of more than one joint. A good example is a lat pulldown in which the upper arm moves about the shoulder joint and the lower arm moves about the elbow joint. The main advantage of a multiple-joint movement is that it engages a relatively large amount of muscle mass in one exercise.

Whenever you do two or more exercises for a large muscle of your torso – your chest, upper back or shoulders – at least one of them should be a single-joint movement. Why is this important?

Multiple-joint movements have a distinct disadvantage, namely a "weak link." When you fatigue in a multiple-joint movement, it's because the resistance has been filtered through a smaller, weaker muscle that exhausts well before a larger, stronger muscle has received a sufficient workload. In an exercise such as the lat pulldown, your biceps are the smaller muscle – the proverbial weak link – and, therefore, will fatigue long before your upper back. In fact, your forearms might fatigue even earlier than your biceps. As a result, your biceps and forearms get an adequate workload but your upper back – which is really the target of the exercise – gets an inadequate workload. So if the exercises that you do for your torso consist entirely of multiple-joint movements, your smaller muscles would receive much more of the workload than your larger muscles.

By including single-joint and multiple-joint movements in your workout, you can obtain the benefits of both types of movements: You get the advantage of a single-joint movement in that you can isolate a large muscle without being hindered by the limited strength of a small muscle. And you get the advantage of a multiple-joint movement in that you can address a relatively large amount of muscle mass in one exercise.

It must be noted that because there's action at more than one joint, multiple-joint movements are more complex than single-join movements. This means that multiple-joint movements have a greater potential for improper technique than single-joint movements. This also means that multiple-joint movements have a greater potential for injury than single-joint movements.

Something else to consider is that multiple-joint movements don't enlist all of the muscles throughout a full range of motion. For instance, the leg press is a multiple-joint movement that involves the hips, quadriceps and hamstrings. When doing this exercise, you'll "feel" it in your hips and quadriceps but not so much in your hamstrings since the range of motion for that muscle is limited. On the other hand, a leg curl is a single-joint movement that stimulates the hamstrings over a much greater range of motion.

This doesn't mean that it would be a major mistake if you only performed multiple-joint movements for a particular muscle. Your workouts will be more efficient and productive, however, if you do a single-joint movement to offset the limitations of a multiple-joint movement.

Sidebar: It's sometimes said that single-joint movements aren't "functional." A definition of functional is useful. This would mean, then, that single-joint movements are non-functional or useless. But if you do the leg curl – a single-joint exercise – and, over time, increase the strength of your hamstrings to produce more force, aren't those muscles now more "functional" (or useful)? Similarly, it's sometimes said that machine exercises aren't "functional." But if you do the lat pulldown – a machine exercise – and, over time, increase the strength of your upper back ("lats"), biceps and forearms to produce more force, aren't those muscles now more "functional" (or useful)?

Order of Exercise

As a reminder, you should train your muscles from largest to smallest. Generally speaking, the order of exercise in a total-body workout would be hips, upper legs (hamstrings and quadriceps), lower legs (calves or dorsi flexors), torso (chest, upper back and shoulders), upper arms (biceps and triceps), abdominals and lower back.

If included, exercises for your neck should be done at the beginning of your workout or just after your lower body (prior to exercises for your torso); exercises for your lower arms (forearms) should be done just after your upper arms.

If you prefer to do a split routine – in which the body is divided or split into parts that are trained over the course of several workouts instead of one total-body workout – the aforementioned order of exercise would still apply. In a workout that targeted your chest, shoulders and triceps, for example, you should still address those body parts from largest to smallest.

Exercise Options

Summaries of exercises that can be done with free weights (barbells and dumbbells), machines (selectorized and plate-loaded) and manual resistance appear in Appendices A, B and C, respectively. Naturally, your exercise options are based on the available equipment.

Given the wide assortment of exercise options, the design of a workout can have almost an infinite number of possibilities. The only limits are the equipment and your imagination.

PROGRAM VARIATION

At some point in your strength training, you'll reach a plateau in your performance. Quite often, this is a result of overtraining. In this case, your volume of training is so great that your musculoskeletal system is overstressed (or overworked). In effect, the demands that you've placed on your muscles have exceeded your ability to recover. Here, you simply need to reduce your volume of training (in terms of the number of workouts, exercises and/or sets).

Sometimes, however, your performance will plateau because you're doing the same thing over and over again for lengthy periods of time. In this case, your strength program has become a form of unproductive manual labor that's monotonous, dull and unchallenging.

Simply checking your records will reveal if you've reached a plateau. You should review your records carefully, however. If you think that you've plateaued in a certain exercise, you must consider your performance in earlier exercises of that workout. For instance, suppose that you did 10 repetitions with 120 pounds on the leg extension for five consecutive workouts. At first glance, it may not seem as if your quadriceps have gotten any stronger. But what if the resistance that you used on the leg press increased from 250 pounds to 275 pounds during those same five workouts? This means that the load on your hips, hamstrings and quadriceps increased by 10% or an average of 2% per workout. In other words, your quadriceps were increasingly more pre-fatigued by the leg press in your workouts each time prior to performing the leg extension. If true, there's little doubt that your quadriceps did get stronger. In fact, simply being able to duplicate your past performances on the leg extension would actually be quite a feat, although that wouldn't be readily apparent. Similarly, if the resistance that you used on the bicep curl plateaus, it could be because your biceps are being exposed to increasingly heavier loads earlier in your workout when you do multiple-joint movements for your torso such as the lat pulldown, seated row or upright row. So, you must examine your entire workout in order to determine whether or not you have indeed reached a plateau.

Keep in mind that unless you're a beginner, you won't be able to improve your performance in every exercise from one workout to the next. Be that as it may, you should observe gradual improvements in your performance over the

course of several weeks. If you fail to make a progression in an exercise by this time – in the amount of resistance and/or the number of repetitions – you should vary some aspect of your strength program.

There are several ways that this may be accomplished. In general, you can vary three main components of your strength program: your workouts, exercises and sets/repetitions.

Varying Workouts

There are a number of ways that you can vary your workouts. For instance, you can change your workouts on a daily basis by doing different workouts on different days such as Workout A on Monday, Workout B on Wednesday and Workout C on Friday. You can also change your workouts on a weekly or monthly basis. Or you can simply change them as needed.

Regardless, the idea is to vary your workouts on a fairly regular basis. Some strength coaches have many different workouts for their athletes with varying themes. For example, the athletes might be assigned to do barbell-only, dumbbell-only, iso-lateral, "no-hands," push-pull, pre-exhaustion or negative-only workouts. (Fast fact: In 1969, Boyd Epley became the first full-time strength coach in history when he was hired by the University of Nebraska.)

Varying Exercises

You have three basic options available to vary your exercises: Specifically, you can rearrange the order, change the equipment and alternate the exercises.

Rearrange the Order

One of the easiest ways that you can integrate variety into your training is to rearrange the order in which you do exercises for a particular muscle. Suppose, for example, that you desire a change in the way that you train your chest. If you've been doing the bench press followed by the bent-arm fly, you can add variety by simply switching the two exercises. In other words, you can perform the bent-arm fly first and the bench press second.

Be aware that whenever you change the order in which you do exercises, you must adjust the levels of resistance. So if you do the bent-arm fly first (instead of second), your chest and shoulders will be fresh and, therefore, you should increase the resistance in that exercise. And if you do the bench press second (instead of first), your chest and shoulders will be fatigued and, therefore, you must decrease the resistance in that exercise.

An additional possibility is to rearrange the order in which you train your muscles. Rather than go from chest to upper back to shoulders, you might start with shoulders, proceed to upper back and then finish with chest. So a six-exercise sequence for your torso of bench press, bent-arm fly, seated row, pullover, shoulder press and shoulder shrug could be changed to shoulder shrug, shoulder press, pullover, seated row, bent-arm fly and bench press. In fact, these six exercises alone could be rearranged for 720 different sequences. [Six exercises can be placed in six different ordered positions. The first exercise that's chosen can be put in six possible spots, the second exercise can be put in one of the five remaining spots, the third exercise can be put in one of the four remaining spots and so on. Therefore, the total number of possible arrangements for six exercises is 6 x 5 x 4 x 3 x 2 x 1 = 720.] Once again, remember that you'll need to adjust the levels of resistance any time that you rearrange the order of exercises.

Change the Equipment

Another way that you can vary the exercises is to change the equipment that you use. Say that you've been doing the bicep curl with a barbell for quite some time and, consequently, desire a change of pace. In this situation, you can perform a bicep curl with another type of equipment such as dumbbells, machines (selectorized or plate-loaded) or manual resistance. There's even variety within selectorized machines since some have one dependent movement arm while others have two independent movement arms (meaning that they function separately). Obviously, the extent to which you can change the equipment depends on what's available.

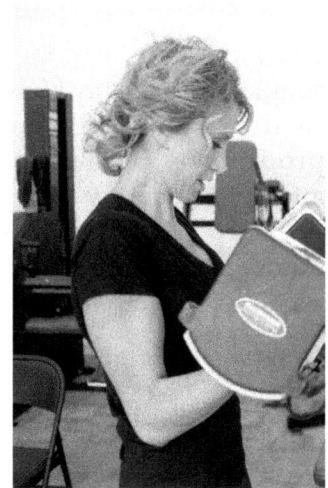

A change of pace from a bicep curl with a barbell is to do the exercise with another type of equipment such as dumbbells, machines or manual resistance. (Photo provided by Luke Carlson.)

Alternate the Exercises

A third means of varying exercises is to alternate them with other ones that employ the same muscles. Consider this: The seated row is a multiple-joint movement that engages your upper back, biceps and forearms. And so do other multiple-joint movements that involve rowing, chinning and pulling. This includes the bench row, bent-over row, chin-up, pull-up, underhand lat pulldown and overhand lat pulldown. Therefore, any of these exercises are potential substitutes for the seated row. Once again, the availability of equipment will determine how much you can alternate the exercises.

Besides providing for variety, periodically alternating your exercises (and/or equipment) has another advantage: It allows you to train your muscles through different ranges of motion. In this way, you can target your muscles in a more complete and comprehensive manner.

Varying Sets/Repetitions

A final component of your strength program that you can vary is the way that you do a set which essentially is the way that you do a repetition. Ordinarily, repetitions are done in a bilateral manner, meaning with both limbs at the same time. But you can do at least six other variations, including negative-only, negative-accentuated, duosymmetric-polycontractile, unilateral, modified-cadence and extended-pause repetitions.

A few words of caution: Although the ensuing ways of varying a repetition may sound simple, a reasonably high level of skill is required to do them in a manner that's safe and productive. Because of this, you shouldn't attempt to employ these advanced applications in your strength program until you can demonstrate proper technique when you do repetitions in a bilateral fashion.

Negative-Only Repetitions

You can perform repetitions in a negative-only manner by having a partner raise the resistance and you lower it. Essentially, the partner does the positive (or concentric) work and the lifter does the negative (or eccentric) work. To illustrate, here's how you'd do negative-only repetitions on the leg curl: With no help from you, your partner brings the movement arm to the mid-range position (your heels near your hips). Then, your partner releases the movement arm and you slowly lower the resistance to the start/finish position (your legs straight). Repeat the procedure for the desired number of repetitions.

As noted in Chapter 4, your eccentric strength is always greater than your concentric strength in the same exercise. In other words, you can always lower more weight than you can raise (again, in the same exercise). This means that you can use more resistance for repetitions that are done in a negative-only manner than you can for repetitions that are done in a traditional manner. How much more? As a starting point, use about 10% more resistance than you normally handle when doing traditional repetitions. So if you most recently used 100 pounds on an exercise, start with about 110 pounds for a set of negative-only repetitions. When you attain the maximum number of negative-only repetitions, you should increase the resistance for your next workout.

To achieve the best results, negative-only repetitions should be done slowly. In general, each negative-only repetition should be performed in about six to eight seconds, depending on the range of motion. (An exercise with a large range of motion should take longer to complete than an exercise with a short one.) Chapter 4 discusses appropriate time frames for training your muscles in the anaerobic domain. For most of the population, this is about 90 to 120 seconds for a hip exercise, 60 to 90 seconds for a leg exercise and 30 to 60 seconds for a torso exercise. Based on these windows of time, then, an eight-second negative-only repetition would translate into repetition ranges of about 11 to 15 for the hips, 8 to 11 for the legs and 4 to 8 for the torso.

Performing negative-only repetitions is extremely demanding. For this reason, they shouldn't be done in any given exercise more than once per week.

Negative-Accentuated Repetitions

The major disadvantage of negative-only repetitions is that at least one other person is almost always required to lift the weight. For the most part, you can do negative-only repetitions without needing help from someone else in a handful of exercises that involve your bodyweight as resistance such as push-ups, dips, chin-ups, pull-ups and abdominal crunches. As an example, you can do negative-only chin-ups by stepping or climbing up to the mid-range position (your arms bent) and lowering your body under control to the start/finish position (your arms completely straight). Stated otherwise, your lower body does the positive work and your upper body does the negative work.

The value of negative-accentuated repetitions is that they emphasize the eccentric component of an exercise yet they can be performed without any assistance from another individual. When doing negative-accentuated repetitions, the positive work is shared by both limbs but the negative work is done by only one limb. In other words, the resistance is raised with both arms or legs and then lowered with only one arm or leg. As a result, the resistance is literally twice as much during the negative phase as it is during the positive phase.

Although it's impossible to perform negative-accentuated repetitions with a barbell, most machines permit you to do so. For instance, you'd perform negative-accentuated repetitions on the leg extension as follows: Using both legs, raise the resistance to the mid-range position (your legs completely straight) and pause briefly. Move your left leg away from the roller pad and hold the resistance momentarily with your right leg. Lower the resistance slowly and steadily to the start/finish position (your leg bent) with your right leg. Raise the resistance to the mid-range position with both legs and continue the preceding sequence using your left leg to lower the resistance. Repeat the procedure for the desired number of repetitions.

Similar to negative-only repetitions, each negative-accentuated repetition should be performed in about six to eight seconds. As a starting point, use about 70% of the resistance that you normally handle when doing traditional repetitions. So if you most recently used 100 pounds on an exercise, start with about 70 pounds for a set of negative-accentuated repetitions. In the case of negative-accentuated exercise, appropriate repetition ranges for most of the population are about 15 to 20 for the hips, 10 to 15 for the legs and 5 to 10 for the torso. (Note that these are the total repetitions for *both* limbs, not the total repetitions for *each* limb.)

One final point: It's important that you maintain a stable position when doing negative-accentuated repetitions. In particular, avoid twisting or turning your torso to safeguard your lower back.

Duosymmetric-Polycontractile Repetitions

The term duosymmetric-polycontractile – or duo-poly, for short – was first introduced in the mid-1970s as a style of performing repetitions with machines that had independent movement arms, something that was fairly unique at the time. Nowadays, many machines are available with independent movement arms thereby giving you the option of executing duo-poly repetitions.

If you have access to a bicep-curl machine with independent movement arms, you can perform duo-poly repetitions in this manner: Using both arms, raise the resistance to the mid-range position (your arms bent) and pause briefly. Lower the resistance to the start/finish position (your arm completely straight) with your right

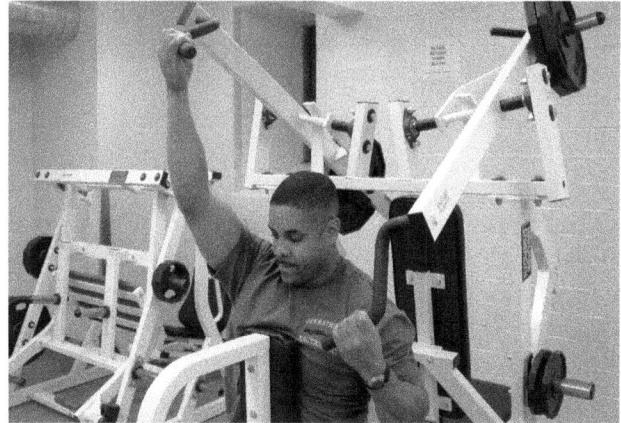

Besides making the exercise more intense, unilateral repetitions are advisable for those who have a strength imbalance between one side of their body and the other. (Photo by Peter Silletti.)

arm while keeping your left arm in the mid-range position. Raise the resistance to the mid-range position with your right arm and pause briefly. Lower the resistance to the start/finish position with your left arm while keeping your right arm in the mid-range position. Repeat the procedure for the desired number of repetitions. Incidentally, you can also perform duo-poly repetitions for your biceps with dumbbells in the manner described here.

Unilateral Repetitions

As a variation in the repetition style, many exercises can be done in a unilateral manner, meaning with one limb at a time. Dr. Ken Leistner – who has been a recognized and respected authority on strength training since the mid-1970s – states, "One-limb work is effective because, in almost all cases, it is more intense than the same exercise done with two limbs working simultaneously."

Besides making the exercise more intense, unilateral repetitions are advisable for those who have a strength imbalance between one side of their body and the other. Unilateral repetitions are also recommended for individuals with hypertension since it dampens the blood-pressure response that's associated with strength training.

Machines that are equipped with independent movement arms allow you to do unilateral repetitions. In addition, you can do unilateral repetitions with dumbbells and manual resistance.

Modified-Cadence Repetitions

Another option is to vary the cadence or speed with which you normally perform your repetitions. One cadence that continues to receive a considerable amount of attention is the SuperSlow® Protocol which was introduced by Ken Hutchins in the early 1980s. The basic cadence for SuperSlow® repetitions is to raise the resistance in 10 seconds and lower it in 5 seconds. (In shorthand, this would be written as a 10/5 speed with the first digit indicating the number of seconds to do the positive phase and the second digit indicating the number of seconds to do the negative phase.)

Effective variations of repetition speed include 4/4, 2/8, 8/8 and 10/10. A single set consisting of one 30/30 repetition can also be done; in other words, one repetition that takes 60 seconds to complete with 30 seconds allotted for the positive phase and 30 seconds for the negative phase. Keep in mind that you'll need to adjust your repetition ranges any time that you modify the duration of a repetition.

Extended-Pause Repetitions

As pointed out in Chapter 4, it's important to pause briefly in the mid-range position of each repetition. There are at least three reasons for emphasizing the mid-range position. First, it enables you to strengthen an otherwise weak position in your range of motion. Second, it allows you to focus your attention on your muscles when they're fully contracted. Third, it permits a smooth transition between the raising and lowering of the weight thereby helping to reduce the influence of momentum.

As a repetition variation, the brief pause in the mid-range position can be done for a slightly longer duration, perhaps in three or four seconds. Using this technique is also an excellent tool to employ with beginners in the initial stages of training in order for them to understand the concept and value of pausing in the mid-range position. Once again, remember that you'll need to adjust your repetition ranges any time that you modify the duration of a repetition.

Note that an extended pause in the mid-range position essentially involves a mild isometric contraction that tends to elevate blood pressure beyond that which is normally encountered in strength training. As such, individuals who have hypertension shouldn't employ this technique.

PRACTICAL APPLICATIONS

Based on the information contained here and in Chapter 4, three sample total-body workouts are shown in Figure 11.1; a sample two-day split routine is shown in Figure 11.2. These sample workouts will give you some ideas for designing and varying your strength program.

How often should a strength program be varied? For the most part, this depends on the individual. But in general, people who are just initiating a strength program or haven't been doing one for too long probably won't require much variety; early on, the program is still too novel to be monotonous or dull. Those who are more experienced will need to vary their strength program in some way on a regular basis.

Figure 11.1: Sample total-body workouts

WORKOUT A	**WORKOUT B**	**WORKOUT C**
Neck Flexion (MR)	Neck Lateral Flexion/R (SM)	Neck Extension (SM)
Neck Extension (MR)	Neck Lateral Flexion/L (SM)	Neck Flexion (MR)
Leg Press (PM)	Hip Adduction (SM)	Hip Abduction (MR)
Prone Leg Curl (SM)	Seated Leg Curl (SM)	Prone Leg Curl (PM)
Leg Extension (MR)	Leg Extension (SM)	Leg Extension (PM)
Standing Calf Raise (DB)	Dorsi Flexion (MR)	Seated Calf Raise (PM)
Dip (BW)	Bent-Arm Fly (DB)	Incline Press (BB)
Bent-Arm Fly (MR)	Bench Press (BB)	Pec Fly (SM)
Chin-Up (BW)	Pullover (EZ)	Bent-Over Row (DB)
Pullover (PM)	Seated Row (PM)	Pullover (DB)
Shoulder Press (BB)	Internal Rotation (MR)	Shoulder Shrug (TB)
Lateral Raise (SM)	External Rotation (MR)	Upright Row (BB)
Bicep Curl (MR)	Bicep Curl (EZ)	Tricep Extension (MR)
Tricep Extension (CC)	Tricep Extension (DB)	Bicep Curl (DB)
Wrist Flexion (BB)	Wrist Extension (DB)	Wrist Flexion (DB)
Side Bend (DB)	Abdominal Crunch (MR)	Torso Rotation (SM)
Back Extension (BW)	Back Extension (SM)	Back Extension (BW)

Equipment Codes: BB = Barbell; BW = Bodyweight; CC = Cable Column; DB = Dumbbells; EZ = EZ Curl Bar; MR = Manual Resistance; PM = Plate-Loaded Machine; SM = Selectorized Machine; TB = Trap Bar

199

Figure 11.2: Sample two-day split routine

WORKOUT A	WORKOUT B
Deadlift (TB)	Neck Flexion (MR)
Seated Leg Curl (PM)	Neck Extension (PM)
Leg Extension (SM)	Chest Press (SM)
Calf Extension (SM)	Bent-Arm Fly (DB)
Pullover (PM)	Shoulder Press (BB)
Pull-Up (BW)	Bent-Over Raise (MR)
Bicep Curl (CC)	Tricep Extension (EZ)
Wrist Flexion (BB)	Torso Rotation (SM)
	Back Extension (SM)

Equipment Codes: BB = Barbell; BW = Bodyweight; CC = Cable Column; DB = Dumbbells; EZ = EZ Curl Bar; MR = Manual Resistance; PM = Plate-Loaded Machine; SM = Selectorized Machine; TB = Trap Bar

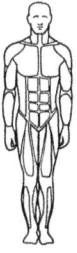

12 Rehabilitative Training

Injuries are an unforeseen, inevitable and unfortunate fact of life. In spite of how much you prepare, many injuries are purely the result of being in the wrong place at the wrong time.

In general, injuries can be either traumatic or non-traumatic. Traumatic injuries are more serious and severe such as fractures of bones and tears of muscle or connective tissue. Quite often, these types of injuries require surgical intervention. On the other hand, non-traumatic injuries are less serious and severe such as tendinitis and bursitis. Sometimes, these types of injuries simply result from overuse. No matter what kind of injury, it's important for you to consult with a qualified sportsmedical specialist such as an orthopedic physician, physical therapist or athletic trainer.

In many instances, an individual who suffers an injury ends up eliminating all forms of physical training, including those that involve uninjured body parts. Yet, it's extremely important to continue some type of physical training whenever possible even in the event of an injury.

According to many authorities, a muscle begins to lose strength (and size) if it doesn't receive an adequate amount of stimulation within about 96 hours of a previous workout. There's some anecdotal evidence suggesting that it may be a bit longer than this time frame, at least for some individuals. But it's clear that a loss of strength (and size) will occur after some period of extended inactivity. Moreover, the rate of strength loss is most rapid during the first few weeks. Because of this, rehabilitative training can prevent a significant loss of not only strength (and size) but also aerobic, anaerobic and metabolic fitness. This, of course, is provided that the training can be done in a pain-free – or nearly pain-free – manner.

Regardless of whether the injury is traumatic or non-traumatic, it will have some degree of impact on your physical training; some injuries – especially those that are traumatic – might not permit any physical training whatsoever. Nevertheless, you can often train parts of your body that aren't related to the afflicted area. And in many cases, you may even be able to address the injured body part directly.

PRUDENT METHODS

There are a number of different options and adjustments that you can use to continue training an injured area or body part in a safe, sensible and pain-free manner. It should be noted that these methods aren't intended for those injuries that are viewed as being very serious or extremely painful. As such, you should receive approval from a qualified sportsmedical specialist before initiating any prescription for rehabilitative training.

You can perform rehabilitative training by applying these 10 prudent methods:

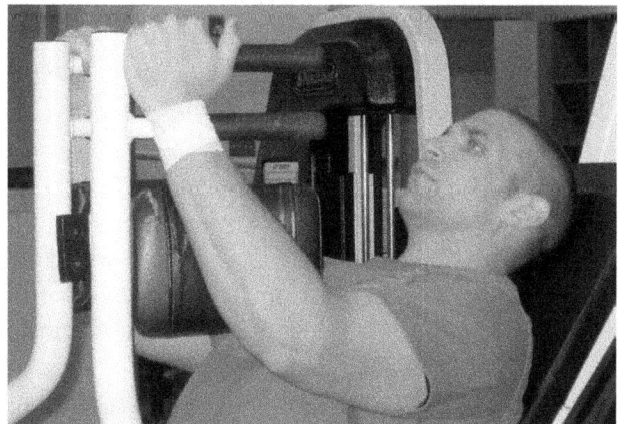

It's extremely important to continue some type of physical training whenever possible even in the event of an injury.

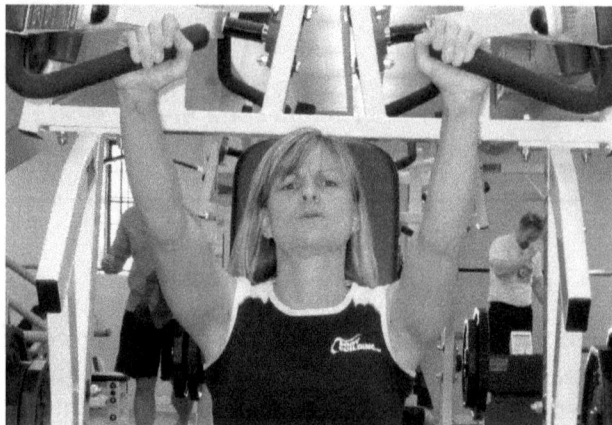

If you want to continue training an injured body part, your first step is to decrease the weight that you normally use in exercises that involve the afflicted area.

1. Decrease the weight.

If you want to continue training an injured body part, your first step is to decrease the weight that you normally use in exercises that involve the afflicted area. This is usually the easiest and most straightforward recommendation. Suppose that you have a knee injury and, as a result, you experience pain in your patellar tendon when doing the leg extension with your usual level of resistance. Decreasing the weight will place less stress on the tendon and perhaps allow you to perform the exercise in a pain-free – or nearly pain-free – manner. The amount that you decrease the weight depends on the extent and nature of your injury.

2. Slow the speed of movement.

Often done in conjunction with decreasing the weight for an exercise is using a slower speed of movement. Slowing the repetition speed decreases the orthopedic stress that's placed on a given joint.

As the injury heals, you can gradually return to your preferred speed of movement. Then again, you may find that the slower speed of movement is more appealing and continue using it after you complete your rehabilitative training. Or perhaps you might even adopt the slower speed of movement to train other body parts that aren't injured. Incidentally, slowing down the speed of movement also requires using a reduced amount of weight thereby lowering the orthopedic stress even further.

3. Change the exercise angle.

If pain persists during certain exercises that involve an injured body part, it may be possible for you to change the angle of the exercise. This essentially alters – and restricts – the angle through which your limb is moved.

You can use this option with many exercises for your torso, particularly those that involve your shoulder joint. This is especially important because the mobility and instability of the shoulder make it highly prone to injury. In fact, one of the most frequently injured body parts is the shoulder. A common problem in this joint is known as shoulder-impingement syndrome, a general term used to describe pain that's often characterized as tightness or pinching in the shoulder.

Suppose that you have slight shoulder impingement when doing the bench press. In some cases, changing the angle of the exercise from supine (flat) to decline – in other words, switching from the bench press to the decline press – will produce significantly less orthopedic stress on your shoulder joint.

Likewise, some people experience pain due to shoulder impingement when moving the bar behind their head/neck during the shoulder press and overhand lat pulldown. Generally speaking, the discomfort in both of these exercises can be lessened considerably by changing the angle of the push and pull. This can be done by performing the exercises with the bar traveling in front of the head/neck rather than behind the head/neck.

This option has limited – though useful – applications for aerobic and anaerobic training. If you have low-back pain, for example, you can pedal a cycle in a recumbent position rather than an upright one. The angle of the seat places the torso in a position that decreases the amount of stress in the lower back. (And the seat itself provides support for the lower back which also decreases the stress.)

4. Use a different grip or hand position.

Many times, there's less orthopedic stress when you use a different grip or hand position. Once again, this is extremely relevant when addressing the shoulder joint. If you have a slight pain in your shoulder when doing an exercise such as the bench press, it's quite possible that there will be a significant reduction in pain by simply changing the position of your hands from that used with a barbell to a parallel grip (palms facing each other) with dumbbells. In exercises for your torso, changing the position of your hands in this way causes the head of your humerus (your upper-arm bone) to rotate laterally which may relieve the stress in your shoulder joint.

As noted in Chapter 8, every exercise that can be performed with a barbell can also be performed with dumbbells. These exercises include the bench press, incline press, decline press, shoulder press, upright row, shoulder shrug, bicep curl, tricep extension, wrist flexion and stiff-leg deadlift. As such, you have an option for varying the position of your hands in exercises for just about every major muscle in your torso. Additionally, some machines offer more than one grip/hand position.

5. Perform different exercises.

Yet another option for rehabilitative training is to perform different exercises that require the same muscle groups. For instance, if you simply can't perform any type of lat pulldown without experiencing shoulder pain or discomfort then perhaps you can employ another exercise that addresses the same muscles albeit in a pain-free manner. In this situation, a seated row or bench row can be substituted for the lat pulldown. Both of these exercises involve the same major muscles, namely your upper back, biceps and forearms.

This guideline can also be applied to aerobic and anaerobic training. If you can't run due to a sprained ankle, for example, you may be able to perform aerobic and anaerobic training with a non-weightbearing activity such as an upright or a recumbent cycle.

6. Bypass the injured area.

Some exercises with machines and manual resistance allow you to apply the resistance above a joint so that it doesn't involve an injured area. Presume that you sprained your wrist and, consequently, exercises for your torso are difficult or uncomfortable – if not impossible – to perform with barbells and dumbbells. In this case, however, you could still use machines and manual resistance to perform a variety of exercises that target the major muscles of your torso without involving your wrist joint. Machine exercises that bypass the wrist area include the pec fly (aka the chest fly), pullover and lateral raise; manual-resistance exercises that bypass the wrist area include the bent-arm fly, front raise, lateral raise and bent-over raise. Actually, you could still perform the aforementioned exercises and others with machines and manual resistance even if your wrist was immobilized in a cast.

Also consider this: If you ruptured your patellar tendon or medial collateral ligament and your leg was placed in a knee immobilizer, it wouldn't be possible for you to perform any multiple-joint movements that address your hips such as the deadlift or leg press. It would be possible, however, to avoid your knee joint and train your hips in a safe and effective fashion – despite the immobilizer – by doing a single-joint movement with machines or manual resistance such as hip abduction or hip adduction.

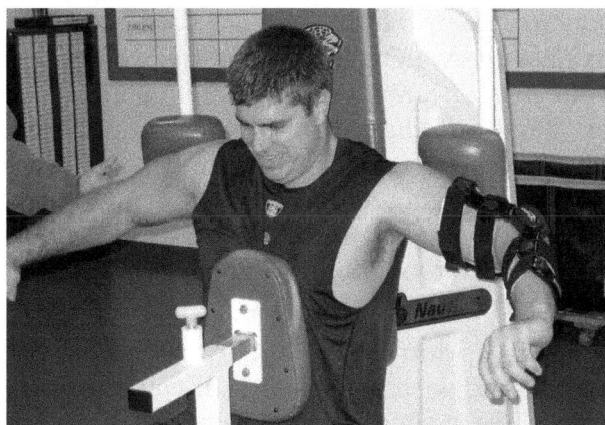

Some exercises with machines and manual resistance allow you to apply the resistance above a joint so that it doesn't involve an injured area. (Photo provided by Mark Asanovich.)

7. Limit the range of motion.

There's a good possibility that pain only occurs at certain points in your range of motion (ROM) such as the start/finish position or mid-range position of the repetition. In either case, you can restrict your ROM for the exercise. For example, an injury such as a hyperextended elbow is especially painful in the start/finish position of the bicep curl. In this instance, you should stop short of completely straightening your arms; by the same token, if pain occurs in the mid-range position of the bicep curl, you should stop short of completely bending your arms. As the injured area heals over a period of time, you can gradually and carefully increase your ROM until it's possible for you to perform repetitions that are pain-free throughout a full ROM.

Nowadays, many machines offer range-limiting devices. This enables you to restrict your ROM in a precise, repeatable manner. As a matter of fact, the ROM can sometimes be adjusted in fractional increments without exiting the machine. By the way, it's a good idea to document your ROM (as well as the resistance and repetitions) during rehabilitative training in order to monitor your progress.

Sometimes, your pain-free ROM may be restricted to a specific joint angle plus or minus a few degrees. In this case, you can perform an isometric contraction of varying durations to train your muscles at pain-free positions. One way to accomplish this is to use your good limb to raise the weight to the pain-free position of your injured limb. At this point, you'd transfer or "hand off" the weight to your injured limb. Then, you'd exert force against this resistance without changing the angle of your injured limb. You can also exert force isometrically against another person who's applying manual resistance.

This option can be incorporated during aerobic and anaerobic training. If you have knee pain while cycling, you can lower the height of the seat thereby reducing the ROM of your knee joint.

8. Exercise the good limb.

If all else fails, you can still train your unaffected limb. Here's an example: Suppose that you had shoulder surgery and, as a result, your right arm was placed in a sling. Obviously, the sling wouldn't allow you to perform any exercises that involved any ROM whatsoever for the right side of your torso. Even so, you could do exercises for the left side of your torso.

This is of great importance to the rehabilitative process because many studies have shown that training a muscle on one side of the body has some effect on the contralateral muscle (the same muscle on the opposite side of the body). This phenomenon – which first came to light way back in 1894 – has been referred to by several different names, including bilateral transfer, cross education and cross transfer.

Although the effect is small, the effect is real. A review and meta-analysis of 13 studies and updated findings of another three studies examined the contralateral effect. After pooling the data of these 16 studies, the researchers determined that strength in the untrained limb improved by an average of 7.6%.

Just how well this bodes for rehabilitative training was graphically demonstrated in a rather novel study. In the study, two groups of subjects had their non-dominant wrist, thumb and hand immobilized in a fiberglass cast for a period of 21 days. During that time, one group trained their dominant (non-casted) arm five days per week and the other group did not. The group that didn't train their non-casted arm showed a 14.7% decrease in the strength of their casted arm. Meanwhile, the group that trained their non-casted arm showed a 2.2% increase in the strength of their casted arm (as well as a 23.8% increase in the strength of their non-casted arm). In addition, the group that didn't train their non-casted arm had a 4.3% decrease in the size of their casted arm. Meanwhile, the group that trained their non-casted arm had a 1.1% decrease in the size of their casted arm (as well as a 2.9% increase in the size of their non-casted arm).

In summary, those who trained their non-casted arm experienced an increase in strength in their casted (untrained) arm and a smaller decrease in size in their casted arm compared to those who didn't train their non-casted arm.

Researchers have explored a number of possible mechanisms – muscular, neural, spinal cord, cortical and subcortical – but don't know the exact reason why the contralateral effect occurs. For instance, support for a muscular mechanism comes from studies that have found some degree of muscle activity in the untrained limb; and support for a neural mechanism comes from studies that have found a significant increase in strength without a significant increase in size. Actually, the collective efforts of two or more mechanisms may be responsible for this phenomenon.

Machines with independent movement arms enable you to do unilateral training – exercising one limb at a time – in a safe and comfortable fashion. You can also use dumbbells and manual resistance for unilateral training.

9. Exercise unaffected body parts.

In the event that you can't train an injured area due to an unreasonable amount of pain or discomfort, you can still perform exercises for your uninjured body parts. So, if you have a hip or knee injury that doesn't allow you to do any exercises for your lower body, you can train your entire torso (provided that the exercises are done while you're sitting or lying and not standing). Likewise, if you have a dislocated shoulder or a torn rotator cuff that doesn't allow you to do any exercises for your torso, you can train your entire lower body along with your arms and mid-section (provided that the exercises don't indirectly produce shoulder pain).

Once again, this guideline is also appropriate for aerobic and anaerobic training. Suppose that you have a hip, a leg or an ankle injury that prohibits you from doing any aerobic or anaerobic training for your lower body. A few commercial devices are available that enable you to do aerobic and anaerobic training exclusively with the muscles of your torso such as a rope-climbing machine or an upper-body ergometer. (An ergometer is a device that measures work.)

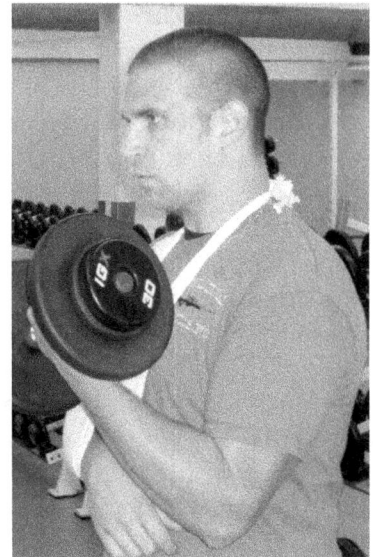

Many studies have shown that training a muscle on one side of the body has some effect on the contralateral muscle (the same muscle on the opposite side of the body).

10. Employ eccentric exercise/activity.

A new and an exciting frontier in rehabilitative training that's being explored by the sportsmedical community is eccentric exercise/activity. In particular, two characteristics of eccentric contractions bode well for use in rehabilitative training.

First, eccentric contractions produce higher muscular force than concentric contractions. When undergoing rehabilitative training, some individuals might not have enough strength to raise even the lightest resistance. But since eccentric strength is greater than concentric strength, they might have enough strength to lower a resistance. In applying this concept, a partner can perform the positive (raising) phase of each repetition while a lifter can perform the negative (lowering) phase. This concept has been put into practice in a number of different ways. For instance, eccentric exercise has shown great promise in treating tendinopathies (tendon disorders) and muscle strains and recovering from anterior cruciate ligament (ACL) injuries.

Second, eccentric contractions have a lower metabolic cost than concentric contractions. More to the point, oxygen intake and caloric expenditure are lower – *a lot lower* – during negative work than during positive work. In one classic study, two subjects pedaled back-to-back on two stationary cycles that were connected with a single chain. One subject did positive work by pedaling forward while the other subject did negative work by resisting the backward-moving pedals. Both subjects applied the same force for about 13 minutes. When pedaling at three different speeds, oxygen intake during positive work was 2.4 to 5.2 times greater than oxygen intake during negative work. In other words, at a given speed, positive work was much more demanding than negative work. Now, here's the kicker: The subject who pedaled forward was J. Murdoch Ritchie, described as "a large, powerful man"; the subject who easily resisted his efforts was Brenda Bigland, described as "a young, petite woman." (Fast fact: Ritchie and Bigland later married.)

In short, the high-force and low-cost properties of eccentric exercise/activity make it a great fit for rehabilitative training. It's an excellent option for individuals who have muscle weakness, muscle strains, tendinopathies, a low or limited tolerance for exercise or a chronic condition, including reduced cardiac function and chronic obstructive pulmonary disease (COPD).

PRUDENT CHOICES

In many instances, you can exercise an injured area or body part in a safe and pain-free manner. This will prevent a significant loss in strength (and size) as well as aerobic, anaerobic and metabolic fitness. And even though you may not be able to exercise an injured area due to an excessive amount of pain or discomfort, you can still train your uninjured body parts. Once the injured area heals, you can reintroduce exercises that were previously painful to perform.

Remember, though, that the critical factor in the administration and application of rehabilitative training is pain-free – or nearly pain-free – exercise/activity. That said, it's important to understand that there's a distinct difference between *muscular* pain and *joint* pain. Muscular pain isn't necessarily cause for alarm; it's an indication that you're doing high-intensity work and your muscles are being fatigued. Joint pain, however, is something else altogether. Localized pain in a joint usually means that there's some type of structural malady. If you experience pain in your joints while exercising, you're merely aggravating your condition and perhaps even causing further damage by brutalizing the joint infrastructure. Simply, an exercise that produces joint pain must be avoided or altered. The key is to make prudent choices.

How important is rehabilitative training? According to Ken Mannie, who has more than 35 years of experience as a strength coach in the collegiate ranks, "Our philosophy . . . has always been that strength training is a vital constituent in the rehab process and that all training options for an injured area will be considered before deciding not to address the area."

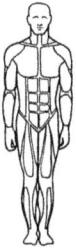

13 Flexibility Training

Flexibility can be defined as the range of motion (ROM) throughout which your joints can move. The best way for you to maintain – or improve – the ROM of your joints is to perform specific stretches to elongate the surrounding muscles.

Flexibility training is undoubtedly the simplest and most effortless type of physical training that you can perform; the exertion level is relatively low and relaxation is an absolute requirement. However, many people often overlook or underemphasize flexibility training.

Increasing flexibility serves at least two purposes. First, being more flexible enables you to exert your strength over a greater ROM. One study compared a group of 22 elite female rhythmic gymnasts to 16 age-matched female athletes from other sports. As would be expected, the group of gymnasts had significantly greater flexibility than the group of other athletes. And the gymnasts "displayed a larger functional ROM," meaning that they produced a high amount of force over a greater ROM than the other athletes. That's an advantage in any sport or activity. Second, improving your flexibility

Improving flexibility is an advantage in many sports and activities, including martial arts. (Photo by John Quigley.)

allows you to move your joints through a greater ROM which makes it easier for you to assume body positions that are otherwise difficult. That's an advantage in many sports and activities, including gymnastics, dancing, diving, figure skating and martial arts.

It should be noted that although stretching after an activity might "feel good," there's no scientific evidence that it reduces muscular soreness. This is also true of stretching before an activity.

FACTORS THAT AFFECT FLEXIBILITY

The most significant contributor to decreased flexibility seems to be inactivity. Obviously, you can avoid at least some loss of flexibility by simply participating in physical training on a regular basis. But besides inactivity, there are many other factors that affect your ROM, some over which you have little or no control.

There's a distinct relationship between your age and your flexibility. The greatest increase in flexibility usually occurs up to and between the ages of 7 and 12. During early adolescence, flexibility tends to level off and thereafter begins to decline with increasing age. Consequently, one of the goals of flexibility training is to slow or perhaps reverse this decline.

Flexibility is also related to gender. Some men are more flexible than some women but, in general, women are more flexible than men (and they retain this advantage throughout life).

In addition, flexibility is influenced by several genetic (inherited) characteristics such as the insertion points of your tendons as well as your percentage of body fat (especially that which is around your mid-section). Your ROM also has genetic limitations that are structural which

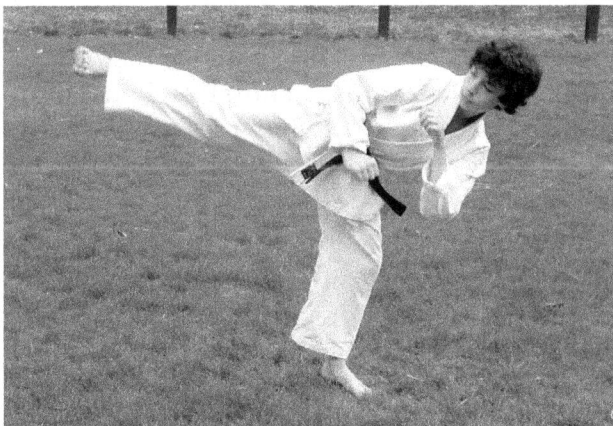

include your bones, tendons, ligaments and skin along with the extensibility of your muscles.

As you may already be painfully aware, previous injury to a muscle or connective tissue can affect your ROM. Furthermore, immobilizing a joint during rehabilitation may cause connective tissue to adapt to its shortest functional length thereby reducing the ROM of the joint.

Finally, your body temperature is another factor that influences your flexibility. Muscles and connective tissue that are warmed up will be more flexible and extensible than muscles and connective tissue that are not. Because of this, some authorities recommend that stretching should be performed after you've completed your physical training when your body temperature is higher.

ASSESSING FLEXIBILITY

It's difficult to assess flexibility in a fair manner. For one thing, some measurements of flexibility can be misleading. A perfect example of this is the traditional sit-and-reach test in which a person sits down on the floor with straight legs and reaches forward as far as possible. This test is often used to measure the flexibility of the lower back and hamstrings. A sit-and-reach test, however, doesn't take into consideration limb lengths. Everything else being equal, those with long arms and/or short legs have a distinct anatomical advantage in a sit-and-reach test. These individuals might appear to be quite flexible but may actually be quite inflexible. Conversely, those with short arms and/or long legs have a distinct anatomical disadvantage in a sit-and-reach test. These individuals might appear to be quite inflexible but may actually be quite flexible. In the case of a sit-and-reach test, using a goniometer to measure the angle of flexion between the lumbar spine and upper legs yields an appraisal of flexibility that's more impartial. (A goniometer is a protractor-like instrument with two movable arms that enable you to measure joint angles.)

It should be noted, too, that flexibility is joint-specific; a high degree of flexibility in one joint

doesn't necessarily indicate a high degree of flexibility in another joint. Along these lines, it wouldn't be unusual for flexibility to vary from one side of the body to the other.

Therefore, the purpose of assessing flexibility shouldn't be to compare your performance to that of someone else. Assessments of flexibility are much more meaningful when your present flexibility is compared to your past flexibility.

STRETCHING AND INJURIES

For many years, it had been thought that pre-activity stretching reduces the risk of injury. This belief wasn't based on any research but it seemed reasonable to assume such. As it turns out, there's scant research on the effects of pre-activity stretching on the risk of injury. And the relatively few studies that have been conducted on the topic show that pre-activity stretching doesn't reduce injuries.

Two of the studies involved Australian Army recruits. The studies were conducted as they went through 12 weeks of basic training.

In the first study, one group of 549 recruits stretched their calves prior to physical training and another group of 544 recruits didn't stretch their calves. Those who stretched before physical training had 23 injuries to their lower leg while those who didn't stretch had 25 injuries to their lower leg.

In the second study, one group of 735 recruits stretched their lower-body muscles (calves, hamstrings, quadriceps, hip adductors and hip flexors) prior to physical training and another group of 803 recruits didn't stretch their lower-body muscles. Those who stretched before physical training had 158 injuries to their lower body while those who didn't stretch had 175 injuries to their lower body.

To summarize, the 1,284 recruits who stretched prior to physical training had 181 injuries and the 1,347 recruits who didn't stretch had 200 injuries. So in both studies, the incidence of injury was very similar regardless of whether or not stretching was done before an activity. Pooling the data from both studies showed that pre-activity stretching reduced the risk of injury by 5% (which wasn't statistically significant). Over the same period of time, the expected risk of injury was 20%. This means that a reduction in the relative risk of injury by 5% translated into a reduction in the absolute risk of injury by only 1%. Based on these data, the researchers calculated that, on average, about 100 people would need to stretch for 12 weeks to prevent one injury. And one person would need to stretch for 23 years to prevent one injury.

So, pre-activity stretching doesn't prevent injury. But pre-activity stretching doesn't cause injury.

STRETCHING AND PERFORMANCE

Another long-time assumption had been that pre-activity stretching improves performance. Again, this belief has been based more on a "gut feeling" than on scientific research. Most studies have shown that stretching prior to an activity can actually hinder a muscle's ability to produce maximum force, at least temporarily. To date, in fact, *no study* has shown that pre-activity stretching improves performance. But there's more to the story.

In one study, 13 subjects did passive stretching of their calves on three separate occasions: for a total of two, four and eight minutes. A fourth occasion served as a control (non-stretching) condition. The calves were stretched on a dynamometer for 30 seconds then released for 20 seconds. This stretch-release sequence was repeated until the muscle was stretched for the assigned duration. For example, two minutes of stretching involved four 30-second stretches. The researchers found that strength decreased by as much as 6% in the immediate aftermath of stretching. However, this wasn't significantly different than the control condition in which stretching wasn't done. Of note was that the decreases in strength were dose dependent in that as the length of the stretching protocol increased so did the reduction in strength.

The researchers found that stretching decreased strength by as much as 6%. However,

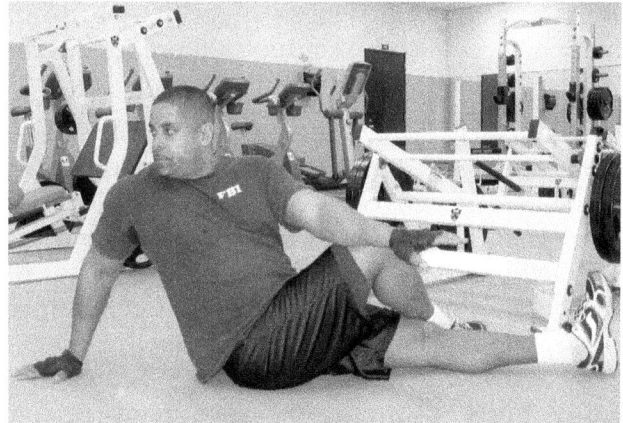

Pre-activity stretching doesn't hurt performance as long as it's not excessive.

this wasn't significantly different than the control condition in which stretching wasn't done. The decreases were dose dependant in that as the length of the stretching protocol increased so did the reduction in strength.

This dose-response effect has been corroborated by a systematic review of more than 100 studies. According to the review, no detrimental effects on performance occur when stretches are held for up to 30 seconds. Decrements in performance are most likely to occur when stretches are held for more than 60 seconds.

So, pre-activity stretching doesn't help performance. But pre-activity stretching doesn't hurt performance as long as it's not excessive.

WARMING UP

The research regarding the need for a warm-up is inconclusive. Some studies have shown that performances with a warm-up are better than those without a warm-up; other studies have shown that performances with a warm-up are worse or no different than those without a warm-up. Nonetheless, a warm-up has both physiological and psychological importance.

For years, warming up was synonymous with stretching. However, warming up and stretching are two separate entities and must be treated as such. Warming up is meant to prepare you for an upcoming session of physical training; stretching is meant to induce a more long-term change in your ROM.

A warm-up should precede flexibility training. Warm-up activities usually consist of low-intensity movements such as light jogging or calisthenics. Regardless of the warm-up activity that you choose, the idea is to systematically increase your body temperature and the blood flow to your muscles. Breaking a light sweat during the warm-up indicates that your body temperature has been raised sufficiently and that you're ready to begin stretching your muscles. As noted previously, muscles and connective tissue that are warmed up have increased flexibility and extensibility. (When the environmental temperature is high, it's likely that your body temperature is already elevated enough for you to start stretching your muscles.)

By the way, there's no need for you to warm-up or stretch prior to strength training, provided that you do a relatively high number of repetitions and lift the weight in a smooth, controlled manner without any explosive or jerking movements. But warming up prior to a physical activity that involves rapid muscular contractions – such as sprinting – is highly advisable to ready your muscles for high-speed movements.

METHODS OF STRETCHING

There are a few methods of stretching that you can employ to improve your flexibility. Here's a thumbnail sketch of four methods of stretching:

Static Stretching

The safest and most effective means of developing long-term improvements in ROM is, arguably, static stretching. With this method, the muscles are stretched slowly to the point of slight discomfort and then that position is held for a prescribed amount of time. It's thought that static stretching might be best suited *after* an activity.

Static stretching can be active or passive. Active static stretching involves holding the stretched position with one or more agonist muscles. (An agonist is a muscle that causes

movement.) An example of this is contracting the quadriceps (here, an agonist) to stretch the hamstrings. Passive static stretching involves holding the stretched position with assistance from another individual, gravity or an object such as a towel or stretch strap.

Ballistic Stretching

Bouncing and jerking movements are inherent to ballistic stretching. These characteristics make ballistic stretching less effective than static stretching. Here's why: When a muscle is stretched quickly, it offers more resistance (more stiffness) and, thus, is *harder* to stretch; when a muscle is stretched slowly, it offers less resistance (less stiffness) and, thus, is *easier* to stretch.

In addition, ballistic stretching produces momentum which aggressively and erratically forces a muscle beyond its natural ROM. Obviously, this increases the potential for injury.

Bottom line: Ballistic stretching is the least preferred method of stretching and shouldn't be considered as a viable option.

Dynamic Stretching

Over time, dynamic stretching has become more and more popular. In particular, it's thought that dynamic stretching might be best suited *before* an activity.

Dynamic stretching can easily be confused with ballistic stretching. The main difference between the two is that dynamic stretching involves a slow and gradual transition from one position to another without the bouncing and jerking movements that are associated with ballistic stretching. Along these lines, it can be difficult to distinguish between dynamic stretching and warm-up movements.

Dynamic stretching often employs specific movements that are involved in an upcoming sport or an activity. For instance, sprinters might perform knee pumps and arm swings as part of their preparation for a race or an interval workout on the track. (You can see now why the line that separates dynamic stretching from warm-up movements is often blurred.) Dynamic stretching can also involve general movements such as arm circles. One of the most common dynamic stretches for the hips is the lateral walk over/ under using a series of 8 to 10 hurdles that are spaced several feet apart. To do this dynamic stretch, you'd position yourself so that either your right or left side faced the first hurdle. Then, you'd step laterally over the first hurdle, under the second hurdle and continue to navigate over/ under the remaining hurdles in the same fashion.

Proprioceptive Neuromuscular Facilitation

Another method of stretching is known as proprioceptive neuromuscular facilitation (which, thank goodness, usually goes by the letters PNF). PNF requires assistance from another individual and consists of three steps. First, a stretched position is held with assistance from a partner (essentially a passive static stretch) for about 30 seconds. Second, an isometric contraction is done in the same stretched position against resistance that's supplied by the partner for about five seconds. And third, the stretched position is held again with assistance from the partner for about 30 seconds. The stretch-contract-stretch cycle can be repeated several times. Note that the isometric contraction should be performed with a high level of effort against a resistance that's great enough such that no joint movement occurs.

To illustrate PNF, consider the butterfly stretch. In the start position, you'd sit on the floor, place the soles of your feet together and bring

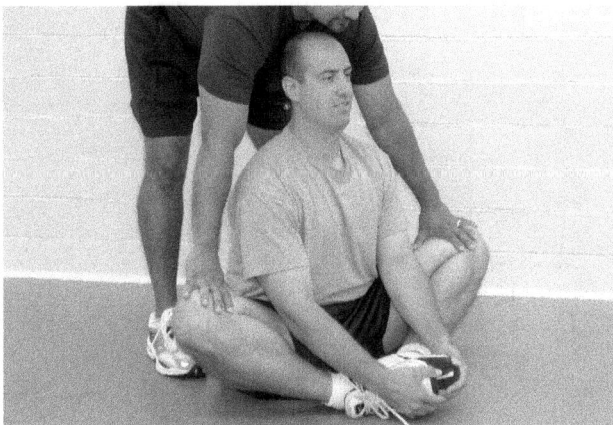

PNF should only be used with assistance from a competent individual. (Photo by Peter Silletti.)

your heels as close to your hips as possible. A partner would place his/her hands on the insides of your knees. To do this stretch using PNF, the partner would assist you by pushing your legs down for about 30 seconds. Next, you'd do an isometric contraction against resistance that's supplied by the partner by trying to bring your knees together for about five seconds. Finally, the partner would assist you again by pushing your legs down for about 30 seconds.

Take heed: An inexperienced partner can unknowingly apply an excessive amount of resistance which could cause an injury. As a result, this type of stretching should only be used with assistance from a competent individual. Even when done correctly, PNF can be uncomfortable for some people. And because it's somewhat complicated and involves the use of another individual, PNF isn't a practical means of stretching.

STRETCHING STRATEGIES

Although your ROM may be limited by the factors that were mentioned previously, it can be improved through flexibility training. Like all other forms of physical training, flexibility training has certain components that must be incorporated to make it safe and productive. These components can be crafted into strategies that will permit you to improve your ROM with a lower risk of injury.

Here are some stretching strategies for your flexibility training:

1. Do a warm-up prior to stretching.

A warm-up in which you break a light sweat will be adequate to elevate your body temperature enough and make your muscles and connective tissue more flexible and extensible.

2. Stretch under control without using any bouncing or jerking movements.

Bouncing or jerking actually makes the stretch more painful and increases your risk of muscular soreness and tissue damage.

3. Inhale and exhale normally during the stretch without holding your breath.

When you hold your breath, it elevates your blood pressure which disrupts your normal breathing pattern and makes it more difficult for you to relax.

4. Stretch comfortably in a pain-free manner.

Since pain is an indication that you're stretching at or near your structural limits, you should only stretch to a point of tightness or slight discomfort.

5. Relax during the stretch.

Relaxing mentally and physically allows you to stretch your muscles throughout a greater ROM.

6. Hold the stretched position for about 10 to 30 seconds.

By gradually stretching your muscles to a point of tightness or slight discomfort, holding that position and then gradually returning them to their pre-stretched length, you can stretch farther with little risk of pain or injury.

7. Attempt to stretch slightly farther than the last time.

In another application of the Overload Principle, progressively increasing your ROM improves your flexibility.

8. Perform stretches on a regular basis.

You should stretch daily and either before or after physical training.

THE STRETCHES

Although your body has roughly 200 joints, it's not necessary to perform a stretch for each one. Your joints range from those that are relatively immovable (such as the sutures of your skull) to those that are freely movable (such as your hips and elbows). You can stretch the muscles of your major joints in a comprehensive manner by performing a little more than a dozen stretches. There are many variations of stretches that involve the same muscle groups. Because of this, your flexibility training can be individualized to meet your personal preferences.

This chapter describes and illustrates the safest and most productive stretches that can be performed. Included in the discussions of each stretch are the muscle(s) stretched, start position, performance description and training tips for making the stretch safer and more productive.

These 16 stretches are described in this chapter: neck forward, neck backward, lateral neck, scratch back, front shoulder, rear shoulder, standing calf, tibia stretch, sit and reach, V-sit, lateral reach, butterfly, spinal twist, knee stack, knee pull and lying quad.

NECK FORWARD

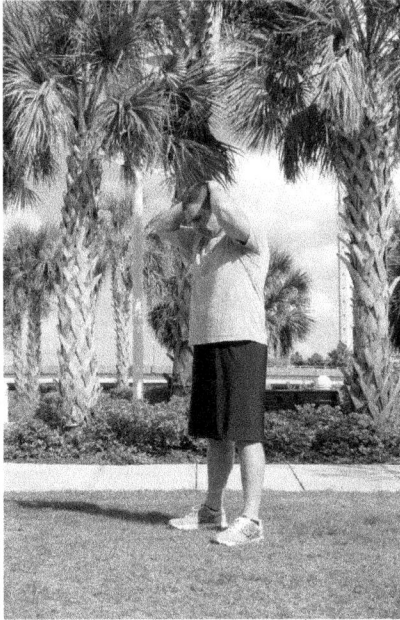

Muscles Stretched: neck extensors and trapezius

Start Position: While standing, spread your feet about shoulder-width apart. Place your hands behind your head and interlock your fingers.

Performance Description: Pull your head to your chest and hold.

Training Tips:

- The stretch must be done carefully since the cervical spine is involved.

- You can also perform this stretch while sitting.

NECK BACKWARD

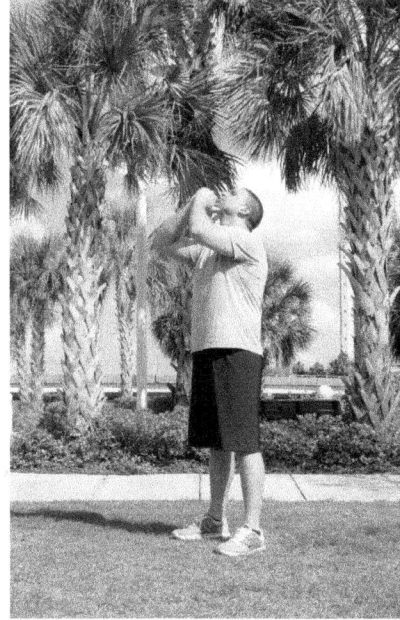

Muscle Stretched: sternocleidomastoideus

Start Position: While standing, spread your feet about shoulder-width apart. Place your thumbs under your chin.

Performance Description: Push your head backward and hold.

Training Tips:

- The stretch must be done carefully since the cervical spine is involved.

- You can also perform this stretch while sitting.

213

LATERAL NECK

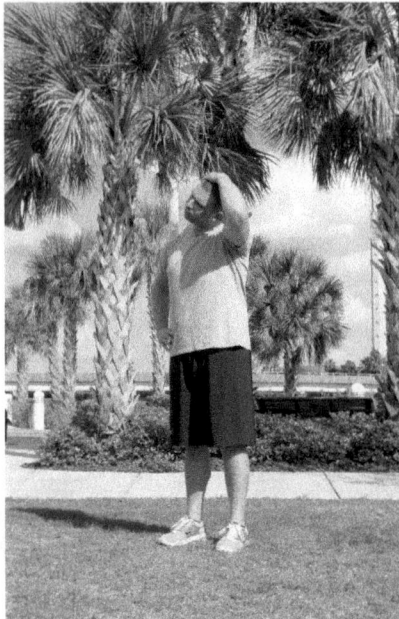

Muscle Stretched: sternocleidomastoideus

Start Position: While standing, spread your feet about shoulder-width apart. Place your left hand on the right side of your head.

Performance Description: Pull your head to your left shoulder and hold. Repeat the stretch for the other side of your body.

Training Tips:

- The stretch must be done carefully since the cervical spine is involved.

- You can also perform this stretch while sitting.

SCRATCH BACK

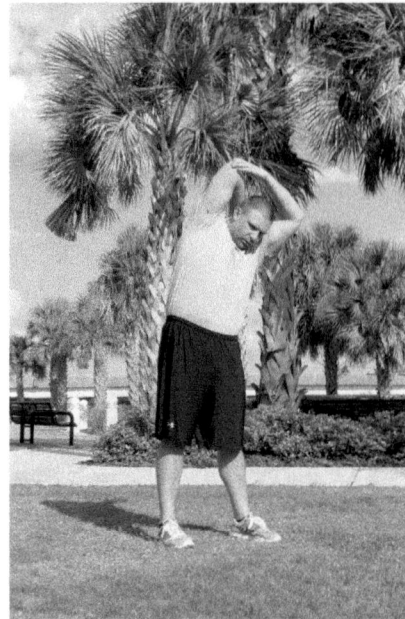

Muscles Stretched: upper back, triceps and obliques

Start Position: While standing, spread your feet about shoulder-width apart. Place your right hand behind your head on the upper part of your back and grab your right elbow with your left hand.

Performance Description: Pull your torso to the left and hold. Repeat the stretch for the other side of your body.

Training Tips:

- Avoid moving your hips.

- You can also perform this stretch while sitting.

- This stretch may be contraindicated if you have shoulder-impingement syndrome.

FRONT SHOULDER

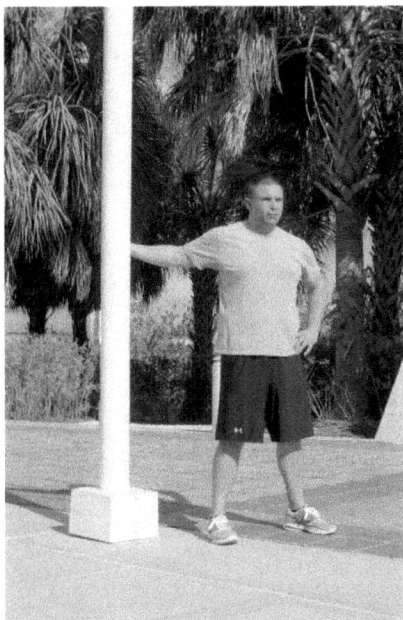

Muscles Stretched: chest and anterior deltoid

Start Position: While standing, spread your feet about shoulder-width apart. Position your right arm so that it's parallel to the floor. Place your right hand on a wall (or something similar that's stable) and your left hand on your hip.

Performance Description: Turn your feet and body to the left and hold. Repeat the stretch for the other side of your body.

Training Tips:

• This stretch may be contraindicated if you have shoulder-impingement syndrome.

REAR SHOULDER

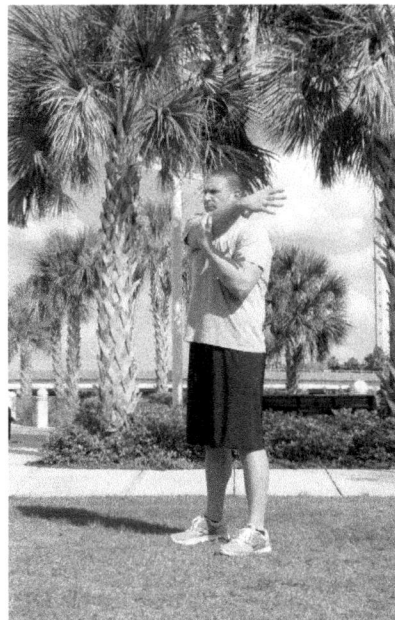

Muscles Stretched: upper back, posterior deltoid, trapezius and rhomboids

Start Position: While standing, spread your feet about shoulder-width apart. Position your right arm so that it's parallel to the floor. Place your left hand above your right elbow.

Performance Description: Pull your upper arm toward your torso and hold. Repeat the stretch for the other side of your body.

Training Tips:

• You can also perform this stretch while sitting.

STANDING CALF

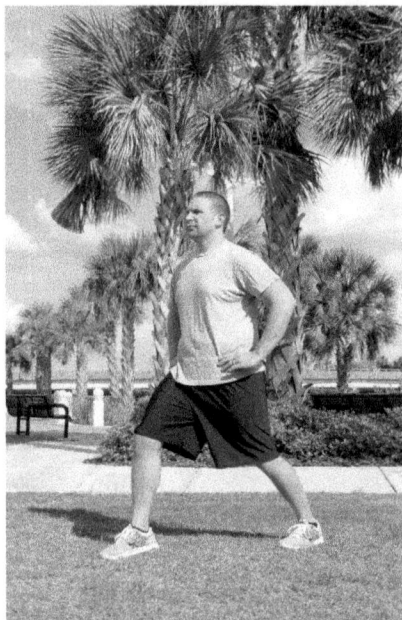

Muscles Stretched: calves and iliopsoas

Start Position: While standing, place your hands on your hips. Step forward with your right foot and bend your right leg. Straighten your left leg and place your left foot flat on the floor. Point your feet straight ahead.

Performance Description: Lean forward and hold. Repeat the stretch for the other side of your body.

Training Tips:

- Keep the heel of your back foot flat on the floor.
- Keep your feet pointed straight ahead.
- Refrain from bending forward at the waist.

TIBIA STRETCH

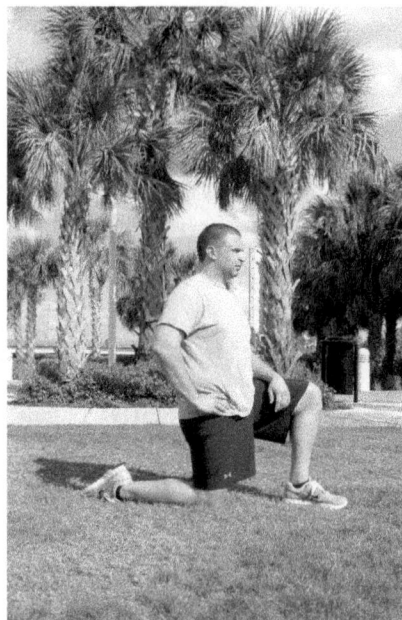

Muscles Stretched: dorsi flexors

Start Position: Kneel down on your right knee. Position your right upper leg so that it's perpendicular to the floor. Point your right toes away from your body. Position your left foot so that your left upper leg is parallel to the floor and your left lower leg is perpendicular to the floor. Place your left foot flat on the floor.

Performance Description: Press your right lower leg and the top part of your right foot flat on the floor and hold. Repeat the stretch for the other side of your body.

Training Tips:

- Keep the top part of the foot that's being stretched flat on the floor.

SIT AND REACH

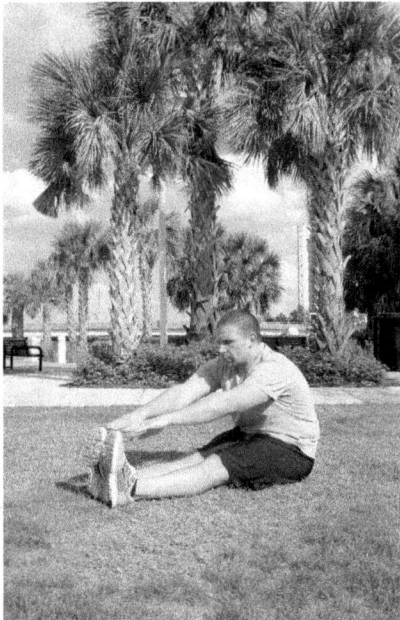

Muscles Stretched: gluteus maximus, hamstrings, calves, upper back and lower back

Start Position: While sitting, straighten your legs and bring them together. Point your toes upward.

Performance Description: Reach forward as far as possible and hold.

Training Tips:

- Keep your legs straight and toes pointed upward.
- A partner can help you obtain a greater stretch by carefully pushing on your upper back.
- You can also perform this stretch while standing (with your torso bent forward at the waist, your legs together and your arms hanging down).

V-SIT

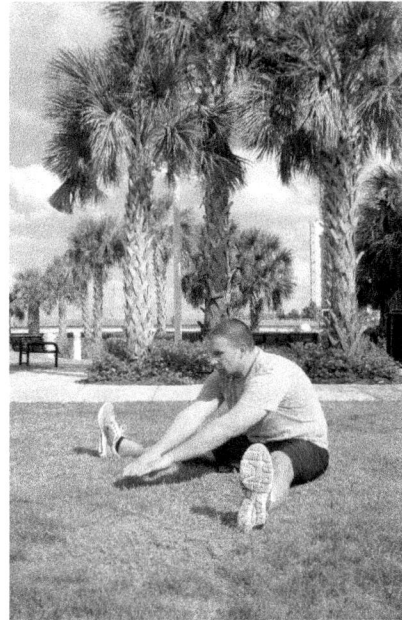

Muscles Stretched: gluteus maximus, hip adductors, hamstrings, calves, upper back and lower back

Start Position: While sitting, straighten your legs and spread them apart as far as possible. Point your toes upward.

Performance Description: Reach forward as far as possible and hold.

Training Tips:

- Keep your legs straight and toes pointed upward.
- A partner can help you obtain a greater stretch by carefully pushing on your upper back.
- You can also perform this stretch while standing (with your torso bent forward at the waist, your legs spread apart and your arms hanging down).

217

LATERAL REACH

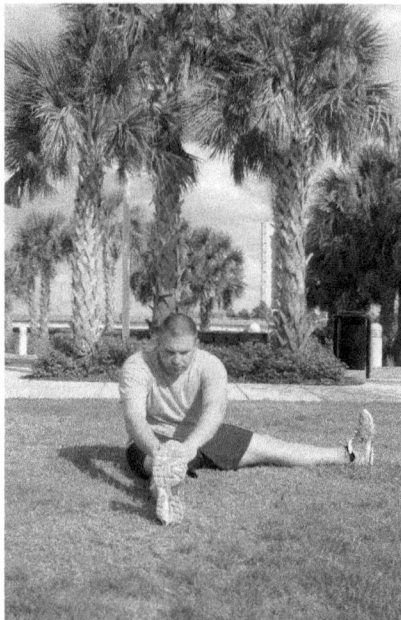

Muscles Stretched: gluteus maximus, hip adductors, hamstrings, calves, upper back, obliques and lower back

Start Position: While sitting, straighten your legs and spread them apart as far as possible. Point your toes upward.

Performance Description: Reach down your right leg as far as possible and hold. Repeat the stretch for the other side of your body.

Training Tips:

- Keep your legs straight and toes pointed upward.

- A partner can help you obtain a greater stretch by carefully pushing on your upper back.

- You can also perform this stretch while standing (with your torso bent laterally at the waist, your legs spread apart and your arms reaching down your leg).

BUTTERFLY

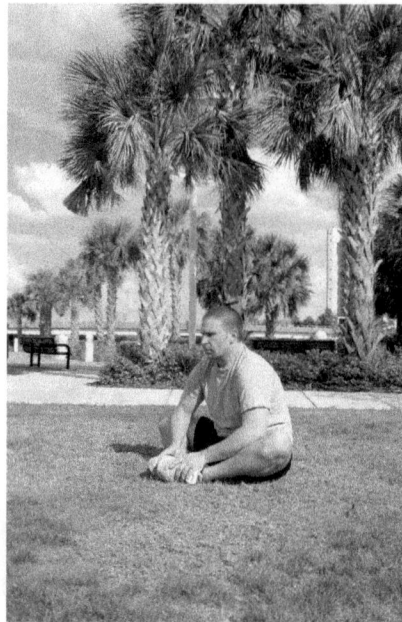

Muscles Stretched: hip adductors and lower back

Start Position: While sitting, place the soles of your feet together. Bring your heels as close to your hips as possible and place your elbows on the insides of your knees.

Performance Description: Push your legs down with your elbows and hold.

Training Tips:

- A partner can help you obtain a greater stretch by carefully pushing on the inside of your knees.

SPINAL TWIST

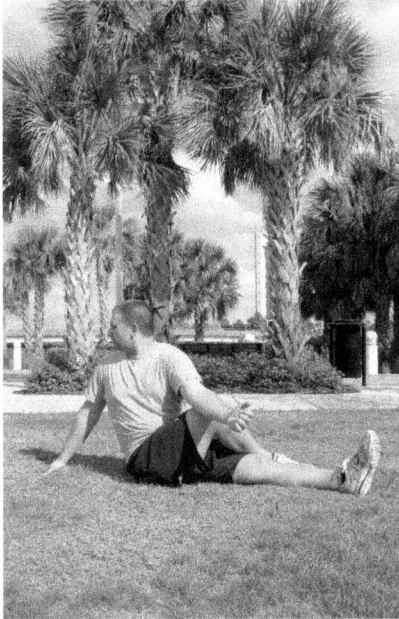

Muscles Stretched: gluteus medius, gluteus minimus, obliques and lower back

Start Position: While sitting, straighten your left leg and position your right foot on the outside of your left knee. Place your left elbow against the outside of your right knee.

Performance Description: Push against the outside of your right knee with your left elbow, look to your right as far as possible and hold. Repeat the stretch for the other side of your body.

Training Tips:

- You can also perform this stretch while lying supine (with your shoulders flat on the floor and rotating one leg to the side).

KNEE STACK

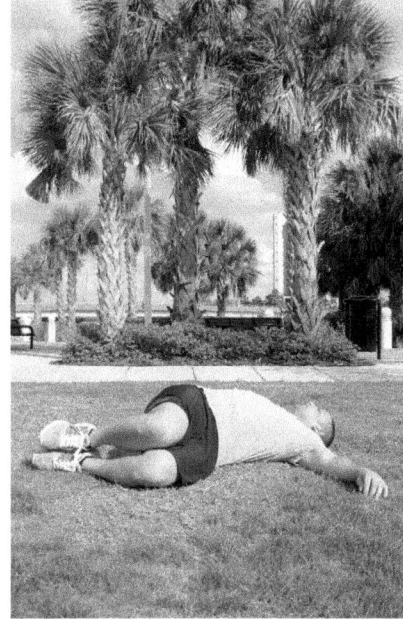

Muscles Stretched: hip abductors, obliques, lower back, chest and shoulders

Start Position: While lying supine, bend your knees. Bring your heels near your hips and position your feet flat on the floor. Keep your shoulders flat on the floor.

Performance Description: Rotate your legs to the left with your right leg "stacked" on top of your left leg and hold. Repeat the stretch for the other side of your body.

Training Tips:

- Keep your shoulders flat on the floor.

KNEE PULL

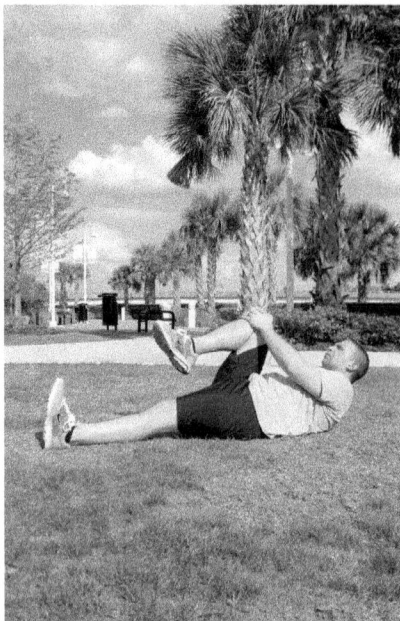

LYING QUAD

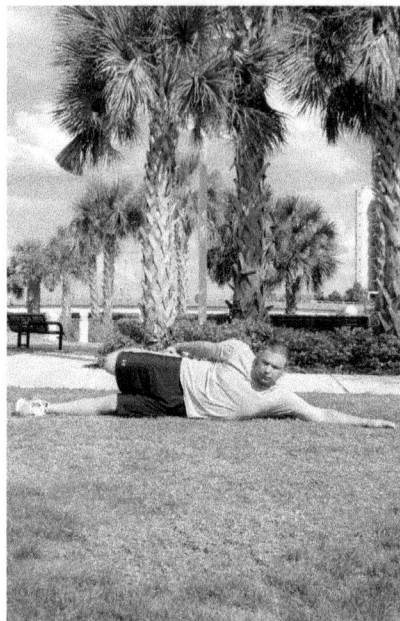

Muscles Stretched: gluteus maximus, hamstrings and lower back

Start Position: While lying supine, straighten your left leg and point your toes upward. Grasp your right leg below your knee.

Performance Description: Pull your right leg toward your chest and hold. Repeat the stretch for the other side of your body.

Training Tips:

• Keep one leg straight and toes pointed upward while the other leg is being stretched.

Muscles Stretched: quadriceps, iliopsoas and abdominals

Start Position: Lie down on your left side and grab your right ankle with your right hand.

Performance Description: Pull your right heel toward your hip and hold. Repeat the stretch for the other side of your body.

Training Tips:

• You can also perform this stretch while lying prone.

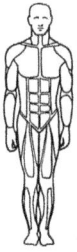

14 Aerobic Training

With the publication of his book *Aerobics* in 1968, Dr. Kenneth Cooper – a physician who achieved the rank of lieutenant colonel in the US Air Force – introduced the idea of aerobic training and, in the process, essentially kicked off the so-called fitness boom. Seemingly overnight, Americans donned running shoes and took to the roads. Prior to this time, if you were outside running down the street – especially in the dark – you were probably up to no good.

The most important aspect of your physical profile is your aerobic fitness. Specifically, your aerobic fitness is a measure of how well your body consumes, transports and uses oxygen during physical exertion. The best way for you to improve these physiological mechanisms is through aerobic training.

The energy system (or pathway) that's responsible for your aerobic fitness is Aerobic Glycolysis (which is vital during long-term, low-intensity efforts). It's no surprise, then, that the main purpose of aerobic training is to improve the functional ability of this energy system. By increasing your aerobic fitness, Aerobic Glycolysis can operate more efficiently and more effectively.

More than any other type of physical training, aerobic training decreases your resting heart rate. This is of utmost importance since resting heart rate is recognized as a predictor of cardiovascular risk and mortality.

Aerobic training helps to modify several factors that contribute to the threat of coronary heart disease. This includes diabetes, hypertension (high blood pressure), overweight/obesity and physical inactivity.

Besides conferring a variety of health-related benefits, aerobic training also has an impact on performance in sports and activities. An athlete who has a higher level of conditioning can work

at greater levels of intensity for longer periods of time at a lower heart rate than an athlete who has a lower level of conditioning. An athlete with this "aerobic advantage" won't expend as much energy as an opponent and can perform skills and activities with less effort.

Case in point: One study involved 12 female cross-country skiers from Norway; six were world-class athletes and six were national-class athletes. As part of the study, the athletes did six five-minute stages of roller skiing, alternating between double poling at a 3% incline and diagonal striding at a 12% incline. When double poling at the same speed, the world-class athletes had a significantly lower heart rate (132 beats per minute versus 160 beats per minute) and lower rating of perceived exertion (11 versus 13 on the Borg RPE Scale®) than the national-class athletes; when diagonal striding at the same speed, the world-class athletes had a significantly lower heart rate (153 beats per minute versus 176 beats per minute) and lower rating of perceived exertion (13 versus 15 on the Borg RPE Scale®) than the national-class athletes. This is to

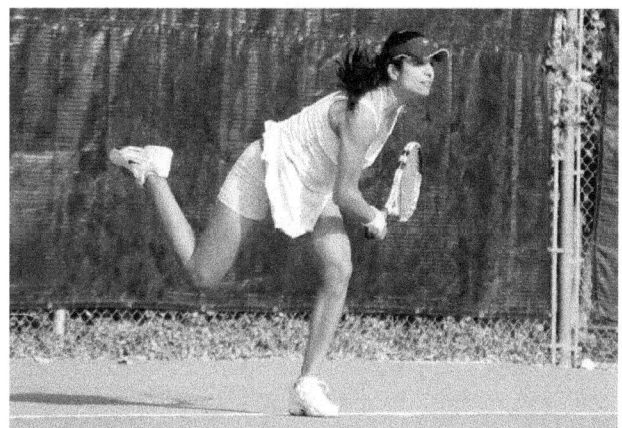

An athlete who has a higher level of conditioning can work at greater levels of intensity for longer periods of time at a lower heart rate than an athlete who has a lower level of conditioning. (Photo provided by Shikha Uberoi.)

221

say, at the same speed, the world-class athletes exerted considerably less effort than the national-class athletes.

In addition, aerobic training improves the speed at which you recover from exercise: After completing the same task, the heart rate of a well-conditioned individual returns to normal more quickly than the heart rate of a less-conditioned individual. This, of course, is an obvious advantage during athletic endeavors.

Aerobic training is also needed to establish a solid foundation of aerobic support in preparation for anaerobic training. The more finely tuned your aerobic pathway becomes, the better your anaerobic pathways are able to function. Clearly, your aerobic pathway must operate as efficiently and as effectively as possible to provide physiological support for your anaerobic efforts.

In addition to the many physiological adaptations, aerobic training – when used in conjunction with sound nutritional training – helps to maintain your percentage of body fat at an acceptable level. This, of course, will improve your appearance.

There are psychological enhancements, too. This includes increased mental alertness, self-confidence and self-esteem.

AEROBIC GUIDELINES

You can improve your aerobic fitness by incorporating several easy-to-follow guidelines that have been adapted from the 2011 position stand by the American College of Sports Medicine (ACSM) on the quantity and quality of exercise for healthy adults. These guidelines can be organized under the acronym FITT which stands for Frequency, Intensity, Time and Type. (Fast fact: A position stand is done by a panel of experts on behalf of an organization or a group; this yields a set of guidelines or "best practices" that's based on the available research that has been published on a specific topic.)

Frequency

In order to improve your aerobic fitness, you should do aerobic training three to five days per week. Training less frequently doesn't appear adequate enough to promote any meaningful improvement in your aerobic fitness; training more frequently may produce a greater improvement in your aerobic fitness but the amount is negligible (which usually isn't worth the time spent).

Having said that, doing aerobic training more frequently may be beneficial if you're a highly competitive athlete. And doing aerobic training more frequently can be beneficial when weight (fat) loss is a goal.

Be advised that beginning with too much activity too soon may very well lead to an overuse injury such as tendinitis. This is especially true of certain populations, including younger children, older adults and those who are inactive or in poor physical condition. Individuals who are susceptible to overuse injuries should initially perform aerobic training two or three days per week to reduce their potential for overuse injuries. As these individuals adjust and adapt to the unfamiliar demands, their dosage of aerobic training can be increased to a frequency of three to five days per week.

Intensity

Other than your genetic (inherited) profile, the most important aspect of aerobic training is your level of intensity (or effort). Your heart rate increases in direct proportion to the demands of an activity. As such, your exercising heart rate is used to gauge your aerobic intensity.

In order to improve your aerobic fitness, it's recommended that you maintain a level of 60 to 90% of your maximum heart rate. This, of course, begs the question, "What's my maximum heart rate?"

Your maximum heart rate can be determined in a clinical setting while performing exhaustive exercise, usually on a treadmill or stationary cycle. Two obstacles are often encountered with this type of testing: availability and expense; many people aren't exactly eager about doing exhaustive exercise, either. However, your maximum heart rate can be easily estimated by using a prediction equation.

In 1938, Dr. Sid Robinson – then of the world-famous Harvard Fatigue Laboratory – compiled data on 93 men and boys who did exhaustive exercise (treadmill running) which showed that their maximum heart rates declined with age. Since then, more than three dozen equations have been proposed as a means of estimating maximum heart rate on the basis of age. (Fast fact: Dr. Robinson competed for the United States in the 1928 Amsterdam Olympics in the 1,500-meter run.)

Of all the prediction equations that have been suggested, none has been more widely used in the fitness industry than "220 - age"; it's firmly entrenched in most textbooks on exercise science and among several equations that are endorsed by the ACSM. In fact, if your heart rate is displayed on some sort of electronic device – such as the console of a treadmill or the screen of a wearable fitness (or activity) tracker – it's more than likely that the device employs "220 - age."

The equation has an intriguing backstory. Dr. Samuel Fox III – a cardiologist who served as a physician to the first group of astronauts in Project Mercury – is credited with devising "220 - age." In 1971, Dr. Fox noted the equation in a study that was published in the *Annals of Clinical Research*. The equation was based on data from 10 studies of North American and European males. Now, here's where the tale of the equation gets a bit murky: In 2001, Dr. William Haskell – an exercise physiologist and co-author of the 1971 study – revealed that the equation was conceived on an airplane by Dr. Fox while they looked over a diagram of data points. (Dr. Fox corroborated this story in 2003.) In other words, no real analysis of the data was done; the equation seemed to be the "best fit" based on a simple observation of the data points. To make matters worse, in 2002, two researchers at the University of New Mexico examined the original study and suggested that the data on which the equation is based doesn't support the equation. Their analysis of the 1971 data derived the equation of "215.4 – (0.9147 x age)."

Crazy, right? Still, no other equation has gained any traction in ousting "220 - age" from its seat. When "220 - age" is compared to other equations, there really isn't much difference between them. For nearly all age groups, most of the equations differ by no more than about five beats per minute (which becomes an even smaller difference when multiplied by 60 to 90% to determine a heart-rate training zone).

The fact of the matter is that *actual* maximum heart rates vary considerably and, thus, are difficult to estimate in a precise manner. So, understand that *every* equation is only an *estimate* or a "prediction" of maximum heart rate. And most equations offer roughly the same degree of accuracy. But the equation "220 - age" is more convenient and less complicated than others and its use continues to be widespread.

To find your age-predicted maximum heart rate in beats per minute (bpm) with this equation, simply subtract your age from 220. For instance, the age-predicted maximum heart rate of an average 30-year-old individual is 190 bpm [220 - 30 = 190]. To find the recommended heart-rate training zone, multiply 190 bpm by 60% and 90% (or 0.60 and 0.90). This means that an average 30-year-old individual needs to maintain an exercising heart rate of about 114 to 171 bpm to improve aerobic fitness [190 bpm x 0.60 = 114 bpm; 190 bpm x 0.90 = 171 bpm].

It must be emphasized that not everyone is average. In the case of maximum heart rate, the equation "220 - age" has a standard deviation of about 11 bpm (which might seem large but it's similar to many other equations). Considering a normal distribution of all 30-year-old individuals, this means that about 68.26% of them are within one standard deviation of the norm with maximum heart rates of about 179 to 201 bpm; 95.45% of them are within two standard deviations of the norm with maximum heart rates of about 168 to 212 bpm; and 99.73% of them are within three standard deviations of the norm with maximum heart rates of about 157 to 223 bpm.

Let's drill down a bit deeper into what this means. Values that are one standard deviation away from the norm indicate that about 15.87% are way below average and 15.87% are way above average. So if you're 30 and in the upper 15.87% of the population, you have a maximum

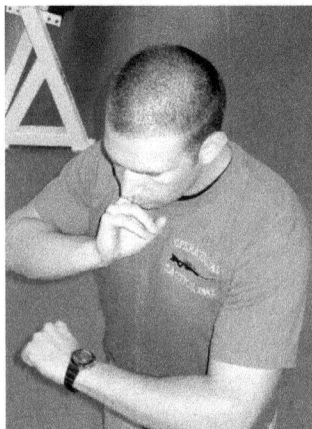

In order to improve your aerobic fitness, it's recommended that you maintain a level of 60 to 90% of your age-predicted maximum heart rate.

heart rate that's more than about 84.13% of all 30-year-olds. This also means that your *actual* maximum heart rate might be more like 200 bpm. Put differently, you'd have the maximum heart rate of an average 20-year-old individual . . . or someone who's *10 years younger than you*; your level of fitness would be above average. Taking this one step further, your recommended heart-rate training zone would be about 120 to 180 bpm [200 bpm x 0.60 = 120 bpm; 200 bpm x 0.90 = 180 bpm].

Of course, this applies to the other extreme as well. If you're 30 and in the lower 15.87% of the population, you have a maximum heart rate that's less than about 84.13% of all 30-year-olds. This also means that your *actual* maximum heart rate might be more like 180 bpm. Put differently, you'd have the maximum heart rate of an average 40-year-old individual . . . or someone who's *10 years older than you*; your level of fitness would be below average. Taking this one step further, your recommended heart-rate training zone would be about 108 to 162 bpm [180 bpm x 0.60 = 108 bpm; 180 bpm x 0.90 = 162 bpm].

Exceptions to using prediction equations for the purpose of estimating maximum heart rate are youths. According to the ACSM, children and adolescents up to the age of about 16 should maintain an exercising heart rate of about 170 to 180 beats per minute. After that age, a prediction equation can be employed to estimate their maximum heart rate.

As intimated earlier, the only way to determine your actual maximum heart rate is to perform exhaustive exercise in a clinical setting;

otherwise, much of this is guesswork. In general, though, some people may need to maintain their heart rates above or below the training zone that's recommended for others of the same age. If you're highly active or have an above-average level of fitness, for example, you should train with a higher percentage of your age-predicted maximum heart rate to produce meaningful results; if you're inactive or have a below-average level of fitness, you should train with a lower percentage of your age-predicted maximum heart rate to avoid potential risks. Using a lower level of intensity may also be necessary in the early stages of aerobic training to increase the likelihood of adherence to the program.

Remember, a favorable response to aerobic training requires an appropriate level of intensity. Intensity is a relative term that depends on your level of fitness. For some people, training with a lower percentage of their age-predicted maximum heart rate may actually represent a high level of intensity and an adequate workload for them. Stated otherwise, exercise of low intensity for an active individual may be of high intensity for an inactive individual. Depending on the initial level of fitness, training with a heart rate that's below the recommended threshold can actually produce some improvement in aerobic fitness.

To determine an appropriate level of intensity, you should adjust your effort based on whether the activity feels too easy or too difficult. If it feels too easy, increase your intensity; if it feels too difficult, reduce your intensity. Also keep in mind that your intensity is influenced by many factors, including the environmental conditions (altitude, temperature and humidity), your body position (seated or upright) and the amount of muscle mass being used (larger muscles produce a higher exercising heart rate than smaller ones).

Sidebar: In the 1960s, Dr. Gunnar Borg – a Swedish psychologist – introduced the concept of perceived exertion. The Borg Rating of Perceived Exertion Scale® – the Borg RPE Scale®, for short – was featured in a 1970 article that he penned for the *Scandinavian Journal of Rehabilitation Medicine*. Dr. Borg actually devised several scales but the one that's used most often in exercise science ranges from 6 to 20. The idea of the scale – which was modified slightly in 1985 and 1998 – is to rate your level of intensity with a number in that range that's accompanied by a "verbal anchor" (or description). For example, an RPE of 6 is "no exertion at all"; 9 is "very light"; 13 is "somewhat hard"; 17 is "very hard"; and 20 is "maximal exertion." The numbers are meant to approximate heart rate in beats per minute (bpm) by multiplying the RPE by 10. So, an RPE of 6 is 60 bpm; 9 is 90 bpm; 13 is 130 bpm; 17 is 170 bpm; and 20 is 200 bpm.

Many people measure (and monitor) their heart rates with some type of chest-strap monitor – which senses the electrical activity of the heart – or wearable fitness tracker. These devices provide varying degrees of accuracy. One study examined six different devices and found that the chest-strap monitor was the most accurate at measuring heart rate based on its agreement with electrocardiograph (ECG) tracings. On average, heart rates differed between the chest-strap monitor and the ECG standard by less than one beat per minute; heart rates differed between other devices and the ECG standard by nearly 20 beats per minute. Also of note is that accuracy varied with the type of activity that was performed: It was highest on a treadmill and lowest on an elliptical with moving handlebars. (Fast fact: In January 2016, consumers in three states filed a fraud class-action lawsuit against the manufacturer of a popular wearable fitness tracker for false advertising, claiming that its device is inaccurate at measuring heart rate which is contrary to how the device is marketed; as of this writing, the case is still pending.)

Thus, "high tech" doesn't necessarily mean "high accuracy." Given the inconvenience of chest-strap monitors and the inaccuracy of many wearable fitness trackers, the best way – and least expensive way – to determine your heart rate is the old-fashioned way and that's to measure it yourself. You can do this by locating your pulse at either the carotid artery (in your neck) or the radial artery (in your wrist). Simply place the tips of your index and middle fingers over one of these sites. (During intense activity, your carotid and radial arteries are easy to find.) Immediately after aerobic training, count your pulse for 10 seconds. Multiplying that number by six yields a good estimate of your exercising heart rate (in beats per minute). You can obtain a similar estimate by counting your pulse for 15 seconds and multiplying that number by four.

Time

In order to improve your aerobic fitness, you should do 20 to 60 minutes of aerobic activity. For years, it was thought that aerobic activities had to be continuous in order to improve aerobic fitness. However, research conducted since the mid-1990s has found that similar benefits can also be derived by doing several bouts of discontinuous activity that are accumulated throughout the course of the day.

In a 2009 review of the literature, researchers looked at 16 studies that involved 836 subjects. In general, the subjects exercised for 20 to 40 minutes per day, three to five days per week, for a period of four to 20 weeks. Those who were assigned to perform discontinuous activity did two to four bouts with each bout lasting 10 to 15 minutes. Most of the studies in the review found no significant differences between equal amounts of discontinuous activity and continuous activity with respect to improving aerobic fitness. There wasn't enough evidence to show that discontinuous activity is as good as continuous activity in other measures such as improving body composition, cholesterol and psychological well-being.

So although 20 to 60 minutes of continuous activity is preferred, you can improve your aerobic fitness by doing multiple bouts of at least 10 minutes in duration that add up to 20 to 60 minutes. For instance, two 15-minute bouts would equal 30 minutes of activity.

Keep in mind, too, that the time of an activity is inversely proportional to the intensity of an activity. This means that the length of your effort can be relatively brief as long as your level of intensity is relatively high. Generally speaking, doing a total of 20 minutes of continuous or discontinuous activity with an appropriate level of intensity is enough for most people to improve their aerobic fitness.

It should also be noted that if the length of your aerobic training is too brief, you might not produce a desirable expenditure of calories. This is an important consideration if one of your primary objectives is to lose or maintain weight. Here, you may need to perform aerobic training for at least 30 minutes (but not more than 60).

When your intensity is low – for whatever reason – your activities should be conducted for a longer period of time to improve your aerobic fitness. Take into account, though, that lengthy workouts may be inappropriate for some people in the initial stages of aerobic training. For one thing, performing too much activity too soon increases the risk of incurring an overuse injury. For another, some individuals may initially have such low levels of fitness that they might only be able to tolerate 5 to 10 minutes of aerobic training. In either case, the length of their aerobic training can be gradually increased as they improve their fitness.

Type

The combined application of the guidelines for the frequency, intensity and time (duration) of aerobic training provides a meaningful workload for your aerobic pathway. If these three ingredients of aerobic training produce the same expenditure of total calories, your physiological adaptations will be similar regardless of the type of aerobic activity that you perform. Therefore, you can use a wide assortment of activities to achieve improvements in your aerobic fitness.

The preferred types of aerobic activities are those that require a continuous effort, are rhythmic in nature and involve large amounts of muscle mass. Outdoor activities that meet these criteria include cross-country skiing, cycling, hiking/backpacking, ice/in-line/roller skating, jogging/running, rowing and walking; indoor activities include dancing, rope jumping and swimming along with exercising on stationary equipment such as cycles (upright or recumbent), ellipticals, rowers, steppers/stairclimbers and treadmills. Most of these aerobic options are activities that can be performed – and enjoyed – throughout a lifetime.

You can also attain improvements in your aerobic fitness from activities such as basketball, soccer and tennis. Remember, though, that your level of intensity can vary a great deal during these activities due to their intermittent nature. The way that these activities are structured also influences your level of intensity: In basketball, playing a full-court game is generally more demanding than a half-court game; in tennis, playing a singles match is generally more demanding than a doubles match.

To avoid boredom, it's important for you to change your activities from time to time. Fortunately, aerobic training allows a considerable amount of variety in terms of your activity selections.

Each aerobic activity has its advantages and disadvantages. For instance, swimming is desirable since it's a non-impact, non-weightbearing activity: The water supports your bodyweight which eliminates compressive forces on your bones and joints. On the other hand, swimming requires a fairly high degree of proficiency. If you have poor swimming skills, your heart rate may exceed your recommended training zone in a struggle just to keep yourself afloat. And if you're not skilled at swimming, you'll also tire very quickly. As such, swimming is a bad option if your skills are inadequate. But it's a good option if your skills are adequate.

In addition, some aerobic activities aren't advisable if you're prone to certain injuries or likely to complicate an existing orthopedic condition. For example, rope jumping is a high-impact activity that carries a greater risk of orthopedic stress and overuse injuries than a low-impact activity. Thus, rope jumping isn't advisable if you're a larger-than-average person – larger due to either fat or muscle – because of the excessive stress that's placed on your ankles, knees and lower back. Furthermore, someone who has chronic low-back pain would be more comfortable cycling in a recumbent position – in which the angle of the seat places the torso in a position that decreases the amount of stress in the lower back – instead of in the traditional upright position. So, the best advice is for you to select suitable aerobic activities that are enjoyable, compatible with your level of skill and orthopedically safe. (Fast fact: In general, a low-impact activity is one in which the feet remain in constant contact with the ground/floor or equipment.)

If you happen to be a competitive athlete who's training for a specific sport or activity – such as running or swimming – the best activities to do are the ones that you're going to perform. In one study, for example, 11 subjects did a 10-week program of running and showed significantly greater improvements in their maximum oxygen intake in running than in swimming (6.3% versus 2.6%). So if you want to become a better runner, you must mainly run; if you want to become a better swimmer, you must mainly swim.

But there's a caveat for runners and other athletes whose sport or activity involves running. As noted, the best activity for them is running. Unfortunately, running is a high-impact activity. In one study, researchers described running as "a series of collisions with the ground." The impact forces that are encountered when running are at least several times bodyweight. (The same holds true for rope jumping, by the way.) And depending on the distance that's run, the number of these "collisions" could easily be *in the thousands*; taking 54-inch steps over the course of a three-mile run amounts to *3,520* "collisions with the ground." What this means is that runners should include at least some non- or low-impact activities as part of their aerobic training to minimize the impact forces that are associated with running.

As long as it's orthopedically appropriate, the type of activity that you choose to improve your aerobic fitness isn't as critical as the frequency, intensity and duration of the activity. Your aerobic pathway doesn't know if you pedaled on a recumbent cycle one day and ran on a treadmill the next. The only thing that really matters is whether or not you applied a meaningful workload to your aerobic pathway.

APPROPRIATE AEROBIC TRAINING

In a nutshell, you should perform your aerobic training with a frequency, intensity and duration that are suitable and safe while using appropriate activities that require a sustained effort. If you're a healthy adult, your specific training prescription is to perform aerobic activities three to five times per week [frequency] at 60 to 90% of your age-predicted maximum heart rate [intensity] for 20 to 60 minutes [time] using preferred activities [type]. Bear in mind that all of these guidelines must be satisfied in order for you to improve your aerobic fitness.

MEANINGFUL AEROBIC TRAINING

Over a period of time, you'll likely find that the same aerobic workout – which was originally difficult – can be performed with less effort. As you improve your aerobic fitness, your exercising heart rate will be lower for a given level of intensity. Because of this, you must increase your intensity as needed so that you're always training with an appropriate percentage of your maximum heart rate. In addition, your ability to maintain a higher exercising heart rate will become easier. As a result, it's important for you to make your aerobic training progressively more challenging in order to produce further improvements in your aerobic fitness.

There are three main ways to overload your aerobic pathway. In comparison to a previous workout, you must attempt to (1) complete the same distance in a shorter duration; (2) cover a greater distance in the same duration; or (3) maintain the same pace for a greater distance or duration. As an example, suppose that you cycled 6.0 miles in 30 minutes (a pace of 12.0 miles per hour). In a future workout, you should try to (1) cycle 6.0 miles in less than 30 minutes; (2) cycle more than 6.0 miles in 30 minutes; or (3) cycle at 12.0 miles per hour for more than 6.0 miles or more than 30 minutes. Regardless of which tactic you employ, you made your aerobic pathway work harder than it's accustomed to working. (Note: With some stationary equipment, you can increase the resistance and/ or incline which also makes your aerobic pathway work harder in comparison to a previous workout.)

For this reason, it's vital that you keep accurate records of your aerobic training. Maintaining records permits you to track your progress thereby making your aerobic workouts more productive and more meaningful. During aerobic training, the key program components to monitor include the date of your workout, the duration of your workout, the distance that you completed and the level of your intensity (your exercising heart rate).

CONCURRENT TRAINING

A comprehensive fitness program includes strength training and aerobic training. When strength training and aerobic training are done as part of a fitness program, the scientific literature refers to it as concurrent training; this term is used regardless of whether the two activities are separated by minutes, hours or days.

The research on concurrent training dates back to 1980. That year, a classic study by Dr. Robert Hickson – then a professor of physical education at the University of Illinois at Chicago – was published in the *European Journal of Applied Physiology*. In his study, 39 subjects were assigned to three experimental groups: One group did strength training for 30 to 40 minutes per day five days per week; the second group did endurance training for 40 minutes per day six days per week; and the third group did concurrent training (strength training and endurance training) with the same duration and frequency as the groups that did strength training or endurance training. After 10 weeks of training, the group that did endurance training and the group that did concurrent training had improvements in maximum oxygen intake that ranged from about 17 to 27%. Meanwhile, the group that did strength training had no significant improvement in maximum oxygen intake. The group that did strength training and the group that did concurrent training had similar

improvements in strength for the first seven weeks of the study. However, during the last three weeks of the study, the group that did strength training continued to improve strength while the group that did concurrent training plateaued then declined. The group that did endurance training had no significant improvement in strength.

The findings of this early study fueled the belief that concurrent training – strength training and aerobic training – produces an interference effect: that one activity would interfere with any improvements that might be made in the other activity. In particular, individuals whose main focus is to increase their muscular strength and size have eschewed aerobic training with the fear that this activity would thwart their efforts. And on the surface, it certainly seems logical to think that strength training and aerobic training would have, so to speak, competing interests. But in the decades that have passed since Dr. Hickson's study was published in 1980, a great deal of research has shown that concurrent training can lead to results that are similar to strength training or aerobic training alone, provided that the volume of training isn't excessive. Indeed, a criticism of Dr. Hickson's study is that the duration and frequency of training was much too high.

One meta-analysis found no significant differences in the improvement of muscular strength and size when comparing groups that did strength training and groups that did concurrent training. The same meta-analysis found no significant difference in the improvement of maximum oxygen intake when comparing groups that did aerobic training and groups that did concurrent training. In fact, there's growing evidence that concurrent training may actually have an *additive effect* – not an interference effect – assisting with increasing strength and aerobic fitness. One study found that after 21 weeks, concurrent training – in which aerobic training and strength training were each done twice per week on separate days – produced nearly twice the increase in quadriceps size than strength training.

SCHEDULING TRAINING

Essentially, there are two options for scheduling strength training and aerobic training: The activities can be done on the same day or on alternate days. The advantage of doing both activities on the same day is that it allows more time for recovery between workouts. If strength training is performed on one day and aerobic training the next, your muscles and energy systems will be constantly stressed and your body may not have adequate time to sufficiently recover. After a while, it may also be very difficult for you to perform these activities several days in a row with a high degree of enthusiasm and requisite level of intensity. Therefore, the recommended way of scheduling strength training and aerobic training is to do both activities on the same day, preferably during the same workout and no more than three times per week on nonconsecutive days.

If strength training and aerobic training are done on the same day, which activity should be done first? It's clear, of course, that doing an activity first will result in better performance than doing it second (due to residual fatigue from the prior activity).

In a study by Dr. Wayne Westcott, eight subjects did strength training, rested for five minutes and then did aerobic training. During a subsequent session that was conducted three days later, the subjects did aerobic training, rested for five minutes and then did strength training. In both conditions, strength training consisted of one set of 8 to 12 repetitions to the point of muscular fatigue in about 20 minutes (11 exercises) and aerobic training consisted of cycling at more than 80% of the age-predicted maximum heart rate for 20 minutes. When strength training was done before aerobic training, the total weight lifted (pounds multiplied by repetitions) – which was used as a metric of strength performance – was 1.46% greater compared to when strength training was done after aerobic training. Therefore, the order of the two activities had a relatively small effect on strength performance. And when strength training was done before aerobic training, the exercising heart rate during aerobic training – which was used as a metric of aerobic performance – was 7.59% higher compared to when strength training was done after aerobic training. Therefore, the order of the two activities had a relatively large effect on aerobic performance. This is to say, the same aerobic workout was much more difficult to perform when it was done after strength training. Based on these findings, Dr. Westcott concluded that strength training has a greater impact on aerobic training than aerobic training has on strength training and that better overall results are obtained when aerobic training is done before strength training.

However, the results of this study must be interpreted with caution. Remember, these are the *short-term effects* of doing strength training and aerobic training in the same workout in a different order. Of far greater importance is what happens over time. In other words, what are the *long-term effects* of doing the two activities in the same workout in a different order?

A 2017 review and meta-analysis evaluated the effects of doing strength training and aerobic training in the same workout for at least eight weeks. Pooling data from seven studies in which concurrent training was done for a period of 8 to 24 weeks, aerobic training before or after strength training had no significant difference in improving maximum oxygen intake. Stated otherwise, the order of the two activities had no effect on aerobic performance.

But the effect that the order of the two activities had on strength performance told a different story. Pooling data from nine studies in which concurrent training was done for a period of 12 to 24 weeks, strength training before aerobic training was significantly better at improving maximum strength in the lower body in comparison to aerobic training before strength training. The effect on maximum strength in the upper body wasn't analyzed since only one study met the inclusion criteria.

Interestingly, a 2018 review and meta-analysis of 10 studies found that in regards to the lower body, strength training before aerobic

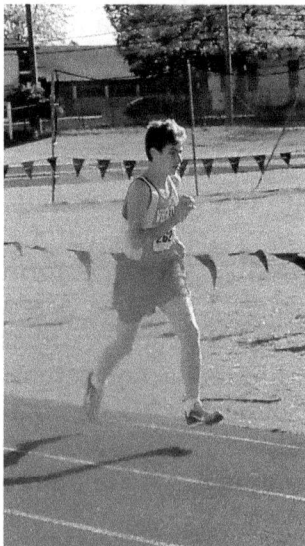

If a sport or an activity has a greater aerobic component then aerobic training should precede strength training. (Photo by Greg Fried.)

training was significantly better at improving dynamic strength but the order of the two activities had no effect on isometric strength. Of equal interest is that the order of the two activities had no effect on muscle size, maximum aerobic capacity and body composition.

In general, then, it appears that when aerobic training is done before strength training, the long-term effect is an impairment of strength performance. A number of variables affect the extent to which this occurs. Obviously, a higher frequency, intensity and/or duration of aerobic training will have a greater effect on strength performance than a lower frequency, intensity and/or duration of aerobic training. Another factor is the muscles that are used during aerobic training. For instance, aerobic training that involves the hips and legs will have a greater effect on strength performance on the leg press than on the bench press. Along these lines, the type of aerobic activity is an important consideration: High-impact activities such as running will have a greater effect on strength performance than low-impact activities such as cycling. In addition, the time (recovery) that's taken between aerobic training and strength training will have an effect on strength performance. Certainly, taking a shorter time between aerobic training and strength training will have a greater effect on strength performance than taking a longer time between aerobic training and strength training.

So what's the bottom line? Based on current evidence, if your primary goal is to increase your aerobic fitness, the order of strength training and aerobic training doesn't matter too much; and if your primary goal is to increase your muscular strength, it's better to do strength training before aerobic training.

There's one final caveat: Dr. Westcott notes that if you're a competitive athlete, whether you do strength training or aerobic training first depends on the nature of your sport or activity. If a sport or an activity has a greater strength component – such as shot putting and high jumping – then strength training should precede aerobic training; if a sport or an activity has a greater aerobic component – such as basketball and soccer – then aerobic training should precede strength training.

In addition to the possibility of doing strength training and aerobic training on the same day, athletes may also be required to do skill training. If these three activities are performed on the same day, better overall results will be obtained if skill training is done first. Of all three activities, the one that's most critical to athletes is skill training. If athletes are exhausted after aerobic training and/or strength training, they'll be drained both physically and mentally. Therefore, they won't practice very hard or work on their technique very well. In fact, they're sure to be inattentive and their performance will probably be quite careless, labored and awkward. Furthermore, athletes are more prone to injury when practicing in a pre-fatigued state. Because of this, it's best for athletes to do skill training before aerobic training and/or strength training.

PREDICTING OXYGEN INTAKE

Oxygen intake (aka oxygen consumption) is perhaps the most widely accepted indicator of aerobic fitness. Like virtually all of your other physiological characteristics, your aerobic potential is greatly influenced by your genetic (inherited) profile (especially as it relates to your predominant muscle fiber type). One of the largest studies on this topic – involving 436 pairs of monozygotic (identical) twins and 622 pairs of dizygotic (fraternal) twins – found that 62%

230

of the difference between individuals in predicted oxygen intake was attributable to genetics. A smaller study – involving 29 pairs of monozygotic twins and 19 pairs of dizygotic twins – found that 66% of the difference between individuals in actual oxygen intake was attributable to genetics. (Fast fact: Dr. AV Hill introduced the concept of maximum oxygen intake in 1923.)

There are a number of ways to accurately measure oxygen intake in a laboratory. One way is to exercise while wearing a mouthpiece or mask that interfaces with a computer which measures and analyzes the amount of oxygen that you inhale and the amount of carbon dioxide that you exhale. The computer is mounted on a compact, portable device that's known as a metabolic cart. (This method can also be used to determine caloric needs.) The most commonly used activity to assess oxygen intake in a laboratory is probably running (or walking) on a treadmill. Other ways include pedaling a cycle ergometer in an upright or recumbent position using your legs and/or arms; stepping up on and down from a bench of a standard height at a fixed rate of stepping; and rowing. Using stationary equipment makes it possible for you to perform at different levels of intensity while maintaining your body in a relatively stable position. This allows you to be instrumented in order to measure not only the respiratory process – the gases that you inhale and exhale – but other physiological responses such as your exercising heart rate, blood pressure and caloric expenditure.

Laboratory tests can provide you with accurate data that are reliable and valid. However, laboratory testing can be impractical, expensive and time-consuming (if this option is even available). Fortunately, there's another way to assess your oxygen intake without the inherent drawbacks of laboratory testing. Since these assessments are performed outside the laboratory, they're referred to as field tests. Certain field tests of oxygen intake have a high correlation to laboratory tests.

One of the most popular field tests that can be used to determine oxygen intake is the 1.5-Mile Running Test. The primary objective of this test is to run 1.5 miles in the least amount of time. For this field test to be as accurate as possible, you must run exactly 1.5 miles and it must be on a level (horizontal) surface. Because of this, running on an indoor or outdoor track is preferred. Generally, the results of the 1.5-Mile Running Test are an excellent predictor of oxygen intake. But it's important to realize that this particular test favors runners since it involves running. (Fast fact: A 1.0-mile run is more appropriate for younger children and older adults.)

Oxygen Intake: Relative

Table 14.1 lists predicted values of oxygen intake based on the time that's taken to complete a 1.5-mile run on a level surface. These values are a relative measure of how much oxygen is consumed in milliliters per kilogram of bodyweight per minute (or mL/kg/min).

Consider a 30-year-old man who weighs 198 pounds and can run 1.5 miles in 12:30 (12 minutes and 30 seconds). Note in Table 14.1 that his oxygen intake for this particular running time is 42.12 mL/kg/min or, simply, 42.12. In other words, he consumed about 42.12 milliliters of oxygen for every kilogram that he weighed during each minute of his 1.5-mile run.

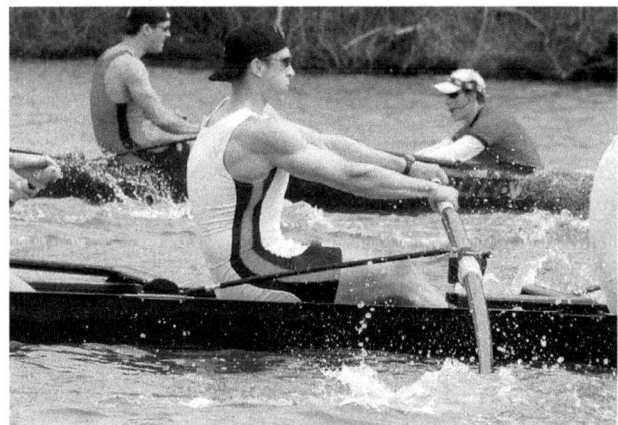

Endurance athletes with high levels of oxygen intake in relative terms include long-distance runners and cyclists and rowers. (Photo by Tom Nowak.)

Table 14.2 shows norms for oxygen intake in relative terms based on age and gender. Note that an oxygen intake of 42.12 mL/kg/min is average for men of his age.

Oxygen intakes of elite endurance athletes typically exceed 80.0 mL/kg/min in men and 70.0 mL/kg/min in women. Among world-class cross-country skiers, for example, average values of 85.6 mL/kg/min for men and 70.1 mL/kg/min for women have been reported. Other endurance athletes with high levels of oxygen intake in relative terms include long-distance runners and cyclists and rowers.

Table 14.1 is only valid for determining oxygen intake during a 1.5-mile run. The ACSM offers this equation for calculating oxygen intake in mL/kg/min for a run of any known distance and duration on a level surface:

oxygen intake = (speed in m/min) x (0.2 mL/ kg/min per m/min) + 3.5 mL/kg/min

As an example, suppose that you just completed a 5K (5,000-meter) race in 20:00. In this scenario, your running speed was 250.0 meters per minute [5,000 m ÷ 20.0 min = 250.0 m/min]. Next, multiply your speed [250.0 m/min] by the oxygen cost of horizontal running [0.2 mL/kg/min per m/min] and add the oxygen cost of resting [3.5 mL/kg/min]. This calculation yields a value of 53.5 mL/kg/min [250.0 m/min x 0.2 mL/kg/min per m/min + 3.5 mL/kg/min = 53.5 mL/kg/min].

For this equation to be accurate, you must run on a level surface at a speed of at least 5.0 miles per hour (mph) or 134.0 m/min. (Note: To convert mph to m/min, multiply the mph by 26.8; to convert miles to meters, multiply the miles by 1,609.)

Oxygen intake can also be calculated for walking speeds between 1.9 and 3.7 mph or 50.0 and 100.0 m/min. (For most people, speeds between 100.0 and 134.0 m/min are too fast for walking and too slow for running.) At low speeds, walking is generally a more efficient process than running. In fact, the oxygen cost of horizontal walking at a given speed is about one half that of horizontal running. Therefore, the only change to the earlier equation is that the oxygen cost of horizontal walking is used which is 0.1 mL/kg/min per m/min. So if you walked 3,000 meters in 30 minutes, your oxygen intake would be 13.5 mL/kg/min [100.0 m/min x 0.1 mL/kg/min per m/min + 3.5 mL/kg/min = 13.5 mL/kg/min].

Oxygen Intake: Absolute

Oxygen intake can also be expressed in absolute terms in liters per minute (L/min). To determine oxygen intake in L/min, you must first convert bodyweight to kilograms (kg). To do this, divide bodyweight in pounds (lb) by 2.2. Using the earlier example of the 30-year-old male, his 198-pound bodyweight is equal to 90 kg [198 lb ÷ 2.2 kg/lb = 90 kg]. Next, multiply his bodyweight (in kilograms) by his oxygen intake (in mL/kg/min). Staying with the same example as before produces a value of 3,790.8 mL/min [90 kg x 42.12 mL/kg/min = 3,790.8 mL/min]. Finally, divide this number by 1,000 (to convert from milliliters to liters). To divide by 1,000, simply move the decimal point three places to the left. This means that a 198-pound individual who ran 1.5 miles in 12:30 would consume about 3.79 liters of oxygen during every minute of his run.

Table 14.3 shows norms for oxygen intake in absolute terms based on age and gender. Note that an oxygen intake of 3.79 L/min is excellent for men of his age. Recall that when bodyweight wasn't considered, his aerobic fitness was average.

Oxygen intakes of elite endurance athletes typically exceed 6.0 L/min in men and 4.0 L/min in women. Among world-class cross-country skiers, for example, average values of 6.38 L/min for men and 4.28 L/min for women have been reported. Other endurance athletes with high levels of oxygen intake in absolute terms include heavyweight rowers (since their bodyweight is a factor here).

A World-Class Application

It's interesting to calculate the oxygen intake of a world-class runner. In 1996, Daniel Komen of Kenya, at the age of 20, set the world record in the men's 3,000-meter run on an outdoor track with a time of 7:20.67. The ACSM equation can be used since the distance and time are known and the performance was done on a level surface without any inclines or declines.

In setting the world record, his running speed was 408.47 meters per minute. (Note: The decimal equivalent of 7:20.67 is 7.3445 minutes.) Multiplying his speed by 0.2 mL/kg/min per m/min and adding the oxygen cost of resting is an oxygen intake of 85.19 mL/kg/min which is literally "off the charts." Multiplying this number by his bodyweight of 55 kilograms (according to the International Association of Athletics Federations) is 4,685.45 mL. Dividing this number by 1,000 reveals an oxygen intake of about 4.69 L/min which is also off the charts but not as impressive because of his low bodyweight.

Expected Oxygen Intake

According to the ACSM, the following regression equations can be used to predict expected oxygen intake (in mL/kg/min) based on activity level, gender and age:

active men: 69.7 - (0.612 x age)

active women: 42.9 - (0.312 x age)

inactive men: 57.8 - (0.445 x age)

inactive women: 42.3 - (0.356 x age)

For instance, an active 30-year-old man would be expected to have an oxygen intake of about 51.34 mL/kg/min [0.612 x 30 = 18.36; 69.7 - 18.36 = 51.34].

Comparing your expected oxygen intake to your actual oxygen intake determines whether or not you have any Functional Aerobic Impairment (FAI). The FAI can be found by subtracting the actual oxygen intake from the expected oxygen intake. This value is divided by the expected oxygen intake and then multiplied by 100 (to convert the number to a percentage).

If the 30-year-old man in this example was found to have an actual oxygen intake of 42.12 mL/kg/min, he would have an FAI of about 18.0% [51.34 mL/kg/min - 42.12 mL/kg/min ÷ 51.34 mL/kg/min x 100 = 17.96%]. A positive percentage indicates that the actual oxygen intake is worse than expected; a negative percentage indicates that the actual oxygen intake is better than expected. It must be reiterated that your genetic profile plays a major role in determining your level of aerobic fitness.

Finally, the purpose of assessing your aerobic fitness shouldn't be to compare your performance to that of someone else. Assessments of aerobic fitness are much more meaningful when your present level is compared to your past level.

Oxygen Intake and Strength Training

As mentioned earlier, your exercising heart rate is a good indicator of your intensity. However, your respiratory and circulatory systems respond much differently while strength training than while aerobic training.

For the same oxygen intake, strength training generates a higher heart rate compared to aerobic training. And for the same heart rate, strength training generates a lower oxygen intake compared to aerobic training.

In a study that was conducted at the Washington University Medical School, researchers examined the physiological responses of 13 males while strength training (one set of 14 exercises to the point of muscular fatigue) and while walking on a treadmill (at 4.0 miles per hour). During strength training, their oxygen intake was 18.3 mL/kg/min and their heart rate was 155 bpm; during treadmill walking, their oxygen intake was 18.4 mL/kg/min – which was virtually identical to that of strength training – but their heart rate was 115 bpm. So according to this study, for roughly the same oxygen intake, strength training produced an exercising heart rate that was nearly 35% higher than aerobic training. And despite training at the same oxygen intake, blood lactate during strength training *was 16 times higher than walking*. This is very telling in that a high level of blood lactate indicates that the primary energy system was Anaerobic Glycolysis; a low level of blood lactate indicates that the primary energy system was Aerobic Glycolysis. On a related note, the RPE was 18 for strength training and 8 for walking.

The study didn't compare oxygen intake for the same heart rate while strength training and treadmill walking. But because there's a linear relationship between heart rate and oxygen intake, the data points can be extrapolated. Remember, a heart rate of 115 bpm while treadmill walking corresponded to an oxygen intake of 18.4 mL/kg/min. From this, it can be estimated that a heart rate of 155 bpm while treadmill walking would correspond to an oxygen intake of about 24.8 mL/kg/min. That same heart rate of 155 bpm while strength training corresponded to an oxygen intake of 18.3 mL/kg/min. So again, this underscores the point that for the same heart rate, strength training generates a lower oxygen intake compared to aerobic training.

ESTIMATING CALORIC EXPENDITURE

In 1824, Nicolas Clement – a French chemist and physicist with no formal education – defined a calorie as a unit of heat. Back then, he used the calorie in reference to fuel efficiency for the steam engine. Nearly 70 years later, the calorie was adopted for use in nutritional science.

In technical terms, a calorie is the amount of heat that's required to raise the temperature of one gram of water by one degree Celsius. In practical terms, a calorie is a measure of your energy intake (eating) as well as your energy output (exercising).

The caloric equivalent of one liter of oxygen ranges from 4.7 calories when fat is used as the sole source of energy to 5.0 calories when carbohydrates are used as the sole source of energy. For all practical purposes – and with little loss in precision – about 5.0 calories are used for every liter of oxygen that's consumed. (Fast fact: The caloric equivalent of one liter of oxygen is 4.4 calories when protein is used as the sole source of energy. Under most circumstances, however, the use of protein isn't significant – it's negligible while resting and minimal while exercising – and, therefore, is usually disregarded.)

To determine the rate of caloric expenditure, simply take oxygen intake in L/min and multiply it by 5.0 calories per liter (cal/L). Recall the earlier example of the 198-pound male whose oxygen intake was 3.79 L/min. In this case, his rate of caloric expenditure would be almost 19.0 calories per minute [3.79 L/min x 5.0 cal/L = 18.95 cal/min].

To determine the total number of calories that he used during his 1.5-mile run, multiply his rate of caloric expenditure (in cal/min) by his running time. In this case, multiplying 18.95 cal/min by 12.5 minutes (12:30 in decimal form) indicates that he used about 237.0 calories during his run [18.95 cal/min x 12.5 min = 236.88 cal].

Remember that when Daniel Komen set the world record of 7:20.67 in the 3,000-meter run, his oxygen intake was about 4.69 L/min. Multiplying this by 5.0 cal/L is a caloric expenditure of 23.45 cal/min. Multiplying this by his time of 7.3445 minutes is about 172.23 calories. Not bad for a little more than seven minutes of exertion.

MET LEVELS

Another way to quantify oxygen intake – and caloric expenditure – during exercise/activity is to use what's technically known as a metabolic equivalent of task (MET) or, for short, a metabolic equivalent. A MET is the amount of oxygen that's consumed while resting in a seated position. Specifically, 1.0 MET is about 3.5 mL/kg/min. In essence, METs are multiples of oxygen intake, so 2.0 METs are about 7.0 mL/kg/min [3.5 mL/kg/min x 2.0 = 7.0 mL/kg/min], 3.0 METs are about 10.5 mL/kg/min and so on.

MET levels can be used to make comparisons. Exercising at 2.0 METs requires twice as much oxygen (or energy) as exercising at 1.0 MET (7.0 mL/kg/min versus 3.5 mL/kg/min); exercising at 6.0 METs requires three times as much oxygen as exercising at 2.0 METs (21.0 mL/kg/min versus 7.0 mL/kg/min).

It's easy to express oxygen intake in METs. To do so, simply divide oxygen intake in mL/kg/min by 3.5 mL/kg/min. For instance, the 198-pound male in the ongoing example had an oxygen intake of 42.12 mL/kg/min when he ran 1.5 miles in 12:30. In this case, his oxygen intake is equal to about 12.0 METs [42.12 ÷ 3.5 mL/kg/min = 12.03 METs]. Or look at it this way:

Running 1.5 miles in 12:30 is about 12 times more demanding than resting in a seated position.

In addition, MET levels can be used to estimate the rate of caloric expenditure in calories per kilogram of bodyweight per minute (cal/kg/min) and calories per minute (cal/min). A value of 1.0 MET is equal to about 0.0175 cal/kg/min. Therefore, caloric expenditure can be estimated in cal/kg/min by multiplying the MET level by 0.0175 cal/kg/min. For example, the 198-pound man who exercised at 12.03 METs used about 0.210525 cal/kg/min [12.03 x 0.0175 cal/kg/min = 0.210525 cal/kg/min]. To estimate cal/min, multiply his bodyweight in kilograms [90] by his cal/kg/min [0.210525]. This produces a value of about 18.95 cal/min [90 kg x 0.210525 cal/kg/min = 18.947 cal/min]. Recall that when a different series of calculations was used in the preceding section, his rate of caloric expenditure was also estimated as 18.95 cal/min.

AEROBIC INTENSITY: HIGH OR LOW?

Energy can be provided by carbohydrates, fat and protein. However, protein isn't a preferred source of energy; its use is negligible while resting and minimal while exercising. In fact, protein is generally used as a last resort. Remember, protein is located in your muscles and if you must rely on it as an energy source, then you're literally cannibalizing yourself.

So that leaves carbohydrates and fat as your main sources of energy. What your body elects to use is dictated by your level of intensity. During activity of lower intensity, your body prefers to use fat; during activity of higher intensity, your body prefers to use carbohydrates. (Carbohydrates are a more efficient source of energy but fat is used because your body doesn't need to be efficient at lower levels of intensity.)

Note that both carbohydrates and fat are used during activity but to different degrees. With low-intensity activity, fat is the main source of energy but carbohydrates are also used; with high-intensity activity, carbohydrates are the main source of energy but fat is also used. So, as an activity becomes more intense, the body shifts to a greater reliance on carbohydrates.

These physiological facts have led to the mistaken belief that low-intensity (or "fat-burning") activity is better than high-intensity (or "carbohydrate-burning") activity when it comes to losing weight, "burning fat" and expending calories. This misconception has also spawned the notion that people should train within their so-called fat-burning zones.

The idea of keeping the intensity low in order to mobilize and selectively use a higher percentage of fat may sound logical but it doesn't hold up mathematically and has never been verified in the laboratory. In truth, even though a greater *percentage* of fat calories are used during low-intensity activity, a greater *number* of fat calories (and total calories) is used during high-intensity activity.

During any activity, the rate of caloric expenditure is directly related to the intensity: The higher the intensity, the greater the rate of caloric expenditure. In the case of running, for example, intensity is directly related to speed: The faster the running speed, the greater the rate of caloric expenditure. The time of activity is also a factor: The longer that a given activity is performed, the greater the total caloric expenditure.

Based on the ACSM equations for calculating oxygen intake and caloric expenditure during walking and running, a 165-pound man who walks 3.0 miles in 60 minutes on a level surface uses roughly 4.33 cal/min. Over the course of his 60-minute walk, then, he'd use about 260 calories. If that same individual ran those 3.0 miles in 30 minutes, he'd use about 13.38 cal/min. (Note the higher rate of caloric expenditure.) Over the course of his 30-minute run, then, he'd use about 401 calories. So, exercising at a higher level of intensity used significantly more calories than exercising at a lower level of intensity [401 calories versus 260 calories]. This is true despite the fact that the activity of lower intensity was performed for twice as long as the activity of higher intensity.

These calculations have been corroborated by research performed in the laboratory. In a study that was conducted by Dr. John Porcari and his colleagues at the University of Wisconsin-Lacrosse, 16 subjects walked on a treadmill at an average speed of 3.8 mph for 30 minutes. In this instance, they used about 8.0 cal/min for a total caloric expenditure of 240 calories. Of these 240 calories, 59% (144 calories) were from carbohydrates and 41% (96 calories) were from fat. As part of the study, the subjects also ran on a treadmill at an average speed of 6.5 mph for 30 minutes. At this relatively higher level of intensity, they used about 15.0 cal/min for a total caloric expenditure of 450 calories. Of these 450 calories, 76% (342 calories) were from carbohydrates and 24% (108 calories) were from fat. In other words, exercising at a higher level of intensity resulted in a greater total caloric expenditure than exercising at a lower level of intensity (450 calories versus 240 calories) and also used a greater number of calories from fat in the same length of time (108 calories versus 96 calories). Other studies have also demonstrated that more calories are expended when running a given distance than walking the same distance. (By the way, this means that walking a mile doesn't use the same number of calories as running a mile as some people have suggested.)

The intent behind advocating low-intensity activity of long duration is to enhance safety and improve adherence, especially in those who are new to training. However, low-intensity activity isn't more effective for fat loss than high-intensity activity. Think about it: The activity that uses the greatest percentage of fat as an energy source is sleeping. And who would recommend sleeping as the best activity to lose fat?

In terms of losing weight, you must expend more calories than you consume in order to produce a caloric deficit. Whether you use carbohydrates or fat to produce this shortfall is immaterial. A caloric deficit that's created by the use of fat as an energy source doesn't necessarily translate into greater loss of fat compared to an equal caloric deficit that's created by the use of carbohydrates as an energy source. The main determinant of fat loss and weight loss is *calories*, not *composition*.

In short, researchers in the area of exercise and weight management generally agree that it probably doesn't matter whether you use carbohydrates or fat while exercising in order to lose weight. (Chapter 22 discusses the subject of weight management in greater detail.) Finally, it should also be noted that low-intensity activity might not elevate the heart rate enough to improve aerobic fitness.

AEROBIC INTENSITY: EFFECT OF CELL PHONES

Using a cell phone while exercising is a distraction that often decreases the intensity and effectiveness of a workout. In one crossover study, 44 students at Kent State University were randomly assigned to walk on a treadmill for 30 minutes on three separate occasions while either texting, talking or listening to self-selected music on their cell phone. On a fourth occasion, they did the same activity but without their cell phone. In each case, the subjects could adjust the speed of the treadmill as they desired but the console was covered so that they couldn't see their walking pace. Speed and heart rate were significantly lower – the intensity was lower – when the subjects used their cell phones for texting and talking compared to when they didn't use their cell phones. Interesting, speed and heart rate were significantly higher – the intensity was higher – when the subjects used their cell phones for listening to music. So although listening to music from a cell phone while exercising can be beneficial, talking and texting on a cell phone is not.

This also applies to strength training, of course. Individuals who exercise their thumbs in between sets are interrupting their concentration. There's no question that doing this greatly interferes with your intensity and makes your workout less effective. If you want to reap the rewards of a fitness program, do yourself a big favor and focus on your workout, not on your cell phone.

Table 14.1: Predicted values of oxygen intake (in mL/kg/min) based on the time to complete a 1.5-mile run on a level surface

TIME	VALUE	TIME	VALUE	TIME	VALUE	TIME	VALUE
8:00	63.84	10:00	51.77	12:00	43.73	14:00	37.98
8:05	63.22	10:05	51.37	12:05	43.45	14:05	37.77
8:10	62.61	10:10	50.98	12:10	43.17	14:10	37.57
8:15	62.01	10:15	50.59	12:15	42.90	14:15	37.37
8:20	61.42	10:20	50.21	12:20	42.64	14:20	37.18
8:25	60.85	10:25	49.84	12:25	42.38	14:25	36.98
8:30	60.29	10:30	49.47	12:30	42.12	14:30	36.79
8:35	59.74	10:35	49.11	12:35	41.86	14:35	36.60
8:40	59.20	10:40	48.75	12:40	41.61	14:40	36.41
8:45	58.67	10:45	48.40	12:45	41.36	14:45	36.23
8:50	58.15	10:50	48.06	12:50	41.11	14:50	36.04
8:55	57.63	10:55	47.72	12:55	40.87	14:55	35.86
9:00	57.13	11:00	47.38	13:00	40.63	15:00	35.68
9:05	56.64	11:05	47.05	13:05	40.39	15:05	35.50
9:10	56.16	11:10	46.73	13:10	40.16	15:10	35.33
9:15	55.68	11:15	46.41	13:15	39.93	15:15	35.15
9:20	55.21	11:20	46.09	13:20	39.70	15:20	34.98
9:25	54.76	11:25	45.78	13:25	39.48	15:25	34.81
9:30	54.31	11:30	45.47	13:30	39.26	15:30	34.64
9:35	53.87	11:35	45.17	13:35	39.04	15:35	34.48
9:40	53.43	11:40	44.87	13:40	38.82	15:40	34.31
9:45	53.01	11:45	44.58	13:45	38.61	15:45	34.15
9:50	52.59	11:50	44.29	13:50	38.39	15:50	33.99
9:55	52.18	11:55	44.01	13:55	38.19	15:55	33.83

Table 14.2: Norms for oxygen intake in relative terms based on age and gender

MEN					
AGE	**LOW**	**FAIR**	**AVERAGE**	**GOOD**	**HIGH**
20 - 29	<38	39 - 43	44 - 51	52 - 56	57+
30 - 39	<34	35 - 39	40 - 47	48 - 51	52+
40 - 49	<30	31 - 35	36 - 43	44 - 47	48+
50 - 59	<25	26 - 31	32 - 39	40 - 43	44+
60 - 69	<21	22 - 26	27 - 35	36 - 39	40+
WOMEN					
AGE	**LOW**	**FAIR**	**AVERAGE**	**GOOD**	**HIGH**
20 - 29	<28	29 - 34	35 - 43	44 - 48	49+
30 - 39	<27	28 - 33	34 - 41	42 - 47	48+
40 - 49	<25	26 - 31	32 - 40	41 - 45	46+
50 - 65	<21	22 - 28	29 - 36	37 - 41	42+

Table 14.3: Norms for oxygen intake in absolute terms based on age and gender

MEN					
AGE	**LOW**	**FAIR**	**AVERAGE**	**GOOD**	**HIGH**
20 - 29	<2.79	2.80 - 3.09	3.10 - 3.69	3.70 - 3.99	4.00+
30 - 39	<2.49	2.50 - 2.79	2.80 - 3.39	3.40 - 3.69	3.70+
40 - 49	<2.19	2.20 - 2.49	2.50 - 3.09	3.10 - 3.39	3.40+
50 - 59	<1.89	1.90 - 2.19	2.20 - 2.79	2.80 - 3.09	3.10+
60 - 69	<1.59	1.60 - 1.89	1.90 - 2.49	2.50 - 2.79	2.80+
WOMEN					
AGE	**LOW**	**FAIR**	**AVERAGE**	**GOOD**	**HIGH**
20 - 29	<1.69	1.70 - 1.99	2.00 - 2.49	2.50 - 2.79	2.80+
30 - 39	<1.59	1.60 - 1.89	1.90 - 2.39	2.40 - 2.69	2.70+
40 - 49	<1.49	1.50 - 1.79	1.80 - 2.29	2.30 - 2.59	2.60+
50 - 65	<1.29	1.30 - 1.59	1.60 - 2.09	2.10 - 2.39	2.40+

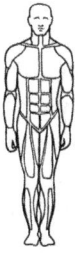

15 Anaerobic Training

Many sports and activities are composed of brief, intense movements that rely heavily on your anaerobic fitness. The best way for you to prepare for these specific physiological demands is through anaerobic training. (Literally, the term anaerobic means in the absence of oxygen.)

The main purpose of anaerobic training is to improve the functional ability of your anaerobic pathways, namely your ATP-PC System and Anaerobic Glycolysis. A second purpose of anaerobic training is to improve your performance potential, especially in "stop-and-go" sports and activities that require short-term, high-intensity efforts such as basketball, football and soccer.

But anaerobic training also produces some unexpected results. As part of a 1996 study that was led by Dr. Izumi Tabata, seven physical-education majors trained five times per week for six weeks. Four of the weekly workouts were anaerobic, consisting of seven to eight repeats of 20 seconds of all-out sprinting on a stationary cycle with 10 seconds of recovery between each sprint. The other weekly workout had aerobic and anaerobic elements, consisting of 30 minutes of continuous exertion along with four repeats of 20 seconds of all-out sprinting on a stationary cycle with 10 seconds of recovery between each sprint. The subjects not only significantly increased their anaerobic capacity by 28% but also significantly increased their oxygen intake by 14%. It's likely that the aerobic training had some influence on the improvement in oxygen intake but it's unclear as to what degree. Nonetheless, since this seminal study, a growing body of research has found that anaerobic training can be highly beneficial.

Sidebar: Doing eight repeats of 20 seconds of all-out effort with 10 seconds of recovery between each effort has become known as the Tabata Protocol or Tabata Method. Although the system bears Dr. Tabata's name, it was actually introduced by Kouichi Irisawa – then the head coach of the Japanese National Speed Skating Team – and had been used for several years by athletes on the team.

In many cases, the results that are attained through anaerobic training are nothing short of spectacular. In one study, for example, Dr. Kirsten Burgomaster and her colleagues assigned eight physically active subjects to an experimental group that did anaerobic training three times per week for two weeks. (A second group acted as a control and didn't train.) Each workout consisted of four to seven repeats of a Wingate Test (30 seconds of all-out effort on a stationary cycle against a fixed resistance that's based on an individual's bodyweight) with four minutes of recovery between each effort. In the two-week period, the subjects in the experimental group did a total of 32 bouts of 30-second efforts, amounting to 16 minutes of sprinting. Their longest "workout" involved 3.5 minutes of sprinting. The subjects improved their time to fatigue while cycling at 80% of their maximum oxygen intake by nearly 100% (from 26 minutes to 51 minutes). The results would've been even more astonishing if the data excluded the results of one subject who had sustained a minor ankle injury (unrelated to the study) the day before the post-test and whose endurance decreased by 16%.

One other study deserves mention since it directly compared aerobic training to anaerobic training. In this study, Dr. Martin Gibala and his colleagues randomly assigned 16 physically active subjects to two groups: One group did aerobic training that consisted of 90 to 120 minutes of continuous exertion while cycling at

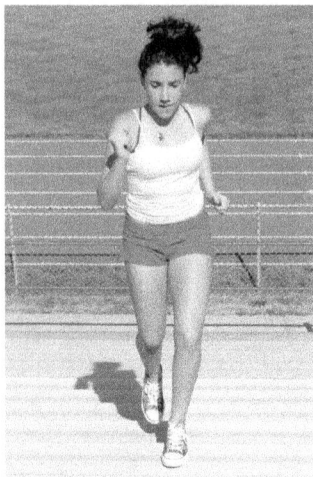

In order to increase anaerobic fitness, anaerobic training should be done one or two days per week. (Photo by Fred Fornicola.)

65% of their maximum oxygen intake. The other group did anaerobic training that consisted of four to six repeats of a Wingate Test on a stationary cycle with four minutes of recovery between each sprint. Both groups did their assigned workout six times over a period of two weeks. In a cycling test that equated to about 30,000 meters (about 18.64 miles), the group that did aerobic training decreased (improved) their time by 7.5% while the group that did anaerobic training decreased their time by 10.1%; in a cycling test that equated to about 2,000 meters (about 1.24 miles), the group that did aerobic training decreased their time by 3.5% while the group that did anaerobic training decreased their time by 4.1%. And get this: Over the two-week period, the total exercise time of the group that did aerobic training was 630 minutes. Meanwhile, the total exercise time of the group that did anaerobic training was *15 minutes* (150 minutes if you count the recovery taken between sprints). So, anaerobic training produced slightly better results than aerobic training and those results were achieved in a fraction of the time.

These studies and others haven't escaped notice by the media. This attention has produced a new-found awareness and appreciation of anaerobic training by the general population.

Note: Before you initiate anaerobic training, you must first establish a solid base of aerobic support through aerobic training. Your anaerobic pathways can't function at optimal levels without assistance from your aerobic pathway.

ANAEROBIC GUIDELINES

Anaerobic training is a bit more complex than aerobic training. The anaerobic pathways play an important role in activities that last anywhere from a split second to roughly three minutes (assuming, of course, that the level of effort is great enough to justify an anaerobic response). Specifically, the ATP-PC System is used for maximum efforts of about 10 seconds or less; the ATP-PC System and Anaerobic Glycolysis for maximum efforts of about 30 seconds or less; Anaerobic Glycolysis for maximum efforts of about 30 to 90 seconds; and Anaerobic Glycolysis and Aerobic Glycolysis for physical efforts of about 1.5 to 3.0 minutes. (Aerobic Glycolysis is used for physical efforts of about three minutes or more.)

You can improve your anaerobic fitness by incorporating several easy-to-follow guidelines. These guidelines can be organized under the acronym FITT which stands for Frequency, Intensity, Time and Type.

Frequency

In order to improve your anaerobic fitness, you should do anaerobic training one or two days per week. The low frequency is required due to the intense nature of anaerobic training.

To be clear, a frequency of three to five days per week that's prescribed for conditioning workouts represents the total frequency of aerobic training *and* anaerobic training. In other words, if anaerobic training is done on two days in a particular week, then aerobic training would be done no more than one to three days for a weekly total of three to five days of conditioning.

Doing anaerobic training a bit more frequently may be beneficial if you're a highly competitive athlete. But if you reach a point where you're no longer making improvements, then you're probably doing too much anaerobic training.

Intensity

With anaerobic training, your efforts must be done in an aggressive and enthusiastic fashion. To engage your anaerobic pathways, then, your intensity must be great enough such that you can't train continuously for much more than about three minutes at a time (which is the upper limit of the anaerobic domain).

Anaerobic intensity can be measured the same way as aerobic intensity: by monitoring your exercising heart rate. But anaerobic training requires a much higher level of intensity than aerobic training. In order to involve your anaerobic pathways, you must elevate your heart rate to near-maximum levels for brief periods of time. Raising your heart rate to 90% or more of your age-predicted maximum is usually a good indication that you're employing your anaerobic pathways. (Chapter 14 describes how you can determine your age-predicted maximum heart rate.)

In general, some people may need to maintain their heart rates above or below the training zone that's recommended for others of the same age. If you're highly active or have an above-average level of fitness, you should train with a higher percentage of your age-predicted maximum heart rate to produce meaningful results; if you're inactive or have a below-average level of fitness, you should train with a lower percentage of your age-predicted maximum heart rate to avoid potential risks.

Remember, the cornerstone of anaerobic training is short-term, high-intensity efforts. Unlike aerobic training – where a decreased level of intensity can be sacrificed for an increased duration of activity – it's an absolute requirement that anaerobic training is performed with a level of effort that's as high as possible.

Time

In determining which energy systems are emphasized, the *duration* of the activity is more critical than the *distance* of the activity. As an example, suppose that two individuals ran 400 meters as fast as possible. Let's say that one of them completed the distance in one minute while the other needed two minutes. So, the distance that was run by the two individuals was the same but the time that was taken by the two individuals was different which means, in this case, that the energy systems were different: The

one-minute, all-out effort involved Anaerobic Glycolysis while the two-minute, all-out effort involved Anaerobic Glycolysis and Aerobic Glycolysis.

That said, it's often more practical to consider distance rather than duration when performing anaerobic training. If a handful of seconds to three minutes is used as the range of time for anaerobic training, you can easily determine a range of distances. For example, an all-out effort that lasts a handful of seconds correlates to running about 40 meters (or 40 yards). And an all-out effort that lasts three minutes correlates to running about 800 meters (or one-half mile), at least for people who are in reasonably good condition. (You can determine a precise range of distances for your anaerobic efforts during rowing, running, swimming and other activities based on the energy continuum and your level of fitness.)

For competitive athletes, the distances (times) that are used during their anaerobic training should approximate the distances (times) that are used during their sport or activity. For example, if a sport or an activity involves a series of intense efforts that are 30 meters or less, then these specific distances should receive the most emphasis during anaerobic training. At least some of the efforts, however, should also consist of distances (times) that are a little beyond those normally encountered in competition.

Type

Most of the same activities that can be used for aerobic training can also be used for anaerobic training. Outdoor activities include cycling, rowing and running; indoor activities include rope jumping and swimming along with exercising on stationary equipment such as cycles (upright or recumbent), ellipticals, rowers, steppers/stairclimbers and treadmills.

If you're a competitive athlete who's training for a specific sport or activity – such as cycling or swimming – the best activities to do are the ones that you're going to perform. So if you want to become a better cyclist, you must mainly cycle; if you want to become a better swimmer, you must mainly swim.

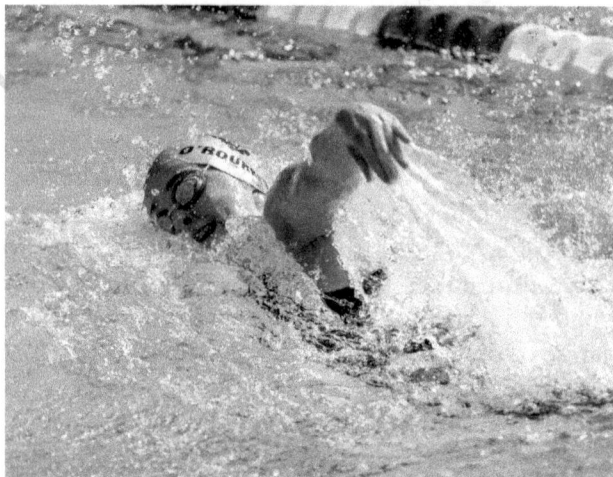

If you want to become a better cyclist, you must mainly cycle; if you want to become a better swimmer, you must mainly swim. (Photo by Mike McLaughlin.)

For runners and other athletes whose sport or activity involves running, the best activity for them is, of course, running. However, they can – and should – include at least some non- or low-impact activities as part of their anaerobic training to minimize the impact forces that are associated with running.

MEANINGFUL ANAEROBIC TRAINING

Over a period of time, you'll likely find that the same anaerobic workout – which was originally difficult – can be performed with less effort. As you improve your anaerobic fitness, your exercising heart rate will be lower for a given level of intensity. Because of this, you must increase your intensity as needed so that you're always training with an appropriate percentage of your maximum heart rate. In addition, your ability to maintain a higher exercising heart rate will become easier. As a result, it's important for you to make your anaerobic training progressively more challenging so that you can produce further improvements in your anaerobic fitness.

There are three main ways to overload your anaerobic pathways. In comparison to a previous workout, you must attempt to (1) complete the same distances in shorter durations; (2) maintain the same pace for greater distances or durations;

or (3) decrease the duration of the recovery between efforts. As an example, suppose that you rowed a series of eight 200-meter sprints in an average time of 1:00 (a pace of 200 meters per minute) and took an average recovery time of 2:30 between your efforts. In a future workout, you should try to (1) row eight sprints of 200 meters in an average time of less than 1:00; (2) row eight sprints of more than 200 meters at an average pace of 200 meters per minute; or (3) take an average recovery time of less than 2:30 between the eight sprints of 200 meters. Regardless of which tactic you employ, you made your anaerobic pathways work harder than they're accustomed to working. (Note: With some stationary equipment, you can increase the resistance and/or incline which also makes your anaerobic pathways work harder in comparison to a previous workout.)

For this reason, it's vital that you keep accurate records of your anaerobic training. Maintaining records permits you to track your progress thereby making your anaerobic workouts more productive and more meaningful. During anaerobic training, the key program components to monitor include the date of your workout, the distances that you completed, the durations of your efforts, the durations of your recovery between your efforts and the level of your intensity (your exercising heart rate).

METHODS OF ANAEROBIC TRAINING

Several different methods can be used to develop your anaerobic pathways. Remember that the parameters for time and intensity must be satisfied in order for an activity to be considered anaerobic. Doing an activity with an intense effort that lasts about three minutes or less is necessary to improve your anaerobic pathways.

For the sake of simplicity, most of the ensuing discussions of anaerobic training use running as the example. However, all of the methods that can be used to increase your running performance can be applied to virtually any type of activity as well as any type of equipment. For instance, if your goal in a particular workout is to run six 400-meter sprints in 90 seconds per sprint, you could cycle, row or do another activity with an intense effort for 90 seconds a total of six times.

The most common method of anaerobic training is to perform a series of intense efforts that last for brief periods of time such as repeated sprints. But in order for your anaerobic training to be as productive as possible, it must be done in an organized manner. Performing anaerobic training on an informal basis can certainly produce favorable results but a formal program that's structured and has a scientific foundation is more precise and more productive.

Three popular methods of anaerobic training are interval training, fartlek training and acceleration sprinting.

Interval Training

Essentially, interval training consists of a series of work intervals (periods of intense exertion) that are alternated with recovery intervals (periods of either reduced activity or complete inactivity). As an example, you'd run a given distance at an intended pace or in a specified time, recover and then repeat the work-recovery sequence until your interval workout is completed.

Interval training has been around since as early as 1910 when it was developed by Lauri Pihkala of Finland as a way to train distance runners. His system was used by Paavo Nurmi – nicknamed "The Flying Finn" – who was one of the most accomplished middle- and long-distance runners in history, setting 22 world records in events that ranged from 1,500 to 20,000 meters. In the 12 events that Nurmi competed during the 1920 Antwerp, 1924 Paris and 1928 Amsterdam Olympics, he won nine gold medals and three silver medals. (Fast fact: Pihkala competed for Finland in the 1908 London Olympics in the high jump and discus and the 1912 Stockholm Olympics in the 800-meter run.)

In the late 1930s, an element of science was woven into the fabric of interval training by Drs. Woldemar Gerschler and Herbert Reindell of Germany. The partnership was a great fit: Dr.

Gerschler was a physician and a track coach while Dr. Reindell was a cardiologist. Their approach to interval training was based largely on the heart rate during the work and recovery intervals. According to what's known as the Gerschler-Reindell Law, the work interval should be of sufficient intensity to increase the heart rate to 180 beats per minute (bpm). The recovery interval should allow the heart rate to decrease to 120 bpm before beginning the next work interval. In this system, then, the duration of the recovery interval isn't pre-determined; rather, it depends on how long it takes the heart rate to recover to 120 bpm. If it takes more than 90 seconds for the heart rate to reach 120 bpm, then the demands are too difficult and an adjustment should be made (such as increasing the length of the recovery interval or simply ending the workout).

In May 1954, Roger Bannister – then a medical student at the University of Oxford – became the first person in history to break the four-minute barrier in the one-mile run, crossing the finish line in 3:59.4 (three minutes and 59.4 seconds). Interval training was a very important part of Dr. Bannister's running program. (More on that point in a bit.)

By the late 1950s, Dr. James "Doc" Counsilman introduced interval training to the sport of swimming at Indiana University (where he coached from 1957 to 1990). Prior to that, swimmers – like their running counterparts – trained using long, continuous efforts. During Dr. Counsilman's tenure, Indiana University was enormously successful in the National Collegiate Athletic Association (NCAA) Swimming and Diving Championships with six consecutive team titles to go along with five second-place finishes.

Interval training remains very popular for running and swimming; it's also used extensively in rowing. However, the principles of interval training can be applied to just about any type of activity and equipment. In fact, these concepts have been promoted as high-intensity interval training, the basis of which had its genesis more than 100 years ago in Finland. And what helped to take these concepts mainstream was the

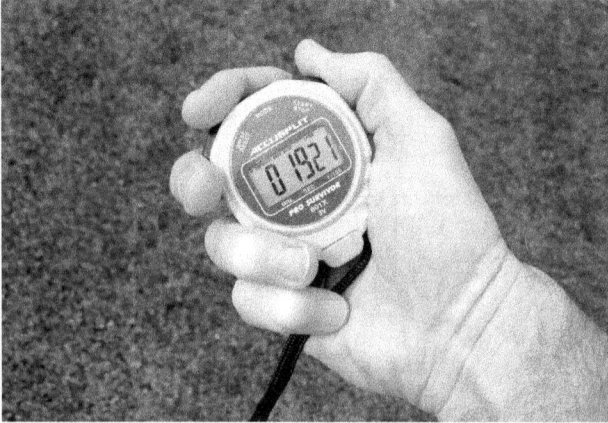

It's important for you to receive a sufficient amount of recovery between your anaerobic efforts.

pioneering research that was done by Dr. Tabata in the late-1990s.

Sidebar: Some researchers distinguish between high-intensity interval training (HIIT) and sprint-interval training (SIT). The basic difference between the two is the level of intensity. There are no universal definitions but in general, HIIT should be efforts that elevate the heart rate to 90% or more of maximum while SIT should be all-out efforts such as doing multiple repeats of a Wingate Test. (Isn't it ironic that something known as SIT would involve an all-out effort?)

The rationale behind interval training is that it allows you to reach and sustain a high level of intensity for a cumulative distance or time that's greater than what you could achieve during continuous training with the same intensity. The reason why you're able to do this is that during the recovery interval, your anaerobic pathways are given the opportunity to return to near-normal function thereby allowing you to make a physiological comeback for the next work interval. So by dividing your training into short, intense intervals of work with intervals of recovery interspersed between those anaerobic efforts, you can perform a greater volume of work than continuous training with the same level of intensity. This concept was demonstrated famously by Dr. Bannister in the early 1950s on his way to breaking the long-coveted four-minute mile. In order to run a mile in less than four minutes, an athlete has to complete each quarter

mile (440 yards) in an average of a little less than 60 seconds. Dr. Bannister regularly did interval training that consisted of 10 440-yard work intervals and each effort was done in about 60 seconds – sometimes less – with a recovery interval of about two minutes between each of the 10 repetitions. In other words, interval training allowed him to run a total of 2.5 miles (10 x 440 yards) at the same pace that he could run one mile continuously. By the way, this entire workout would have taken about 30 minutes to complete. Whew.

An interval program consists of seven different variables that you can manipulate to effectively overload your anaerobic pathways. These variables are dependent on your level of fitness; someone who has a low level of fitness won't be able to perform as much volume of training as someone who has a high level of fitness. The seven variables are:

1. Number of Repetitions

One variable to consider during interval training is the number of repetitions (or times) that the anaerobic efforts are performed. For example, you might do eight repetitions of a specified distance during your interval workout.

2. Repetition Distance

A second variable during interval training is the distance of the repetitions – the anaerobic efforts – such as running 800 meters or swimming 200 meters in a specified time. An interval workout usually begins with longer efforts and tapers down to shorter ones. For instance, you'd complete all of the 400-meter sprints followed by all of the 200-meter sprints and so on.

If you're an athlete who's interested in improving your anaerobic fitness to better prepare yourself for competition, the distance of your intense efforts should approximate the requirements of your sport or activity. So, a softball player who's looking to get down the base path more quickly should emphasize intense efforts of 20 yards (60 feet; the distance from home plate to first base).

3. Work Interval

The intended time of the anaerobic effort is the work interval. Your goal, for example, might be to row a specified distance in a work interval of 30 seconds or less.

4. Recovery Interval

The time that's allotted to recuperate between the work intervals is the recovery interval. It's important for you to receive an adequate amount of recovery between your anaerobic efforts. This allows your depleted anaerobic pathways enough time to recover so that you can make another intense effort. As an example, the recovery intervals between your work intervals might provide 90 seconds of recuperation.

In general, the duration of the recovery interval is related to the time that it takes to complete the work interval. You can also customize the duration of your recovery interval by using your heart rate to determine when you're physiologically ready to perform your next work interval. For instance, you can apply the Gerschler-Reindell Law where you begin your next work interval when your heart rate drops to 120 bpm. Or to make it even more individualized, you might begin your next work interval when your heart rate drops to a predetermined level such as 60% of your age-predicted maximum heart rate. An appropriate decrease in heart rate depends on several factors, including the length of the last work interval and your level of fitness.

The recovery interval can consist of either reduced activity (that ranges from light to moderate) or complete inactivity. For anaerobic efforts that last about 10 seconds or less, the recovery interval should consist of complete inactivity. This gives your ATP-PC System the opportunity to replenish much of its stores. Moderate activity hinders this process which places greater demands on your other anaerobic pathway, Anaerobic Glycolysis. For anaerobic efforts that last about 30 seconds or more, the recovery interval should consist of light activity (such as walking) or moderate activity (such as jogging). This doesn't significantly impact the

recovery of your ATP-PC System and allows for the partial removal of blood lactate.

Incidentally, most sports and activities have built-in recovery intervals because of their intermittent nature. Though these inherent respites are unofficial, unscientific and unpredictable, they permit a fairly successful replenishment of your stockpiles of ATP and PC.

5. Work:Recovery Ratio

The recovery interval is usually expressed in relation to the work interval. This is known as the work:recovery ratio and is most often designated as 1:1, 1:2, 1:3 or 1:4. These particular ratios state that the recovery interval should be one, two, three or four times the duration that it took you to perform the work interval. As a rule of thumb, the shorter the duration of effort – and the higher the intensity of effort – the greater the work:recovery ratio.

Because of the high level of intensity, an all-out effort that's done in 30 seconds or less requires a work:recovery ratio of at least 1:3. As an example, a work interval that takes you 15 seconds to perform should be followed by a recovery interval of about 45 seconds or more. An all-out effort that's done in 30 to 90 seconds requires a work:recovery ratio between 1:3 and 1:2. Finally, an all-out effort that's done in 90 to 180 seconds requires a work:recovery ratio between 1:2 and 1:1. (Interestingly, Dr. Bannister's preferred interval workout consisted of work intervals that took him about 60 seconds to perform and recovery intervals of about two minutes which is a work:recovery ratio of 1:2 which fits into the recommendations that are presented here.) Table 15.1 shows a summary of times, running distances and their accompanying work:recovery ratios.

6. Workout Distance

The sum of all the distances that are performed in an interval workout is the workout distance. When performing work intervals that last between about 1.5 and 3.0 minutes, the total distance of your workout shouldn't exceed about 2.0 to 2.5 miles (or 3,200 to 4,000 meters) of running; when performing work intervals that

Table 15.1: Summary of times, running distances and work:recovery ratios

WORK/TIME (sec)	DISTANCE (m)	WORK:RECOVERY RATIO
0 to 30	0 to 200	1:4 to 1:3
30 to 90	200 to 400	1:3 to 1:2
90 to 180	400 to 800	1:2 to 1:1

Note: The ranges of time apply to both the highly and poorly conditioned; the running distances are for those who are in reasonably good condition.

last less than about 90 seconds, the total distance of your workout shouldn't exceed about 1.5 to 2.0 miles (or 2,400 to 3,200 meters) of running. (Note: Swimming distances equate to roughly 20% of running distances.)

7. Workout Frequency

A final variable to consider is the frequency of the interval workouts. Except for highly competitive athletes, interval training shouldn't be done more than once or twice a week. The low frequency is required due to the intense nature of interval training.

A prescription for interval training can be written in shorthand. In the language of interval training, for example, "8 x 100 m (0:20/1:00)" indicates that you're to perform eight 100-meter work intervals and that each effort should be done in 20 seconds (or less) with a recovery interval of one minute between each of the eight repetitions. (Note that the work:recovery ratio is 1:3 because each effort is less than 30 seconds in duration.)

Table 15.2 is a detailed example of a nine-week interval program for running that has an anaerobic emphasis. As mentioned earlier, interval training that's designed for running can be easily adapted to virtually any type of activity and equipment.

Fartlek Training

A modified version of interval training is fartlek training, a method that was developed in Sweden by Gustaf ("Gösta") Holmér in or around 1937. Legend has it that Holmér designed fartlek training for use by Swedish long-distance runners to make them more competitive against their Finnish counterparts. Fartlek training made its way to the United States in the 1940s.

The Swedes are famous in physical-education circles for developing systems of training that were basic in structure and used the outdoors as much as possible. It's no surprise, then, that fartlek training is usually performed outside over natural but varied terrain that ranges from flat surfaces to steady inclines and declines. For this reason, fartlek training was probably a precursor of the hill training that's often used by modern runners. Fartlek training can also be done indoors using a wide variety of equipment.

Fartlek is formed from the Swedish words fart (speed) and lek (play) which is why it's sometimes referred to as speed play. Fartlek training is less formal and less exact than interval training; otherwise, the two are quite similar. Fartlek training improves anaerobic fitness by employing different combinations of effort such as walking, jogging and running. The work and recovery intervals are left entirely up to the individual; you can change your pace and recover at your own discretion. So, there's a clear intent to "play" with speed.

A sample fartlek workout for running that emphasizes your anaerobic pathways might look like this:

1. jog 400 meters

2. walk 200 meters

3. jog 400 meters

4. walk 200 meters

5. sprint 100 meters uphill and walk 100 meters downhill in an alternating fashion for six minutes

6. jog 400 meters

7. walk 400 meters

8. sprint 50 meters and walk 50 meters in an alternating fashion for three minutes

Sidebar: Holmér competed in the 1912 Stockholm Olympics in the decathlon, finishing fourth. (Sweden finished first in the medal standings.) In 1913, Holmér was awarded the bronze medal after the winner – Jim Thorpe of the United States who also won the pentathlon – was disqualified when it was found that he had played two seasons of semi-professional baseball. In those days, professional athletes weren't allowed to compete in the Olympics. In 1982, Thorpe – one of the greatest all-around athletes in history – was reinstated as the winner but Holmér retained his bronze medal. Holmér also competed in the 1920 Antwerp Olympics in the 110-meter hurdles and decathlon (in which he was fourth).

Acceleration Sprinting

An effective technique that's used by many runners to increase their speed is acceleration sprinting. This technique, however, can also be used to increase speed in other activities such as cycling, rowing and swimming.

As the name implies, acceleration sprinting is characterized by a gradual increase in speed until a full, all-out effort is reached. When running, for example, you'd begin by jogging then increase to striding and finally accelerate to sprinting the intended distance or duration. Between work intervals, the recovery intervals can consist of either reduced activity or complete inactivity.

Gradually increasing your speed throughout your effort allows you to concentrate on your technique which is enormously important in speed development. Acceleration sprinting also provides a smooth transition towards an all-out sprint thereby minimizing the potential for a muscle strain or pull.

A series of 100-meter acceleration sprints for running might look like this:

1. jog 20 meters, stride 30 meters and sprint 50 meters

2. walk 50 meters and repeat the series for a total of 10 times

SCHEDULING TRAINING

Similar to strength training and aerobic training, there are two options for scheduling strength training and anaerobic training: The activities can be done on the same day or on alternate days. The advantage of doing both activities on the same day is that it allows more time for recovery between workouts. Therefore, the recommended way of scheduling strength training and anaerobic training is to do both activities on the same day, preferably during the same workout and no more than one or two times per week on nonconsecutive days. (As a reminder, a frequency of three to five days per week that's prescribed for conditioning workouts represents the total frequency of aerobic training *and* anaerobic training.)

Studies that have investigated the scheduling of strength training and anaerobic training are scarce. However, the same considerations that were discussed in the previous chapter with respect to aerobic training would also hold true for anaerobic training.

In one study that did examine strength training and anaerobic training, 57 elite-level soccer players were randomly assigned to three experimental groups: One group did strength training before anaerobic training; the second group did strength training after anaerobic training; and the third group did strength training and anaerobic training on alternate days. (A fourth group acted as a control and didn't train.) The groups that did strength training and anaerobic training on the same day trained twice per week and the group that did the activities on alternate days trained four times per week so that the volume of training was equal. The groups that did strength training and anaerobic training on the same day were given 15 minutes of recovery between the two activities. (The researchers used the term endurance training which suggests that the activity was aerobic. However, the groups actually did high-intensity interval training which is anaerobic.) After 12 weeks, doing strength training and

A Practical Approach to Strength and Conditioning

Table 15.2: Sample nine-week interval program for running

WEEK	SPRINT REPS	DISTANCE (m)	WORK: RECOVERY RATIO	WORK TIME	RECOVERY TIME	WORKOUT DISTANCE	WORKOUTS PER WEEK
1	4	800	1:1	3:00	3:00	3,200	1
2	3	800	1:1	3:00	3:00	3,200	1
	2	400	1:2	1:30	3:00		
3	2	800	1:1	2:55	3:00	3,200	1
	4	400	1:2	1:30	3:00		
4	1	800	1:1	2:55	3:00	3,200	1
	6	400	1:2	1:25	2:45		
5	4	400	1:2	1:25	2:45	2,400	2
	4	200	1:3	0:40	2:00		
6	3	400	1:2	1:20	2:45	2,400	2
	4	200	1:3	0:40	2:00		
	4	100	1:3	0:20	1:00		
7	2	400	1:2	1:20	2:45	2,400	2
	6	200	1:3	0:39	2:00		
	4	100	1:3	0:20	1:00		
8	1	400	1:2	1:15	2:30	2,400	2
	6	200	1:3	0:39	2:00		
	8	100	1:3	0:19	1:00		
9	1	400	1:2	1:15	2:30	2,400	2
	4	200	1:3	0:38	1:45		
	8	100	1:3	0:19	1:00		
	8	50	1:4	0:10	0:45		

anaerobic training on the same day produced similar results in a variety of fitness tests as doing strength training and anaerobic training on alternate days. Stated differently, performing the activities on alternate days offered no advantage compared to performing the activities on the same day.

If strength training and anaerobic training are done on the same day, which activity should be done first? It's clear, of course, that doing an activity first will result in better performance than doing it second (due to residual fatigue from the prior activity). Nothing is clear beyond that since studies on this topic are lacking. Making it more difficult to determine the best sequence of strength training and anaerobic training is the fact that strength training is a type of anaerobic training.

At any rate, if your primary goal is to increase your anaerobic fitness, the order of strength training and anaerobic training *probably* doesn't matter too much; and if your primary goal is to increase your muscular strength, it's *probably* better to do strength training before anaerobic training.

HOW AEROBIC IS ANAEROBIC?

It's interesting to delve deeper into the nature of anaerobic training. Let's say that you did eight work intervals of one minute each and in between those eight work intervals you did seven two-minute recovery intervals. This workout fits the general definition of anaerobic training: a series of brief, intense efforts that are alternated with periods of recovery. Note, too, that the total exercise time for this workout was 22 minutes. Let's also say that during the work intervals, you elevated your heart rate to 95% of your age-predicted maximum. This satisfies the FITT guideline of intensity for anaerobic training. Finally, let's say that during the recovery intervals, your heart rate decreased to 60% of your age-predicted maximum. Okay, now let's connect the dots. During this anaerobic workout, you exercised at 60 to 95% of your age-predicted maximum heart rate for 22 minutes of continuous effort. What does that sound like? It sure sounds a lot like the FITT guidelines of intensity and time for *aerobic* training.

The point is that anaerobic training has an element of aerobic training. This could also explain why research consistently shows that anaerobic training can improve aerobic fitness.

TESTING AND MEASURING ANAEROBIC FITNESS

Evaluating anaerobic fitness is complicated. The difficulty arises because no single test serves as a reliable indicator of your anaerobic fitness. Remember, the two anaerobic pathways – the ATP-PC System and Anaerobic Glycolysis – contribute in varying ways to a wide range of efforts that last from an instant up to about three minutes. But since your aerobic pathway begins to assist your anaerobic pathways with intense efforts that are beyond about 90 seconds in duration, a measurement of your *unassisted* anaerobic fitness should involve efforts of less than about 90 seconds. To obtain a true picture of your anaerobic fitness, then, it's necessary to perform several tests across this anaerobic spectrum. (Needless to say, measuring an instantaneous effort has plenty of room for error.)

One way to test your anaerobic fitness is to measure your power output. Before discussing how you can measure your power output, it's important for you to understand the meaning of the power. In physics, power is defined as the amount of work done per unit of time or, more simply, work divided by time. Since work is defined as force multiplied by distance, it follows that power is also defined as force multiplied by distance divided by time. Example: If you can move 100 pounds [lb] a distance of three feet [ft], you did 300 foot-pounds [ft-lb] of work [100 lb x 3 ft = 300 ft-lb]; and if you performed this effort in 0.25 seconds [sec], your power output is 1,200 ft-lb/sec [300 ft-lb ÷ 0.25 sec = 1,200 ft-lb/sec].

In a laboratory setting, a popular test of anaerobic fitness is the Margaria-Kalamen Power Test. The test was developed by Dr. Rodolfo Margaria and two of his colleagues in 1966 at the University of Milan and later modified by Dr. Jerome Kalamen. At the start of this test, you're to stand six meters in front of a staircase. Initiating movement on your own, you'd run up the stairs as fast as possible, contacting every third step (in other words, taking three steps at a time). To calculate your power output, multiply your bodyweight times the vertical distance between the third and ninth step and divide by the time of your effort (to the nearest hundredth of a second). For instance, suppose that you weigh 198 pounds and covered a vertical distance of four feet in 0.75 seconds. In this case, your power output would be 1,056 foot-pounds per second [198 lb x 4 ft ÷ 0.75 seconds = 1,056 ft-lb/sec]. (Fast fact: The power output of some heavier athletes can exceed 2,000 ft-lb/sec.)

In a field setting, there are several popular tests of anaerobic fitness. Field tests that are employed to evaluate all-out efforts that last a mere instant include the vertical jump (aka the Sargent Jump Test), standing long jump and medicine-ball put. (Think of this as doing the shot put with a medicine ball.) A field test of anaerobic fitness that's a little farther up the energy continuum is a 40-yard dash.

The tests that have been mentioned so far involve maximum efforts of 10 seconds or less which employ the ATP-PC System. Of slightly longer duration – though still in the anaerobic realm – is the Wingate Anaerobic Test or, simply, the Wingate Test. This highly popular test is conducted in a laboratory setting. As noted earlier in this chapter, the test is 30 seconds of all-out effort on a stationary cycle against a fixed resistance that's based on an individual's bodyweight. Maximum efforts of about 30 seconds or less rely on the ATP-PC System and Anaerobic Glycolysis. (Fast fact: The Wingate Test – described by some as "the longest 30 seconds of your life" – is named after the Wingate Institute for Physical Education and Sport in Netanya, Israel, where it was developed in 1974.)

Maximum efforts of about 30 to 90 seconds involve Anaerobic Glycolysis. Field tests that are within this window of time are a 400-meter sprint and 100-meter swim.

As a reminder, even though the upper edge of the anaerobic spectrum is around three minutes, your aerobic pathway begins to assist your anaerobic pathways with intense efforts that are beyond about 90 seconds in duration. Therefore, a measurement of your *unassisted* anaerobic fitness should involve efforts of less than about 90 seconds.

HIIT IS HOT

When Dr. Tabata conducted a study of anaerobic training in 1996, few people would've imagined how popular it would eventually become; at the present time, more than 200 studies per year are published on different aspects – and different interpretations – of anaerobic training.

Research has found that HIIT can be highly beneficial in a wide range of clinical and non-clinical populations. In particular, there's an abundance of research in treating conditions that are related to overweight/obesity. A recent review and meta-analysis of 65 studies found that when done for less than 12 weeks, HIIT significantly improved maximum oxygen intake and diastolic blood pressure in overweight/obese populations; when done for 12 weeks or more, HIIT significantly improved waist circumference, percentage of body fat, maximum oxygen intake, resting heart rate, systolic blood pressure and diastolic blood pressure in overweight/obese populations.

But doing short, intense intervals of work alternated with intervals of recovery isn't for everyone. Some individuals have little or no interest in training with that level of effort. In addition, HIIT won't produce a significant expenditure of calories so it's not ideal for individuals whose main goal is to lose weight.

Be that as it may, HIIT is hot. And it doesn't seem likely that HIIT will cool off anytime soon.

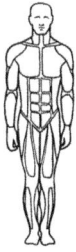

16 Metabolic Training

Most people typically perform their strength training separate from their aerobic training. Yet, many people – especially athletes – are required to integrate their muscular strength with their aerobic fitness. Good examples of this are basketball, boxing, crew, football and wrestling in which athletes perform a series of brief, intense efforts that occur within the aerobic domain (this is to say, anything that lasts about three minutes or more). Being able to merge your muscular (or anaerobic) fitness with your aerobic fitness is a true measure of your metabolic fitness.

Essentially, metabolic training (aka metabolic conditioning) is a union of strength training (or other anaerobic efforts) and aerobic training such that it requires the collective efforts of the musculoskeletal, respiratory and circulatory systems. These three systems can be developed at the same time by doing exercises/activities that engage a large amount of muscle mass with efforts that are short-term and intense while taking very little recovery between the exercises/activities.

Metabolic training might seem like a recent idea but it really isn't. In October 1975, the *Athletic Journal* published an article that was penned by Arthur Jones – who had earlier founded Nautilus® Sports/Medical Industries and later MedX® Corporation – called "Flexibility and Metabolic Condition." This appears to have been the first time that metabolic training was mentioned and discussed in print.

Lately, there has been a renewed interest in metabolic training. A thorough understanding of metabolic training and an application of specific methods can enhance your performance in exercises/activities that involve muscular strength and aerobic fitness.

Sidebar: Metabolism refers to the chemical reactions that occur within the body. The term can be subdivided into catabolism (breaking down) and anabolism (building up). In the animal kingdom, the three-toed sloth has the lowest metabolism and the ruby-throated hummingbird has the highest metabolism.

PROJECT TOTAL CONDITIONING

In the spring of 1975, research designated as Project Total Conditioning was conducted at the US Military Academy in West Point, New York. The subjects were drawn from the Corps of Cadets who were athletes at the academy. Project Total Conditioning actually consisted of several different studies. For instance, one study examined the effects of a strength program on the neck strength and size of rugby players; another study examined the effects of two different training protocols on the vertical jump of volleyball players.

However, the main portion of Project Total Conditioning was a study that investigated metabolic training (though it wasn't referred to as such). In this study, 19 football players did strength training three times per week for six weeks. The workouts were done on nonconsecutive days with two days of recovery after the third workout of the week. (The subjects did 17 workouts during the six-week period.) Each workout consisted of 10 exercises; six exercises for the neck were also performed twice per week. One set of each exercise was done to the point of muscular fatigue within a repetition range of 5 to 12. The subjects took a minimum amount of recovery between exercises.

Prior to the study, the subjects followed the training protocol for two weeks in order to reduce the influence of the learning effect. Pre-testing was done after those first two weeks to collect baseline data. (Fast fact: The learning effect refers to the dramatic increases that are often attained

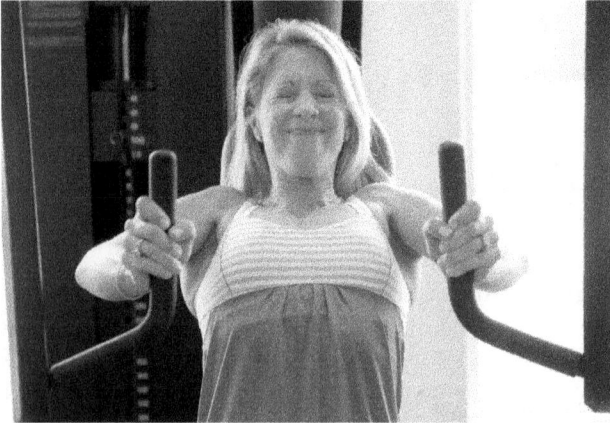

A form of metabolic training that has seen continued interest is high-intensity training or, simply, HIT. (Photo provided by Luke Carlson.)

by individuals in the initial stages of a training program that are attributable to improvements in neurological function rather than muscular function.)

The study produced very compelling results. After six weeks of training, the subjects increased the resistance that they used by 58.54%. The minimum improvement in strength was 45.61% while the maximum improvement was 69.70%. The subjects also increased the number of repetitions that they performed by 6.59%.

Interestingly, the time that the subjects needed to complete their workouts decreased substantially. The subjects reduced the duration of their workouts by 24.09% – from 37.73 minutes to 28.64 minutes. Two subjects almost literally cut their workout times in half – one from 49 minutes to 25 minutes and the other from 43 minutes to 22 minutes – yet they increased their strength by 68.32% and 65.59%, respectively. A third subject reduced his workout time from 42 minutes to 27 minutes and increased his strength by 66.32%.

Besides the tremendous improvements in strength, the subjects also decreased their time in the two-mile run by 88 seconds, from 13:18 to 11:50. This represented an improvement of 11.03% . . . without having performed any running except during the course of spring football practice (which occurred during the first four weeks of training). The subjects also had

lower resting heart rates and lower exercising heart rates at various workloads on a stationary cycle. Moreover, they were able to perform more work before reaching heart rates of 170 beats per minute.

The subjects decreased their time in the 40-yard dash from 5.15 seconds to 5.09 seconds, an improvement of 1.17%. Their vertical jump increased from 22.60 inches to 24.07 inches, an improvement of 6.50%. And they improved their range of motion in torso flexion by 5.57%, shoulder flexion by 11.62% and torso extension by 15.58%.

The results are even more startling when you consider the fact that they were accomplished in such a time-efficient manner: The total amount of actual training time performed by each subject during the six-week study was less than 8.5 hours which is less than 30 minutes per workout. It should be noted, too, that the subjects were highly conditioned football players who were already quite strong and fit at the start of the study. Nonetheless, this study demonstrated the far-reaching effects of short-duration, high-intensity strength training on metabolic fitness.

TYPES OF METABOLIC TRAINING

You can improve your metabolic fitness by simply doing your strength training with a high level of intensity while taking very little recovery between exercises/sets (à la Project Total Conditioning). When performed in this fashion, the shared demands that are placed on your musculoskeletal, respiratory and circulatory systems create improvements in metabolic fitness that can't be approached by traditional methods of strength training.

There are a number of different types of metabolic training; some types are formal, others are informal. Three of the most popular types of metabolic training are circuit training, high-intensity training and CrossFit®.

Circuit Training

One of the oldest and most popular types of metabolic training is circuit training. The birth of circuit training can be traced back to Ronald

Morgan and Graham Adamson who developed the system at the University of Leeds in the early 1950s. It wasn't long before circuit training made its way across the Atlantic where it became all the rage in the United States, especially in high schools and colleges.

With circuit training, the idea is to perform a series (or circuit) of exercises/activities with a very brief recovery interval between each exercise/activity. In a sense, therefore, circuit training is a form of interval training.

Circuit Strength Training. The traditional version of circuit training is essentially strength training with a fast pace between exercises/sets. (To be clear: The *pace* between the exercises/sets should be quickened, not the *speed* of the repetitions.) This can be referred to as circuit strength training (CST).

A popular way of doing CST is on a multi-station machine (aka multi-station gym). This offers several advantages. First of all, the exercises of a multi-station gym are in close proximity to each other which allows you to move quickly around the circuit. Secondly, the selectorized weight stacks of a multi-station gym enable you to make quick and easy adjustments in the resistance. But CST can also be performed with single-station equipment and/or free weights provided that the distance between the exercises isn't too great.

CST is very versatile; you can manipulate the number of exercises in the circuit, the number of repetitions for each exercise and the amount of recovery that's taken between the exercises. The number of exercises that you do in the circuit and the amount of recovery that you take between the exercises are a function of your level of fitness. However, a comprehensive workout of CST involves a series of about 12 to 14 exercises that address your major muscles.

Many multi-station gyms don't offer exercises for the hips, legs and mid-section. In this case, a multi-station gym would need to be augmented with some single-station machines and/or free weights in order to target all of the major muscles. An example of a total-body circuit that incorporates a multi-station gym and a few supplemental exercises is the ball squat, leg curl,

leg extension, bench press, push-up, chin-up, overhand lat pulldown, upright row, scapulae adduction, bicep curl, tricep extension, wrist flexion, side bend and back extension.

At each station, you can either perform a given number of repetitions or do as many repetitions as possible during a specified time frame (in a smooth, controlled manner). Allotting 60 seconds to perform each exercise (the work interval) and 30 seconds to recuperate between each exercise (the recovery interval; this includes the set-up for the next exercise), a circuit of 12 to 14 exercises can be completed in as little as 18 to 21 minutes. It should be noted that the resistance you use at each station should permit you to reach – or at least approach – the point of muscular fatigue by the end of the allotted work interval.

With CST, there are three main ways of overload. In comparison to a previous workout, you must attempt to (1) increase the resistance that you use at a given station; (2) increase the length of the work interval (thereby doing more repetitions); or (3) decrease the length of the recovery interval that's taken between stations. Though well intended, you shouldn't try to increase the number of repetitions that you do in a certain amount of time since this encourages improper technique.

To summarize CST: You begin at a particular station and complete one set of an exercise. After this, you move to the next station in the circuit where you set up for your next exercise and recuperate for the remainder of the recovery

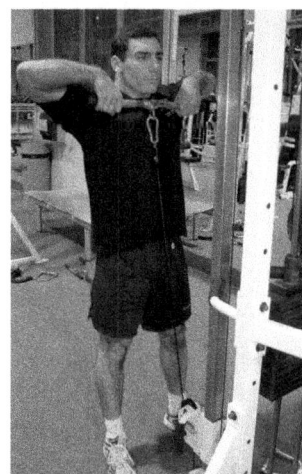

A popular way of doing CST is on a multi-station machine. (Photo by Peter Silletti.)

interval. This process is repeated until the entire circuit is completed.

Circuit Strength and Anaerobic Training. A second version of circuit training is to integrate strength training with another type of anaerobic training. This can be referred to as circuit strength and anaerobic training (CSAT).

For instance, you might do the chest press, pedal a stationary cycle for one to two minutes, do the underhand lat pulldown, pedal a stationary cycle for another one to two minutes and so on. The goal is to perform the equivalent of about 20 to 30 minutes of total activity.

In 1969, Dr. Patrick O'Shea – a researcher and competitive weightlifter – advanced a version of CSAT that he referred to as interval weight training. In brief, O'Shea proposed a two-phase protocol. The first phase was a work interval that consisted of one set of "an athletic type core lift" (such as the squat, push press, power snatch or power clean) followed immediately by 90 to 180 seconds of a "free [anaerobic] exercise" (such as pedaling a stationary cycle, running on a treadmill or jumping rope) that would elevate the heart rate to 90 to 95% of the age-predicted maximum. An "active rest interval" of 90 to 180 seconds was then given that involved walking and stretching. This series of exercises/activities was repeated three or four times with the same core lift. Thereafter, the process was replicated for one or two additional core lifts. Following a five-minute recovery, the second phase consisted of four sport-specific exercises for the upper body done in a circuit. Each exercise was performed for 12 to 15 repetitions with 30 to 45 seconds of recovery between each exercise. The circuit was repeated two or three times with 120 to 180 seconds of anaerobic exercise done at the end of each series.

Along these lines, a basic but brutal form of CSAT can be done by alternating dips and chin-ups with sprinting. In other words, you might do a set of dips, sprint a specified distance, do a set of chin-ups, sprint a specified distance and repeat this circuit several times. (If performed indoors, you can run on a treadmill as long as its location is convenient.)

Circuit Aerobic Training. Since the term cross training came into vogue in the mid-1990s, there has been a growing interest in circuit aerobic training (CAT). Although the emphasis of CAT is more on aerobic fitness than metabolic fitness, it's a version of circuit training and, thus, merits note here.

CAT involves a series of aerobic activities or stations. It can be designed many different ways; you can vary the number of activities, the duration and intensity of each activity and the amount of recovery that's taken between activities.

As with all other types of physical training, most of these variables are dependent on your level of fitness. Your goal, however, is to perform the equivalent of about 20 to 60 minutes of aerobic activity with an appropriate level of intensity. Keep in mind that 30 minutes of activity can be done as two 15-minute bouts, three 10-minute bouts or even six 5-minute bouts. So, you can exercise for 10 minutes on a stationary cycle, 10 minutes on a rower and 10 minutes on a stepper/stairclimber for a total of 30 minutes of activity. Or, you might perform each of those same three activities for five minutes but repeat the circuit twice for a total of 30 minutes of activity. Regardless, your level of intensity should be as high as possible during each of your efforts.

The Fitness Trail. Originating in several of the Scandinavian countries, the so-called fitness trail is a type of circuit training that's performed outdoors in a natural environment such as a park. A typical fitness trail consists of numerous stations that are positioned at various points along a circuitous route. You'd run or sprint to a station, stop and perform some kind of exercise or activity that may be for agility (such as hurdles, log walks or vaults), strength (such as push-ups, abdominal crunches, dips or chin-ups) or flexibility (such as a calf stretch) and then proceed to the next station.

High-Intensity Training

A type of metabolic training that has seen continued interest is high-intensity training or, simply, HIT. The term high-intensity training appears in trade publications as early as 1973.

(The acronym HIT became fashionable in 1988 with the publication of the *HIT Newsletter*.) HIT can be effective for anyone – regardless of lifting experience or aspiration – as long as it encourages progressive overload and allows sufficient recovery between workouts. The past four decades have provided literally tens of thousands of examples of individuals – both male and female with various levels of experience ranging from untrained beginners to highly trained athletes – as empirical evidence that HIT can be extremely productive.

Since it was first popularized in the early 1970s, there have been endless interpretations, variations and applications of HIT. Nevertheless, most versions of HIT have a number of common denominators. As the name implies, HIT is characterized by intense, aggressive efforts. Each set is typically performed to the point of muscular fatigue. Another characteristic of HIT is the emphasis on progressive overload. Whenever possible, an attempt is made to increase either the resistance that's used or the repetitions that are done in comparison to a previous workout. A minimum number of sets are performed, often only one set of each exercise but sometimes several sets. With safety and efficiency in mind, the repetitions are done in a smooth, controlled manner so that momentum doesn't play a significant role in raising the resistance. Additionally, HIT is comprehensive; addressing all of the major muscles is a priority.

HIT involves very brief workouts with a minimum amount of recovery between exercises/sets. The abbreviated recovery interval enables you to maintain a fairly high exercising heart rate for the duration of your workout. Like other types of metabolic training, the length of the recovery interval that's taken between exercises/sets depends on your level of fitness. The recovery interval isn't usually structured, timed or predetermined. Initially, however, a recovery interval of perhaps several minutes may be necessary between efforts; with improved fitness, your pace should be quickened to the point where you're moving as rapidly as possible between exercises/sets. (To be clear: The *pace* between the exercises/sets should be quickened, not the *speed* of the repetitions.)

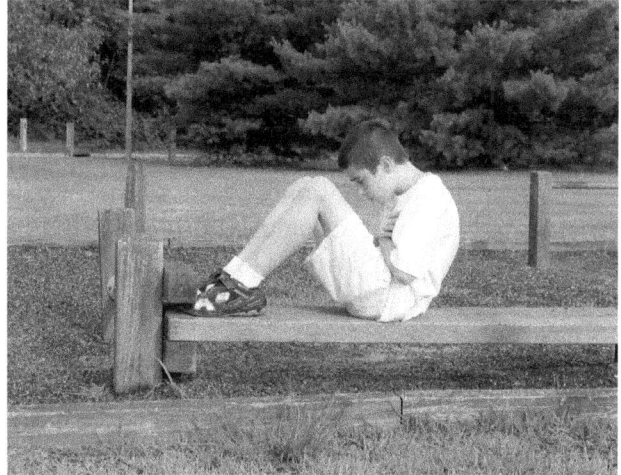

A typical fitness trail consists of numerous stations that are positioned at various points along a circuitous route.

In short, HIT can place large demands on your musculoskeletal, respiratory and circulatory systems. Furthermore, HIT can be used to improve your metabolic fitness in a safe and time-efficient manner.

The 3x3 Workout. A simple but effective type of HIT workout that deserves special note is a 3x3 Workout or, for short, a 3x3 (read as "three by three"). Bob Rogucki has been credited with developing the 3x3 Workout in the late 1980s when he was the Strength Coach at the US Military Academy. The workout was detailed in December 1996 when *Coach and Athletic Director* published an article (by this author) called "Metabolic Conditioning with the 3x3 Workout."

A 3x3 Workout involves a series (or circuit) of three multiple-joint movements: one for the hips, one for the chest and one for the upper back. This series of three exercises is repeated a total of three times; essentially, it's doing three sets of three exercises (thus the moniker 3x3). Virtually every major muscle in your body is addressed in a 3x3 Workout, including your hips, hamstrings, quadriceps, chest, upper back, shoulders, biceps, triceps and forearms.

There are numerous options for multiple-joint movements that can be used in a 3x3 Workout. The safest and most effective multiple-joint movements for your hips are the deadlift, leg press and ball squat. Any multiple-joint movement that

255

involves a pushing motion – such as the bench press, incline press, decline press, dip and push-up – can be used to target the muscles of your chest (as well as those of your shoulders and triceps); any multiple-joint movement that involves a pulling motion – such as the bench row, seated row, underhand lat pulldown, chin-up and pull-up – can be used to target the muscles of your upper back (along with your biceps and forearms).

The first time that the series of three exercises is done, you should reach muscular fatigue by about 20 repetitions for the hip exercise and 10 for the chest and upper-back exercises. The second time through the series, you should reach muscular fatigue by about 15 repetitions for the hip exercise and 8 for the chest and upper-back exercises. And the third time though the series, you should reach muscular fatigue by about 12 repetitions for the hip exercise and 6 for the chest and upper-back exercises. In summary, a 3x3 Workout uses descending repetitions in each of the three sets: 20, 15 and 12 for the hips; 10, 8 and 6 for the chest; and 10, 8, 6 for the upper back.

As you might imagine, there are countless variations of a 3x3 Workout. Without a doubt, the most demanding series of exercises is the deadlift, dip and chin-up. Another version is a series of the leg press, bench press and seated row. Not to belabor a point but in both of these examples, the series of three exercises would be done three times (for a total of nine sets in the workout). As a side note, each of the three series can contain different exercises. For instance, a 3x3 Workout could be one set of the deadlift, incline press, pull-up, leg press, bench press, seated row, ball squat, decline press and underhand lat pulldown.

In doing a 3x3 Workout, you should take as little recovery as possible between exercises/sets. This will yield excellent improvements in your metabolic fitness. Plus, it makes a 3x3 Workout extremely time-efficient; most variations can be performed in about 20 minutes or less.

The simplicity of this type of HIT workout can be deceptive. Though it may not appear so, a 3x3 Workout – if done as outlined here – can be incredibly challenging and demanding. Remember, you're doing exercises that engage a large amount of muscle mass while training to the point of muscular fatigue and taking as little recovery as possible between each of the nine sets.

CrossFit®

Simply mention CrossFit® to a group of individuals who are avid exercisers and many of them will quickly and vehemently make known their allegiance as either fans or foes. Clearly, no other type of training has ever been more polarizing – or more controversial – than CrossFit®.

Legend has it that in the early 1990s, Greg Glassman – a former gymnast – developed and implemented workouts that got him banished from (by his count) *seven* gyms. Glassman branched out on his own, opening the first CrossFit® gym in Santa Cruz (CA) in 1995 and founding the company – CrossFit®, Inc. – in 2000. Since that time, CrossFit® has experienced an unparalleled growth in popularity, first as an exercise program and later as a competitive sport. There's no scientific data to support this contention but at the present time, CrossFit® – with more than 13,000 gyms (or "boxes") in more than 120 countries – has probably motivated more people to exercise than any other type of training.

CrossFit® has become synonymous with metabolic conditioning (aka metcon in CrossFit® lingo), a topic that Glassman first wrote about in the October 2002 issue of the *CrossFit Journal*. This, of course, came *27 years after* Arthur Jones wrote about metabolic conditioning in the *Athletic Journal*. And though not described as such, metabolic conditioning really dates back to the early 1950s when circuit training was developed. CrossFit® workouts are certainly packaged much differently but the underlying concepts of metabolic conditioning have been employed for more than 60 years.

A CrossFit® workout is a series (or circuit) of exercises/activities that are done with a very high level of intensity while taking very little recovery between the exercises/activities. Workouts consist of "functional" movements that can include (examples in parentheses) calisthenic-type and bodyweight exercises (the air squat, lunge, "burpee," box jump, push-up, pull-up, muscle-up and dip); Olympic-style lifts (the snatch and clean and jerk) and their derivatives (the power clean, push jerk and push press); powerlifts (the squat, bench press and deadlift) and their derivatives (the front squat and overhead squat); and certain aerobic activities (rowing, running/sprinting and swimming).

Fran. One of the oldest and best-known CrossFit® workouts is named Fran. First publicized on the CrossFit® website in August 2003, the workout is a series of three exercises: the "thruster" (a combination of two exercises namely, the front squat and push press) and pull-up. This series of exercises is repeated a total of three times; essentially, it's doing three sets of three exercises. Fran uses descending repetitions in each of the three sets: 21, 15 and 9. In other words, the workout is 21 thrusters, 21 pull-ups, 15 thrusters, 15 pull-ups, 9 thrusters and 9 pull-ups. As you can see, the protocol for Fran – three sets of three exercises with descending repetitions – is a lot like that of a 3x3 Workout (which was developed at least 14 years earlier).

Safety. It would be remiss not to mention the potential for injury from CrossFit® workouts. Indeed, nothing is more heavily and heatedly debated about CrossFit® than the topic of injuries.

Two surveys collected data on injuries from CrossFit® workouts. In one survey, 75 individuals reported at least one injury during CrossFit® in the six months prior to the survey, citing 89 injuries. The survey found that the most frequently injured areas were the shoulder, lower back, knee and arm/elbow. The other survey appeared as a poster presentation that was shown in 2014 at the 61st Annual Meeting of the American College of Sports Medicine in Orlando. In this survey, 376 individuals reported at least one injury during CrossFit® in the year prior to the survey (with 60 injuries requiring some form of hospitalization). The most frequently injured areas were the shoulder, back and hand.

It's often pointed out that the injury rates in CrossFit® are similar to those of sports such as Olympic-style weightlifting, powerlifting and gymnastics. Well, there's a problem with this

rationale: The vast majority of individuals who do CrossFit® use it as an exercise program. And an exercise program – done to improve strength and fitness – shouldn't be a risky venture. Comparing injury rates of exercise programs to injury rates of competitive sports is, as they say, like comparing apples to oranges.

In most CrossFit® workouts, the goal is to do the exercises/activities as quickly as possible – in the shortest amount of time – or for "as many rounds as possible" (AMRAP) in a designated time. The emphasis is on doing the repetitions quickly, not strictly.

There's no question that in speeding through a series of exercises/activities, technique is compromised. And when technique is compromised, bad things can happen. This is especially true of the competitive lifts and their derivatives which are the most complicated things that you can do with a barbell. For those exercises to be safe and effective, using proper technique is extremely critical.

Doing the competitive lifts while racing against the clock and/or when fatigued is a recipe for disaster. When high repetitions are performed in complex lifts, technique will quickly deteriorate. With the clean and jerk, for example, the technique becomes "get the weight from the floor to overhead any way you can." This is in stark contrast to competitive weightlifters who mostly do low-repetition sets – singles, doubles and triples – and don't lift when fatigued. They never sacrifice proper technique by speeding through their sets or repetitions.

To underscore how much injuries are a part of CrossFit®, look no further than the company website where one of the forums is dedicated exclusively to injuries. The very existence of such a forum says a lot. Granted, this is anecdotal evidence but the sheer volume of injuries that are reported in the forum – and elsewhere on the Internet – is far too much to ignore.

METABOLIC DYNAMICS

Metabolic training presents an enormous physiological challenge to your musculoskeletal, respiratory and circulatory systems. In response to the demands, these three systems make a number of sudden – and sometimes dramatic –

257

adjustments that gradually return to resting levels once the activity is completed.

Detailing your specific responses to metabolic training is impossible. Your responses can vary a great deal based on your intensity and the duration of the activity as well as the type of metabolic training that was done. Other factors that determine your response include your size, gender and level of fitness. Therefore, what follows is an overview of your general responses to metabolic training.

In going from rest to intense activity, these metabolic responses occur:

- An increase in the rate and depth of breathing. Labored breathing is an unmistakable indicator of intense activity. This leads to a heightened sense of respiratory distress, general discomfort and widespread fatigue.

- An increase in tidal volume (the amount of air that you inhale or exhale in a single breath, measured in liters per breath).

- An increase in minute ventilation (the amount of air that you inhale or exhale each minute, measured in liters per minute). Minute ventilation is calculated by multiplying the rate of your breathing by your tidal volume.

- An increase in oxygen intake and the rate of caloric expenditure.

- An increase in the involvement of the respiratory muscles, specifically the abdominals and internal intercostal muscles (which reside between your ribs along with your external intercostal muscles). During intense activity, your respiratory muscles may require 25% or more of your oxygen intake.

- An increase in heart rate. During intense activity, your heart beats faster to meet the demands for more blood and oxygen. (Your heart rate actually increases above resting levels *prior* to your effort due to the so-called anticipatory response.)

- An increase in stroke volume (the amount of blood that's pumped by your heart, measured in milliliters per beat).

- An increase in cardiac output (the amount of blood that's pumped by your heart in a given amount of time). Cardiac output is calculated by multiplying your heart rate by your stroke volume. Once your stroke volume reaches your physiological limit, further increases in your cardiac output are only possible through increases in your heart rate.

- An increase in blood flow to more active muscles and organs and a decrease in blood flow to less active muscles and organs. At rest, about 20% of your blood flow goes to your muscles; the majority of the blood goes to your digestive organs, kidneys and brain. During intense activity, about 70% or more of your blood flow goes to your exercising muscles. In addition, there's an increase in the volume of blood flow to your heart as well as to your skin in order to dissipate heat. (The volume of blood flow to your brain is unchanged.)

- An increase in systolic blood pressure and no change or a slight decrease in diastolic blood pressure (measured in millimeters of mercury). Maximum blood pressure usually occurs at maximum heart rate.

- An increase in body temperature, especially in hot, humid conditions. Your body has a temperature-regulatory mechanism that acts in the same manner as a thermostat, trying to maintain its temperature at a relatively constant value of roughly 98.6 degrees Fahrenheit (about 37 degrees Celsius).

- An increase in the production of carbon dioxide and lactate (lactic acid). This decreases your muscle pH. The lactate spreads from your muscles into the surrounding tissues and eventually spills into your blood. When lactate enters your blood at a greater rate than it leaves, it accumulates and becomes more concentrated. This decreases your blood pH. High accumulations of lactate produce an acidic environment that can irritate your nerve endings and cause pain, discomfort and distress; it's also believed to cause feelings of heaviness in your muscles, labored breathing and fatigue.

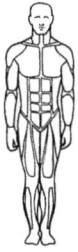

17 Power Training

An important aspect of athletic performance is power. It's no surprise, then, that coaches and athletes are continually looking for ways to improve this valuable physical commodity.

It has long been thought that in order to improve power, it was necessary to do the Olympic-style lifts (the snatch and clean and jerk) and/or their derivatives (the power clean, push jerk and push press) and high-speed repetitions. But power training doesn't have to incorporate this approach.

POWER DEFINED

Before discussing how you can improve your power output, it's important for you to understand the meaning of power. In physics, power is defined as the amount of work done per unit of time or, more simply, work divided by time. Since work is defined as force multiplied by distance, it follows that power is also defined as force multiplied by distance divided by time.

Another definition of power is force multiplied by velocity. The term velocity is defined as distance divided by time. Once again, it follows that power is force multiplied by distance divided by time.

So, power has three variables: force, distance and time. Manipulating any of these three variables will affect power.

METHODS FOR IMPROVEMENT

Based on the equation "power equals force multiplied by distance divided by time," you can improve your power output three different ways: (1) increase the force that you produce; (2) increase the distance over which you produce force; and (3) decrease the time that it takes you to produce force.

Let's take a closer look at how this can be accomplished.

Increase the Force

If you increase the force that you produce and keep the other two variables in the equation the same – namely, the distance over which you produce force and the time that it takes you to produce force – you'll generate more power. Example: If you can bench press 160 pounds a distance of 18 inches (1.5 feet) in two seconds, your power output is 120 foot-pounds per second [160 lb x 1.5 ft ÷ 2.0 sec = 120 ft-lb/sec]. Suppose that at some point in the future, you increased your bench press to 180 pounds. Assuming that the distance you moved the resistance (18 inches) and the time it took you to move the resistance (two seconds) remained the same, your power output is now 135 foot-pounds per second. So by increasing the force that you produced, you've improved your power output.

How do you increase the force that you produce? One way is to increase the strength of your muscles. If you increase the strength of your muscles, they can produce more force; if your muscles produce more force, you'll have the potential to generate more power.

How do you improve your strength so that you can produce more force? While there's no shortage of opinions, any strength program will be productive if – and only if – it incorporates the Overload Principle. Arguably, this principle is the most important underlying construct for improving physical performance, whether it's training for strength, aerobic fitness or even flexibility. As far as strength training is concerned, the principle states that your musculoskeletal system must be overloaded or made to work harder than it's accustomed to

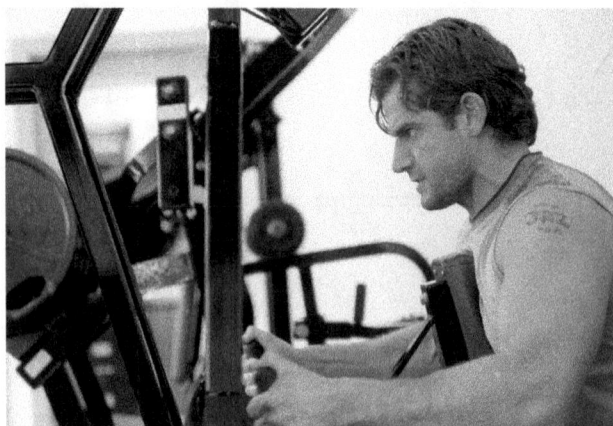

If you increase the strength of your muscles, they can produce more force; if your muscles produce more force, you'll have the potential to generate more power. (Photo provided by Luke Carlson.)

working by being exposed to progressively greater demands.

In order to overload your muscles, every time that you train you should try to increase the resistance that you use and/or the repetitions that you do in comparison to a previous workout. This can be viewed as a double-progressive technique. Stated otherwise, you must expose your muscles to demands that they haven't previously encountered by using more resistance and/or doing more repetitions. Exposing your muscles to progressively greater demands triggers compensatory adaptation in response to the unaccustomed workload. Your muscles adapt to such demands by increasing in strength (and size).

Also remember that it really doesn't matter whether your muscles are "loaded" with resistance from machines, barbells, dumbbells, resistance bands, sandbags, bricks or even another human being. Your muscles don't possess the ability to distinguish between different types of resistance; they simply respond to being loaded.

Increase the Distance

If you increase the distance over which you produce force and keep the other two variables in the equation the same – namely, the force that you produce and the time that it takes you to produce force – you'll generate more power. Example: If you can squat 300 pounds a distance of 21 inches (1.75 feet) in two seconds, your power output is 262.5 foot-pounds per second [300 lb x 1.75 ft ÷ 2.0 sec = 262.5 ft-lb/sec]. Suppose that at some point in the future, you increased your range of motion in the squat so that you're now moving the resistance a distance of 24 inches. Assuming that the resistance you lifted (300 pounds) and the time it took you to move the resistance (two seconds) remained the same, your power output is now 300 foot-pounds per second. So by increasing the distance over which you produced force, you've improved your power output.

How do you increase the distance over which you produce force? One way is to become more flexible. If you become more flexible, you can increase the range of motion of your joints; if you increase the range of motion of your joints, you'll have the potential to generate more power.

How do you improve your flexibility so that you can produce force over a greater distance? Like strength training, there's no shortage of opinions. But any method of flexibility training will be effective if it adheres to several strategies. To reduce your risk of injury, you should stretch under control without using any bouncing or jerking movements. Moreover, you should hold the stretched position for about 10 to 30 seconds. Similar to strength training, you must make your flexibility training progressively more challenging. You can do this by attempting to stretch slightly farther than the last time. Finally, it's important to stretch daily and either before or after physical training.

Decrease the Time

If you decrease the time that it takes you to produce force and keep the other two variables in the equation the same – namely, the force that you produce and the distance over which you produce force – you'll generate more power. Example: If you can deadlift 400 pounds a distance of 18 inches (1.5 feet) in two seconds, your power output is 300 foot-pounds per second [400 lb x 1.5 ft ÷ 2.0 sec = 300 ft-lb/sec]. Suppose that at some point in the future, you increased your speed of movement in the deadlift to 1.5 seconds (you did the repetition faster). Assuming that the resistance you lifted (400 pounds) and the distance you moved the resistance (18 inches) remained the same, your power output is now 400 foot-pounds per second. So by increasing the speed at which you produced force, you've improved your power output.

How do you decrease the time that it takes you to produce force? One way is to perfect your technique in a given skill. If you perfect your technique, you can perform the skill more quickly; if you perform the skill more quickly, you'll have the potential to generate more power.

How do you improve your technique so that you can decrease the time that it takes you to produce force? The scientific literature is in general agreement as to how this can best be achieved. First, it's important that you learn how to do the skill correctly. Second, you must perform the skill over and over again until you can execute it with little or no conscious effort. The skill must be practiced perfectly and exactly as it would be used during a sport or an activity. Remember, practice makes perfect . . . but only if your practice is perfect.

MORE POWER TO YOU!

As demonstrated earlier, your power output can be improved by three different means: (1) increase the force that you produce; (2) increase the distance over which you produce force; and (3) decrease the time that it takes you to produce force. This can be accomplished by improving your strength, flexibility and technique.

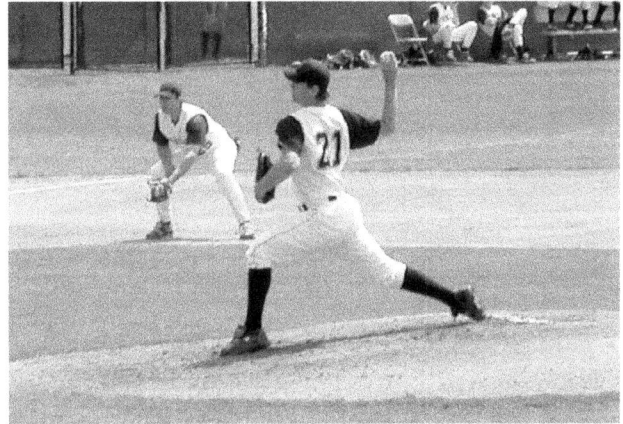

If you perfect your technique, you can perform a skill more quickly; if you perform a skill more quickly, you'll have the potential to generate more power. (Photo by Melanie Silletti.)

Be forewarned, however, that just because you can generate more power during a given exercise inside the fitness center doesn't mean that you'll automatically generate more power during a given skill outside the fitness center. Despite an abundance of anecdotal claims, there's no legitimate, scientific evidence to suggest that generating power can transfer from one activity to another.

Think about it: If doing the power clean (or an Olympic-style lift or its derivative) improves your performance in the vertical jump, for example, then doing the vertical jump should improve your performance in the power clean. But it doesn't.

The bottom line is that producing power inside the fitness center is one thing and producing power outside the fitness center is another.

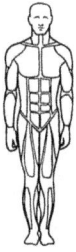

18 Skill Training

Motor learning is the study of how motor skills are acquired, applied and refined. Motor control is the study of how the neuromuscular system works to coordinate the nerves, muscles and limbs that are involved in motor skills. Together, motor learning and motor control investigate the improvement and performance of skills.

Naturally, this information is highly important for those who are trying to learn skills. With skill training, however, there are a number of practices that are well meaning but are often unsupported by the scientific literature.

SKILLS AND ABILITIES

The terms skill and ability are often used interchangeably and are somewhat related. However, skills are much different than abilities.

A skill refers to the level of performance in one specific action. Examples of skills include hitting a baseball, shooting a basketball, throwing a football and kicking a soccer ball. Skills can be improved through practice and experience.

An ability, on the other hand, refers to a general trait. In the early 1950s, Dr. Edwin Fleishman – then the branch chief of the Perceptual and Motor Skills Research Laboratory at Lackland Air Force Base in San Antonio – began studying human performance. Based on this and later research, he advanced the theory that there are two different types of abilities: perceptual motor and physical proficiency.

Included among perceptual-motor abilities are multi-limb coordination, response orientation, reaction time, arm-hand steadiness and aiming; included among physical-proficiency abilities are static flexibility, dynamic flexibility, balance, coordination, static strength, dynamic strength, explosive strength, speed of limb movement and stamina.

Although abilities aren't specific skills, they establish the foundation of specific skills. Doing a specific skill such as a handstand, for instance, requires the general abilities of balance and static strength. Abilities are thought to be genetically determined and, as a result, can be improved but only within inherited limits. Physical-proficiency abilities likely have a greater potential for improvement than perceptual-motor abilities.

Different skills – no matter how alike they seem – require different abilities. For instance, throwing two balls of different size, shape and/or weight – say, a baseball and football – would involve different abilities. Furthermore, abilities are thought to be independent of each other; the quality of one ability isn't dependent on the quality of another. So, an individual who can perform well in some skills doesn't necessarily perform well in others.

A perfect example of this is when Michael Jordan – perhaps the greatest basketball player of all time – took his world-class abilities from the basketball court to the baseball diamond. In 1994, while playing for the Class AA Birmingham Barons of the Southern League, he stole 30 bases

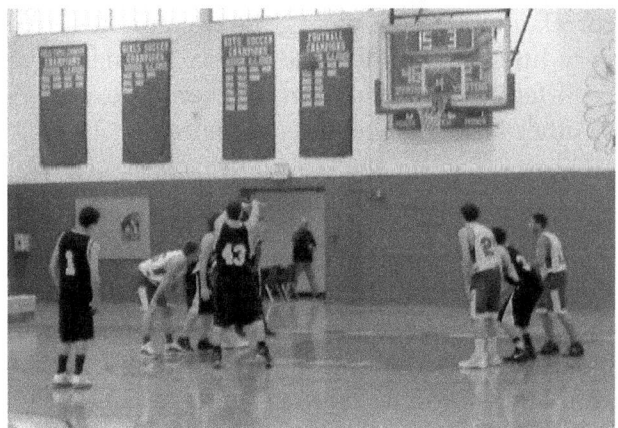

An example of a skill is shooting a basketball. (Photo by Mark Brzycki.)

(in 48 attempts) and drove in 51 runs. But Jordan only hit .202 – the lowest batting average of any regular player in the league – and whiffed 114 times in 436 at bats. On defense, he led all outfielders in the league with 11 errors. He couldn't return to the basketball court fast enough.

Quickness and Balance Exercises

Athletes often do drills for quickness and balance. The expectation, of course, is that executing drills that involve quickness or balance will transfer to skills that require quickness or balance and, thus, improve athletic performance.

Numerous studies have investigated this possibility. According to Dr. Richard Schmidt – a renowned researchers in motor learning and motor control – there's little evidence that practicing a skill that requires a certain ability will improve another skill that requires the same ability.

Being quick is advantageous in most sports and activities. Dr. Schmidt notes that at least three abilities are used to be quick: (1) reaction time (the interval of time between an unanticipated stimulus and the start of the response); (2) response orientation (where one of many stimuli is presented, each of which requires its own response); and (3) speed of limb movement (the interval of time between the start of a movement and its completion). These three abilities are separate and independent of each other. For example, studies have shown that reaction time and speed of limb movement have essentially no correlation. In other words, the two abilities have very little in common. Additional studies have reported no transfer from quickening exercises to other tasks that require quickness.

In short, being quick depends on the circumstances under which quickness is required.

Having balance is also advantageous in most sports and activities. As with quickness, balance that's required for one activity isn't related to balance that's required in another. In a classic study from 1961, 320 subjects were tested on two different balance devices: a stabilometer and ladder climb. The two balance tasks were found

to be contingent on separate and independent abilities. The researcher concluded that the correlation between the two balance tasks was "little more than zero." In a classic study from 1967 that involved 50 subjects, researchers examined six tests of static and dynamic balance that were commonly used in physical education. They found that the abilities supporting one test of balance were separate from those supporting another.

In a more recent study, 40 subjects were pre-tested on two different balance devices: a tilt board and a movable platform. Tests were done with both devices in two different directions so that there were a total of four tasks. The subjects were then matched and divided into two experimental groups: One group trained on one device and the other group trained on the other device. (A third group acted as a control and didn't train.) The subjects in the experimental groups did each of the four tasks five times. The first two times were for familiarization; the last three times were used for assessment. The subjects did their assigned training six times in a two-week period. Post-tests showed that the subjects performed better only in the tasks of balance that they practiced. In other words, there was no transfer of balance from one task to another. This was true even when two different tasks were done on the same device.

In short, having balance depends on the circumstances under which balance is required.

Open and Closed Skills

Skills can be classified as either open or closed. Both types of skills differ in several areas that pertain to the context of the environment (which consists of the playing field or surface, objects and other individuals).

Open skills occur in an environment that's variable and unpredictable. An individual reacts to a situation and initiates a response that can match the constantly changing environmental conditions. Since the conditions may vary from one response to another, the individual must have a variety of responses available to accomplish the skill. Examples of open skills are hitting a pitched baseball, rebounding a basketball and heading a soccer ball. Baseball, basketball and soccer are sports in which open skills dominate. In fact, this is true of most team sports.

Closed skills occur in an environment that's stable and predictable. Because the environment doesn't fluctuate, an individual can plan or predict a response well in advance. The individual initiates movement and isn't required to begin until ready to do so. With a closed skill, an object waits to be acted upon by the performer. Examples of closed skills are putting a golf ball, doing a cartwheel and throwing a discus. Golf, gymnastics and track and field are sports in which closed skills dominate. By the way, weightlifting – whether it's competitive or recreational – is an activity in which closed skills dominate.

Designations of open and closed actually mark the extreme points on a continuum. Skills that have assorted degrees of environmental variability and predictability reside between the two extremes.

Open and closed skills demand entirely different strategies for learning. With open skills, diversification is required. This means that open skills should be practiced in a variable environment to learn adaptability. With closed skills, fixation is required. This means that closed skills should be practiced in a stable environment to learn consistency.

Interestingly, the National Football League (NFL) "combine" – the world's best-known evaluation of athletic ability – includes the 225-pound bench press, 40-yard dash, 20-yard shuttle, 60-yard shuttle, three-cone drill, vertical jump and standing broad jump, all of which are closed skills. This, despite the fact that football is a sport in which open skills dominate. It's no surprise, then, that the usefulness of these tests in predicting success as a football player has been questioned for many years.

Proprioception and Kinesthetic Awareness

Related to this discussion is the topic of proprioception and kinesthetic awareness. Though closely related and used interchangeably, proprioception and kinesthetic awareness are different. Proprioception – the so-called "sixth

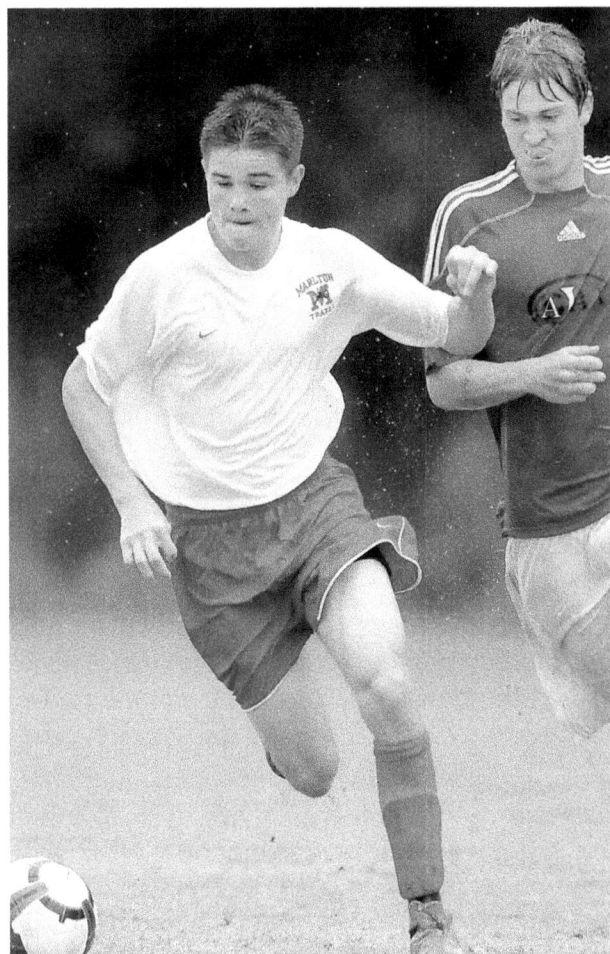
Soccer is a sport in which open skills dominate. (Photo by Karl Wright.)

sense" – is internal and cognitive and has to do with the sense or awareness of body and limb position; kinesthetic awareness – or kinesthia – is external and behavioral and has to do with the sense or awareness of body and limb motion. To simplify things, proprioception refers to position (static) while kinesthetic awareness refers to motion (dynamic).

For example, hanging from a bar involves proprioception; doing a chin-up or pull-up involves kinesthetic awareness.

Can proprioception and kinesthetic awareness be trained or improved? This is highly debatable. See how long you can stand on one leg with your eyes closed. Repeat that every day for a few weeks and it's likely that you'll be able to do it for a longer period of time. Did you improve your proprioception? Or did you improve your *skill* at standing on one leg with your eyes closed? (Fast fact: A field sobriety test – which can involve standing on one leg, walking heel-to-toe in a straight line and touching the nose with the eyes closed – essentially evaluates impairment of proprioception and kinesthetic awareness.)

THE TRANSFER OF LEARNING

The transfer of learning refers to the effects of past learning on the acquisition of a new skill. Many individuals take the transfer of learning for granted. They assume that the learning of one skill always and automatically transfers or "carries over" to the learning of another.

Types of Transfer

The acquisition of skills depends on the correct use of the transfer of learning principles. In reality, the transfer of learning from one skill to another may be positive, negative or neutral (absent altogether).

Positive transfer occurs when the learning of one skill facilitates the learning of another skill. Example: Learning to position yourself to field a baseball would probably facilitate learning to position yourself to field a softball.

Negative transfer occurs when the learning of one skill inhibits the learning of another skill. Example: Learning to shoot free throws on either a nine-foot rim or an 11-foot rim would probably inhibit learning to shoot free throws on a 10-foot rim, at least initially.

Neutral (no) transfer occurs when the learning of one skill has a negligible influence on the learning of another skill. Example: Learning to swim would have no effect on learning to accurately tap a volleyball (as was demonstrated in one study).

It's interesting to note that the transfer of learning is greater from the non-dominant (non-preferred) arm/leg to the dominant (preferred) arm/leg than the other way around. Say that you're right-handed, for example. Dribbling a basketball with your left (non-dominant) hand will have greater transfer of the skill to your right

(dominant) hand than dribbling a basketball with your right hand will have to your left hand.

THE USE OF WEIGHTED OBJECTS

It's widely believed that using weighted objects contributes to the learning of specific movement patterns and sport skills. This has led to the practice of trying to simulate skills in the fitness center using a variety of implements. In the scientific literature, practicing a skill with a weighted object or additional resistance is known as overload training. Barbells, dumbbells, medicine balls and other weighted objects are used during overload training with the expectation of improving performance.

The basis for mimicking skills with weighted objects is mostly anecdotal, having very little support from the scientific literature. In one study, for instance, 37 subjects were assigned to two groups: One group threw a weighted softball and the other group threw a regulation softball. (The weighted softball was two ounces heavier than the regulation softball.) Both groups performed a series of lob throws from various distances ranging from 30 to 70 feet with their assigned softball. After six weeks of training, there were no significant differences between the groups in throwing velocity. The researchers concluded: "Training with a weighted ball resulted in essentially the same effect as training with the regulation ball."

Along these lines, many individuals insist that certain weightlifting skills transfer to other skills. If there were a correlation between weightlifting skills and other skills, then highly successful weightlifters would excel at literally every skill that they attempted. And we know that this isn't true.

The Kinesthetic Aftereffect

Research in motor control refers to a kinesthetic aftereffect which is defined by Dr. George Sage as "a perceived modification in the shape, size, or weight of an object . . . as a result of experience with a previous object." Individuals experience the kinesthetic aftereffect during overload training. This phenomenon is exemplified by a person who runs with a weighted vest and after removing it, has the perceived ability to run faster. Essentially, the kinesthetic aftereffect is nothing more than a sensory illusion.

So after doing a skill with a weighted object, an individual might "feel" faster or more powerful but research indicates that there's no measurable improvement in those areas. One study had subjects do elbow flexion with and without resistance. There was no change in the speed of movement shortly after the overload (although the subjects reported "feeling faster"). Another study had subjects perform vertical jumps with a weighted vest followed by jumps without the extra weight. There were no improvements in the vertical jump shortly after the overload. Yet another study had groups sprint with a weighted sled, sprint with a weighted vest or sprint without any additional resistance. After seven weeks of training, those who ran with added resistance performed no better in sprinting than those who ran without added resistance. Many other studies have reported similar results from the use of weighted objects.

Dr. Sage states, "Any attempt to improve performance by utilizing objects that are slightly heavier than normal while practicing gross motor skills that will be later used in sports competition seems to be hardly worth the time spent and the money paid for the weighted objects." Dr. Schmidt adds, "Teaching a particular Skill A simply because you would like it to transfer to Skill B, which is of major interest, is not very effective, especially if you consider the time spent on Skill A that could have been spent on Skill B instead."

Problems with Using Weighted Objects

According to Dr. Wayne Westcott, four problems occur when practicing sport skills with weighted objects. The problem areas relate to neuromuscular confusion, incorrect movement speed, orthopedic stress and insufficient workload.

1. **Neuromuscular confusion.** Every skill involves a movement pattern that's specific to that skill alone. Introducing anything foreign to the pattern – such as a sled,

weighted vest, barbell, dumbbell, medicine ball or ankle weights – will only serve to confuse the neuromuscular pathways and produce negative transfer. Watch someone swing a weighted racquet or shoot a weighted basketball and you'll quickly notice that the effort used to direct the unfamiliar weight results in a movement pattern that's labored and awkward; in reality, it's a very different motion altogether. Studies of competitive swimmers consistently show that their stroke mechanics are altered as a result of resisted swimming.

2. **Incorrect movement speed.** To facilitate learning, a skill should be practiced with the speed at which it will be performed. Practicing a skill at a slower or a faster speed than actually would be used in performing the skill will produce negative transfer. In addition, doing a skill at slower speeds – which would occur when doing it with a weighted object – may train the neuromuscular system to function at slower speeds.

3. **Orthopedic stress.** Another problem is the added stress that a weighted object places on the joints. Practicing a skill with an object that's heavier than normal puts orthopedic stress on the joints that's greater than normal. Structural stress is most evident in the shoulder, elbow and wrist.

4. **Insufficient workload.** A weighted object doesn't increase the strength of the involved musculature. The reason is that the extra resistance provided by a weighted object isn't sufficient enough to surpass the threshold for strength development; it's a fraction of what's necessary to overload the muscles.

SPECIFICITY VERSUS GENERALITY

In 1901, Drs. Edward Thorndike and Robert Woodworth – then instructors of psychology and physiology, respectively, at Columbia University – proposed their Identical Elements Theory of Transfer. In 1958, Dr. Franklin Henry – a professor of physical education at the University of California, Berkeley – advanced his Specificity

Hypothesis. Both theories are forerunners of what's widely known as the Principle of Specificity. The underlying fundamentals of this principle are documented extensively in the scientific literature. Even so, the Principle of Specificity continues to be misinterpreted and misused almost as often as it's referenced. (Fast fact: Dr. Thorndike is known as the father of educational psychology; Dr. Henry is known as the father of motor-behavior research.)

The Principle of Specificity states that activities must be specific to an intended skill in order for a maximum transfer of learning – or carryover – to occur. Specific means exact or identical, not similar or just like. Indeed, Dr. Sage states, "Transfer is highly specific and occurs only when the practiced movements are identical."

Movement patterns for different skills are never identical. According to Dr. Schmidt, two movement patterns – although outwardly appearing to use the same muscular actions – are actually quite different and require learning and practicing each skill separately. Performing an overhead smash with a tennis racket involves a different movement pattern than performing an overhead smash with a badminton racket. Swinging a golf club involves a different movement pattern than swinging a hockey stick. And throwing a baseball involves a different movement pattern than throwing a javelin.

Case in point: Shortly after the 1996 Atlanta Olympics, the Atlanta Braves hosted a tryout for Jan Zelezny, an athlete from the Czech Republic who was a two-time Olympic champion (1992

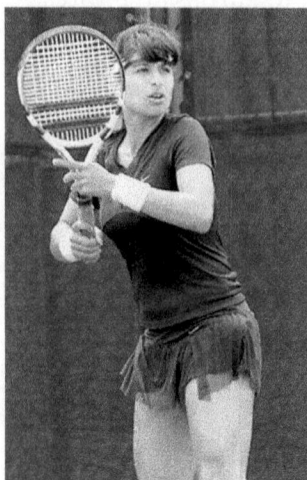

Performing an overhead smash with a tennis racket involves a different movement pattern than performing an overhead smash with a badminton racket. (Photo provided by Shikha Uberoi.)

and 1996) and world-record holder in the javelin. (He would later win an unprecedented third gold medal in the javelin at the 2000 Sydney Olympics.) According to one account, the international scouting director for the Braves reasoned that "the motions of throwing a javelin and a baseball were not all that different." No doubt, he also felt that the strength of Zelezny's arm and shoulder coupled with his capacity to throw a javelin farther than anyone on the planet – having tossed the spear 323 feet in Germany a few months before the tryout – made him a great candidate for pitching in the major leagues. After a few warm-up throws, Zelezny took the mound. His third pitch reportedly sailed over the head of the catcher . . . and also *over the eight-foot backstop*. He threw some additional pitches but the results weren't impressive. Several of his pitches were clocked at around 80 miles per hour which isn't bad but not major-league stuff. At the end of the tryout, Zelezny uncorked a throw for distance that was estimated to be 275 feet but he took a running start. Unfortunately, pitchers don't throw for distance. And they don't take a running start. Don't forget, too, that differences in the weight and shape of a javelin and baseball require different throwing motions; a javelin is a 28.22-ounce spear while a baseball is a five-ounce sphere. The moral of the story: Skills are highly specific and not necessarily transferable. (Fast fact: At the present time, Zelezny still owns five of the top six javelin throws in history.)

Exercises that are very similar don't even transfer to each other. In one study, 24 subjects performed three sets of five repetitions of the bicep curl in the standing position three times per week for six weeks. Their strength increased by 14.38 pounds when the bicep curl was measured in the standing position. But their strength increased by only 3.37 pounds when the bicep curl was measured in the supine position. In other words, the strength gained from doing a standing bicep curl didn't transfer to a supine bicep curl, an exercise that's very similar . . . but not identical. Exercises that are performed in the fitness center are even less similar to other skills and, therefore, won't transfer to other skills.

One exercise that has been thought to be specific to a wide range of skills is the power clean. Over the span of about five years, a variety of articles that were published in a "journal" for strength coaches stated that the power clean was specific to the following skills (and others): shooting a basketball; long-snapping a football; spiking a volleyball; rowing a boat; forehanding a tennis ball; pedaling a bicycle; tackling a football player; hitting a golf ball; swimming the backstroke, butterfly and breaststroke; throwing a javelin, discus and hammer; putting a shot; sprinting; playing baseball; Nordic skiing; pole vaulting; and sled racing. Really? In which of those skills does an athlete grasp an inanimate object that's resting on the ground and then pull it to shoulder level and drop under it all in one motion?

Obviously, it's impossible for the power clean – or any other exercise, for that matter – to be specific to such a broad range of differing skills. In fact, *no exercise* that's done in the fitness center – with free weights or machines – will expedite the learning of a skill. So, doing power cleans may be similar to driving off the line of scrimmage and doing lunges may be just like going for a layup but the truth is that power cleans will only help you to get better at doing power cleans and lunges will only help you to get better at doing lunges. Likewise, heaving medicine balls around is great for improving your skill at heaving medicine balls around and nothing else. And jumping off boxes will only perfect your skill at jumping off boxes. Remember, it's the Principle of *Specificity*, not the Principle of *Similarity*.

On a related note, if Skill A is specific to Skill B, then Skill B should be specific to Skill A. So if the power clean is specific to the pole vault, then the pole vault should be specific to the power clean. In other words, if doing the power clean helps your performance in the pole vault, then doing the pole vault should help your performance in the power clean. But it doesn't.

Elements of Specificity

There are four elements of specificity that define the rules for determining whether or not an exercise is specific to a skill:

1. **Muscle specificity.** The muscles used in the exercise must be exactly the same as in the skill.

2. **Movement specificity.** The movement pattern used in the exercise must be exactly the same as in the skill.

3. **Speed specificity.** The speed of movement used in the exercise must be exactly the same as in the skill.

4. **Resistance specificity.** The resistance used in the exercise must be exactly the same as in the skill.

In order for an exercise to be specific to a skill, all four of these elements would have to be true. An exercise may resemble a skill in terms of exact muscles, movement pattern, speed of movement and resistance. However, at best an exercise can only *approximate* a skill, not *duplicate* it.

Refer back to the laundry list of skills for which the power clean is thought to be specific. Those skills involve different muscles, different movement patterns, different speeds of movement and different resistances. Indeed, just consider the obvious differences between hitting a golf ball and rowing a boat. How, then, can the power clean be specific to such vastly different skills? Answer: It can't.

By the way, specificity doesn't only apply to the learning of sport skills. A guitar and banjo are stringed instruments but if you want to get better at plucking a guitar, don't practice with a banjo. An M16 and AK-47 are assault rifles but if you want to get better at shooting an M16, don't practice with an AK-47.

THE STAGES OF MOTOR LEARNING

Skill development is accomplished in stages (or phases) of learning. It's important to understand that the learning of a skill is a continuous process. Therefore, the stages don't have a distinct beginning or end and shouldn't be viewed as being separate or unconnected elements.

In their book *Human Performance*, Drs. Paul Fitts and Michael Posner identified three stages

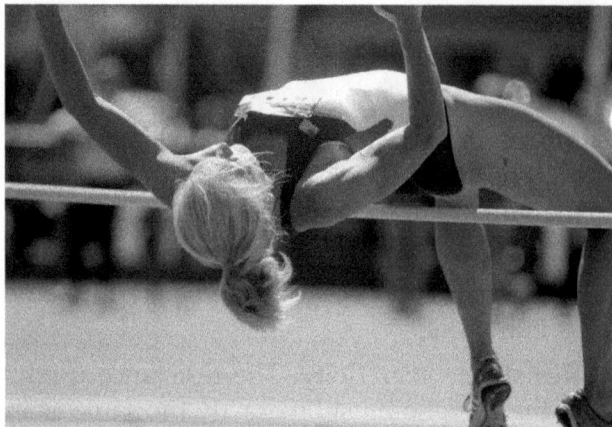

The first requirement for improving a skill is to literally practice the intended skill for thousands and thousands of task-specific repetitions. (Photo by Ken Stone.)

of motor learning. (Dr. Fitts – a professor of psychology at the University of Michigan – penned a few chapters before his untimely death in 1965; Dr. Posner – a professor of psychology at the University of Oregon – completed the book in 1967.) According to these two researchers, the three stages are an early or Cognitive Stage, an intermediate or Associative Stage and a final or Autonomous Stage. Let's take a closer look at these stages.

The Cognitive Stage

In the first stage of motor learning, the skill is completely new to the performer. The performer seeks an understanding of the skill and its demands. During this stage, the attention requirements are high and movements are jerky and fragmented. Gains in proficiency are very rapid but performance is usually very inconsistent. Good strategies are retained and poor ones are discarded. The Cognitive Stage may last anywhere from several moments to several weeks, depending on the complexity of the skill, the frequency of practice and so on.

The Associative Stage

During the second stage of motor learning, the performer organizes more effective and efficient movement patterns that are more coordinated and consistent. The enhanced movement efficiency reduces the energy costs of the skill. Performance improvements in the Associative Stage are rapid, though not as rapid as in the Cognitive Stage. The length of this stage varies considerably and may last several weeks or months.

The Autonomous Stage

In the third stage of motor learning – after many months and possibly years of painstaking practice – the skill becomes highly organized and well-developed. Now, the skills are performed with little or no conscious effort. In other words, the skill becomes automatic. For learning an open skill, the emphasis is on adapting the movement to a variety of environmental conditions and possibilities; for learning a closed skill, the emphasis is on refinement of technique. Because of the high degree of skill, performance improvements are slowest in the Autonomous Stage. At this point, there's simply "not much room for improvement."

IMPROVING SKILLS

The improvement of skills is a process in which an individual develops a set of responses into an integrated and organized movement pattern. In order for you to improve a skill, there are two requirements: Practice the skill and strengthen the muscles that are used to perform the skill.

Practice the Skill

The first requirement for improving a skill is to literally practice the skill for thousands and thousands of task-specific repetitions. Each repetition must be done with perfect technique so that its specific movement pattern becomes firmly ingrained in your "motor memory." The skill must be practiced perfectly and exactly as it would be used during a sport or an activity. Remember, practice makes perfect . . . but only if your practice is perfect. And as noted earlier, the skill shouldn't be practiced with weighted objects.

Strengthen the Muscles

The second requirement for improving a skill is to strengthen the major muscles that are used during the performance of the skill. Remember, strength training shouldn't be done in a manner that tries to mimic or replicate the skill so as not to confuse the neuromuscular pathways or impair the intended movement pattern. A stronger muscle can produce more force; if you can produce more force, you'll require less effort and be able to perform the skill more quickly, more accurately and more efficiently. But again, this is provided that you've practiced enough in a correct manner so that you'll be more skillful in applying that force.

SPORT-SPECIFIC EXERCISES

Are there sport-specific exercises or even position-specific exercises? Should a basketball player do different exercises than a football player or a swimmer? Should a pitcher do different exercises than a catcher or an outfielder?

All athletes have the same muscles that are used in the same manner. For example, the main function of the quadriceps is knee extension (straightening the legs). This is true for a diver, shot putter, quarterback, point guard and softball player. It follows, then, that there's no such thing as sport-specific exercises or position-specific exercises. For that matter, there's no such thing as gender-specific exercises, either.

Some athletes need to perform certain exercises as a precautionary measure against injury to a joint that receives a great deal of stress in their particular sport such as wrestlers who

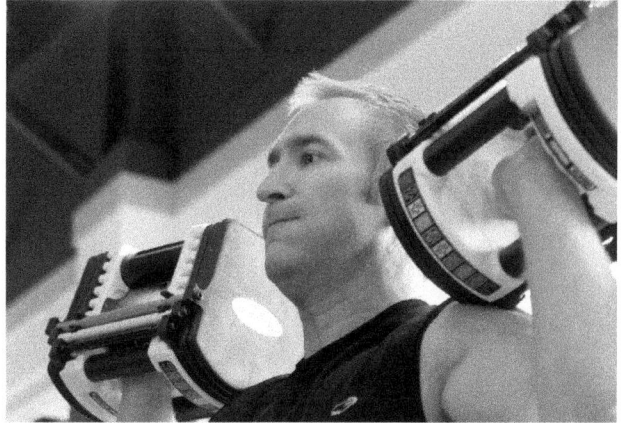

Skill training is specific to a sport or an activity but strength training is general. (Photo provided by Luke Carlson.)

do exercises for their neck which other athletes might not need to perform. Some athletes need to perform certain exercises to focus on a muscle that's essential to their sport such as golfers who do exercises for their grip which other athletes might not need to perform.

Aside from that, you should select exercises that train your muscles in the safest and most efficient way possible. Skill training is specific to a sport or an activity but strength training is general. In other words, the development of strength is general but the application of strength is specific.

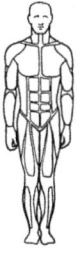

19 Nutrional Training

Nutrition is the process by which you select, consume, digest, absorb and utilize food. Unfortunately, this important aspect of a fitness program is either inadequately addressed or entirely overlooked.

Nutritional training includes being able to recognize and choose desirable foods and understanding the recommended intakes of those foods. This is essential for several reasons.

In general, nutritional training promotes good health. For example, decreasing the intake of cholesterol and sodium will reduce the risk of heart disease and hypertension (high blood pressure), respectively. Moreover, becoming familiar with the caloric contributions of the various nutrients and estimating your caloric needs – the number of calories that you require to maintain your weight – can assist in weight management.

From an athletic perspective, nutritional training plays a crucial part in your capacity to perform at optimal levels and assists in the improvement of your strength, endurance and fitness. Consuming the right foods/fluids before and after an activity allows you to maximize your performance. Pre-activity foods/fluids affect your ensuing performance; post-activity foods/ fluids affect your recovery from that performance. And because so many meals are eaten away from home – especially at fast-food restaurants – it's important to be aware of healthy options.

THE SIX NUTRIENTS

Everything that you do requires energy. The energy is obtained through the food that you consume and is measured in calories (which, technically, are units of heat). Essentially, the food that you eat is fuel for your body. Food is also necessary for the ongoing growth, maintenance and repair of your biological tissues such as muscle and bone.

In order to be considered nutritious, your food intake must contain the recommended amounts of nutrients. No single food satisfies this requirement. As a result, variety is the key to a healthy diet. (Here and in other discussions that follow, the term diet simply refers to a normal food intake, not a specialized regimen of eating.)

Foods have varying proportions of six nutrients. These nutrients can be divided into macronutrients and micronutrients based on the relative amounts that you should consume. Macronutrients are needed in relatively large amounts and include carbohydrates, protein, fat and water; micronutrients are needed in relatively small amounts and include vitamins and minerals.

Carbohydrates

The primary function of carbohydrates (or carbs) is to furnish you with energy, especially during intense activity. Your body breaks down carbohydrates into glucose which can be used as an immediate form of energy during activity

Nutritional training plays a crucial part in your capacity to perform at optimal levels and assists in the improvement of your strength, endurance and fitness. (Photo provided by Luke Carlson.)

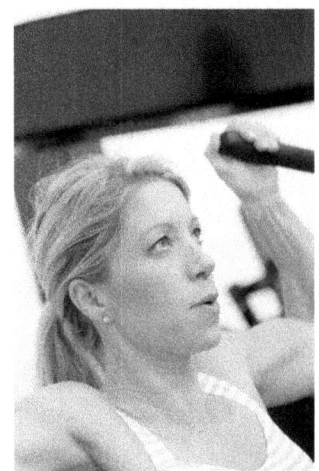

or stored as glycogen in your liver and muscles for later use. Highly conditioned muscles can stockpile more glycogen than poorly conditioned muscles. If your glycogen stores are depleted, you'll feel overwhelmingly exhausted. Having greater glycogen stores can give you a significant physiological advantage thus the enormous importance of carbohydrates.

But not all carbohydrates are created equal. Indeed, carbohydrates run the gamut from potatoes to pastries, from corn to cola and from peas to pies. Most nutritional authorities recognize two types of carbohydrates: simple and complex.

Simple carbohydrates – made of one or two sugars – are digested more quickly than complex carbohydrates. This means that simple carbohydrates enter your bloodstream more quickly and raise your blood glucose (blood sugar) more quickly.

Foods and beverages that are high in simple carbohydrates – including cake, candy, cookies and soda – use refined ingredients such as white sugar, white flour and high fructose corn syrup and have no nutritional value. Consequently, these products are considered sources of "empty calories." Simple carbohydrates are also found in milk and milk products, fruits, vegetables, honey and yogurt. These foods and beverages have a greater nutritional value, making them more favorable sources of carbohydrates.

Complex carbohydrates – made of three or more sugars though often referred to as starches – are digested more slowly than simple carbohydrates. This means that complex carbohydrates enter your bloodstream more slowly and raise your blood glucose more slowly (providing you with a sustained level of energy throughout the day). Complex carbohydrates also offer you a wealth of vitamins and minerals.

Foods that are high in complex carbohydrates include certain vegetables (broccoli, corn and potatoes), breads, cereals, grains, legumes (which include kidney beans, pinto beans, black beans, lima beans, chickpeas, split peas and lentils), yams, rice, spaghetti and macaroni.

Fiber – a category of complex carbohydrates – only comes from plant-based foods and passes through your system undigested. There are two types of fiber: soluble and insoluble.

Soluble fiber can be dissolved in water. It binds to fatty substances and escorts them out of your body as waste. Soluble fiber is found in legumes, nuts, oat bran and various fruits and vegetables. Insoluble fiber can't be dissolved in water. It ushers food through your intestinal tract and promotes regular bowel movements. Insoluble fiber is found in brown rice, wheat bread, whole wheat, whole grains and certain fruits and vegetables.

About 50 to 65% of your daily calories should be from carbohydrates. (Active individuals should be at the higher end of this range.) This includes no more than about 10% from added sugars. It's preferable that your intake is comprised of more complex carbohydrates and less simple carbohydrates.

Protein

The term protein is derived from the Greek word protos which means first. That's an apt description since protein is the major functional and structural component of every cell in your body; it's necessary for the growth, maintenance and repair of your biological tissues, particularly muscle tissue. Additionally, protein regulates water balance and transports other nutrients. Protein can also be used as an energy source in the event that adequate carbohydrates and fat aren't available (although this is generally as a last resort).

The "building blocks" of protein are amino acids. Nine amino acids must be provided in your diet and are considered essential (or indispensable) amino acids. Five amino acids can be synthesized by the body and are considered non-essential (or dispensable) amino acids. And six amino acids can be synthesized by the body but this process may be limited by certain diseases or conditions (such as severe bodily stress from a burn injury) and are considered "conditionally indispensable" amino acids. (Fast fact: As it relates to nutrition, the term essential is used to describe nutrients that must be provided by the diet because your body can't make them endogenously.)

Like carbohydrates, not all proteins are created equal. There are two types of protein: complete and incomplete.

A complete protein contains all of the essential amino acids in amounts that facilitate the growth, maintenance and repair of biological tissues. Proteins that are found in animal sources – such as meat, poultry, fish, eggs, milk, cheese and yogurt – are complete proteins. (Soy is also regarded as a complete protein.) An incomplete protein lacks at least one of the essential amino acids. Proteins that are found in plants, legumes, grains, nuts, seeds and vegetables are incomplete proteins.

Another term that's sometimes used in the discussion of protein is biological value (BV). This is an index in which all protein sources are compared to whole eggs which are the most complete protein and have a BV of 100. Animal sources (complete proteins) have a high BV, meaning that a large portion of the protein is absorbed and retained. (An exception is gelatin.) Vegetable sources (incomplete proteins) have a low BV, meaning that a small portion of the protein is absorbed and retained. Some examples of BVs for foods are 79 for chicken/turkey, 74 for beef, 64 for rice and 55 for peanuts.

About 15 to 20% of your daily calories should be from protein. It's preferable that your intake is comprised of protein from quality sources such as lean or low-fat meat and poultry.

Fat

It may be difficult to believe but fat is actually an important part of a balanced diet. First, fat serves as the preferred source of energy during low-intensity activities such as sleeping, reading and walking. Second, fat helps in the absorption and transportation of certain vitamins. Third, fat adds considerable flavor to foods. This makes food more appetizing . . . and also explains why fat is craved so much.

Like carbohydrates and protein, not all fats are created equal. There are several types of fats: saturated fatty acid, unsaturated fatty acid, essential fatty acid and trans fatty acid.

Saturated fatty acid – or saturated fat – is found in red meats, certain oils (such as coconut and palm oils), high-fat dairy products (such as butter and lard) and many processed foods. Unsaturated fatty acid – or unsaturated fat – is found in fish (such as halibut, mackerel, salmon and trout), nuts, olives, seeds and a variety of oils (such as canola, corn, olive, peanut, sesame, soybean and sunflower oils). Unsaturated fat can be subdivided into monounsaturated and polyunsaturated fats.

What differentiates saturated fat from unsaturated fat? From a technical standpoint, saturated means that the fatty acid contains the maximum amount of hydrogen; in other words, it's "saturated" with hydrogen. Unsaturated means that the fatty acid lacks the maximum amount of hydrogen. (More on that point in a bit.) From a practical standpoint, there are at least two ways that unsaturated fat can be distinguished from saturated fat. For one thing, unsaturated fat is vegetable fat (oil) and saturated fat is animal fat. And at room temperature, unsaturated fat tends to be liquid (think olive oil) and saturated fat tends to be solid or semi-solid (think butter and whipped cream). There are a few exceptions, though, most notably coconut oil, palm oils and whole milk which are liquid at room temperature but high in saturated fat.

Essential fatty acid (EFA) – a type of unsaturated fat – is so named because this fat can't be made endogenously and, therefore, must be provided by the diet. There are two types of EFAs: omega-3 and omega-6 fatty acids. The main omega-3 fat is alpha-linolenic acid and the main omega-6 fat is linoleic acid. (Two other fatty acids – omega-7 and omega-9 – aren't classified as essential because these fats can be made endogenously.)

Omega-3 and omega-6 fats are polyunsaturated fats. (Omega-7 and omega-9 fats are monounsaturated fats.) The best sources of omega-3 fats are fish (such as cod, flounder, halibut, pollock, salmon, sardines, scallops, swordfish and trout). Other sources include walnuts, flaxseeds, flax oil and eggs that are fortified with omega-3s. Omega-6 fats are found in seeds and nuts – and the oils extracted from them – but the main sources are refined vegetable oils which are used in most snack foods, cookies and crackers.

In general, omega-3 fats decrease inflammation (pain and swelling) and blood clotting while omega-6 fats increase those responses. Moreover, a high ratio of omega-6 fats to omega-3 fats is associated with overweight/obesity. Most Americans consume far too many omega-6 fats and far too few omega-3 fats. It becomes apparent, then, that an emphasis should be placed on eating foods that are high in omega-3s with the goal of achieving a balanced ratio – that is, a 1:1 ratio – of omega-3 fats to omega-6 fats.

Some studies have found that consuming omega-3 fats can decrease the risk of heart disease – which is the leading cause of death worldwide – but other studies have found no benefit. These contradictory findings might be best summed up by the US Food and Drug Administration (FDA) which notes that there's "supportive but not conclusive research" that omega-3 fats "may reduce the risk of coronary heart disease." (Fast fact: When essential fatty acids were discovered in 1923, they were referred to as Vitamin F.)

Trans fatty acid – or trans fat – is another type of fat. Manufacturers can create artificial trans fat through hydrogenation, a process in which hydrogen is added to liquid oil to make it more solid. Essentially, this converts unsaturated fat into saturated fat. The process dates back to 1901 when Dr. Wilhelm Normann – a German chemist – became the first person to hydrogenate liquid oil. (Fast fact: In 1903, Dr. Norman was granted a German patent – retroactive to 1902 – for the process which he referred to as fat hardening.)

Scientists can manipulate the extent to which liquid oils are hydrogenated (or saturated). In general, hydrogenation can be complete or incomplete (partial). When hydrogenation is incomplete, it forms partially hydrogenated oils which are the main source of artificial trans fat in foods.

Unsaturated fat is less harmful than saturated fat and trans fat. (Although trans fat is a type of unsaturated fat, its chemical structure is different than the unsaturated fat that occurs naturally in vegetables.) It's well known that saturated fat and trans fat increase low-density lipoprotein (the "bad" cholesterol) and decrease high-density lipoprotein (the "good" cholesterol). This clogs arteries and raises the risk of heart disease.

Sidebar: The FDA has determined that partially hydrogenated oils are no longer "generally recognized as safe." Manufacturers must eliminate artificial trans fat from their products by June 2018. Artificial trans fat had been used extensively by the food industry since the mid-1950s because it's cheaper than animal fat and has a longer shelf life. It was used in baked goods (cakes, cookies, crackers, doughnuts and pies), snack foods, fried foods, vegetable shortenings, stick margarine and coffee creamer. Trans fat won't completely disappear, however, since small amounts of natural trans fat are found in the fatty parts of meat and dairy products. Plus, manufacturers can petition the FDA to use artificial trans fat in small amounts.

About 20 to 25% of your daily calories should be from fat. This includes about 10 to 15% from unsaturated fat and no more than about 10% from saturated fat. It's preferable that your intake is comprised of unsaturated fat and food sources that provide high levels of omega-3 fats. (The Institute of Medicine recommends that your intake of trans fat should be "as low as possible.")

Water

Since it's needed in rather large quantities, water is classified as a macronutrient. Incredibly, almost two thirds of your bodyweight is water.

Unlike the other three macronutrients, water doesn't have any calories and, thus, doesn't provide you with any energy. However, water does have significant roles in your body. For one thing, it regulates your body temperature. This is especially critical when exercising in hot, humid conditions. Also, water helps to lubricate your joints. And water helps to carry nutrients to your cells and waste products from your cells.

Water can be obtained from a variety of sources. This includes fruits, fruit juices, vegetables, vegetable juices, milk, soup and, of course, drinking water. Caffeinated beverages – including coffee, tea, soda and energy drinks – are sources of water, for sure, but aren't good ones because of their diuretic effects which can, ironically, cause a *loss* of water.

The volume of water that's needed can vary greatly from one person to the next based on such factors as age, size, level of fitness and the duration and intensity of activity as well as the environment. (Cold, heat, humidity and altitude all increase the need for water.) According to the Food and Nutrition Board of the Institute of Medicine, an "adequate intake" of water per day for sedentary individuals is 3.7 liters (about 125 ounces) for men and 2.7 liters (about 91 ounces) for women. That might sound like a lot but this is *total water from all fluids and foods*. The actual breakdown is about 81% from fluids – drinking water and beverages – and 19% from foods. Considering fluids alone, an "adequate intake" of water per day is 3.0 liters (about 101 ounces) for men and 2.2 liters (about 74 ounces) for women. In addition, you should consume about 16 ounces of water for every pound of bodyweight that you lose while training, practicing or competing.

Vitamins

Dr. Kazimierz (Casimir) Funk – a Polish biochemist – is credited with discovering vitamins. In 1912, Dr. Funk penned an article for *The Journal of State Medicine* in which he first used the term vitamines – a portmanteau word that blends "vital" and "amines" – to describe "preventive substances" that, when consumed in adequate amounts, could prevent and cure several deficiency diseases such as beriberi and scurvy. (Fast fact: Around 1920, the "e" was snipped from the end of vitamine after it was shown that some vitamins don't have an amine component.)

Vitamins are potent compounds that are required in very small amounts. They're found in a wide assortment of foods, especially in fruits and vegetables. You can get an adequate intake

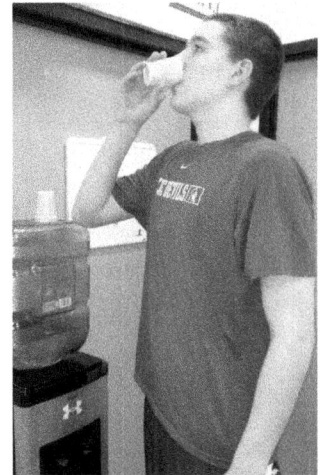

Water regulates your body temperature which is especially critical when exercising in hot, humid conditions. (Photo by Fred Fornicola.)

of vitamins from a balanced diet that contains a variety of healthy foods and sufficient calories.

Even though vitamins have no calories and, therefore, aren't a source of energy, they perform many different functions that are vital to an active lifestyle. There are two types of vitamins: fat soluble and water soluble.

Vitamins A, D, E and K are considered fat-soluble vitamins because they require the presence of adequate amounts of fat before transportation and absorption can take place. Excessive amounts of fat-soluble vitamins are stored in your body. Table 19.1 lists the fat-soluble vitamins along with their functions and sources.

The eight B vitamins (biotin, cobalamin, folate, niacin, pantothenic acid, pyridoxine, riboflavin and thiamine) and vitamin C are considered water-soluble vitamins because they're found in foods that have a naturally high content of water. There's minimal storage of water-soluble vitamins in your body; excess amounts are generally excreted in your urine. Table 19.2 lists the water-soluble vitamins along with their functions and sources.

Minerals

Minerals are required in very small amounts, too. Like vitamins, you can get an adequate intake of minerals from a balanced diet that contains a variety of healthy foods and sufficient calories. Also like vitamins, minerals have no calories but have many different functions that are vital to an active lifestyle. There are two types of

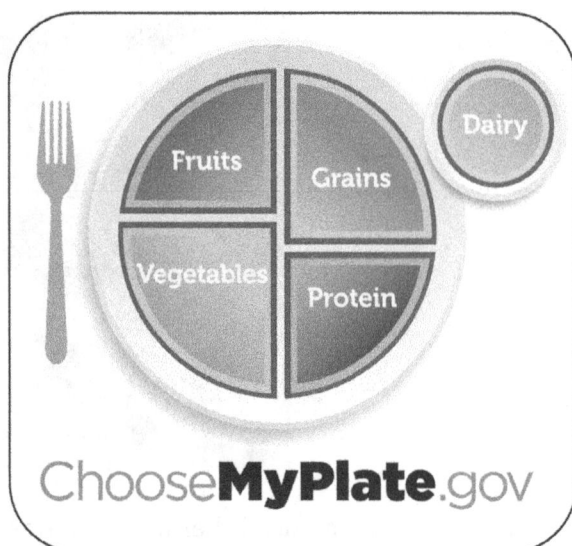

The current recommendations for a healthy diet are to fill 50% of your plate with fruits and vegetables, 25% with grains and 25% with protein. (Icon provided by the US Department of Agriculture.)

minerals: macrominerals (aka major minerals) and microminerals (aka trace minerals).

As the name implies, macrominerals are needed in larger amounts than microminerals specifically, more than 250 milligrams per day. The macrominerals are calcium, chloride, magnesium, phosphorus, potassium, sodium and sulfur. Table 19.3 lists the macrominerals along with their functions and sources.

As you might suspect, microminerals are needed in smaller amounts than macrominerals specifically, less than 20 milligrams per day. The microminerals are chromium, copper, fluoride, iodine, iron, manganese, molybdenum, selenium and zinc. (A number of other minerals – including arsenic, boron, cobalt, lithium, nickel, silicon, tin and vanadium – are probably essential in very small amounts but their roles in the human body are unclear and recommended intakes haven't been established.) Table 19.4 lists the microminerals along with their functions and sources.

THE PYRAMID AND THE PLATE

After nearly 20 years of service as a tool to educate people about a healthy diet, the Food Pyramid was retired in 2011. Introduced jointly in 1992 by the US Department of Agriculture and US Department of Health and Human Services, the Food Pyramid showed four food groups in the shape of a pyramid – thus the name – with the number of recommended servings that should be eaten from each group. Residing at the widest part – the base – were breads, cereals, rice and pasta (6 to 11 servings per day); at the narrowest part – the tip – were fats, oils and sweets ("use sparingly"). In 2005, a revision added two more food groups, renamed some food groups and depicted a person walking up steps on the left side of the pyramid to symbolize the need for exercise.

The Food Pyramid has been replaced with a much simpler concept known as MyPlate or the Food Plate. At the present time, the US Department of Agriculture recognizes five food groups. MyPlate has four colored sections that represent four of the food groups: fruits (red), grains (orange), protein (purple) and vegetables (green). Think of a circle that's divided into four parts of equal size. In other words, the current recommendations for a healthy diet are to fill 50% of your plate with fruits and vegetables, 25% with grains and 25% with protein. (An "athletic" food plate should have more carbohydrates and less protein.) Near the plate is a smaller circle that represents the fifth food group: dairy (blue).

THE FIVE FOOD GROUPS

Since the basis of the Food Plate is the five food groups, it's important to discuss them in greater detail.

The Grain Group

This group consists of foods that are made from wheat, rice, oats, cornmeal, barley or another cereal grain. Examples include bread, pasta, oatmeal and breakfast cereals.

There are two sub-groups of grains: whole grains and refined grains. Whole grains contain the entire grain kernel. Examples include whole-wheat flour, oatmeal and brown rice. Refined grains have been milled which eliminates parts of the grain kernel (the bran, germ and endosperm). This process removes dietary fiber, iron and many B vitamins. Examples include white flour, white bread and white rice.

The Vegetable Group

Any vegetable and any 100% vegetable juice is included in this group. The vegetables can be raw, cooked, fresh, frozen, canned, dried/dehydrated, whole, cut or mashed. There are five categories of vegetables (examples in parentheses): dark green (broccoli, spinach and romaine lettuce); red and orange (carrots, sweet potatoes and tomatoes); beans and peas (black beans, kidney beans and split peas); starchy (corn, green peas and potatoes); and other (beets, celery and cucumbers).

The Fruit Group

Any fruit and any 100% fruit juice is included in this group. The fruits can be fresh, frozen, dried/dehydrated, canned, whole, cut or pureed. Examples include apples, berries, grapes, melons, peaches and pears.

The Dairy Group

This group consists of all fluid milk products and foods that are made from milk that retain their calcium content. (For this reason, cream cheese and butter are excluded from the Dairy Group.) Examples include milk, milk-based desserts, calcium-fortified soy milk, cheese and yogurt.

The Protein Foods Group

This group consists of a wide range of foods in six different sub groups (examples in parentheses): meats (beef, ham and liver); poultry (chicken, duck and turkey); eggs; beans and peas; nuts and seeds (almonds, peanut butter and sesame seeds); and seafood (salmon, lobster and sardines). Note that beans and peas are also part of the Vegetable Group.

DIETARY REFERENCE INTAKES

The most recent approach for assessing and planning diets is the use of the Dietary Reference Intake (DRI). The DRIs include these four "reference values":

Estimated Average Requirement (EAR): The average daily nutrient intake level estimated to meet the needs of 50% of all healthy individuals for a particular age or gender.

Recommended Dietary Allowance (RDA): The average daily nutrient intake level estimated to meet the needs of 97.5% of all healthy individuals for a particular age or gender.

Adequate Intake (AI): The average daily nutrient intake level based on observed or experimentally determined approximations or estimates by a group of healthy individuals.

Tolerable Upper Intake Level (UL): The highest average daily nutrient intake level that's unlikely to produce any adverse effects in almost all individuals in the general population.

The RDA is the recommended goal for everyone. First published in 1943 and updated regularly, the RDAs were developed by the Food and Nutrition Board of the National Academy of Sciences/National Research Council. The RDAs are set by first determining the floor below which deficiency occurs and then the ceiling above which harm occurs. A margin of safety is included to meet the needs of nearly all healthy people. In other words, the RDAs exceed what most people require in order to meet the needs of those who have the highest requirements. So, the RDAs aren't minimum standards. And failing to consume the recommended amounts doesn't necessarily indicate that you have a dietary deficiency. (Note: The AI is used when the RDA for a nutrient can't be determined.)

FOOD LABELS

In deciding whether or not to buy a product in a supermarket or convenience store, do you use the food label to make your decision? According to the 2014 FDA Food and Diet Survey, about 77% of Americans said that they use food labels "always," "most of the time" or "sometimes." On the other hand, about 22% said that they "never" or "rarely" use food labels. Of those 22%, 7% said that food labels were difficult to use and more than half of those people said that they didn't know what to look for even if they could read the food labels.

Clearly, then, simply being able to read food labels isn't good enough. In order to make healthy choices, it's important for you to interpret the information that's on food labels.

Thanks to the Nutrition Labeling and Education Act (NLEA) of 1990 – which amended the 1938 Federal Food, Drug and Cosmetic Act – food labels are required for most packaged foods. This includes breads, cereals, canned/frozen foods, snacks, desserts and beverages. (Food labels on raw fruits, vegetables and fish are voluntary.) In addition, any health claims that are made on food labels must comply with specific regulations.

The Nutrition Facts Panel

Located on the food label is an area that's known as the Nutrition Facts panel. Introduced in May 1993 as part of the NLEA – and required on food labels as of May 1994 – the facts panel (aka facts label) had the same basic design until May 2016 when it was revised by the FDA. Manufacturers with more than $10 million of annual food sales must use the new facts panel on their products by January 2020; manufacturers with less than that have an additional year to comply. A side-by-side comparison of the old (left) and new (right) facts panel in a vertical format is shown in Figure 19.1. (Unless otherwise noted, the ensuing discussion refers to the new facts panel.)

Near the top of the facts panel are the servings per container and serving size. Note that the order of this information is reversed and much more prominent in the newer version, bringing much more attention to the servings per container. Previously, this information was easily overlooked and, as a result, some people could unknowingly consume an excessive amount of calories.

In order to compare similar foods, serving sizes are standardized in an amount of food "customarily consumed" and use a "common

Figure 19.1: Sample Nutrition Facts panels, side-by-side comparison of old (left) and new (right). (Images provided by the US Food and Drug Administration.)

household measure that is appropriate to the food." Household measures include cups, tablespoons, teaspoons and ounces; metric measures include grams, milligrams and milliliters. What's more, some of the measures incorporate fractions (such as 1/2, 1/3, 2/3 and 1/4). Do you know the difference between a tablespoon and a teaspoon? Or what 1/2 cup of potatoes actually looks like? How about three ounces of chicken? Most people don't know the answers to these questions. (Fast fact: One tablespoon equals three teaspoons; 1/2 cup of potatoes looks like half of a tennis ball; and three ounces of chicken are about the size of a deck of cards.)

Remember, the servings per container and serving size influence the quantity of the ingredients that are listed on the facts panel. Key point: Unless it's a single-serving package, the amount of each ingredient is only for a portion of the contents. If a food has two servings per container, then eating the entire contents literally doubles the amount of calories and nutrients. For this reason, the FDA now requires manufacturers to use a dual-column label when a product has more than one serving but the entire contents could reasonably be consumed in one sitting.

With a dual-column label, one column indicates the amount of calories and nutrients *per serving* and the other column indicates the amount of calories and nutrients *per container*.

After the servings per container and serving size is the amount of calories per serving. This information is also much more prominent in the newer version. Also note that the calories from fat have been removed from the facts panel which is an acknowledgement that the *type* of fat is a more important consideration than the *amount* of fat. If you want to determine the percentage of fat in a food, multiply the total fat in grams by nine calories per gram and then divide this number by the calories per serving. Referring to the new facts panel in Figure 19.1, for example, one serving of the food has eight grams of fat. Multiplying this number by nine calories per gram is 72 calories. Dividing 72 calories by 230 calories – the amount of calories in one serving – means that the food is about 31.3% fat. (Caloric contributions are discussed in greater detail later in this chapter.)

Directly below the information on calories is a section on nutrients. At the top of this list is total fat which is subdivided into saturated fat and, as of January 2006, trans fat.

Sidebar: As mentioned earlier, manufacturers must eliminate artificial trans fat from their products by June 2018. If a product contains less than 0.5 grams of trans fat, the number can be rounded down to zero on the label. However, any ingredient that has "partially hydrogenated" in its name is a telltale sign of hidden trans fat.

Appearing next on the facts panel is an area that's devoted to cholesterol and sodium. Cholesterol is linked to heart disease and sodium is linked to hypertension. Your intake of cholesterol should be less than 300 milligrams per day; your intake of sodium should be less than 2,300 milligrams per day.

Following cholesterol and sodium are total carbohydrate and protein. Total carbohydrate is subdivided into dietary fiber and total sugars. Listed right below total sugars are added sugars (in grams). This includes sugars that have been put in during the processing or packaging of a food.

The final nutrients that are listed on the facts panel are vitamins and minerals. Information on vitamin D, calcium, iron and potassium is required on the facts panel. (Other vitamins and minerals can be declared voluntarily.) The older version required information on vitamin A, vitamin C, calcium and iron. Vitamin A and vitamin C were removed because deficiencies are rare. Vitamin D and potassium were added because these two micronutrients aren't always consumed in the recommended amounts and, thus, demand greater awareness. (Fast fact: Blood pressure can be reduced by either decreasing sodium intake or increasing potassium intake.)

Percent Daily Value

An important concept that's used on the facts panel is Percent Daily Value or % Daily Value (% DV). It appears at the bottom of the facts panel as a standard footnote (provided that the label is large enough).

The new version simplifies the meaning of the % DV. According to the footnote, the % DV "tells you how much a nutrient in a serving of food contributes to a daily diet" and that "2,000 calories a day is used for general nutrition advice."

The % DVs appear on the right-hand side of the facts panel across from the corresponding nutrients. As suggested by the footnote, the % DVs are representative of a 2,000-calorie diet. But even if your daily caloric needs are less than or more than 2,000, you can still take advantage of the information that's provided by the %DVs. Specifically, you can determine at a glance if a serving of a food is low or high in a given nutrient. As a rule of thumb, a DV that's 5% or less is low; a DV that's 20% or more is high. In Figure 19.1, for instance, you can see that saturated fat is 5% which is low and added sugars are 20% which is high. Note, too, that this food is high in calcium and iron, checking in at 20% and 45%, respectively. (Fast fact: Sugar and trans fat don't have % DVs; a % DV isn't required to be listed for protein unless a claim is made such as "high in protein.")

Now remember, the % DVs apply to one serving. In Figure 19.1, sodium is 7% which is relatively low. But again, that's for one serving. If you downed three servings, the % DV would be 21% which is high. (In consuming three servings, the amount of sodium triples, going from 160 milligrams to 480 milligrams.) Or look at it this way: You just consumed 21% of your daily allowance for sodium. Does this mean that you should toss this particular food into someone else's shopping cart? No. It simply means that for the remainder of the day, you'd have to pay closer attention to the sodium content of foods and make better choices.

Sidebar: The DV represents a diet that consists of about 60% carbohydrates, 10% protein and 30% fat. A better guideline for active individuals, however, is a diet that consists of about 65% carbohydrates, 15% protein and 20% fat.

Ingredient Lists

If a food has more than one ingredient, they must be listed on the food label. What many individuals don't realize is that the ingredients on the food label are listed in "descending order of predominance by weight." In other words, the first ingredient weighs the most and the last ingredient weighs the least. So a food or beverage that has some form of sugar among its first few ingredients probably has low or no nutritional value and, in that case, would do little or nothing to improve health.

And while on the subject, understand that sugar can appear in many forms. Ingredients that end in the suffix "-ose" – such as dextrose, fructose, lactose, maltose and sucrose – are sugars but not all sugars have that ending. Other sugars or sugar-based ingredients include caramel, corn sweetener, corn syrup, dextrin, honey, malt syrup, maltodextrin, mannitol, molasses, nectar and sorbitol.

CALORIC CONTRIBUTIONS

As stated earlier, carbohydrates, protein and fat are sources of energy; in this regard, energy is expressed as calories. Investigations into the caloric contributions of these three macronutrients date back to 1884 when Dr. Max Rubner – a German physiologist – determined that the energy yield of carbohydrates and protein was 4.1 calories per gram (cal/g) and fat was 9.3 cal/g. About a decade later, Dr. Wilbur Atwater – an American chemist – and his colleagues at the Storrs Agricultural Experiment Station in Connecticut found nearly identical energy yields: about 4.0 cal/g for carbohydrates and protein and about 9.0 cal/g for fat. (By the way, the energy yield for alcohol is about 7.0 cal/g.) First published in 1896, the values – referred to as Atwater general factors – are derived from an "average diet" that was consumed in the late 1800s. So the values are actually averages of mixed foods – not single foods – from many decades ago which has led to repeated criticism. Nonetheless, the values are easy to use and reasonably accurate. After well more than a century, the Atwater general factors continue to be employed throughout the world. (Fast fact: Dr. Atwater is regarded as the father of American nutrition; for a brief time, he and Dr. Rubner were co-workers in the same laboratory in Munich, Germany.)

Armed with the Atwater general factors, you can approximate the caloric contributions of the three energy-providing macronutrients for any food, provided that you know how many grams of each macronutrient are in a serving.

As an example, consider Lays® Classic Potato Chips (Frito-Lay, Incorporated). Examining the facts panel reveals that a one-ounce serving of this snack food has 15 grams of carbohydrates, 2 grams of protein and 10 grams of fat. To find the exact number of calories that are supplied by each macronutrient, simply multiply its number of grams per serving by its corresponding energy yield. Therefore, each serving has 60 calories from carbohydrates [15 g x 4 cal/g], 8 calories from protein [2 g x 4 cal/g] and 90 calories from fat [10 g x 9 cal/g]. So, this food has a total of 158 calories per serving (which is rounded to 160 on the facts panel). In this product, then, about 56.96% of the calories (90 of the 158) are supplied by fat.

Now consider Lay's® Baked Original Potato Crisps, another product by the same manufacturer. A one-ounce serving of this snack food has 22 grams of carbohydrates, 2 grams of protein and 3.5 grams of fat. Therefore, each serving has 88 calories from carbohydrates [22 g x 4 cal/g], 8 calories from protein [2 g x 4 cal/g] and 31.5 calories from fat [3.5 g x 9 cal/g]. So, this food has a total of 127.5 calories per serving (which is rounded to 130 on the facts panel). In this product, then, about 24.71% of the calories (31.5 of the 127.5) are supplied by fat.

In comparing these two snack foods, the potato crisps have 6.5 less grams of fat and 30.5 less calories than the potato chips. That might not seem like much of a difference but remember, *that's per ounce.* And the stark reality is that most people eat a lot more than one ounce of a snack food.

On a related note, some products carry a statement on the packaging that they're a certain percent fat free. It's important for you to determine the exact fat content of these foods so that this statement isn't misinterpreted. Case in point: A package that proclaims a product to be 99% fat free leads many consumers to believe that only 1% of its calories come from fat. But the designation of 99% fat free means that it's 99% fat free by *weight*, not by *calories*. How critical is this distinction? Very. Placing one gram of fat in 99 grams of water forms a product that, in terms of weight, is 99% fat free. Since water has no calories, however, this particular 99% fat free product, in terms of calories, is actually *100% fat.*

The preceding example is hypothetical. But if you think that this doesn't occur with real products, think again. Here are three examples:

A can of Progresso® Chicken Noodle Soup (General Mills, Incorporated) states that it's "99% fat free." But one serving of this product (1 cup; 237 grams) has 90 calories of which 18 are from fat, meaning that it's 20.00% fat.

A package of Oscar Mayer®'s Franks (The Kraft Heinz Company) states that it's "95% fat free." But one serving of this product (1 link; 50 grams) has 58.5 calories of which 22.5 are from

The designation 99% fat free means that a product is 99% fat free by weight, not by calories.

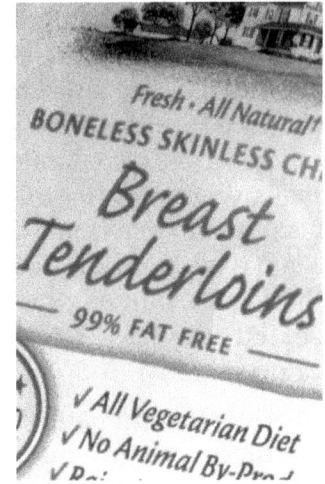

fat, meaning that it's 38.46% fat. (The numbers on the facts panel are rounded to 50 calories per serving with 20 calories from fat.)

A package of Perdue® Ground Turkey (Perdue Farms) states that it's "7% fat" (or in other words, "93% fat free"). But one serving of this product (112 grams) has 156 calories of which 72 are from fat, meaning that it's 46.15% fat. (The numbers on the facts panel are rounded to 160 calories per serving with 80 calories from fat.)

The percentage of fat in these three products isn't terribly bad. But it's certainly a far cry from how the statements on the package can be interpreted.

ESTIMATING YOUR CALORIC NEEDS

Your caloric needs are the number of calories that you require to maintain your weight. This is determined by several factors, including your age, gender, size, body composition, metabolic rate (the rate at which you use calories) and level of activity.

The most accurate way to ascertain your caloric needs is through either direct or indirect calorimetry. Remember, a calorie is a unit of heat. And the heat that your body produces can be measured both directly and indirectly. Direct calorimetry is a direct measurement of the heat that's produced by the body while inside a small, sealed, insulated room – known as a metabolic (or respiration) chamber – for a specified period of time (usually 24 hours); indirect calorimetry is an indirect measurement of the heat that's produced by the body based on the amount of oxygen that's consumed and carbon dioxide that's produced. (Fast fact: Direct calorimetry is also used to determine the number of calories in a food based on the heat that's produced when the food is burned; this is done within a small, sealed device that's known as a bomb calorimeter.)

Direct calorimetry isn't practical because it requires access to a metabolic chamber and there aren't too many of those around. And even if a metabolic chamber is available, it comes at no small expense. (A metabolic chamber is usually about the size of a dorm room with "all the comforts of home": a bed, desk, chair, television, computer, sink and toilet.) Indirect calorimetry is more common and less expensive but requires access to elaborate equipment often in a university or clinical setting. During indirect calorimetry, an individual wears a mouthpiece or mask that interfaces with a computer which measures and analyzes the gases that are inhaled and exhaled. The computer is mounted on a compact, portable device that's known as a metabolic cart. (This method can also be used to determine oxygen intake.)

Direct and indirect calorimetry can provide you with accurate data that are reliable and valid. However, as noted, laboratory testing can be impractical, expensive and time-consuming (if these options are even available). Fortunately, there's another way to assess your caloric needs without the inherent drawbacks of laboratory testing.

A number of equations can be used to estimate caloric needs albeit with varying degrees of complexity. The Institute of Medicine, for example, offers a rather complicated equation that considers gender, age, activity level, weight and height.

For a quick and reasonably accurate estimate of your daily caloric needs, you can multiply your bodyweight by a number that corresponds to your gender and approximate level of activity.

Essentially, this number represents your energy requirement in calories per pound of bodyweight per day (cal/lb/day). For women, the values are 14 if sedentary, 18 if moderately active and 22 if very active; for men, the values are 16, 21 and 26, respectively. To illustrate, a 200-pound man who's very active requires approximately 5,200 calories per day (cal/day) to meet his caloric needs [200 lb x 26 cal/lb/day].

Be advised that this equation has gray areas; most notably, the terms moderately active and very active are subject to a wide range of interpretations. Though imperfect, it still results in a fairly good estimate of your caloric needs. And remember, any other equation that's used in this regard is just that: an estimate.

At first blush, 5,200 calories seems like a lot. And it is. But don't forget that at a bodyweight of 200 pounds, this man is significantly heavier than the average man. Plus, this man is very active which requires a greater caloric consumption to compensate for a greater caloric expenditure. It wouldn't be unusual for many football and basketball players – who are big and active, for sure – to consume 6,000 or more calories per day to meet their caloric needs. And they'll need even more calories if they're trying to increase their lean-body mass. (Fast fact: The "reference man" stands 5'10" and weighs 154 pounds while the "reference woman" stands 5'4" and weighs 126 pounds.)

Researchers have investigated the caloric consumption of athletes and found some intakes to be ridiculously high. One study involved eight cross-country skiers (four male and four female) from the Swedish national teams. The women completed seven days of "normal training" and the men, arriving one day later, completed six days of "normal training." On average, the female skiers consumed about 4,347 cal/day (one woman consumed 4,872 cal/day) and used 4,371 cal/day (one woman used 4,825 cal/day); on average, the male skiers consumed about 7,213 cal/day (one man consumed 8,598 cal/day) and used 7,213 cal/day (one man used 8,336 cal/day). That's an intake of about 36.3 cal/lb/day for the women and 43.6 cal/lb/day for the men!

(Incidentally, their diet consisted of about 58.0% carbohydrates, 13.0% protein and 28.0% fat.)

Individuals whose bodyweights are average or lighter than average may need to consume an unusually high number of calories, too, if they're very active. One study involved nine male Kenyan middle- and long-distance runners who competed in events ranging from 1,500 meters to the marathon; the group included world, Olympic and junior champions. They completed seven days of heavy training about five months prior to the 2004 Athens Olympics. On average, the runners consumed about 3,164 cal/day and used about 3,492 cal/day (which, by the way, resulted in a weight loss of about 0.7 pounds, decreasing from about 123.5 to 122.8 pounds). That's an intake of about 25.6 cal/lb/day. (Their diet consisted of about 67.3% carbohydrates, 15.3% protein and 17.4% fat.)

That's nothing: One study involved six male professional cyclists who competed in the 2009 Tour of Andalusia. During this Spanish road race, they covered about 400 miles in four days at an altitude as high as 1.1 miles. On average, the cyclists consumed about 5,644 cal/day which enabled them to maintain their bodyweight of 149 pounds. That's an intake of about 37.9 cal/lb/day! (Their diet consisted of about 62.3% carbohydrates, 14.5% protein and 23.2% fat.)

Once you've estimated your caloric needs, you can determine how many of these calories should come from carbohydrates, protein and fat. For a diet that consists of 65% carbohydrates, 15% protein and 20% fat, someone who requires about 5,200 cal/day should consume roughly 845 grams of carbohydrates, 195 grams of protein and 115 grams of fat [5,200 cal/day x 0.65 ÷ 4 cal/g = 845 g; 5,200 cal/day x 0.15 ÷ 4 cal/g = 195 g; 5,200 cal/day x 0.20 ÷ 9 cal/g = 115.56 g].

To be clear: There's no need to count calories or calculate grams of each macronutrient. The preceding discussion of caloric needs with respect to consumption and expenditure is only meant to demonstrate the dynamics of weight management as it pertains to estimating a caloric budget and maintaining weight.

GLYCEMIC INDEX AND GLYCEMIC LOAD

A 1981 study by a group of Canadian and British researchers determined the glycemic index (GI) of 62 foods and sugars. Their research was done to learn the effects that different foods have on blood glucose in order to assist people with diabetes. The first table of GI was published in 1995 and had 565 entries that were collected from the scientific literature. The table was updated in 2002 and had almost 1,300 entries. The most recent table was published in 2008 and boasts nearly 2,500 entries.

The GI is a system of quantifying the carbohydrates in foods based on how they affect blood glucose compared to a reference food (either glucose or white bread). A value is assigned to a food that correlates to the magnitude of the increase in blood glucose. For instance, a food with a GI of 50 means that it elevates blood glucose to a level that's 50% as great as consuming the same amount of pure glucose which has a GI of 100. (Note: A GI of 55 or less is considered low, 56 to 69 is medium and 70 or more is high.)

A limitation of the GI is that it's not related to portion size. So, the GI is the same whether an individual consumes 50 grams of a particular food or 150 grams. And that's where the glycemic load enters the picture.

The concept of glycemic load (GL) was introduced in 1997 by researchers at the Harvard School of Public Health. It's a measure of the quality *and* quantity of carbohydrates. To calculate the GL of a food, multiply the carbohydrate content in grams by the GI and divide by 100. For example, eating a food that has 20 grams of carbohydrates and a GI of 50 yields a GL of 10 [20 x 50 ÷ 100 = 10]; eating a food that has 10 grams of carbohydrates and a GI of 80 yields a GL of 8 [10 x 80 ÷ 100 = 8]. So in this example, the food with the lower GI would actually raise blood glucose more than the food with the higher GI because a larger portion size was consumed. (Note: A GL of 10 or less is considered low, 11 to 19 is medium and 20 or more is high.)

PRE-ACTIVITY FOODS/FLUIDS

Foods and fluids that are consumed before an activity – whether it's some type of physical training, practice or competition – have several purposes. Pre-activity foods/fluids remove your hunger pangs, ready your body with fuel for the upcoming activity, put you in a relaxed state and ease any anxiety that you might have.

There's no food that you can consume prior to an activity that will improve your performance. But there are some foods that you can consume prior to an activity that can impair your performance and, for this reason, should be avoided. For instance, foods that are high in fiber, protein and fat are digested slowly and, therefore, shouldn't be eaten before training, practicing or competing. Other foods to omit include those that are greasy, highly seasoned and flatulent (gas-forming) along with any specific foods that you may personally find distressful to your digestive system. If anything, what you select for your pre-activity foods should be almost bland yet appetizing enough so that you want to eat it.

Before an activity, you should also avoid eating foods and drinking beverages that cause a sharp increase in your blood glucose (blood sugar). Here's why: Your body tries to maintain a relatively stable internal environment – referred to as homeostasis – whether it's in regards to your core temperature, blood acidity or blood glucose. When a level of blood glucose is detected that exceeds a certain limit, your pancreas reacts and releases a hormone known as insulin. As a result of this biochemical balancing act, your blood glucose is decreased which can lead to hypoglycemia or low blood glucose. (When low blood glucose occurs after eating, it's referred to as reactive – or rebound – hypoglycemia.) If this happens during exercise, it reduces the availability of blood glucose as a fuel and might cause you to feel fatigued. Effectively, the body is decreasing blood glucose at the same time that the exercising muscles are using blood glucose. That's a bad combination. (Fast fact: The concept of homeostasis was introduced in 1865 by Dr. Claude Bernard, a French physiologist; however, the term wasn't coined until 1926 by Dr. Walter Cannon – a physiologist and graduate of the Harvard Medical School – who also coined the phrase "fight or flight" in 1916.)

One crossover study involved 10 competitive cyclists who were very fit, averaging 9.7% body fat and a maximum oxygen intake of 58.1 milliliters per kilogram of bodyweight per minute. The subjects performed an endurance test to exhaustion on three separate occasions 30 minutes after consuming one liter of a beverage that contained either glucose (40 grams), galactose (40 grams) or a placebo. Glucose and galactose are sugars, of course, but with different effects on blood sugar: Glucose has a very high GI (100) while galactose has a very low GI (about 20). The researchers found that the subjects produced worse times to exhaustion after receiving glucose (58.5 minutes) than either galactose (68.7 minutes) or the placebo (63.9 minutes). They also found that glucose increased blood sugar to a higher level before the endurance test than galactose and the placebo and decreased blood sugar more rapidly during the endurance test than galactose and the placebo. In fact, after receiving glucose, 30% of the cyclists were susceptible to reactive hypoglycemia during the first 20 minutes of the test; one of the cyclists was unable to continue the test.

So although everyone doesn't experience reactive hypoglycemia, it remains an important consideration when choosing pre-activity foods/fuels, especially for those who are "sugar sensitive."

The idea, then, is to consume foods that elevate or maintain blood glucose without triggering a dramatic response by the pancreas. At one time, it was believed that simple carbohydrates (sugars) increase blood glucose more rapidly than complex carbohydrates (starches). A more recent trend of thought has been to take into account the GI of a food.

Before an activity, it's best to consume foods that are easy to digest and rich in carbohydrates that have a low GI. These foods help to keep your blood glucose within a desirable range.

Don't simply assume that a sugary food raises blood glucose more than a starchy food. Indeed, an apple (40) has a lower GI than a white bagel (72) and, given these two options, would be a better choice for a pre-activity food.

Foods with a relatively low GI include peanuts (13), cherries (22), plums (24), grapefruit (25), peaches (28), low-fat yogurt (33), pears (33), low-fat chocolate milk (34), tomato juice (38), apples (40), apple juice (40), oranges (40), grapes (43), white spaghetti (44), macaroni (45), orange juice (46) and bananas (51).

Water is perhaps the best liquid for you to drink before training, practicing and competing. Your fluid intake should be enough to guarantee optimal hydration during the activity.

The timing of a pre-activity meal is also crucial. To ensure that your digestive process doesn't impair your performance, you should eat your pre-activity meal at least three hours prior to training, practicing or competing. So if you have a workout, practice or competition that starts at 6:00pm, it's best to finish your pre-activity meal by about 3:00pm. (Closer to an activity, you can eat a small snack such as fruit.) In short, your pre-activity meal should include foods that are familiar to you and well tolerated, preferably carbohydrates with a low GI.

POST-ACTIVITY FOODS/FLUIDS

Foods and fluids that are consumed after an activity – whether it's some type of physical training, practice or competition – have several purposes. Post-activity foods/fluids accelerate your recovery and prepare you for your next physical challenge. Following an activity – especially one that requires intense efforts – the amount of carbohydrates in your body is depleted; the needle on your "gas gauge" is pointing toward "E" and your "gas tank" – your glycogen depot – needs refilling. It makes a great deal of sense, then, to consume carbohydrates in order to refill your "gas tank" in preparation for the next time that you train, practice or compete. And the sooner that you refuel with carbohydrates, the better. Delaying the consumption of carbohydrates significantly reduces the rate at which your glycogen stores

are replenished. This will impede the recovery process and impact your future performance.

One crossover study involved 12 cyclists who were very fit, averaging a maximum oxygen intake of 4.19 liters per minute. Prior to the study, the subjects did the training protocol for two weeks in order to become familiar with it. The subjects performed 70 minutes of continuous and exhaustive exercise on a stationary cycle on two separate occasions: One time they consumed a carbohydrate supplement immediately after the activity and the other time they consumed it two hours after the activity. The researchers found that after an activity, a delayed intake of carbohydrates resulted in a slower rate of glycogen storage in comparison to an immediate intake of carbohydrates.

After an activity, it's best to consume foods that are rich in carbohydrates that have a high GI. These foods will help to restore muscle and liver glycogen in the quickest fashion.

In another crossover study, seven men ran on a treadmill at a constant speed for 90 minutes on two separate occasions. This was followed by a four-hour recovery period during which they were fed a meal. (The meal came 20 minutes into the recovery period.) One time the meal had a high GI (77) and the other time the meal had a low GI (37). After the four-hour recovery, they ran to exhaustion at the same speed as in the 90-minute run. The subjects ran 15.2% longer after consuming the high GI meal than after consuming the low GI meal (86.6 minutes compared to 75.2 minutes). In other words, the subjects recovered more quickly from 90 minutes of running after they ate foods with a high GI.

Foods with a relatively high GI include whole-grain bread (59), Kellogg's Raisin Bran® (61), raisins (64), pineapples (66), white bread (71), watermelon (72), white bagels (72), waffles (76), Gatorade® (78), jelly beans (80), pizza (80), Kellogg's® Rice Krispies® (82), puffed rice cakes (82), pretzels (83), Kellogg's Corn Flakes® (92), baked russet potatoes (94), buckwheat pancakes (102) and dates (103).

There are a few reasons why fluids might be a better choice than foods to deliver carbohydrates immediately after an activity. For one thing, in the aftermath of an activity – especially one that's intense – your appetite is suppressed, at least initially (a phenomenon that has been dubbed exercise-induced anorexia). This makes fluids more appealing than foods or a meal. In addition, after an activity, fluids help to rehydrate your body; and cold fluids help to cool your body. Finally, fluids tend to be more readily accessible than foods.

Commercial sports drinks can be excellent post-activity fluids. In terms of recovery, there are two important components of a sports drink: carbohydrates and electrolytes (sodium and potassium). Since all sports drinks are different, you should read the facts panel to be sure of their exact contents.

A good rule of thumb is to consume about 0.5 grams of carbohydrates per pound of your bodyweight (g/lb) within 30 minutes of completing an activity. This should be repeated again within two hours of completing the activity. Say, for instance, that the 200-pound man in the continuing example finished his training at 8:00am. He should consume about 100 grams of carbohydrates – or 400 calories of carbohydrates – by 8:30am and another 100 grams of carbohydrates by 10:00am [0.5 g/lb x 200 lb = 100 g].

As stated previously, delaying the consumption of carbohydrates significantly reduces the rate at which the glycogen stores are replenished. This will impede the recovery process and impact your future performance.

There's some evidence to suggest that combining carbohydrates with a small amount of protein can expedite recovery by improving the rate at which your glycogen stores are replenished. However, it appears that simply increasing the quantity of post-activity carbohydrates will yield the same result. Nonetheless, consuming a small amount of protein following an intense activity may aid in the repair of muscle tissue. If carbohydrates and protein are consumed in combination after an activity, it should be in a 4:1 ratio, meaning that 80% of the calories should be from carbohydrates

and 20% of the calories should be from protein. To use the earlier example, instead of consuming 100 grams of carbohydrates within 30 minutes of completing an activity, the man would consume 80 grams of carbohydrates and 20 grams of protein.

In this regard, an easy, inexpensive and effective way to get protein after training, practicing or competing is to drink low-fat chocolate milk. This beverage contains all nine essential amino acids and has a near-perfect ratio of carbohydrates and protein. (Eight ounces of most low-fat chocolate milk have about 26 grams of carbohydrates and eight grams of protein for 3.25:1 ratio.) An added bonus is that chocolate milk has a number of key nutrients, including several vitamins (vitamin A, vitamin D, cobalamin and riboflavin) and minerals (calcium and potassium). And there's no need to splurge on a nutritional product or supplement; low-fat chocolate milk from a supermarket is less expensive and works fine. (Fast fact: Research has shown that consuming 20 to 30 grams of protein at any one feeding is the maximum amount that can be used by the body.)

Finally, it's also important to rehydrate after an activity. You should consume about 16 ounces of water for every pound of bodyweight that you lose while training, practicing or competing.

FAST FOODS, SLOW CHOICES

If you eat at fast-food restaurants on a regular basis, you're not alone. In 2013, a Gallup Poll of 2,027 American adults found that about 47% eat fast food at least once per week. No wonder: Statistics from the US Department of Agriculture show that there were 228,677 fast-food restaurants in the United States in 2014. According to the National Restaurant Association, sales at limited-service (or quick-service) restaurants were $221.9 billion in 2016 (plus another $544.1 billion throughout the restaurant industry). And Americans spend 48% of their "food dollar" eating away from home. (Fast fact: A limited-service restaurant is one in which a consumer selects items to eat and drink before paying; a fast-casual restaurant is very similar but slightly more upscale.)

The good news is that fast food is inexpensive, convenient and, of course, fast. But the bad news is that, for the most part, it's not very healthy or nutritious. Fast food tends to be high in calories, fat and sodium. In fact, research has shown that on the days that people eat fast food, they tend to consume more calories and fat than on other days.

Healthy Tactics

Believe it or not, there are healthy tactics that you can employ when eating fast food. Since fast foods are so widespread and can vary so much from one restaurant to another, it's well beyond the scope of this chapter to offer you a detailed list of specific suggestions. However, here are some general suggestions that you'll find useful in your quest to make healthy choices at fast-food restaurants (and, in many cases, full-service restaurants as well):

1. Reduce fat.

Fast food is often synonymous with fat food. In general, you should limit your intake of fat, especially saturated fat.

Perhaps the most ubiquitous item on a fast-food menu is an order of French fries. Indeed, it's estimated that the average American eats about 30 pounds of French fries per year. Unfortunately, French fries are very high in fat. A medium serving can have 17 grams of fat of which 3 grams are saturated fat. Do you still want fries with that burger?

Onion rings are actually worse. A medium serving can have 21 grams of fat of which 3.5 grams are saturated fat. A better choice to accompany your meal is a baked potato which has no fat whatsoever.

Here's another helpful hint to reduce your intake of fat: If you like to eat toast with your breakfast, use jelly or jam instead of butter.

2. Watch sodium.

As noted previously, your intake of sodium should be less than 2,300 milligrams per day. This is the equivalent of about one teaspoon of table salt per day.

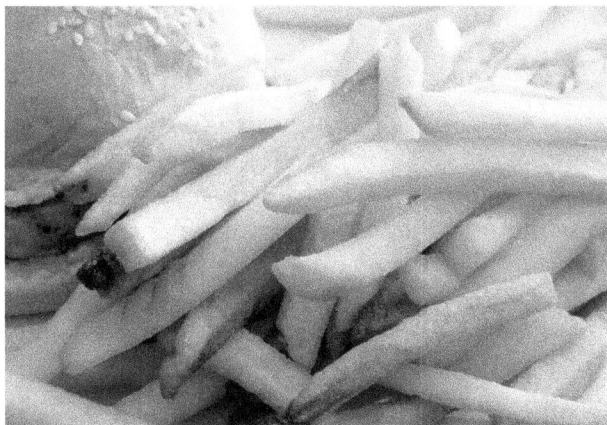
It's estimated that the average American eats 28 pounds of French fries per year.

Fast food is notorious for being high in sodium. If you're not careful, you can easily get more than an entire day's worth of sodium in just one meal. An example of this is eating a ham-and-cheese omelet, two pancakes, sausage, bacon, hash browns and a biscuit for breakfast. Add to this a cheeseburger, medium fries and a medium milkshake for lunch and a few slices of pizza for dinner and you'll have a great head start on establishing your very own salt mine (as well as clogging your arterial pipeline).

Most people know that French fries are high in sodium; a medium serving can have 570 milligrams. But a medium serving of onion rings can have 1,080 milligrams. How about a side order of chili? One small serving can have 780 milligrams. A medium serving of hash browns can have 1,140 milligrams.

The fact of the matter is that sodium shows up in a number of startling places. For instance, a medium chocolate milkshake can have 500 milligrams. Another unexpected surprise is that squirt of ketchup on your burger; a small packet can have 125 milligrams. And those seemingly harmless dill pickles can check in at about 200 milligrams. Salad dressings can be loaded with sodium: Fat-free Italian dressing has a whopping 390 milligrams. Cole slaw, surprisingly, is also high in sodium.

Sidebar: Although sea salt and table salt differ in flavor, texture and processing, both are made of the same two minerals: sodium and chloride.

It's thought that sea salt has less sodium than table salt. This misconception stems from the fact that sea salt is flaky so it weighs less than the same volume of table salt. Given the same volume, sea salt has less sodium than table salt. But in reality, sea salt and table salt have the same amount of sodium: about 390 milligrams per gram or, for a standard serving (one-quarter teaspoon or 1.5 grams), about 590 milligrams. A potential problem is that individuals who think that sea salt is healthier might use it more liberally on their foods. Finally, table salt usually has added iodine; sea salt does not. Iodine, of course, is a good preventive measure against goiter.

3. Think green.

Many fast-food restaurants now offer salads and some even have salad bars. However, just because it's salad doesn't automatically mean that it's healthy. You can't go wrong with ingredients such as lettuce, tomatoes, cucumbers and carrots. But you can sabotage an otherwise excellent choice of food with the dressing.

In general, salad dressings are almost all fat and quite high in sodium. So rather than drown your salad in dressing, order it on the side. Or better yet, use a fat-free or reduced-fat dressing. Remember, though, that using a reduced-fat dressing doesn't give you the license to pour it on *ad libitum*. Be aware, for example, that a packet of reduced-fat creamy ranch dressing can still have 100 calories of which 70 are from fat (along with 550 milligrams of sodium).

Something else to avoid on salads are croutons which can be 30% fat or more (and high in sodium). Along these lines, skip the bacon bits. Also, a garden salad is much healthier than a Caesar salad.

4. Limit toppings/sauces.

A traditional topping for a sandwich is mayonnaise. Choosing to "hold the mayo" could save you 150 calories or more . . . and they're all from fat. If you need to put something on a sandwich, try using mustard instead of mayonnaise.

As noted earlier, a baked potato is a better choice than French fries or onion rings. But get it sans butter, sour cream or other toppings/stuffings. Having a baked potato "stuffed" with bacon and cheese can increase the calories from about 300 to 580, the fat calories from 0 to 200 and the milligrams of sodium from 25 to 950. Yikes!

Few foods are as inextricably linked with toppings more than the ever-popular pizza. It's important to understand that a cheese pizza has more calories from fat than you might think. One medium slice of cheese pizza can have 240 calories of which 10 grams are from fat, including 5 grams of saturated fat (plus 650 milligrams of sodium). And seriously, who eats just one slice? Add meat toppings and it only gets worse. Consider this: One medium slice of sausage pizza can have 340 calories of which 18 grams are from fat, including 8 grams of saturated fat (plus 910 milligrams of sodium). All in one slice! So if you're going to have pizza, order it plain or with vegetable toppings. An even healthier option is to get pizza with whole-wheat dough.

Ketchup is a popular condiment but, again, it's high in sodium. Sauces, too, are usually high in sodium. Get tarter, barbeque and other sauces on the side. The same is true of gravy: If you want it with mashed potatoes or anything else, order it on the side.

5. Go grilled.

A good rule of thumb when eating at fast-food restaurants – or anywhere else, actually – is to limit your intake of fried foods. Everything else being equal, grilled food is *always* healthier than fried (or breaded) food. Other healthier ways to prepare food are to have it baked, broiled, charbroiled, roasted or steamed. In addition to avoiding foods that are fried or breaded, steer clear of foods that are dubbed crispy.

6. Choose poultry/fish.

Here's another good rule of thumb: Lighter meats are healthier than darker meats. So instead of ordering beef, choose chicken, turkey or fish. For breakfast, ham is a healthier choice than bacon or sausage.

As mentioned previously, the way that a food is prepared has an enormous impact on its nutritional content. Grilled chicken is a better choice than fried chicken. If the chicken that you ordered has skin, remove it; the skin has plenty of calories and fat. Interestingly, some parts of a chicken are healthier than others. A drumstick, for instance, has much less calories and fat than a thigh. (Fast fact: The darker meats of a turkey – such as those of the leg and thigh – have a high percentage of slow-twitch muscle fibers which allows for greater endurance; the lighter meats – such as those of the breast – have a higher percentage of fast-twitch muscle fibers which allows for greater strength and speed.)

7. Eat fruit.

Like vegetables, fruits are very low in calories and fat and packed with nutrients. In an effort to provide healthier choices, many fast-food restaurants offer choices of fruit. Hint: Apple pies, blueberry muffins, cherry turnovers and strawberry shakes aren't charter members of the Fruit Group.

Besides a garden salad, you might be able to get a fruit salad. Another healthy option is yogurt.

8. Drink responsibly.

What do you drink at fast-food restaurants? Two beverages to avoid are milkshakes and sodas. Besides being high in sodium, milkshakes are high in calories and fat: A medium vanilla shake can have 17 grams of fat of which 11 grams are saturated fat. Gulp. A better choice is low-fat milk. Non-diet sodas are very high in sugar which has virtually no nutritional value. Couple that with free, unlimited, help-yourself refills and you have a recipe for dietary disaster. If you simply have to drink soda, choose a diet version.

Of course, an excellent choice for a beverage is water which has no calories. Another healthy option for a beverage is some type of juice.

9. Get substitutes.

When you order your food, you have the right to ask for substitutes. Just because a value meal comes with soda doesn't mean that you can't ask for low-fat milk; just because a value meal comes with French fries doesn't mean that you can't

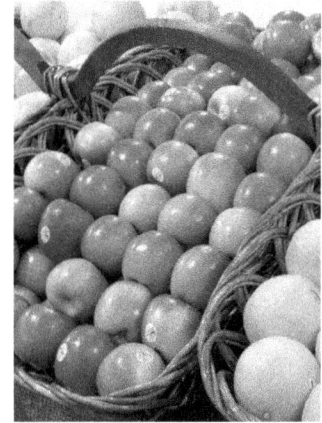

Like vegetables, fruits are very low in calories and fat and packed with nutrients.

ask for a baked potato (plain, of course); just because the sandwich comes with a sesame-seed bun doesn't mean that you can't ask for a whole-grain bread/roll. Remember, you can "have it your way."

10. Control portions.

Value meals sure sound tempting, right? But remember, the "value" is *economical*, not *nutritional*. Yeah, you do get a lot of food for your money but what you usually get is a lot of bad food for your money: more calories, more fat and more sodium. Some bargain.

One of the most important things that you can do when eating fast food is to exercise portion control. Get the smallest burger, not the largest one (and get it minus cheese). Get the smallest order of fries, not the largest one. In short, you'd be very wise *not* to "supersize." Also keep in mind that there are no standards throughout the restaurant industry for portion sizes. So, a small size at one restaurant can be larger than a small size at another restaurant.

11. Share food.

Just because you sprung for a value meal, there's nothing that says that you have to eat it by yourself. You can save some calories by getting a large-size value meal and then splitting it with another individual. Or, you can get part of it wrapped and eat it later.

12. Become knowledgeable.

A food at one restaurant can be dramatically different from the same food at another. For example, researchers from the Consumer Union

291

– the non-profit publishers of *Consumer Reports* magazine – compared the nutritional profiles of 36 chicken sandwiches from 16 fast-food chains. They found that a chicken sandwich at one fast-food restaurant had 360 calories of which 7 grams were from fat, including 2 grams of saturated fat. And a chicken sandwich at another fast-food restaurant had 950 calories of which 56 grams were from fat, including 10 grams of saturated fat. For that matter, a restaurant can offer different types of chicken sandwiches with vastly different nutrients.

You should become familiar with the menus and nutritional information of the fast-food restaurants at which you typically visit. At this point in time, all of the major fast-food chains have their own websites that contain very detailed information about the nutritional content of their foods. Sometimes, you can even find nutritional information conveniently posted right on menu boards in restaurants.

RECIPE FOR SUCCESS

Nutrition is a critical part of a fitness program. The proper application of nutritional training can help you to improve your health and maximize your performance.

Table 19.1: Summary of fat-soluble vitamins and their functions and sources

FAT-SOLUBLE VITAMIN	FUNCTIONS	SOURCES
Vitamin A (retinol)	is required for normal vision (especially at night) and promotes bone growth, healthy hair, skin and teeth	organ meats, dairy products, fish, eggs, carrots, spinach and sweet potatoes
Vitamin D (calciferol)	enhances calcium absorption and is vital for strong bones and teeth	fish, fortified milk products and cereals, dairy products and egg yolks
Vitamin E (tocopherol)	acts as an antioxidant, aids in the formation of red blood cells and helps to maintain muscles and other biological tissues	poultry, seafood, eggs, vegetable oils, nuts, fruits, vegetables and meats
Vitamin K	assists in blood clotting and bone metabolism	green leafy vegetables, Brussels sprouts, cabbage, potatoes, plant oils, oats, margarine and organ meats

Table 19.2: Summary of water-soluble vitamins and their functions and sources

WATER-SOLUBLE VITAMIN	FUNCTIONS	SOURCES
biotin	helps to synthesize glycogen, amino acids and fat	liver, fruits, vegetables, nuts, eggs, poultry and meats
cobalamin (B_{12})	forms and regulates red blood cells, prevents anemia and maintains a healthy nervous system	fortified cereals, meats, fish, poultry and dairy products
folate (folic acid and folacin)	is needed to manufacture red blood cells and aids in the metabolism of amino acids	enriched cereal grains, fruits, dark green leafy vegetables, meats, fish, liver, poultry, enriched and whole-grain breads and fortified cereals
niacin (B_3)	promotes normal appetite, digestion and proper nerve function and is required for energy metabolism	meats, fish, poultry, eggs, potatoes, enriched and whole-grain breads and bread products, orange juice, peanuts and fortified cereals
pantothenic acid (B_5)	helps in the metabolism of carbohydrates, protein and fat	chicken, beef, potatoes, oats, cereals, tomato products, liver, kidney, yeast, egg yolks, broccoli and whole grains
pyridoxine (B_6)	assists in the formation of red blood cells and the metabolism of carbohydrates, protein and fat	fortified cereals, organ meats, lean meats, poultry, fish, eggs, milk, vegetables, nuts and bananas
riboflavin (B_2)	aids in the maintenance of skin, mucous membranes and nervous structures	organ meats, poultry, beef, lamb, fish, milk, dark green leafy vegetables, bread products and fortified cereals
thiamine (B_1)	maintains a healthy nervous system and heart and helps to metabolize carbohydrates and amino acids	enriched, fortified and whole-grain products, bread and bread products, ready-to-eat cereals, meats, poultry, fish, liver and eggs
Vitamin C (ascorbic acid)	promotes healing, helps in the absorption of iron and the maintenance and repair of connective tissues, bones, teeth and cartilage	citrus fruits, tomatoes, tomato juice, potatoes, Brussels sprouts, cauliflower, broccoli, strawberries, watermelon, cabbage and spinach

Table 19.3: Summary of macrominerals and their functions and sources

MACROMINERAL	FUNCTIONS	SOURCES
calcium	is essential in blood clotting, muscle contraction, nerve transmission and the formation of bones and teeth	milk, cheese, yogurt, oysters, broccoli and spinach
chloride	is an electrolyte that regulates body fluids in to and out of cells and helps to maintain a proper acid-base (pH) balance	table salt, milk, canned vegetables and animal foods
magnesium	is essential for healthy nerve and muscle function and bone formation	green leafy vegetables, nuts, meats, poultry, fish, oysters, starches, milk and beans
phosphorus	maintains pH, helps in energy production and is essential for every metabolic process in the body	milk, yogurt, ice cream, cheese, peas, meats, poultry, fish and eggs
potassium	is an electrolyte that regulates body fluids in to and out of cells and promotes proper muscular contraction and the transmission of nerve impulses	citrus fruits, bananas, deep yellow vegetables and potatoes
sodium	is an electrolyte that regulates body fluids in to and out of cells, transmits nerve impulses, maintains normal blood pressure and is involved in muscle contraction	table salt, milk, canned vegetables and animal foods
sulfur	is needed to make hair and nails	beef, peanuts, clams and wheat germ

Table 19.4: Summary of microminerals and their functions and sources

MICROMINERAL	FUNCTIONS	SOURCES
chromium	functions in the metabolism of carbohydrates and fat and helps to maintain an appropriate level of blood glucose	meats, poultry, fish and peanuts
copper	stimulates the absorption of iron and has a role in the formation of red blood cells, connective tissues and nerve fibers	organ meats, seafood, nuts, beans, whole-grain products and cocoa products
fluoride	prevents dental caries and stimulates the formation of new bones	fluoridated water, teas and marine fish
iodine	is necessary for proper functioning of the thyroid gland and prevents goiter and cretinism	seafood, processed foods and iodized salt
iron	is involved in the manufacture of hemoglobin and myoglobin (two proteins that transport oxygen to the tissues) and has a role in normal immune function	liver, fruits, vegetables, fortified bread and grain products, meats, poultry and shellfish
manganese	is involved in the formation of bones and the metabolism of carbohydrates	nuts, legumes, coffee, tea and whole grains
molybdenum	helps to regulate the storage of iron	dark green leafy vegetables, legumes, grain products, nuts and organ meats
selenium	protects cell membranes	organ meats, chicken, seafood, whole-grain cereals and milk
zinc	has a role in the repair and growth of the biological tissues	fortified cereals, meats, poultry, eggs and seafood

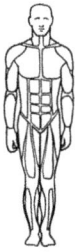

20 Nutritional Supplements

According to National Health and Nutrition Examination Survey (NHANES) data from 2013 to 2014, about 54% of American adults reported taking at least one dietary supplement during the previous 30 days; 10% reported taking more than five. Because their use is so widespread – particularly among active individuals – no detailed discussion of nutrition would be complete without an examination of nutritional supplements.

At the present time, there are *about 29,000 nutritional supplements* on the market. The most popular nutritional supplements include protein and vitamins/minerals. But many people also use herbal supplements and a wide variety of other nutritional supplements. As a result, it's important to know what the research says about the safety and effectiveness of these pills, powders and potions.

PROTEIN AND VITAMIN/MINERAL SUPPLEMENTS

As noted, protein and vitamin/mineral supplements are highly popular. There are many misconceptions about these products, however. Let's take a peek behind the curtain to learn more.

Protein Supplements

Many individuals think that they need to consume large amounts of protein in order to increase their strength (and size) and, for that reason, take protein supplements. A number of studies have shown that the protein needs of active individuals are higher than those of their inactive counterparts. But this need has been drastically exaggerated by the manufacturers of protein supplements.

The fact of the matter is that individuals who consume adequate calories generally obtain adequate protein. Remember, your caloric needs are determined by several factors, including your size and level of activity. Larger, more active individuals require and consume more calories than the average person. With these additional calories comes additional protein. In other words, the increased protein need of active individuals is met by an increased caloric consumption.

For adults, the Recommended Dietary Allowance (RDA) for protein is 0.8 grams per kilogram of bodyweight per day (g/kg/day) or about 0.36 grams per pound of bodyweight per day (g/lb/day). According to the Academy of Nutrition and Dietetics, the Dieticians of Canada and the American College of Sports Medicine, active individuals should consume 1.2 to 2.0 g/kg/day or about 0.55 to 0.91 g/lb/day. Assuming a sufficient caloric consumption, this amount of protein is present in any normal diet that contains 15% of its calories as protein.

In Chapter 19, it was estimated that a 200-pound man who's very active requires approximately 5,200 calories per day (cal/day) to meet his energy needs. If 15% of these calories came from protein, he'd be getting 780 calories from protein or 195 grams [780 cal ÷ 4 cal/g]. This amount of protein represents about 2.15 g/kg/day which is more than the recommended maximal intake of 2.0 g/kg/d for active individuals. And don't forget, this is without the person making any effort to consume extra protein. So even if the requirement for active individuals is greater, it's likely that they're already consuming enough protein to ensure proper levels of consumption. If you're concerned that you're not getting enough protein in your diet, you can obtain adequate amounts by simply consuming more foods that are high in protein such as lean or low-fat meat and poultry.

Discussions of protein supplements often include a specific group of essential amino acids

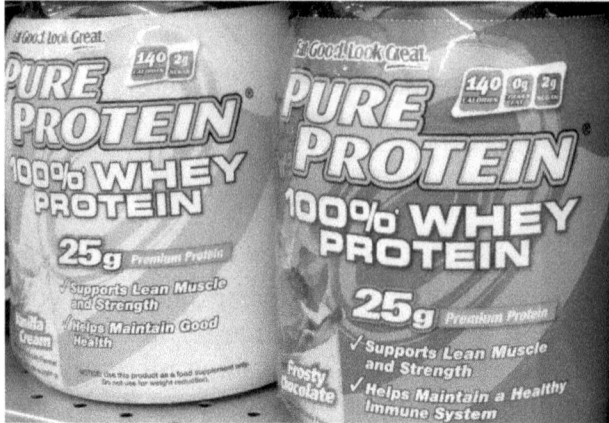

The increased protein need of active individuals is met by an increased caloric consumption.

known as branched chain amino acids (BCAAs). There are three BCAAs: isoleucine, leucine and valine. For a 20-year-old individual, the RDAs for isoleucine, leucine and valine are 19, 42 and 24 milligrams per kilogram of bodyweight per day (mg/kg/day), respectively. For a man who weighs 200 pounds, that works out to a daily intake of about 1,727 mg of isoleucine, 3,818 mg of leucine and 2,181 mg of valine. These amounts can be easily met by consuming a normal diet that contains 15% of its calories as protein, paying particular attention to lean or low-fat meat and poultry. For instance, one chicken breast (140 g) has about 2,293 mg of isoleucine, 3,259 mg of leucine and 2,155 mg of valine. (Fast fact: Most studies haven't found any evidence that BCAAs enhance performance; there's limited evidence to suggest that BCAAs reduce muscle soreness or improve recovery.)

It must be understood that an excessive intake of protein carries the potential for many adverse effects. An intake of protein that's greater than the needs for the growth, maintenance and repair of biological tissues is either stored as fat or excreted in the urine. When a large amount of protein is excreted, it can place a heavy burden on the liver and kidneys and the stress may damage those organs. A high intake of protein also increases the risk of dehydration which, in turn, increases the risk of developing a heat-related disorder such as heat exhaustion, heat stroke or heat cramps. Other potential adverse effects from a high intake of protein include diarrhea, cramps, gastrointestinal upset and an excessive loss of calcium in the urine.

Vitamin/Mineral Supplements

Many individuals think that foods don't provide them with enough micronutrients and, therefore, take vitamin/mineral supplements. In fact, according to a report in the *Nutrition Business Journal*, vitamins and minerals made up 31% and 8%, respectively, of the $41.4 billion worth of supplements that were sold in 2016 in the US alone. Yet, there's no unbiased, scientific evidence to suggest that those who consume a balanced diet that contains a variety of healthy foods need vitamins and minerals in excess of the RDA. And there's no unbiased, scientific evidence to suggest that an intake of vitamins and minerals that's in excess of the RDA confers any extra benefits or improves performance.

As noted earlier, active individuals require and consume more calories than the average person. With these additional calories comes additional vitamins and minerals. In truth, even a marginal diet provides adequate vitamins and minerals. Understand, too, that your liver is a storehouse for vitamins and minerals. This organ can quickly compensate for a temporary dietary shortfall by releasing its stored micronutrients as needed and then replenishing its reservoirs when the opportunity arises.

That being said, some individuals may need a multi-vitamin/mineral supplement. For example, a nutritional supplement may be warranted for vegetarians and women who are pregnant or lactating. A nutritional supplement may also be appropriate for athletes who restrict their caloric consumption in order to "make weight" to compete in sports such as boxing, competitive weightlifting, judo, lightweight crew and wrestling. And since women have an increased risk of iron and calcium deficiency, nutritional supplements may be justified for those two minerals.

Whenever possible, though, it's better to get vitamins and minerals from foods rather than pills because the high concentration of these micronutrients in pill form may interfere with the absorption of other nutrients. Also keep in mind that nutritional supplements containing more than 150% of the RDA are for disease treatment and should never be used unless a physician has diagnosed their need.

There's nothing wrong with taking a low-dose multi-vitamin/mineral supplement on a daily basis. When consumed in reasonable doses, vitamins and minerals pose no health or safety risks. The Academy of Nutrition and Dietetics is the largest organization of food and nutrition professionals in the world. According to this group, high doses of vitamins and minerals pose a risk of toxicity that can lead to serious medical complications. When taken in megadoses – defined as any dose that's greater than 10 times the RDA – vitamins that are in excess of those needed to saturate the enzyme systems function as free-floating drugs instead of receptor-bound nutrients. Like all drugs, high doses of vitamins and minerals have the potential for adverse effects.

Of greatest concern is an excessive intake of the fat-soluble vitamins – particularly vitamins A and D – which can be extremely toxic. Consuming high doses of vitamin A can result in decalcification of bones (resulting in fragile bones), an increased susceptibility to disease, enlargement of the liver and spleen, muscle and joint soreness, nausea, vomiting, diarrhea, drowsiness, headaches, double vision, irritability, amenorrhea (cessation of menstruation), stunted growth, loss of appetite, loss of hair and skin rashes; consuming high doses of vitamin D can result in decalcification of bones, nausea, vomiting, diarrhea, drowsiness, headaches, loss of appetite, loss of hair, loss of weight, hypertension and elevated cholesterol.

Excessive amounts of the B vitamins and vitamin C are generally excreted in the urine (which has prompted some authorities to suggest that consuming a high amount of water-soluble vitamins leaves a person with nothing more than expensive urine). When a large amount of these vitamins is excreted, it can place a heavy burden on the liver and kidneys and the stress may damage those organs. Though mainly excreted, high amounts of water-soluble vitamins can still

There's no unbiased, scientific evidence to suggest that those who consume a balanced diet that contains a variety of healthy foods need vitamins and minerals in excess of the RDA.

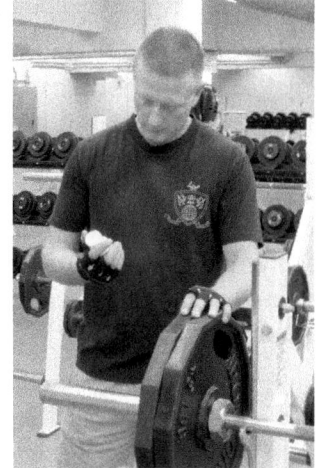

produce adverse effects while in the body. Consuming high doses of pyridoxine (vitamin B_6) can damage sensory nerves; consuming high doses of niacin (vitamin B_3) can result in nausea, vomiting and what has been dubbed niacin flush (a skin disorder that's characterized by a burning, tingling and itching sensation along with a reddened flush that appears mainly on the face, arms and chest); consuming high doses of vitamin C can result in nausea, diarrhea, stomach cramps, kidney stones, bladder irritation, intestinal problems, destruction of red blood cells, gout, elevated cholesterol, ulceration of the gastric wall and leaching of calcium from bones.

Sidebar: Did you ever have or know anyone who had beriberi? How about scurvy? Pellagra? Rickets? These are vitamin deficiency diseases that have been eradicated in our country and other civilized nations. If Americans consumed inadequate amounts of vitamins, these diseases would be widespread.

HERBAL SUPPLEMENTS

Many herbal and other botanical (plant-derived) supplements are marketed for specific medical purposes for which there often isn't any valid proof. The truth is that a large number of herbal supplements have no recognized role in nutrition.

Additionally, there are concerns about the safety of many herbal supplements. For instance, chaparral, comfrey, germander, kava, ma huang (ephedra), pennyroyal and sassafras have been linked to liver toxicity; germander, kava and mistletoe to hepatitis; ma huang to seizures, heart attacks and stroke; ginseng to hypertension, insomnia, depression and skin blemishes; and yohimbine to kidney failure, seizures and death. There are similar fears with high-potency enzymes and glandular extracts from dried animal organs such as the pituitary gland, thyroid gland and testicles.

MISCELLANEOUS SUPPLEMENTS

A host of nutritional supplements have been publicized as ergogenic aids (or performance enhancers). Others have been touted for a variety of reasons, including fat loss, weight reduction, muscle gain and strength improvement. Here's a critical look at some of the notable nutritional supplements that have been promoted in recent years:

Aspartate

Aspartate is a non-essential amino acid. Like most amino acids, aspartate has been investigated as an ergogenic aid. In fact, the first known study on aspartate was conducted more than 50 years ago.

The majority of the research on aspartate has examined its effect on aerobic endurance, almost all of which involved rats swimming to exhaustion. This has yielded a mixed bag of results with some studies showing a positive effect and roughly an equal number of studies showing no effect. Even then, results from animal studies can't always be generalized to humans. A handful of studies have been conducted on humans, most of which involved cycling to exhaustion. Again, the findings are inconsistent. Research has shown that aspartate has no effect on muscular endurance or strength.

Several studies have looked at the effects of aspartate in combination with other nutritional supplements, most often arginine (another amino acid). These studies offer no direct support for the use of aspartate as an ergogenic aid.

Take note: Researchers caution that adverse effects are possible when aspartate is used alone or with other amino acids.

Beta-alanine

Beta-alanine is a non-essential amino acid. Along with histidine – an essential amino acid – beta-alanine is involved in the synthesis of carnosine, a molecule that's highly concentrated in skeletal muscle. Carnosine can buffer the acidity in exercising muscles thereby delaying the onset fatigue and, in theory, improve performance. It's thought that the level of carnosine in muscles is affected more by the availability of beta-alanine than histidine.

In one study, 55 men were randomly assigned to groups that received either beta-alanine, creatine, beta-alanine and creatine or a placebo. The researchers examined eight indices of cardiorespiratory endurance. After 28 days, the group that received beta-alanine improved significantly in just one of the eight indices. (The group that received beta-alanine and creatine improved significantly in five of the eight indices.) There were no significant differences between groups in their improvements. A caveat is that the study was sponsored by a manufacturer of nutritional supplements.

In another study, 15 400-meter sprinters – who had an average personal-best time of 50.45 seconds – were randomly assigned to groups that received either beta-alanine or a placebo. After four weeks, the group that received beta-alanine significantly increased the carnosine content of the gastrocnemius and soleus more than the group that received the placebo. But this didn't translate into better performance. The group that received beta-alanine improved dynamic fatigue significantly – though *slightly* – more than the group that received the placebo. Both groups significantly improved their isometric endurance and their time to run 400 meters. There were no significant differences between groups in their improvements in those two measures. In other words, their improvements were similar in both tests.

Boron

Individuals have used boron thinking that it will improve their strength (and size). However, there's little or no proof to support this belief.

In one study, 12 subjects who received boron for a period of 48 days increased their level of testosterone by as much as 268%. But these subjects were post-menopausal women, aged 48 to 82, whose testosterone levels were naturally low. What's more, as part of the study, the women had been fed a diet that was deficient in boron for the previous 119 days.

In another study, 19 male bodybuilders were randomly assigned to groups that received either boron or a placebo. After seven weeks of strength training, boron had no significant effect on total testosterone, lean-body mass or strength.

Low doses of boron are generally safe. But high intakes can cause nausea, vomiting, diarrhea and a loss of appetite.

Calcium

Many nutritional supplements have been promoted as an effective means to lose weight. One of the latest to garner attention as a weight-loss product is calcium.

In one study, 340 overweight/obese subjects were randomly assigned to groups that received either calcium or a placebo. After two years, calcium didn't produce significantly better results than the placebo in any measure, including changes in bodyweight, body fat and Body-Mass Index. Nor did calcium yield any significantly better improvements than the placebo in abdominal circumference, hip circumference and tricep skinfold thickness.

Calcium is an important macromineral that's essential in blood clotting, muscle contraction, nerve transmission and the formation of bones and teeth. But there's no evidence that it promotes weight loss. And there's no scientific evidence that it has any ergogenic value.

Chromium

As a micromineral, chromium functions in the metabolism of carbohydrates and fat and helps to maintain an appropriate level of blood glucose. It's believed that chromium can promote fat loss and muscle gain.

Most of the claims regarding the benefits of chromium are based on two poorly designed,

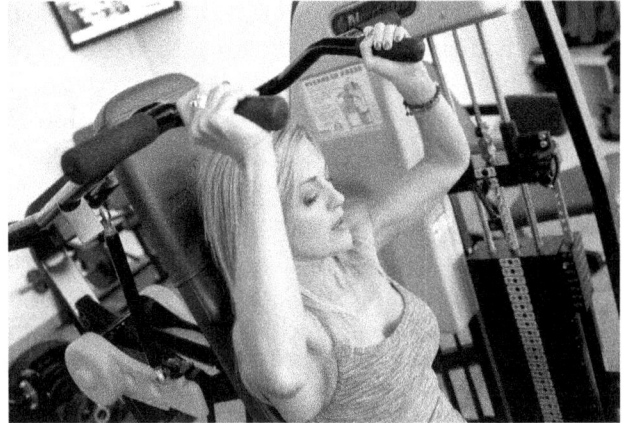

There's no scientific evidence that calcium promotes weight loss or has any ergogenic value. (Photo provided by Luke Carlson.)

unpublished studies. These two studies were referenced in a review article that was written by a chemist who was consulting for a manufacturer of nutritional supplements. In 1996, the Federal Trade Commission ordered the manufacturer (and two others) to stop making unsubstantiated claims that chromium decreases body fat and increases muscle mass. Nevertheless, misconceptions about chromium still persist.

The vast majority of studies on chromium have been conducted with animals. Most of the studies that have been conducted with humans have shown that the use of chromium doesn't decrease body fat or promote fat loss in any way. In one study, 95 Navy personnel were alternately assigned to groups that received either chromium or a placebo. Both groups did supervised aerobic training for a minimum of three times per week for at least 30 minutes. After 16 weeks of training, chromium didn't significantly reduce body fat or increase lean-body mass more than the placebo. A meta-analysis of 10 studies found that chromium produced a weight loss of about 2.4 to 2.6 pounds over the course of 6 to 14 weeks which isn't very impressive.

To date, only one study has reported that chromium increases muscle mass. And in that study, muscle mass was estimated from anthropometric measurements which can be unreliable.

It appears as if chromium doesn't increase strength, either. In one study, 16 men were randomly assigned to groups that received either chromium or a placebo. After 12 weeks of strength training, the placebo actually increased strength more than chromium. No improvements in percentage of body fat, lean-body mass or skinfold thickness were made by either group. Interestingly, another study found that those who received chromium had urinary chromium excretions that were *60 times higher* than those who received a placebo.

Cobalamin

Largely because many athletes have said that they've received injections (or "shots") of cobalamin (vitamin B_{12}) – perhaps most famously, former major-league pitcher Roger Clemens – it's thought that this vitamin has some ergogenic value. But there's no research to support this contention.

In one study, 16 marksmen were randomly assigned to groups that received either a combination of three B vitamins (cobalamin, pyridoxine and thiamin) or no treatment for eight weeks. Those who were given the B vitamins significantly improved their shooting accuracy with a pistol more than those who were given nothing. The study was repeated the next year in which 19 marksmen were randomly assigned to groups that received either the same B vitamins or a placebo for eight weeks. The results of the second study were similar to the first study. However, since the subjects used cobalamin in combination with two other B vitamins, it's impossible to tell if their performance was enhanced by the cobalamin. In other words, these studies offer no direct support for the use of cobalamin as an ergogenic aid. Although a case could be made that the three B vitamins had an ergogenic benefit, improvements in pistol marksmanship have no relevance to other sports.

Conjugated Linoleic Acid

In studies of animals, conjugated linoleic acid (CLA) has been shown to decrease body fat and increase lean-body mass. But studies of humans have found conflicting results. Some studies have shown that CLA decreases body fat and/or increases lean-body mass while others have shown no effect. Many of the studies that found positive effects had small numbers of subjects and were of short duration which makes it difficult to draw any meaningful conclusions.

In one study, 180 obese subjects were randomly assigned to three groups: Two groups received different types of CLA and another group received a placebo. In comparison to the placebo group, the CLA groups significantly decreased body fat and increased lean-body mass. One CLA group lost 3.74 pounds of fat and gained 1.54 pounds of lean-body mass; the other lost 5.28 pounds of fat and gained 1.32 pounds of lean-body mass. So the results weren't exactly breathtaking, especially considering that this was after taking CLA for 12 months.

Also worth mentioning is that all three groups reduced their caloric consumption over the course of the study. By the 12th month, the CLA groups were consuming at least 105 calories per day less than the placebo group. This, of course, could easily account for much of the difference in the results.

Creatine

For many years, creatine has received a great deal of attention within the athletic, scientific and medical communities. It may very well be the most studied nutritional supplement in history.

There are many anecdotal reports that creatine is effective but scientific research is, at best, inconclusive. Much of the research that has investigated creatine has been conducted in a laboratory. In this controlled setting, the best evidence for performance enhancement from the use of creatine is in repeated, maximal, short-term sprints on a stationary cycle. And even then, some studies have shown no improvements. Of the research that has been conducted outside a laboratory, very few studies have shown that creatine improves performance in realistic activities such as running and swimming. In one study that involved nine highly trained sprinters – all were among the top 10 men and women in their country in the 100- and/or 200-meter dash – creatine proved no better than a placebo on

302

single or repeated 40-meter sprint times. In two studies that involved a total of 52 elite male and female swimmers, creatine didn't improve performance in 25-, 50- and 100-meter swim sprints more than a placebo. In some studies, creatine actually *worsened* performance. In short, research has found that any improvements that may occur in laboratory settings don't translate into improvements in realistic activities.

It appears as if using creatine in the recommended dose is safe. However, many individuals – thinking that more is better – typically exceed the recommended dose, undoubtedly putting them at greater risk for incurring adverse effects. At this point in time, the long-term effects of creatine are unknown.

Adverse effects are rarely reported in studies. But most studies don't include any formal way of assessing adverse effects. While few adverse effects have been reported in studies that were done in a laboratory, there have been endless accounts from individuals who have experienced adverse effects. Although these observations are anecdotal, their sheer volume is such that they can't be ignored. In a study that surveyed 52 collegiate athletes who voluntarily took creatine, 38 (73.1%) reported at least one adverse effect. There are numerous reports of water retention, muscle cramping, dehydration/heat-related disorder, muscle strains/dysfunction, gastro-intestinal distress (such as an upset stomach, gastrointestinal pain, nausea and vomiting) and liver and kidney dysfunction.

Dehydroepiandrosterone

A precursor (or prohormone) is a substance that the body can convert into a hormone. Dehydroepiandrosterone (DHEA) is a precursor to many hormones, including testosterone. Because of this, it's believed that DHEA can increase the production of testosterone in the body which could yield the same effects as steroids. This hasn't been corroborated by research, however.

In one study, 20 male soccer players were randomly assigned to groups that received either DHEA or a placebo. After four weeks, DHEA increased total testosterone more than the placebo

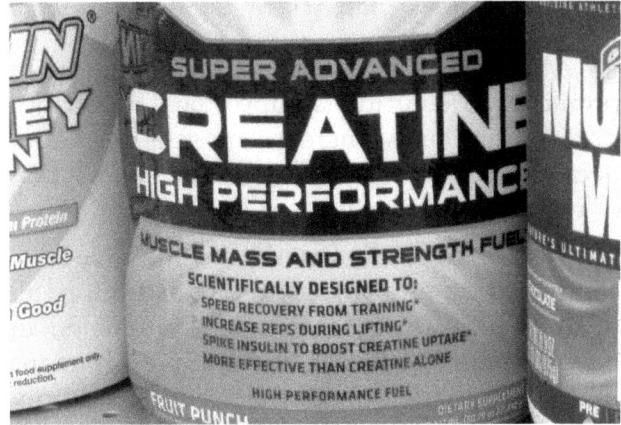

There are many anecdotal reports that creatine is effective but scientific research is, at best, inconclusive.

but no significant improvements in body composition were made by either group.

Since DHEA is a precursor to testosterone, it's no real surprise that it has the potential for the same adverse effects as steroids. For instance, women can experience growth of facial hair and a deepening of the voice; men can experience gynecomastia (the appearance of female-like breasts on the male physique). DHEA may also increase the risk of uterine and prostate cancer.

Understand that DHEA or any other testosterone precursor – or "booster" – could cause an individual to fail a test for steroids. A highly publicized example of this happened in 2017 when Joakim Noah – then a center for the New York Knicks – was suspended 20 games by the National Basketball Association after failing a drug test for Ligandrol, a supplement that's marketed as a "testosterone booster" and banned by the league. (Fast fact: As a result of his suspension, Noah lost at least two million dollars of his salary.)

Of no small importance is that many DHEA products have been shown to contain inaccurate doses. Independent testing of 16 DHEA products found that only eight (50%) had the exact amount of DHEA that was stated on the labels; the actual levels varied *as much as 150%*. Amazingly, three (18.75%) of the products didn't contain any DHEA whatsoever.

Ecdysterone

A plant sterol, ecdysterone has been promoted as a nutritional supplement to enhance protein synthesis, increase muscle mass and decrease body fat. But there's no evidence that ecdysterone is effective.

Most of the studies on ecdysterone have been conducted on animals. With one exception, all of the studies on humans were published in obscure journals. In the lone study on humans that's legitimate, 45 subjects were randomly assigned to receive either methoxyisoflavone, ecdysterone, sulfo-polysaccharide or a placebo. After eight weeks of strength training, there were no significant differences between any of the three supplements and the placebo in percentage of body fat, maximum strength (the bench press and leg press), power and level of testosterone.

Glutamine

Glutamine is a non-essential amino acid. Like other amino acids, glutamine plays a role in protein synthesis. As a result, it's billed as an ergogenic aid.

In one study, 31 subjects were randomly assigned to groups that received either glutamine or a placebo. After six weeks of strength training, both groups increased their strength and lean-body mass. But there were no significant differences between glutamine and the placebo in those two measures.

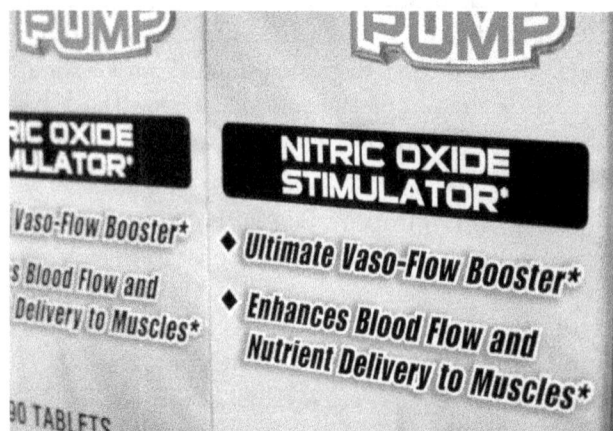

At the present time, no studies have shown that nitric oxide taken as a nutritional supplement improves physical performance or any biological functions.

Hydroxy Methylbutyrate

A relative newcomer to the ranks of nutritional supplements is hydroxyl methylbutyrate which, thankfully, goes by the letters HMB; it's a metabolite of leucine, an essential amino acid. (Fast fact: A metabolite refers to any substance that's produced during metabolism; examples are lactic acid, pyruvic acid and carbon dioxide.)

HMB has been promoted as a nutritional supplement that increases strength and lean-body mass, supposedly by preventing the breakdown of muscle tissue. This has no scientific merit, however. One study did support the theory that HMB may prevent muscle damage. But the study didn't examine whether or not HMB had any effect on strength or lean-body mass. In a crossover study that did look at this aspect, 35 collegiate football players were randomly assigned to groups that received either HMB or a placebo for four weeks. After a one-week washout period, the subjects were switched to the other treatment for four weeks. There were no significant differences between HMB and the placebo in strength and body composition.

Research on HMB has found minimal improvements in performance in untrained individuals and almost none in trained individuals. One meta-analysis pooled data from nine studies that involved 394 subjects. In untrained subjects, HMB produced small improvements in lower-body strength and negligible improvements in upper-body strength; in trained subjects, HMB produced "trivial" improvements in lower-body and upper-body strength. In both untrained and trained subjects, the effect on body composition was also described as trivial.

Nitric Oxide

Recently, nitric oxide has been promoted as an ergogenic aid. Nitric oxide is actually a gas, though not to be confused with nitrous oxide (aka "laughing gas"). Years ago, strange as it may seem, nitric oxide was best known as an air pollutant (formed when nitrogen and oxygen react with each other during combustion and are emitted into the air à la car exhaust). Needless to say, it came as quite a shock when the biological functions of nitric oxide were discovered in the 1980s. In fact, *Science* magazine named it Molecule of the Year in 1992. And three pharmacologists from the United States were awarded the 1998 Nobel Prize in Physiology or Medicine for discovering the role of nitric oxide as a "signaling molecule in the cardiovascular system."

In the body, nitric oxide has numerous roles. For one thing, it's an important neurotransmitter that relays messages between nerve cells. In addition, nitric oxide signals the body to dilate blood vessels thereby increasing blood flow. In theory, this could improve performance. (Fast fact: Though at first it sounds bizarre, heart conditions are often treated with nitroglycerin – yes, the active ingredient in dynamite; nitroglycerin releases nitric oxide which widens the arteries and veins that supply the heart, making it easier for the organ to pump blood.)

Be that as it may, this doesn't mean that there are any benefits in taking nitric oxide as a nutritional supplement. At the present time, no studies have shown that nitric oxide improves physical performance or any of the aforementioned biological functions.

Pangamic Acid

The use of pangamic acid (aka calcium pangamate and vitamin B_{15}) dates back to at least the mid-1970s. In that Cold War era, there was an enormous fascination with the sport system of the Soviet Union – comprised of 15 republics, including Russia – especially as it pertained to training. It was said that Soviet athletes used pangamic acid to reduce fatigue and improve stamina. However, there's no legitimate scientific evidence to support those claims or any others about pangamic acid. In fact, much of the research is from the 1960s and hails from the Soviet Union. Besides being poorly designed, most of those studies involved animals and those results can't always be generalized to humans.

In one study that was well designed, 16 track athletes were randomly assigned to groups that received either pangamic acid or a placebo. After

three weeks, there were no significant differences between pangamic acid and the placebo in endurance and recovery heart rate when the subjects ran to exhaustion on a treadmill.

There's no RDA for pangamic acid. That's because pangamic acid hasn't been shown to be essential in the diet and isn't associated with any deficiency diseases. In fact, if you look in any nutrition textbook, you'll discover that there's little or no mention whatsoever of pangamic acid. Why not? Well, there are 13 recognized vitamins and vitamin B_{15} isn't among them. (Fast fact: The Food and Drug Administration has ruled that it's illegal to sell pangamic acid as a nutritional supplement in the United States.)

Ribose

As noted in Chapter 2, the breakdown of adenosine triphosphate (ATP) releases chemical energy that's converted into mechanical energy which is used to perform muscular work. Since the body has a limited stockpile of ATP, it must be rebuilt over and over again. One of the components of ATP is ribose (a sugar). In theory, then, ribose supplements could increase the inventory of ATP and improve performance.

In one crossover study, 11 cyclists and strength-trained individuals were randomly assigned to groups that received either ribose or a placebo 30 minutes prior to a bout of exercise. Each session consisted of three repeats of a Wingate Test (30 seconds of all-out effort on a stationary cycle against a fixed resistance that's based on an individual's bodyweight) with two minutes of recovery between each test. After a one-week washout period, the subjects were switched to the other treatment and repeated the same protocol. There were no significant differences between ribose and the placebo in any measure, including peak power, average power and percent decrease in power.

In fact, the majority of research hasn't found any significant ergogenic benefits from ribose; in at least one study, ribose produced less improvement than a placebo. In this study, 31 collegiate rowers were randomly assigned to receive either ribose or a placebo. After eight weeks of training, the placebo produced significantly greater improvement in rowing 2,000 meters than ribose.

Sodium Bicarbonate

Sodium bicarbonate (aka baking soda) has a wide range of applications such as treating acid indigestion, whitening teeth and absorbing odors in refrigerators. But it's also been promoted as a substance that delays the onset of fatigue by buffering the buildup of lactic acid. Sodium bicarbonate is one of the few nutritional supplements that seem to be effective as an ergogenic aid.

A great deal of research has shown that sodium bicarbonate improves performance. In one study, 16 female subjects were randomly assigned to groups that received either sodium bicarbonate or a placebo (sodium chloride) prior to a bout of exercise. After eight weeks of interval training on a stationary cycle, sodium bicarbonate had significantly greater improvements in lactate threshold and endurance than the placebo.

Adverse effects from sodium bicarbonate include gastrointestinal disturbances such as nausea, vomiting, diarrhea and flatulence. Sodium citrate is thought to have the same ergogenic value as sodium bicarbonate without the adverse effects. But in one study, eight of nine subjects (elite athletes) who received sodium citrate experienced gastrointestinal distress.

Vanadyl Sulfate

A micromineral that's also known as vanadium, vanadyl sulfate has been investigated as an ergogenic aid. There's no proof that it has any effect on muscle mass or strength.

In one study, 40 subjects were paired together based on gender, age, bodyweight, height and training program. One subject from each pair was randomly assigned to receive either vanadyl sulfate or a placebo. After 12 weeks of strength training, there were no significant differences between vanadyl sulfate and the placebo in bodyweight, body composition and muscle circumference. Both groups had significant improvements in strength and muscular endurance. However, were no significant differences between groups in their improvements. (Those who consumed vanadyl sulfate had a significantly better increase in their maximum strength in the leg extension than those who consumed the placebo but this was attributed to their lower level of strength during the pre-testing.)

TAINTED PRODUCTS

There's no shortage of athletes who have tested positive for banned substances. Many of the athletes who have been in this predicament blame it on tainted products and, therefore, assert that the banned substance was taken unknowingly. Nonetheless, athletes are responsible for what they put into their bodies; using the defense of "I didn't know" after a positive test for any performance-enhancing drug isn't grounds for immunity.

You don't have to be an athlete for this to be a concern; other jobs often require drug testing. Case in point: According to *The New England Journal of Medicine*, a police sergeant who worked "in one of the most dangerous cities in the United States" was fired after a drug test showed the presence of amphetamines. He had been taking a weight-loss product that contained fenproporex, a Schedule IV controlled substance that's used as an appetite suppressant. Inside the body, fenproporex is converted into amphetamines, thus the positive test.

Many scientific investigations of nutritional supplements have unearthed a large number of tainted products. In one study, researchers bought 634 nutritional supplements from 215 companies in 13 countries. The products were purchased in stores, from the Internet and over the phone. The researchers found that 94 of the 634 nutritional supplements (14.8%) contained steroids. Some of the products had enough steroids to result in a positive test.

In another study, researchers bought 58 nutritional supplements from retail outlets and the Internet. A total of 54 nutritional supplements were successfully analyzed of which 13 (25%) had low levels of steroids and six (11%) had banned stimulants. Of note, 67% of the products that were categorized as testosterone boosters contained steroids and/or stimulants; 29% of the products that were categorized as weight loss contained steroids and/or stimulants.

In yet another study, researchers examined 64 nutritional supplements. They found that eight (12.5%) of the nutritional supplements contained steroids and/or ephedrine, a banned stimulant.

Even products that are as seemingly innocuous as vitamin/mineral supplements can contain banned substances; one study found stanozolol (trade name: Winstrol) – one of the most popular steroids in history – in multi-vitamin tablets. Other nutritional supplements have been shown to contain heavy metals and pesticides. Laboratory analyses found trace amounts of one or more potentially hazardous contaminants in 37 of the 40 herbal supplements that were tested. All 37 tested positive for trace amounts of lead; of those, 32 also contained mercury, 28 cadmium, 21 arsenic and 18 residues from at least one pesticide.

There are two likely reasons why a high percentage of nutritional supplements are tainted. First, it could be the result of cross-contamination. This occurs when the same machines are used to process different types of products without proper cleaning of the equipment. In other words, it's due to poor quality

control. Second, manufacturers may deliberately "spike" the nutritional supplement with an illegal or banned substance with the hope that it will work better. Obviously, a product that works better can lead to greater sales.

The moral of the story is that you may be consuming unknown substances that could pose a significant threat to your health. If you choose to take nutritional supplements, make sure that the products have been tested for undeclared ingredients and certified by an independent, third-party laboratory such as Banned Substances Control Group, ConsumerLab.com, United States Pharmacopeia and NSF International.

FOOD FOR THOUGHT

Most of the claims concerning nutritional supplements are purely speculative and anecdotal with little or no scientific or medical basis. These products offer more hype than hope.

As long as you consume a balanced diet that contains a variety of healthy foods and sufficient calories, there's no need for you to take nutritional supplements. And it makes more sense to invest your money in high-quality foods than spend it on expensive nutritional supplements. Remember, there are no shortcuts on the road to proper nutrition.

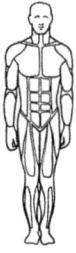

21 Nutritional Quackery

The health and fitness industry continues to be overrun by hordes of unscrupulous and unsavory entrepreneurs who seek to make quick and easy profits on the naiveté of consumers. Many individuals are easily tempted by seductive promises that nutritional supplements can help them to decrease fat, increase muscle, lose weight, get fit, improve appearance and enhance performance.

When nutritional supplements are promoted that are unproven and/or ineffective, it constitutes nutritional quackery. Each year, millions of Americans spend billions of dollars on nutritional supplements that are worthless and sometimes dangerous. But nutritional quackery isn't anything new.

SNAKE OIL SALESMEN

No other product is more closely associated with nutritional quackery than snake oil. In China, snake oil has been used for centuries as a medicinal product. In the United States, its use dates back more than 150 years. Legend has it that in the mid-1860s, Chinese laborers gave snake oil to co-workers who suffered from aches and pains while building the First Transcontinental Railroad. Over time, the term snake oil was used to describe a health product that was fraudulent. And anyone who sold such a product was subsequently referred to as a snake oil salesman.

During the late 1800s, snake oil salesmen thrived in the Midwest and rural areas of the South. This early form of consumer rip-off combined free amusement with the sale of "secret" goods that supposedly had curative powers. Traveling by horse and wagon, these "medicine shows" began innocently enough with complimentary entertainment – ranging from musical acts to magical tricks – that was given by various performers to entice an unsuspecting audience. Soon afterward, a "doctor" (or "medicine man") peddled his elixirs and tonics in colorful glass bottles as remedies for a wide assortment of ills, aches and pains to the gullible and all-to-eager masses using a spellbinding sales pitch.

A shill was often planted among the spectators who offered convincing – and scripted – testimony about how the product cured his condition. To get things moving, it wasn't unusual for the shill or another accomplice to purchase the first bottle. Thereafter, the performers circulated throughout the crowd to sell the "doctor's" product. Once money and "medicine" exchanged hands, it was only a matter of time until the showmen decided to load up their wagon and "git outta Dodge" before people realized that they had been swindled.

The products that were sold in those days – many of which were advertised as "cure-alls" – included salves, liver pads, hair growers, electric belts, powdered herbs, common forms of liniment or laxative, bunion and corn remedies and, of course, snake oil. Few could resist the alluring names and assorted purposes. For instance, Dr. Kilmer's Swamp-Root was touted as a "kidney, liver and bladder remedy"; Renne's Magic Oil was promoted for "pain killing"; Dr. McClintock's Dyspeptic Elixir was advertised as "effectual for combating dyspepsia" and a cure for "heartburn, nervousness, indigestion and all other symptoms arising from want of tone in the stomach"; McDonald's Cough Annihilator was sold to remove "the most fearful cold in a few hours"; Hamlin's Wizard Oil was said to treat "pneumonia, cancer, diphtheria, earache, toothache, headache and hydrophobia" using the marketing motto of "there is no sore it will not heal, no pain it will not subdue"; and Clark

Stanley's Snake Oil Liniment was billed as a cure for bruises, frost bite, sore throat, lumbago and sciatica and "good for man or beast." Who could refuse?

Some of the best showmen of that era were actually women: Madame DuBois had a brass band, sold medicine and pulled teeth; Princess Lotus Blossom – who was portrayed as an immigrant from China but was really Violet McNeal, a farm girl from Minnesota – sold Vital Sparks which she described as a "rejuvenator for lost manhood" that was made from male turtles and could restore "health, virility and happiness." Alas, Vital Sparks was actually aloe-coated candy.

Fast forward to the present day and only a few things have changed. The promises of combating dyspepsia and curing heartburn have shifted to "burning" fat and building muscle; the touring medicine shows and ubiquitous newspaper advertisements that were used to hawk products have been replaced by infomercials, websites and emails (spams); and, of course, there's considerably more money to be made. But today, as in the past, snake oil salesmen still prey on naïve consumers, targeting them with products that pledge miracles.

THE ART OF THE SEDUCTION

Make no mistake about it: The sale of nutritional supplements is a big business. The

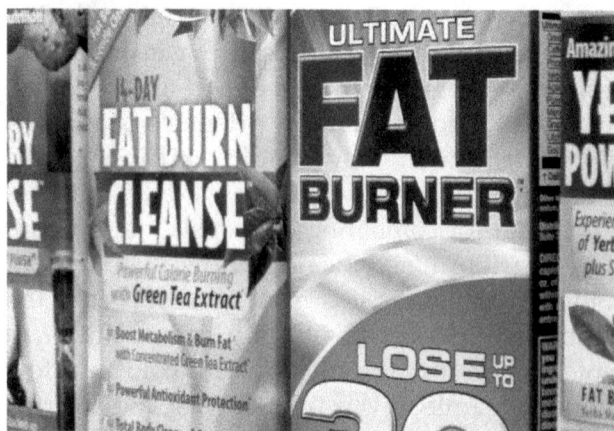

Today, as in the past, snake oil salesmen still prey on naïve consumers, targeting them with products that pledge miracles.

highly sophisticated marketing tactics used to seduce consumers are very appealing and cunning while the advertisements for products are often misleading, if not pure fabrication. Here are 10 characteristics that are common to the sales pitch for nutritional supplements:

Alluring Names

Most nutritional supplements have catchy brand names to bait consumers. Consider this random sampling of real-life products: Mega Mass, Monster Mass, Serious Mass, Elite Mass, True-Mass, Re-Built Mass, Carnivor Mass, H.U.G.E. Mass, Amplified Mass XXX, Iso Mass Extreme Gainer, Hyperbolic Mass Gainer, Mass-Tadon, Bulk Up Weight Gainer, Russian Bear 5000 Weight Gainer, CytoGainer, N-Large^2, Muscle Juice, Black All Natural Testosterone Booster, TestostroGROW, TestoJack 100, TestoRipped, Test Freak, T-Bomb, T-Up, Anabolic Freak, Anabolic Pump, Anabolic Prescription, Animal Pak, PowerFULL, Bullet Proof, Androbolix, MyoBuild, Platinum Hydro Builder, D4 Thermal Shock, Amplified Muscle Igniter 4X, Physio-Burn, Beta Burn, MethylBurn Extreme, Thermo Burst Hardcore, Thermo Detonator, Arson, Nuke, Jet Fuel, Ripped Fuel, Ripped Abs, Ripped Fast, Meltdown Fat Assault, UltraLean, AdrenaLean, Sculpted Abs, Monster Amino, Amino Burst 3000, Amino Freak and Amino Fuel. Again, this is just a sample; the list is practically endless.

Many of the names employ terms or their derivatives that connote aggressive action (amplify, grow, boost, build, bomb, shock, ignite, detonate, nuke, assault) with bodybuilding lingo (mass, ripped, pump, burn, sculpted) and scientific – or pseudoscientific – terminology (anabolic, hyperbolic, physio). The idea is to make the product sound unique, irresistible and absolutely essential for your nutritional needs.

Bodybuilding Magazines

For the most part, "muscle mags" are catalogs for nutritional supplements that are neatly packaged with some articles on training. Advertisements for a nutritional supplement are often strategically placed adjacent to articles that promote the very same nutritional supplement. Plus, having photographs of bodybuilders with heavily muscled physiques throughout the magazine – and usually accompanying the advertisements – implies that you can achieve the same results.

For the most part, "muscle mags" are catalogs for nutritional supplements that are neatly packaged with some articles on training.

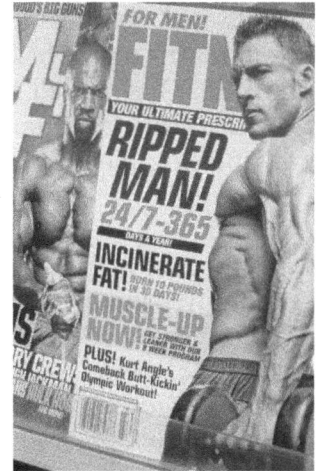

Unrecognized Credentials

Support for nutritional supplements often comes from individuals with degrees or titles that aren't nationally recognized. These types of credentials are substandard – or even meaningless – often having been self-conferred or received through some type of diploma mill or dubious organization. In the early 1980s, a physician famously obtained a "professional membership" for his dog in the American Association of Nutrition and Dietary Consultants and his cat in the International Academy of Nutritional Consultants merely by submitting the animal's name, address and 50 bucks.

The most reputable and recognized individual for dispensing nutritional information is a registered dietician (RD). These professionals must earn a four-year degree from an accredited college or university, complete an internship of at least eight months in a supervised setting – getting *at least 1,200 hours of experience* – and pass a national exam. In some states, licensure may also be required. And to maintain their credentials, RDs must update their accreditation on an annual basis.

Remember, not even an MD or a PhD guarantees that a person is qualified as an authority on nutrition (or exercise). For example, a PhD who dispenses information on nutrition (or exercise) may have a degree in an unrelated field such as sport sociology or endocrinology.

Natural Products

Many nutritional supplements claim to be natural (or even legal). One study found that there's no scientific evidence to support the promotional claims for 42% of the natural products that were reviewed. Another 32% of the products had some scientific evidence to support their claims but were judged to be marketed in a misleading manner. In other words, 74% of the natural products either had no scientific evidence to support their claims or were marketed in a misleading manner.

Keep in mind, too, that because a product has natural ingredients doesn't necessarily mean that it's safe. Few things are more natural than dirt but you wouldn't want to sprinkle it on your breakfast cereal. And, in fact, a number of natural substances can cause serious harm, including high doses of certain vitamins, minerals and herbs. (Chapter 20 discusses the safety aspect of nutritional supplements in more detail.)

Nebulous Terminology

Scientific-sounding names can be confusing and, at the same time, appealing. This is particularly true for those who seek quick and easy results. Many advertisements contain ambiguous language and rely upon the inability of consumers to understand complex terms. For instance, one product is said to contain adaptogens, metabolic intermediates, exogenous anabolic activators and energetics. Try to find those terms in any nutrition textbook.

Patent Numbers

Stating that a nutritional supplement is patented or "patent pending" can give the false impression that the US Patent and Trademark Office (USPTO) has approved the effectiveness of the product. A patent is a way to protect an inventor so that no one else makes, uses or sells the same product. Moreover, a patented product indicates that it's new and useful. New means that it's not identical to anything done before; useful means that it has a use, not that it works. The USPTO is tasked with distinguishing one product from another, not in evaluating or guaranteeing the effectiveness of a product.

Personal Testimonials

The use of personal testimonials from seemingly ordinary people is highly effective. Maybe even more effective is the use of celebrity testimonials from actors and athletes. For the right price, some individuals can be pretty eager to offer testimonials to promote practically any product.

It's fairly standard practice for testimonials to employ what's become known as before-and-after photographs. These photographs can be easily faked or "photoshopped," especially nowadays. Also, there's no evidence that the "after" photograph is truly the result of using the product.

Testimonials also come from those whom consumers trust or hold in high regard such as scientists and physicians. But reputable scientists and physicians aren't in the business of selling nutritional supplements; their testimonials should immediately raise skepticism.

Phony Endorsements

Some manufacturers make claims about their products by implying or falsely stating endorsement by professional groups. For instance, some products are said to be "university tested" which may actually mean that someone at a university was merely involved. In other cases, university testing may not have even occurred.

Since the mid-1980s or earlier, there have been commercials in which actors have said, "I'm not a doctor but I play one on TV." Then, the actors endorsed some type of product but at least they gave full disclosure. Many endorsements come from individuals who wear a white lab coat and stethoscope. Naturally, consumers assume that these people are physicians. However, if they're not referred to as physicians, they probably aren't. That's because it's illegal to impersonate a physician.

Product Labels

The label of a nutritional supplement rarely contains false claims. Untruthful or misleading information could trigger federal action since only factual data is allowed on labels. As a way around this, some manufacturers place misleading information in their advertisements – rather than on their labels – where it may be overlooked by regulators.

While on the subject, the exact content of many nutritional supplements is unknown and may not be represented accurately on the list of ingredients. In one study, for example, researchers bought 12 brands of nutritional supplements from various stores in Los Angeles. Only one of the 12 brands contained 90 to 110% of the amount of ingredients that were declared on the label; the others had significantly more or less. Such poor quality control would be unacceptable in a medication.

Some products may even contain small amounts of banned substances such as steroids or may actually be steroids but not labeled as such. Researchers bought 58 nutritional supplements from retail outlets and Internet sites. Of the 54 nutritional supplements that were successfully analyzed, 13 (25%) had low levels of steroids and six (11%) had banned stimulants.

Questionable Research

In their advertisements, many manufacturers claim to have conducted scientific research, done breakthrough research or had secret research results. An advertisement might say that "in a university study, subjects increased their muscular strength by 20%" or "more than 20 studies have proven the effectiveness of the key ingredients."

The mere mention of studies makes it sound as if there's credible evidence that a nutritional supplement is effective. But if you peak behind the curtain, you'll see that the "scientific research" that's used by manufacturers to hype their products is often so unscientific that it's basically useless. (Chapter 24 discusses how to evaluate research.)

CONSUMER PROTECTION

Fortunately, consumers aren't alone in confronting nutritional quackery. The two main federal agencies that are tasked with protecting consumers are the Federal Trade Commission (FTC) and the Food and Drug Administration (FDA). Both organizations have been safeguarding the public for more than a century.

In 1903, the Bureau of Corporations was created by Congress. In 1914, the bureau became the FTC when President Woodrow Wilson signed the Federal Trade Commission Act into law. The primary duty of the FTC is to protect the public against unfair methods of competition – such as monopolies – but the agency is also sanctioned to move against false and deceptive advertising; mislabeling; and misrepresentation of quality, guarantee and terms of sale.

In 1906, President Theodore Roosevelt signed the Pure Food and Drug Act into law which authorized the federal government to oversee the safety and quality of food. The responsibility for enforcing this act was given to the US Department of Agriculture and its Bureau of Chemistry. The bureau was renamed the Food, Drug and Insecticide Administration in 1927 and shortened to its present name in 1930. In 1938, the Federal Food, Drug and Cosmetic Act replaced the Pure Food and Drug Act of 1906. This new act was signed into law a little more than six months after Elixir Sulfanilamide – an untested "wonder drug" – killed 107 people in 15 states. The act extended the range of commodities that came under federal control – to include cosmetics and medical devices – and increased penalties for violators. It also prohibited statements in food labeling that were false or misleading

The Dietary Supplement Health and Education Act of 1994 amended the Federal Food, Drug and Cosmetic Act of 1938. This act – co-authored by Senator Orrin Hatch of Utah, a state that's home to many manufacturers of nutritional supplements – has had a drastic impact on the way that the FDA does business. Essentially, it shifted the role of the FDA from pre-market approver to post-market enforcer. Under this act,

manufacturers can send a nutritional supplement directly to the market without submitting any proof about its safety or effectiveness to the FDA. Essentially, the FDA can take action against a nutritional supplement only after it's proven to be unsafe. The lone exception is when a nutritional supplement contains a "new dietary ingredient" (which is defined as one that wasn't marketed in the United States in a nutritional supplement prior to October 15, 1994 when the act became law).

Manufacturers of nutritional supplements are allowed to make specific claims of health benefits – referred to as structure/function claims – on the label of a product. However, a claim that's made on the label that a specific nutrient or ingredient has an effect on the structure or function of the body requires this disclaimer: "This statement has not been evaluated by the Food and Drug Administration. This product is not intended to diagnose, treat, cure or prevent any disease."

The FTC and FDA in Action

Besides protecting the public against nutritional quackery, the FTC and FDA have a myriad of other responsibilities as well as limited resources to review the vast amount of nutritional supplements that proliferates on the market. Nonetheless, the FTC and FDA have flexed their regulatory muscles for decades.

In 1927, the FTC filed its first weight-loss case. Action was taken against McGowan Laboratories, Incorporated for advertisements that the company had placed in *True Romances* magazine for a product known as McGowan's Reducine. It was claimed that after applying the cream, "the excess fat is literally dissolved away" and it will "slenderize" any part of the body "quickly, surely and permanently." Fast-forward more than 90 years and it's more of the same story. Most recently, in 2017, the FTC settled charges against three affiliate marketers to the tune of $500,000. The individuals were charged with using illegal spam email, false weight-loss claims and phony celebrity endorsements to sell weight-loss products, including Original Pure Forskolin, Original White Kidney Bean and Mango Boost Cleanse.

Since 1990, the FTC has been especially active in investigating weight-loss products. Several of the cases were particularly newsworthy. In 2004, for example, the FDA banned the sale of products that contained ephedra (aka ma huang) because research showed that it was associated with an increased risk of hypertension, stroke, heart palpitations and psychiatric symptoms. And in 2009, the FDA questioned the safety of Hydroxycut® – yet another weight-loss product and "fat burner" – after 23 cases of liver toxicity were reported in a seven-year period, including one death and one liver transplant. The FDA ordered the manufacturer to cease distribution and recall the product from the marketplace. However, the product was reformulated and is back on store shelves. (Fast fact: In 2009, a class-action lawsuit was filed against the manufacturer of Hydroxycut® for making false and misleading statements in its labeling and advertising in regards to the effectiveness of more than 30 Hydroxycut® products; in 2014, a federal judge approved a settlement of $14 million.)

In 2009, the FDA questioned the safety of Hydroxycut after 23 cases of liver toxicity were reported in a seven-year period.

CAVEAT EMPTOR

Although the source of the quote is the subject of debate, a very bright person once said, "There's a sucker born every minute." Then the person added, "And two to take his money." Unfortunately, this is probably an underestimate on both counts.

Translated from Latin, caveat emptor means "Let (or may) the buyer beware." This advice certainly holds true for nutritional supplements. Don't fall prey to nutritional quackery.

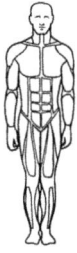

22 Weight Management

Weight management refers to gaining, losing or maintaining bodyweight. Managing your weight boils down to the mathematical interplay of two variables: caloric consumption (aka caloric intake) and caloric expenditure (aka caloric output). If you consume (eat) more calories than you expend (use), you'll gain weight. If you expend (use) more calories than you consume (eat), you'll lose weight. And if you consume (eat) the same number of calories as you expend (use), you'll maintain the same weight. The dynamics of weight management can be summarized below.

weight gain: calories in > calories out

weight loss: calories in < calories out

weight maintenance: calories in = calories out

A CLOSER LOOK

While the end result of caloric consumption and caloric expenditure boils down to simple arithmetic, there's a right way and a wrong way to manage your weight. Let's take a closer look at the proper approach to weight management.

To be clear: Calories count but there's no need to count calories. The ensuing discussion of calories with respect to consumption and expenditure is only meant to demonstrate the dynamics of weight management as it pertains to gaining and losing weight.

Gaining Weight

Some people will look, feel and perform better if they gained weight. Technically, the main goal of weight gain isn't merely to gain *weight*; rather, it's to gain *muscle*.

A mistake that's often made is gaining weight too quickly. There's a limit as to how much muscle an individual can gain in a given amount of time. And it's not as much as many people think.

In order to gain weight, a caloric surplus must be produced. The daily caloric surplus shouldn't be more than about 350 calories above the amount that's necessary for weight maintenance. If the weight gain is more than about 0.5% (one-half percent) of your bodyweight per week, it's likely that at least some of the increase was in the form of fat, not muscle. In practical terms, this means that the weight gain shouldn't exceed about one pound per week. For most people, an increase of about one-half pound per week is probably more realistic. If the weight gain isn't too great and the result of a demanding fitness program in conjunction with a moderate increase in caloric consumption, then it will probably be in the form of increased muscle.

One pound of muscle has about 2,500 calories. Therefore, if you consume 250 calories per day (cal/day) above the amount that you need to maintain your weight – a 250-calorie surplus – it will take you 10 days to gain one pound of muscle [2,500 cal ÷ 250 cal/day]. So if a 200-pound man who's very active requires 5,200 cal/day to maintain his bodyweight [200 lb x 26 cal/lb], he must consume 5,450 cal/day – 250 calories above his need – to gain one pound of muscle in 10 days. This estimate must be recalculated on a regular basis to account for changes in bodyweight. After increasing his bodyweight to 201 pounds, for example, he'll now require 5,226 cal/day to meet his energy needs [201 lb x 26 cal/lb]. In order to gain another pound of muscle in 10 days, he must increase his caloric consumption to 5,476 cal/day – 250 calories above his need.

Specific Tips

There are many tactics that you can employ to gain weight. What follows are 10 tips for gaining weight in a manner that's effective, practical, sustainable and safe.

1. Eat at least three meals per day.

In order to gain weight, you need to consume more calories. It's that simple. To get enough calories, you'll need to eat at least three meals per day on a regular basis.

Your body doesn't absorb one or two large meals very well; most of these calories are jammed through your digestive system. As a matter of fact, if you consume a large number of calories at one time, the sudden and severe rush of food will wreak havoc on the digestive process and cause some of those calories to be stored as fat. A better approach, then, is to spread the calories over three or more regular-sized meals.

2. Eat at least three nutritious snacks per day.

Besides getting at least three meals per day, you'll need to get at least three snacks per day. But it shouldn't be any kind of snacks just for the sake of getting more calories; the snacks should have some nutritional value. Examples are low-fat yogurt, whole-grain crackers and certain energy/snack bars.

If you have a hectic or an unpredictable schedule, you'll probably find this tough to accomplish without good planning. For instance, you can pre-package nutritious snacks that you could eat at work or school.

Note: Consuming three meals intermingled with three snacks essentially amounts to eating every three hours or so.

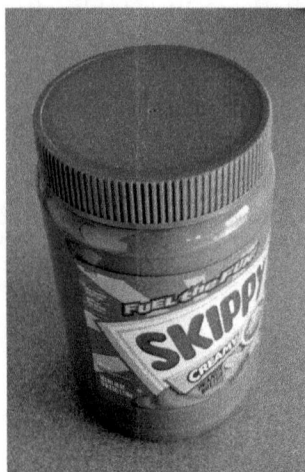

To gain weight, you can "get more bang for your buck" by choosing foods with a high caloric density.

3. Consume foods that are high in calories (but not too high in fat).

You can "get more bang for your buck" by choosing foods with a high caloric density. These foods have a relatively large number of calories in small portions. A bagel with peanut butter, a peanut butter and jelly sandwich and nuts (such as almonds, peanuts and walnuts) are good examples of calorie-dense foods.

4. Eat calorie-dense fruits and vegetables.

Not to belabor a point but to gain weight, you need to consume more calories. This means eating calorie-dense fruits (such as bananas, pineapples and raisins) and vegetables (such as peas, corn and carrots). An added bonus is that fruits and vegetables are rich sources of vitamins and minerals.

5. Drink calorie-dense beverages.

A great way to gain weight is by drinking calorie-dense beverages such as low-fat milk and fruit juice. These beverages contain more calories – and more nutrients – than water or unsweetened beverages.

6. Eat a healthy breakfast.

If you're the type of person who frequently skips meals, then it will be all the more difficult for you to get the amount of calories that you need to gain weight. Perhaps no other meal is skipped more than breakfast. Pass on breakfast and you'll spend a good part of the day trying to compensate for the hundreds of calories that you didn't get earlier.

7. Increase the size of your portions.

If you're already consuming a balanced diet that contains a variety of healthy foods and trying to gain weight, you've got most of the battle won. Here, an easy and effective way to get more calories is to increase the size of your portions.

Increasing portion sizes is fairly simple: You can use a larger plate/bowl for your food and a larger glass/cup for your beverage. This helps you to increase the number of calories that you consume.

8. Make a dedicated effort.

Gaining weight requires total dedication for seven days each week. Additional calories must be consumed on a regular basis until you achieve the desired increase in weight. You won't gain weight by making a half-hearted attempt or applying these tips every now and then.

9. Do strength training on a regular basis.

Most people who try to gain weight also engage in a strength program. However, some people overemphasize the muscles of their torso and arms and underemphasize the muscles of their hips and legs (or they ignore these muscles altogether). Neglecting your hips and legs means that an enormous amount of muscle mass isn't receiving any stimulus for growth.

10. Get adequate recovery.

Doing any type of physical training with a high level of intensity requires an adequate amount of recovery. This has even greater importance when trying to gain weight.

Make sure that you schedule enough time between your workouts. And make sure that you get adequate rest (sleep), preferably at least eight hours of uninterrupted sleep each night.

Those two aspects are certainly a large part of the recovery process but there's a nutritional aspect that must be considered. Just remember the three Rs of nutritional recovery: Refuel with carbohydrates, rehydrate with fluids and repair with protein. (The details of nutritional recovery are discussed in Chapter 19.)

Losing Weight

Some people will look, feel and perform better if they lost weight. Technically, the main goal of weight loss isn't merely to lose *weight*; rather, it's to lose *fat*.

A mistake that's often made is losing weight too quickly. There's a limit as to how much fat an individual can lose in a given amount of time. And similar to gaining weight, it's not as much as many people think.

In order to lose weight, a caloric deficit must be produced. The daily caloric deficit shouldn't

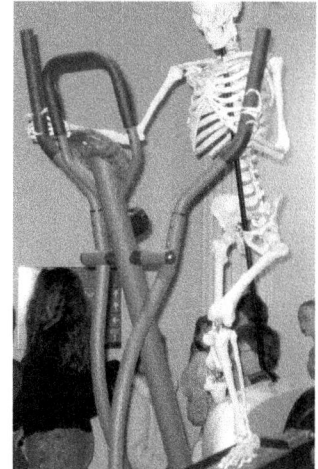

When losing weight too quickly, a significant amount of the loss can be in the form of muscle.

be more than about 1,000 calories below the amount that's necessary for weight maintenance. If the weight loss is more than about 1% of your bodyweight per week, it's likely that at least some of the decrease was in the form of water and/or muscle, not fat. In practical terms, this means that the weight loss shouldn't exceed about two pounds per week. For most people, a decrease of about one pound per week is probably more realistic. If the weight loss isn't too great and the result of a demanding fitness program in conjunction with a moderate decrease in caloric consumption, then it will probably be in the form of decreased fat.

One pound of fat has about 3,500 calories. Therefore, if you consume 250 cal/day below the amount that you need to maintain your weight – a 250-calorie deficit – it will take you 14 days to lose one pound of fat [3,500 cal ÷ 250 cal/day]. So if a 200-pound man who's very active requires 5,200 cal/day to maintain his bodyweight, he must consume 4,950 cal/day – 250 calories below his need – to lose one pound of fat in 14 days. Remember, this estimate must be recalculated on a regular basis to account for changes in bodyweight. After decreasing his bodyweight to 199 pounds, for example, he'll now require 5,174 cal/day to meet his energy needs [199 lb x 26 cal/lb]. In order to lose another pound of fat in 14 days, he must decrease his caloric consumption to 4,924 cal/day – 250 calories below his need.

Actually, there are three ways to lose weight: You can (1) decrease the number of calories that you consume and maintain the same amount of activity that you do; (2) maintain the same number of calories that you consume and increase the amount of activity that you do; or (3) decrease the number of calories that you consume and increase the amount of activity that you do.

The third way – decrease the number of calories that you consume (eat less) and increase the amount of activity that you do (exercise more) – is the preferred way. Why? Well, suppose that your goal is to lose 10 pounds of fat in 10 weeks. This represents a rate of one pound of fat per week. Since one pound of fat has 3,500 calories, you'd need to create a deficit of 500 calories per day. Eating 500 less calories per day can be quite a challenge; the same can be said about using 500 more calories per day. And don't forget, this 500-calorie deficit would need to be achieved every day for 70 consecutive days.

The best way, then, is to do a combination of the two: Eat a little less and exercise a little more. And it doesn't have to be a 50-50 split. In this example, you could achieve a deficit of 500 calories by eating 200 less calories and using 300 more calories. Same result but less overwhelming. Or, perhaps a 250-calorie deficit is a more realistic pursuit for you than a 500-calorie deficit.

Sidebar: In a 2016 public-service announcement concerning overweight and obesity, Dr. Stephen Hawking – one of the greatest scientific minds in history – stated, "We eat too much and move too little. Fortunately the solution is simple: More physical activity and change in diet. It's not rocket science."

Several problems are associated with losing weight too quickly. For one thing, a significant amount of the weight loss can be in the form of muscle. Consider a 200-pound man with 20.00% fat. This means that he has 40 pounds of fat [200 lb x 0.20] and 160 pounds of fat-free (lean-body) mass. If he lost 10 pounds, he'd weigh 190 pounds. But if it was done too quickly, it's possible that only one pound of the weight loss came from fat. In this case, he'd have 39 pounds of fat and 151 pounds of fat-free mass . . . meaning that he's now *20.53% fat.* So, he lost weight but his percentage of body fat actually increased.

This scenario was demonstrated by AJ Perez – a reporter for *USA Today* – who chronicled his attempt to lose 20.0 pounds in 21.5 days to simulate what mixed martial arts fighters, boxers and wrestlers might do to "make weight." Although his bodyweight decreased from 175.8 to 154.9 pounds, the 20.9-pound loss in weight – *nearly one pound per day* – came from 7.44 pounds of fat and 13.46 pounds of lean-body mass. What's a bit surprising is that his body fat dropped from 14.1% to 11.2%. But the fact remains that he lost a very large amount of lean-body mass in a very short period of time.

A loss of muscle isn't desirable since muscle is functional tissue: Muscle acts across your joints to produce movement of your bones which enables you to perform mechanical work. In addition, muscle is a metabolically active tissue. Having less muscle decreases your metabolic rate (the rate at which you use calories). In other words, you'll be less efficient at "burning" calories which will make it more difficult for you to lose weight. Remember, you want to lose *fat weight,* not *muscle weight.*

And when you lose weight too quickly, it's often temporary because your body can't sustain such extreme changes. It's not unusual for people to regain much of the weight that they lost. Case in point: Researchers at the National Institutes of Health in Bethesda (MD) studied contestants from Season 8 of *The Biggest Loser*, a reality show in which obese/overweight contestants vie for cash prizes that are awarded to the person who loses the greatest percentage of bodyweight. Of the original 16 contestants, 14 agreed to participate in the study. At baseline, the 14 contestants (six men and eight women) weighed 328.27 pounds. By the end of the 30-week contest, they weighed 199.74 pounds, meaning that they lost 128.53 pounds or 4.28 pounds per week. (The winner shed 239 pounds or 7.97 pounds per week.) Six years after the show ended, the contestants weighed 290.13 pounds, meaning that they *regained 90.39 pounds.* Of the 14 contestants, only one didn't regain any weight. Something else happened: As an adaptation to the lighter bodyweight, their metabolic rates had "slowed" by 275 calories per day. In other words, they used 275 less calories per day than would be expected for their age and size. And six years later – after they regained much of that bodyweight – their metabolic rates had slowed even further. At that point, they used about *500 less calories per day* than would be expected, making it much more difficult for them to lose weight.

Look at it this way: If you're 10 pounds overweight, you probably didn't get that way in a week. So you shouldn't expect to lose 10 pounds in a week, either.

In general, it's rarely a good idea to pursue a "quick fix." In order to realize long-term success, you must install changes in your lifestyle and behavior. By losing weight too quickly, you won't change any bad habits. At best, you'll only experience short-term results.

It's worth mentioning that the numbers on bathroom scales and height/weight charts are poor indicators of whether or not someone should lose weight. The need for weight loss should be determined by *body composition*, not *bodyweight*. This is especially true for active individuals. For the most part, active individuals tend to be larger and have more lean-body mass than the general population. Think about it: Two people could be same height and weight but have markedly different body compositions. For example, one might have 15% body fat and the other might have 30% body fat. If this was the case, then only one person might need to lose weight: the one with the higher percentage of body fat.

A variety of methods can be used to measure body composition such as air displacement plethysmography, bioelectrical impedance analysis, computerized tomography, dual energy x-ray absorptiometry, hydrostatic (underwater) weighing and near infrared reactance. But perhaps the most popular method of measuring body composition is to use skinfold calipers. In general, this is considered to be the most practical and least expensive method of assessment without sacrificing much in the way of accuracy (assuming that the person who takes the measurements is reasonably skilled and the equation that's used is valid).

Sidebar: In most sports, a low percentage of body fat is desirable; in some sports, however, a high percentage of body fat is actually desirable. In long-distance swimming, for example, athletes obtain increased buoyancy and thermal insulation from higher levels of body fat. And, of course, a high percentage of body fat is desirable in sumo wrestling.

Specific Tips

There are many tactics that you can employ to lose weight. What follows are 20 tips for losing weight in a manner that's effective, practical, sustainable and safe.

1. Read food labels.

Whenever you purchase food in a supermarket or convenience store, examine the food label. Based on federal law, food labels are required for most packaged foods. This includes breads, cereals, canned/frozen foods, snacks, desserts and beverages.

An important part of the food label is the Nutrition Facts panel. With respect to weight loss, pay particular attention to the servings per container, serving size, amount of calories per serving and total fat per serving.

Also be wary of the fine print. For example, a container of food that has 100 calories per serving means that the container has 100 calories if – and only if – it has one serving. If a container of food has 100 calories per serving but has four servings per container, eating the entire contents will give you 400 calories.

With respect to weight loss, pay particular attention to the servings per container, serving size, amount of calories and total fat per serving.

2. Become more knowledgeable.

Most full-service and limited-service restaurants don't readily disclose the nutritional information of their foods . . . and for good reason. For instance, value meals – which are standard fare at limited-service restaurants – typically include a burger or sandwich, fries and a soda. This combo has plenty of calories, fat and sodium. But "upgrade" that to a larger size and the meal balloons to much more. Add a dessert and wash everything down with a refill of soda and this can result in a staggering amount of calories, fat and sodium. If you're not careful, you can easily get a day's worth of those nutrients all in one meal.

Value meals are tempting but understand that the "value" is *economical*, not *nutritional*. Although you get a lot of food for your money, it's usually a lot of *bad food* for your money: more calories, more fat and more sodium.

Needless to say, the gory nutritional details aren't made too obvious at the majority of full-service and limited-service restaurants. More knowledge is only a few clicks away, though, since the major establishments have websites that list their nutritional information.

3. Eat more frequently.

The notion that eating more meals can help you to lose weight seems counterintuitive. Indeed, how is it possible to eat more and weigh less? Well, the *number* of meals should be higher but the *size* of those meals – in terms of calories – should be smaller. By spreading calories over more meals – rather than by stuffing calories into less meals – you're better able to keep your hunger at bay.

In one crossover study, 15 subjects were randomly assigned to eat all of their calories in either three meals per day for eight weeks or two meals per day for two weeks and then one meal per day for six weeks. After an 11-week washout period, the subjects were switched to the other diet for eight weeks. Both diets consisted of roughly the same number of calories. The researchers found that eating three meals per day produced lower ratings of hunger and higher ratings of satiety (fullness) compared to eating one meal per day. And as time went on, those ratings became more pronounced.

One of the worst things that you can do is skip a meal. In this case, you'll be ravenous and the next time that you have a meal, you'll probably satisfy your appetite by eating anything that doesn't move.

4. Decrease the size of your portions.

If you're already consuming a balanced diet that contains a variety of healthy foods and trying to lose weight, you've got most of the battle won. Here, an easy and effective way to get less calories is to decrease the size of your portions.

Decreasing portion sizes is fairly simple: You can use a smaller plate/bowl for your food and a smaller glass/cup for your beverage. This helps you to decrease the number of calories that you consume. And it certainly makes sense that if you decide to eat an entire bowl of potato chips, for example, a smaller bowl would yield fewer calories than a larger bowl.

However, you can use a larger plate/bowl and a larger glass/cup to your advantage. With these items, you can give yourself bigger servings of healthier foods such as fruits and vegetables.

5. Sit away from the serving area.

When you sit near a serving area – whether it's at home or a buffet-style restaurant – the food is readily available and easily accessible, tempting you to eat more than you should. It doesn't require much effort to reach across the table or get up and take a few steps to grab second – or third – helpings. And don't forget something else about sitting away from food: Out of sight, out of mind, out of mouth.

6. Avoid doing activities while eating.

Certain activities are associated with eating. This includes watching television, playing a board game and reading a book. When engaged in such activities, people focus on what they're doing rather than what they're eating. Therefore, it's a good idea to refrain from eating while doing these and other activities.

If you do get caught in those types of situations or anything similar, use your non-dominant hand to pick up food. It sounds strange but the added effort makes it less likely that you'll overeat.

7. Confine eating to a designated area.

People tend to eat more when they're distracted. And as just mentioned, eating is triggered by some activities such as watching television. A great way to keep you from doing this is to restrict your eating to a designated place or room (and not in front of something with a screen).

8. Chew your food slowly.

At first glance, this tip might seem odd. If you chew your food slowly, however, you're less likely to mindlessly inhale it as if you're the defending champion in an eating contest.

In one crossover study, 30 subjects were randomly assigned to eat as much food as they wanted either quickly or slowly. When they ate quickly, they consumed 646 calories in 8.6 minutes or about 75.1 calories per minute; when they ate slowly, they consumed 579 calories in 29.2 minutes or about 19.8 calories per minute. Besides eating fewer calories when they chewed their food slowly, the subjects reported greater feelings of satiety and lower feelings of hunger. And they enjoyed the meal more.

The fact of the matter is that by chewing your food slowly, your brain is given adequate time to receive a signal from your stomach that it's full. In addition, taking the time to chew your food facilitates the digestive process.

To help you slow down, you can place your fork or spoon on the table between bites. So, pay attention to the food that you eat and take the time to really savor the flavor.

Sidebar: On July 4, 2017, Joey "Jaws" Chestnut claimed his 10th victory at the annual Nathan's® Famous International Hot Dog Eating Contest in Coney Island, New York. Chestnut set a world record by downing 72 hot dogs and buns. Here's something to chew on: One Nathan's® all-beef dog and bun has a nutritional profile that includes 280 calories, 18 grams of fat (of which 6 grams are saturated fat and 0.5 grams are trans fat), 10 grams of protein and 780 milligrams of sodium. So Chestnut – who's listed as having a bodyweight of 230 pounds – consumed about 20,160 calories, 1,296 grams of fat (of which 432 grams were saturated fat and 36 grams were trans fat), 720 grams of protein and 56,150 milligrams of sodium. Among other things, that's 8.6 times the Recommended Dietary Allowance for protein per day (or 8.6 day's worth of protein) and 24.4 times the recommended maximum amount of sodium per day (or 24.4 day's worth of sodium). Oh, yeah: He ate the 72 hot dogs in 10 minutes or about 2,016 calories per minute.

8. Start your meals with soup and/or salad.

This is a very simple and easy tactic for you to implement. Because they're comprised mostly of water, soups and salads provide you with relatively few calories but give you a feeling of satiety. If you lead off with soup and/or salad, then, you're less likely to consume as many calories during the remainder of your meal.

Key point: Broth-based soups usually have fewer calories (and less fat) than cream-based ones. And even though they're both salads, a garden salad usually has fewer calories (and less fat) than a Caesar salad.

10. Eat foods that are low in fat.

A food that's high in fat is loaded with calories. Packed with nine calories per gram, fats are more than twice as dense as carbohydrates and protein which have four calories per gram. Or look at it this way: A food that's high in fat has more calories for the same weight than a food that's low in fat.

In particular, you should reduce your intake of saturated fat (found in red meats, certain oils, high-fat dairy products and many processed foods) and trans fat (found naturally in the fatty parts of meat and dairy products). Limiting your consumption of fat dramatically decreases the number of calories that you eat. Plus, your food choices are much healthier.

Eating less fat and more carbohydrates will help you to lose weight, provided that it's a gram-for-gram swap or thereabouts. Let's say that you've been consuming 100 grams of fat per day. Now, decrease your fat intake by 50 grams per day and increase your carbohydrate intake by 50 grams per day. That's still a total of 100 grams but the number of calories in those 100 grams goes from 900 to 650. Do that for two weeks and you'll have consumed 3,500 fewer calories which would produce a loss of one pound of fat (everything else being equal).

This concept has been corroborated by research. For instance, one study determined that a 1% decrease in the percentage of calories from fat coupled with a corresponding 1% increase in the percentage of calories from carbohydrates (or protein, for that matter) led to a reduction in the number of calories that were consumed. The idea is to choose foods that are less dense in calories. And seriously, does it really make sense that in order to lose fat you should eat more of it?

This isn't to say that you should eliminate fat completely; fat does perform several functions that are vital to your health. In the context of losing weight, however, you must reduce your intake of calorie-dense foods.

Studies have shown that people tend to eat about the same weight of food each day; not the same calories of food, the *same weight of food*. So choosing foods with a low caloric density – those that have the smallest number of calories in the largest portions – means that you'll consume fewer calories without sacrificing satiety.

Consider, for example, grapes and raisins. Essentially, raisins are dried grapes. In terms of weight and volume, 100 calories of grapes are more food – and more filling – than 100 calories of raisins.

11. Eat more fruits and vegetables.

Foods (and beverages) that offer very few calories along with a feeling of satiety are great choices for those who are trying to lose weight. Fruits and vegetables meet these criteria because they contain exceptionally high amounts of water and water has no calories.

Moreover, fruits and vegetables have an added bonus: They're jam-packed with vitamins and minerals. Truly, nothing on the planet comes closer to being a magical food than fruits and vegetables.

Yet, many people struggle with getting enough fruits and vegetables. An effective way to meet this challenge is to keep fruits and vegetables on hand and available. Then, you can incorporate different tactics to increase your intake. For example, you can eat an apple as a snack. You can add carrots to soup. Or, you can put sliced tomatoes and/or lettuce on a sandwich. In short, use your imagination.

And while on the subject, it's important for you to consume a variety of fruits and vegetables. Since fruits and vegetables come in such a wide range of colors, just follow this simple directive to ensure variety: Eat a rainbow.

12. Get more fiber.

Fiber is a type of complex carbohydrate that can't be digested. Foods that are high in fiber tend to have fewer calories, an obvious advantage for weight loss. Also, fiber slows the rate at which food passes through your digestive system thereby increasing satiety. You can boost your intake of fiber by eating fruits, vegetables and whole-grain products (such as breads and cereals).

13. Eat spicy foods.

This tip might sound as if it originated from a headline in a supermarket tabloid. However, there's some scientific evidence that eating spicy foods can help you to lose weight.

For one thing, spicy foods can increase your metabolic rate by raising your body temperature. The greatest increase in body temperature is triggered by capsaicin, a molecule that's found in chili peppers; it's what makes hot peppers hot. (Fast fact: Capsaicin is also the active ingredient in pepper sprays that are used for self-defense.)

With that said, the thermogenic effect of capsaicin on metabolic rate is temporary and small. Keep in mind, too, that eating *any* food will increase your metabolic rate. The reason is that the body uses calories in the digestion, absorption and assimilation of the nutrients in food. For a mixed diet of carbohydrates, protein and fat, this thermic effect of food – first documented more than 200 years ago and referred to scientifically as specific dynamic action – is roughly 10% of caloric consumption. So if you consumed 400 calories, for instance, your body would use about 40 calories to digest, absorb and assimilate those nutrients.

But the real benefit of eating spicy foods is the fact that capsaicin seems to curb appetite. In a study that was conducted in The Netherlands, 15 subjects were randomly assigned to receive four treatments: 100% of their estimated daily caloric needs with and without capsaicin (from red chili pepper) and 75% of their estimated daily caloric needs with and without capsaicin. On the day after each treatment, the subjects were fed dinner that they ate *ad libitum*. When the subjects consumed 100% of their caloric needs with capsaicin included, they had significantly greater feelings of satiety compared to when they consumed 100% of their caloric needs without capsaicin included. And in the meal that was consumed the day after each of those two treatments, the subjects ate 30% fewer calories when capsaicin was included.

A few words of caution: Some individuals experience gastrointestinal distress from spicy foods. Therefore, spicy foods should be avoided by those who suffer from ulcers and chronic heartburn.

14. Decrease your intake of sweetened beverages.

Included among sweetened beverages are non-diet soda, fruit drinks, lemonade and iced tea. Essentially, sweetened beverages are liquid sugar. The problem here is twofold: Sweetened beverages provide a significant amount of calories and no nutritional value whatsoever. Also, numerous studies have found a strong association between the intake of sweetened beverages and obesity.

The average non-diet soda has about 100 calories per eight ounces. Drinking one 12-ounce can of soda on a daily basis translates into about 54,750 calories in a year . . . or *about 15.6 pounds.*

15. Drink more water.

It's a wise move for you to drink plenty of water before, during and after meals. Remember, water has weight but no calories. Therefore, drinking water creates a feeling of satiety without adding anything to your caloric budget.

Here's something of interest: In one study, subjects ate the same food for lunch but drank a different type of beverage (either regular cola, diet cola or water). Regardless of the beverage, the subjects ate the same number of calories. So, the calories from the beverage were added to the calories from the meal. This means that when water was the beverage that accompanied the meal, fewer calories were consumed.

16. Choose healthy snacks.

There's nothing inherently wrong with snacking. It becomes problematic, however, when poor choices are made. As a rule of thumb, unhealthy snacks are those that are high in calories and fat (as well as sodium and sugar) and have little or no nutritional value.

But a food that's loaded with calories and fat without much in the way of nutrients – such as cookies, cake and ice cream – isn't necessarily bad as long as it's consumed in moderation. In other words, something like ice cream is

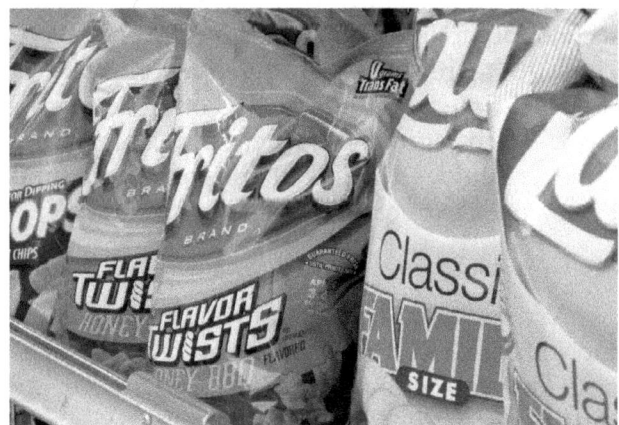

Unhealthy snacks are those that are high in calories and fat (as well as sodium and sugar) and have little or no nutritional value.

323

generally okay provided that it's not eaten in large quantities and/or on a habitual basis.

Healthy snacks include fruit, raw vegetables, low-fat yogurt, popcorn (sans butter), whole-grain crackers, pretzels, cereal and certain energy/snack bars.

Energy/snack bars must be carefully vetted. Some energy/snack bars are reasonably healthy, meaning low in calories and fat (as well as sodium and sugar) with at least some nutritional value. But some energy/snack bars are little more than glorified – and expensive – candy bars. To tell, check the Nutrition Facts panel on the wrapper. Remember, the ingredients are listed by weight from highest to lowest. If the first few ingredients include sugar in one or more of its many forms, it's basically a candy bar. Ingredients that end in the suffix "-ose" are sugars; other sugars or sugar-based ingredients include caramel, corn sweetener, corn syrup, dextrin, honey, malt syrup, maltodextrin, mannitol, molasses, nectar and sorbitol.

To illustrate, let's take a look at a Nature Valley™ roasted mixed nut sweet & salty nut granola bar. How can this bar not be healthy? What image comes to mind when you think of nature valley? Listen very carefully and you can almost hear birds chirping in the background. The word granola also arouses feelings of health. Once the euphoria subsides, take a glimpse at the ingredients of this "granola bar." The first four are roasted peanuts, corn syrup, whole grain oats and sugar. Huh? Yes, that's right: Among its first four ingredients are corn syrup and sugar. Hold up, there's more. Scattered among the rest of the list are no less than five other sugars or sugar-based ingredients: fructose, tapioca syrup, honey, maltodextrin (linked units of glucose) and barley malt extract (aka malt syrup). Whoa.

17. Minimize unhealthy foods in your home.

As noted previously, unhealthy foods include those that are high in calories and fat (as well as sodium and sugar) and have little or no nutritional value. When there are little or no healthy options in your home, it's virtually impossible for you to make healthy choices. To add to an earlier point: Out of house, out of sight, out of mind, out of mouth.

18. Restrict the number of meals that you eat in limited-service restaurants.

It's estimated that about 47% of American adults eat fast food at least once per week. In 2014, there were 228,677 fast-food restaurants in the United States. Sales at limited-service (or quick-service) restaurants were $221.9 billion in 2016 (plus another $544.1 billion throughout the restaurant industry).

Fast food is inexpensive, convenient and fast. But for the most part, it's not very healthy or nutritious. Fast food tends to be high in calories and fat (and sodium). Research has shown that on the days that people eat fast food, they tend to consume more calories and fat than on other days.

19. Make activities less sedentary and more physical.

Studies have reported that an increase of sedentary activities and a decrease of physical activities are contributing factors to the steady rise of obesity. Obviously, you should do less sedentary activities and more physical activities. But whenever possible, sedentary activities should be made more physical. For example, use the steps, not the elevator; at a mall or work, park farther from the building, not closer.

20. Do strength training and aerobic training.

Like all types of physical training, strength training and aerobic training use calories. Strength training is unique, though, in that it can decrease fat and increase muscle thereby improving body composition and enhancing appearance. Muscle tissue is more metabolically active than fat tissue, meaning that it requires more calories to function. As a result, those with more muscle are more efficient at using calories. (Each pound of muscle that you gain will increase your caloric expenditure by about 10 more calories per day.) Aerobic training is also important since it can produce a sustained and significant use of calories.

Gaining and Losing Weight: General Tips

There are several tactics that you can employ to gain or lose weight. What follows are three general tips for gaining or losing weight in a manner that's effective, practical, sustainable and safe.

1. Set SMART goals.

Many individuals who try to manage their weight aren't very successful. Often at the root of their failure is that they either didn't set any effective goals or didn't set any goals whatsoever. Effective goals are SMART: Specific, Measurable, Attainable, Realistic and Timed.

Specific: One of the main reasons why people fail to achieve their goals is because they're not specific. The truth is that those who have specific goals in mind are more likely to reach them. A general goal is to get fit; this is abstract and has numerous interpretations. A specific goal is to increase the number of repetitions that you do in the leg press in your next workout; this is concrete and has one clear objective.

Measurable: If a goal can't be measured, it can't be assessed. And if a goal can't be assessed, how do you know if you've achieved it? So rather than have an ambiguous goal to exercise more, a measurable goal is to do strength training an average of two days per week; rather than have an ambiguous goal to eat more vegetables, a measurable goal is to consume three servings of vegetables per day. Goals that can be measured are more likely to be met.

Attainable: Although some people have goals that are specific and measurable, they're often far too difficult to achieve. A goal of losing 50 pounds of fat in three months, for example, can't be attained. An attainable goal is to lose one pound of fat per week for the next two months. Remember, too, that a successful outcome is more likely when a goal is within reach.

Realistic: Having realistic goals is closely related to having attainable goals. Don't set your sights on running a six-minute mile if the last time that you did so was 10 years and 20 pounds ago. Don't think about trimming your mid-section by a few inches if you get your three daily

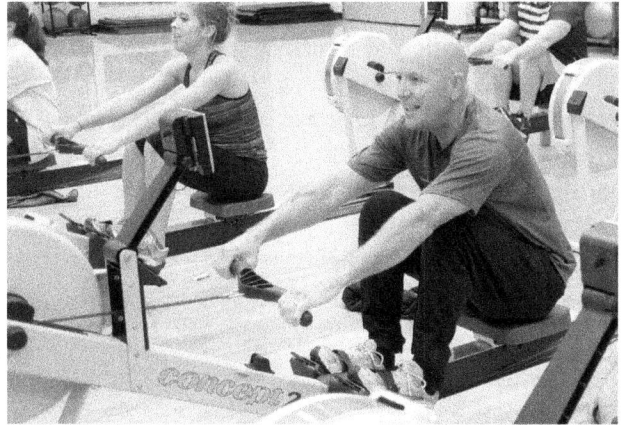

Aerobic training is important since it can produce a sustained and significant use of calories. (Photo provided by Greg Hammond.)

servings of fruit from a blueberry muffin, an apple pie and a banana split. In making realistic goals, it's important to be honest with yourself. Take into consideration things like your age, situation and motivation.

Timed: This means that you should put a time requirement on achieving your goal. A goal to gain five pounds of muscle has good intentions but when is it supposed to be attained? In two months? Six months? Whenever? The point is that it's easy to put off goals unless a deadline is attached. The deadline could be weeks or months or a specific date. For instance, a timed goal might be to gain 10 pounds of muscle by June 30. Or it might be to run a 5K by your 40th birthday.

2. Keep a food/activity diary.

Another important tactic for weight management is to keep a food/activity diary. Chronicling your efforts helps you to stay focused on your goals and progress (or lack thereof). Essentially, using a food/activity diary holds you accountable to yourself.

One study found that people who used a food/activity diary for at least six days per week lost about twice as much weight in six months as those who didn't use such a diary. There's no reason to think that this wouldn't also work for those who are interested in gaining weight.

You should record the specific foods that you eat as well as a rough idea of the quantity. By documenting this information, you may discover that you actually eat a different amount of food – either less or more – than you thought. You should track good choices (such as the servings of fruits and unsweetened beverages) and bad ones (such as the number of cookies and sweetened beverages). Although calories count, there's no need to literally count calories. You do need to be mindful of calories, however, without it being obsessive.

Since engaging in a fitness program is also an integral aspect of weight management, it's a good idea to maintain a record of your activities as well. Note the types of activities that you do along with the duration of the activities and, if applicable, the distances that you complete. Participation in formal activities (such as strength training and aerobic training), informal activities (such as walking, skiing and playing "pick-up games") and organized sports should be included.

3. Implement a few changes at a time.

There are a plethora of changes that you can employ to manage your weight. Although they have the best intentions, many people are often unsuccessful in their attempts for two reasons: One is trying to make changes that are too big; another is trying to make changes that are too numerous.

Dr. James Hill – the Director of the Center for Human Nutrition at the University of Colorado Denver and an authority in weight management – is an advocate of what's known as the small-changes approach. He and his colleagues have calculated that 90% of the population gets a surplus of about 50 calories per day which, of course, results in weight gain. Because of the metabolic costs that are associated with storing fat, 50 calories result from an excess of about 100 calories. Stated differently, decreasing caloric consumption, increasing caloric expenditure or a combination of the two that adds up to about 100 calories each day is enough to prevent weight gain in 9 out of 10 individuals.

If you're trying to lose weight, you'd need to produce a caloric deficit that's more than 100 calories per day. But the point is that a small-scale change can be effective and accomplished with relative ease. A good strategy is to limit yourself initially to three small, easy, doable changes that you can make without much sacrifice or effort. Once these three changes become part of your dietary routine, you can add more.

The effectiveness of a small-changes approach has been demonstrated in a number of studies and is endorsed by many organizations. This includes the Academy of Nutrition and Dietetics, the American Heart Association and the American Cancer Society.

The fact of the matter is that making a few changes at a time that are small, easy and doable increases the likelihood that those changes will become habits. And that's what you need to do: Get to the point where a change becomes a habit. Clearly, small changes can lead to big results.

THE RIGHT "WEIGH"

According to the World Health Organization, the number of adults aged 18 and older who are either overweight or obese was more than 1.9 billion in 2016; this represented about 52% of all adults on the planet. The term globesity has been used to indicate the global prevalence of obesity.

In an attempt to lose weight, many individuals resort to unhealthy and/or unsafe practices. This includes fasting and excessive exercise as well as the use of laxatives, weight-loss supplements and diet pills.

Many individuals also try fad diets. The list of fad diets seems endless, literally running from A (Atkins) to Z (Zone).

As the name suggests, fad diets are those that are trendy for a while and then fade away only to resurface at some point in the future (sometimes with a new name). Fad diets have at least four things in common. All fad diets (1) promise quick results (specifically, a rapid loss of weight); (2) offer short-term fixes, not long-term results; (3) fail to teach people the right way to eat; and (4) restrict one or more food groups or macronutrients.

Weight loss can be achieved in a manner that's effective, practical, sustainable and safe by following the approach as outlined in this chapter.

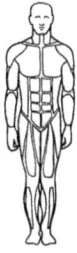

23 A Primer on Steroids

Strength training is done to increase muscular strength and size. Steroids are used as a means to accelerate these increases. As a result, strength training and steroids are inexorably linked. Therefore, any detailed discussion of strength training should include information about steroids.

MAJOR MOMENTS IN HISTORY

In some regards, the history of steroids began thousands of years ago with the belief that certain organs and their glandular extracts had medicinal and performance-enhancing qualities. The ancient Egyptians and Romans, for example, thought that the testicles had special healing powers; the ancient Greeks actually ate the raw testicles of animals. (Evidently, ass and sheep were favorite choices.)

Scientific investigations of glandular extracts – which come from the hormone-producing glands of animals – can be traced back to the late 19th century. In June 1889, at a meeting of the Paris Biological Society, Dr. Charles-Edouard Brown-Sequard – a French neurologist and physiologist – announced that he had given himself 10 injections with a liquid that included a small amount of water mixed with testicular blood, seminal fluid and "juice" that was extracted from the crushed testicles of a "perfectly healthy" dog (the first five injections) and a number of guinea pigs (the second five injections). Dr. Brown-Sequard, then 72, claimed that the injections, given over a three-week period, increased the maximum strength of the forearm flexors in his right arm by about 18.9% – as measured with a hand dynamometer – from 81.4 pounds to 96.8 pounds. (He also claimed that the injections improved his "intellectual labour," relieved his constipation and lengthened "the jet" of his urine.) Although these changes were

almost certainly the result of a placebo effect, he was the first scientist to associate glandular extracts with physical strength. (Fast fact: In a case of "who's your daddy," some consider Dr. Brown-Sequard to be the father of endocrinology while others consider Dr. Thomas Addison to have paternity rights.)

In the late 1890s, two scientists from what was then Austria-Hungary – Dr. Oskar Zoth, a physiologist, and Dr. Fritz Pregl, a chemist and physician – injected themselves with a liquid extract of bull testicles. In 1896, they concluded that daily injections of this extract coupled with daily exercise using "heavy dumb-bells" delayed the onset of fatigue, improved muscular power and increased the circumference of the upper arm. (Oddly enough, their conclusions were based on measuring the strength of their middle fingers.) Dr. Zoth may have been the first person to suggest giving these injections to athletes as a way to test the effects of testicular extracts.

The Emergence and Use of Testosterone

In 1935, within the span of about three months, three groups of scientists working for three pharmaceutical companies that were located in three countries made significant contributions to the research and development of steroids. The three companies who funded the groups were Organon (the Netherlands), Schering (Germany) and Ciba (Switzerland). In May, the Organon researchers isolated 10 milligrams (0.00035 ounces) of testosterone from 100 kilograms (220 pounds) of bull testicles (and, in the process, coined the name testosterone from the words testis, sterol and ketone). In August, the Schering researchers synthesized testosterone from cholesterol. And exactly one week after this breakthrough, the Ciba researchers accomplished the same thing and subsequently applied for a patent on their method. (Fast fact: In 1939, two of the researchers – Dr. Adolf Butenandt of Schering and Dr. Leopold Ruzicka of Ciba – shared the Nobel Prize in Chemistry.)

Several rumors about Germany and its association with testosterone date back to this period of time. (These rumors might be due to the fact that much of the early research on testosterone was conducted in Germany.)

The first rumor is that testosterone was given to some German athletes to prepare for the 1936 Berlin Olympics in which Germany garnered 89 medals, including 33 gold which was far more than any other country. (The United States was a distant second with 56 medals, including 24 gold.) This was an enormous improvement by Germany in comparison to the 1932 Los Angeles Olympics where the country finished ninth with 20 medals, including 3 gold. (That year, the United States led the way with 103 medals, including 41 gold.) A second rumor is that steroids were given to Nazi Schutzstaffel (SS) Troops during World War II to make them more aggressive and less fearful of violence. Although rumors of giving testosterone to German athletes and soldiers in this era are juicy, neither one has ever been confirmed. (It does appear as if German soldiers received some sort of stimulant to prevent fatigue on the battlefields, however.) A third rumor is that Adolf Hitler received injections of testosterone. Hitler was a drug addict who – according to Dr. Theodor Morell, his personal physician – used *roughly 80 different drugs*, including amphetamines, barbiturates, cocaine and opiates. Also on his laundry list were extracts from bull testicles and Testoviron, a compound consisting of two forms of testosterone – testosterone propionate and testosterone enanthate – that was developed by Schering (and is still available today). So this particular rumor does have a factual basis.

Sidebar: In the 1936 Berlin Olympics, Jesse Owens of the United States won four gold medals, setting world records in the 200-meter dash, long jump and 4 x 100 relay and tying the world record in the 100-meter dash. But his performance in the 1935 Western Conference (now the Big 10 Conference) Track and Field

Championships was even better. Owens – then a sophomore at Ohio State – achieved what must be the greatest feat in the history of sports. He set or tied four world records, first tying the world record in the 100-yard dash then setting world records in the long jump, 220-yard dash and 220-yard low hurdles . . . all of which were achieved *in the span of 45 minutes.*

In the late 1930s, testosterone was available for purchase in the United States in drugstores without a prescription. By the early 1940s, researchers started to investigate the effects of testosterone on muscular growth. It was only natural that there was a rising interest in testosterone as a performance enhancer. In fact, the first documented case of using testosterone to increase athletic performance was in 1941 . . . with an 18-year-old racehorse named Holloway. After testosterone pellets were implanted under its skin by Dr. Walter Kearns, the horse – which had been castrated a number of years before – quickly developed "a great deal of spirit and anxiety to exercise" and "firm muscles." The horse improved its performance such that in 23 races, it finished first five times, second five times and third three times. After one testosterone pellet was implanted under its skin, White Front – another racehorse that had been castrated – "did the best running of his career." (Interestingly, a racehorse named Calvin Dillon also received testosterone pellets but as its appetite, weight and training improved, it became "more fractious and disagreeable" and the experiments were discontinued.)

By the late 1940s, testosterone had muscled its way into the bodybuilding community on the west coast. From there, testosterone and its derivatives – collectively referred to as steroids – quickly infiltrated the athletic community.

Steroids and the "York Gang"

As early as the 1950s, athletes from Eastern Bloc countries were administered steroids – or steroid-like drugs – as part of government-sponsored programs. The first reported use among athletes was by Soviet weightlifters at the 1954 World Weightlifting Championships in Vienna, Austria (where the Soviet Union and

United States tied for first with each country winning seven medals). There, supposedly over "a few drinks," Dr. John Ziegler, the American team physician, was told by the Soviet team physician that some of his country's weightlifters were using testosterone.

In 1958, Ciba – a pharmaceutical company that was based in Switzerland – introduced a steroid known as methandrostenolone (trade name: Dianabol) to the United States. Originally, the steroid was intended for medical purposes. But in what has been described as "a patriotic response" to the drug-inspired success of the Soviet athletes, Dr. Ziegler – who was working with a Ciba laboratory in Summit, New Jersey – began testing the effects of the steroid by offering it to several competitive weightlifters at the legendary York Barbell Club in York, Pennsylvania.

To put this into perspective, it's important to understand the lofty status that was held by the York Barbell Club in that era. From around 1930 to the mid-1970s, the York Barbell Club – previously known as the York Oil Burner Athletic Club – was a juggernaut in American weightlifting. As a result, the town of York was considered the "mecca" of competitive weightlifting in America and nicknamed Muscletown USA. The United States, in fact, was consistently one of the top two or three teams in the world from the mid-1930s to the late 1950s with many of its weightlifters coming from the York Barbell Club (who were also employees of the York Barbell Company).

The first weightlifters from the "York Gang" to use Dianabol included Tony Garcy, Bill March and Louis Riecke. Others soon followed and the experiment quickly spun out of control. The weightlifters consumed far more than the recommended doses; it's said that they were "eating [the pink pills] like candy." It didn't help matters that when supplies of Dianabol ran low, prescriptions could be filled at Schultz's Drug Store which was located just a few blocks away from the gym. (Fast fact: Riecke later served as the strength coach of the Pittsburgh Steelers from 1970 to 1980, a period in which the team won four Super Bowls.)

Dr. Ziegler – who served as an officer in the US Marine Corps during World War II and was wounded in the historic assault on Tarawa – would later regret his role in introducing steroids to the weightlifters. To set the record straight about Dr. Ziegler, he didn't create Dianabol. And he isn't the person who's responsible for the extensive use of steroids in America.

Up until the early 1960s, steroids were mostly used by American and Soviet weightlifters. But that would soon change. In 1963, Alvin Roy became the first strength coach in professional football when he was hired by the San Diego Chargers of the American Football League (which merged with the National Football League in 1969). Roy had close ties to the York Barbell Club. Likely influenced by what had transpired at York, Roy introduced steroids to the football players, one of whom later stated that in the pre-season training camp, Dianabol was "mandatory" and on the table at every meal "in cereal bowls." Just before the season began, some players protested about having to take the steroid and it became optional. (It's important to understand that the laws, ethics and attitudes regarding the use of steroids were totally different in that era than today.)

The rampant use of steroids – along with a new generation of growth-stimulating drugs and so-called designer steroids – has been escalating ever since.

State Plan Theme 14.25

In 1949, a few years after the end of World War II, Germany was split into two countries: East Germany (the German Democratic Republic; controlled by the Soviet Union) and West Germany (the Federal Republic of Germany; allied with the United States, the United Kingdom and France). The two countries were physically separated by the "inner German border," an intricate system of heavy fortifications and security zones that stretched about 880 miles; it included metal fences and walls, electrified barbed wire, alarms, floodlights, anti-vehicle barriers and ditches, watchtowers, booby traps and minefields. Just in case these measures weren't enough to keep the border secure, there were also armed border guards and guard dogs. You get the idea. The purpose of the border wasn't to keep people from *entering* East Germany but to keep people from *exiting* it.

East Germany debuted at the 1968 Mexico City Olympics where the country finished fifth with 25 medals, including 9 gold. In the 1972 Munich Olympics, East Germany improved to third with 66 medals, including 20 gold. East Germany continued its meteoric rise to athletic prominence in the 1976 Montreal Olympics, 1980 Moscow Olympics and 1988 Seoul Olympics where the country finished second each time, collecting a total of 318 medals, including 124 gold. These were stunning achievements, especially considering that East Germany was roughly the size of Virginia with a population of about 17 million. (Fast fact: The United States and about 60 other countries boycotted the 1980 Moscow Olympics to protest the Soviet invasion of Afghanistan in 1979; in response to the American-led protestation, East Germany boycotted the 1984 Los Angeles Olympics as did 13 other Eastern Bloc countries and allies.)

Germany remained divided – literally and figuratively – until November 1989 with the fall of the inner German border and the better-known Berlin Wall (which had surrounded West Berlin, separating it from East Berlin and isolating it from West Germany). Following the reunification of Germany a year later, information began to surface that would ultimately reveal the most extensive and egregious use of steroids in history. It was discovered that from 1966 to 1990, an estimated 10,000 East German athletes or more were given steroids – some of whom were 14 years old or younger – as part of a highly organized program that was sponsored by the government. Among other things, the government – which took full control of the program in 1974 – distributed performance-enhancing drugs and encouraged research on developing and administering new drugs. Cryptically named Staatsplanthema 14.25 – translated as State Plan Theme 14.25 – the clandestine research program was overseen by the much-feared Ministry for State Security (aka the Stasi or secret police) and involved hundreds

of government officials, scientists, professors, physicians and coaches. The program was viewed as an "official state secret" and those involved were literally sworn to secrecy. Essentially, the athletes were experimented on like guinea pigs, being told that the blue pills they swallowed were vitamins and the injections they received were necessary medications. (In reality, the blue pills were oral-turinabol, the favored steroid of East Germany.) As a direct result of the steroids that the athletes were given, many of them suffered long-term damage, including liver disease, heart disease and cancer.

The revelation that East German athletes had used steroids came as little surprise to most people. Suspicions had been aroused for years because of their sudden success and dominant performances accompanied by numerous accounts of East German women who sported deep voices and facial hair. One of the more memorable anecdotes occurred at the 1976 Montreal Olympics. Legend has it that Kathy Heddy, a US swimmer, ran up to her coach, Jack Nelson, and informed him that there were men in the women's locker room. Coach Nelson famously responded, "No, dear, those are the East Germans."

PREVALENCE OF STEROID USE

Up to around 1980, steroids were mainly used by athletes to improve their performance. At that point in time, many underground handbooks and guides on steroids began to surface which spawned greater use by non-athletes. Since then, the vast majority of individuals who use steroids do so to improve their *appearance*, not their *performance*. In a survey of 500 steroid users, 78.4% (392 of 500) were non-competitive bodybuilders and non-athletes.

A 2014 study estimated that 2.9 to 4.0 million people in the United States (age 13 to 50) have used steroids for nonmedical reasons. About one million of those individuals have experienced dependence on steroids.

According to the 2015 Youth Risk Behavior Survey, about 3.5% of American high-school students (grades 9 through 12) have taken steroids without a prescription at least once in their lifetime. That might seem like a small percentage until you consider the fact that there are about 15 million students in public high schools. Do the math and that amounts to *about 525,000 students* who have used steroids without a prescription at least once. And remember, that's not counting those students who attend private schools.

According to the 2014 National Study of Substance Use Habits of College Student-Athletes in which about 21,000 individuals were surveyed, 0.5% used steroids during the previous 12 months (0.7% men; 0.1% women). In men's sports, usage was highest in soccer (1.2%), ice hockey (1.1%), football (0.9%), baseball (0.8%) and lacrosse (0.7%); in women's sports, usage was highest in gymnastics (0.7%), ice hockey (0.5%), crew (0.4%), field hockey (0.3%) and track (0.3%).

The use of steroids for nonmedical purposes occurs outside of the United States as well. A 2014 meta-analysis of 187 studies found that 3.3% *of the global population* took steroids in their lifetime for nonmedical reasons. This includes a prevalence rate of 6.4% in men and 1.6% in women. Also of note is a prevalence rate of 18.4% in "recreational sports people," 13.4% in athletes and 12.4% in prisoners and arrestees.

Interestingly, a web-based survey of 1,955 men who used steroids for nonmedical reasons determined a profile of a steroid user. The typical user was Caucasian, about 31 years old, using steroids since the age of about 26, well-educated (46% had at least a Bachelor's degree), employed as a full-time "white-collar" professional (3.9% were working in the fitness industry, by the way) and earning an above-average income (50% had an annual household income between $40,000 and $99,999). Moreover, the typical user was never involved in organized sports and took steroids to increase muscle mass, strength and physical attractiveness.

Any sport in which athletes rely on size, strength, speed and power will have a high prevalence of steroid use. For example, one study of 380 competitive bodybuilders found that 54% of the men and 10% of the women used steroids

on a regular basis. Besides bodybuilding, steroids are prevalent in competitive weightlifting (powerlifting and Olympic-style weightlifting), American football and track and field.

WHAT ARE STEROIDS?

Steroids are synthetic (lab-made) derivatives of testosterone that have anabolic as well as androgenic properties (thus the technical term of anabolic-androgenic steroids or AAS). The anabolic (growth-promoting) effects of testosterone include increases in strength, muscle mass, bone density, protein synthesis and nitrogen retention; the androgenic (masculinizing) effects include the development of male secondary sexual characteristics such as an increase in facial and body hair, a deepening of the voice and a heightened libido ("sex drive"). Scientists who develop steroids try to maximize the anabolic effects and minimize the androgenic effects.

Steroids can be taken by ingestion, injection, transdermal patch, cream, gel, lotion and subcutaneous pellet. By far, the most common way of self-administration is injection. And the most common site for injections is the buttocks; it's a relatively big target with a considerable amount of muscle mass that can accommodate larger doses and has a vast network of blood vessels that allows the steroid to be absorbed and transported faster to other tissues.

Several terms are frequently used in discussing the administration of steroids. This includes "stacking" (using two or more different types of drugs at the same time); "cycling" (alternating periods in which the drugs are used with periods in which the drugs aren't used); and "pyramiding" (increasing doses of the drugs for the first half of a cycle and then decreasing doses of the drugs for the second half).

Street names for steroids include 'roids, arnolds, gym candy and "the juice." Popular steroids (trade names in parentheses) are methandrostenolone (Dianabol), nandrolone decanoate (Deca-Durabolin), fluoxymesterone (Halotestin), oxandrolone (Anavar) and stanozolol (Winstrol). Also of note are designer steroids that are made in such a way as to avoid detection in drug testing. Two classic examples are "The Cream" (a semi-solid preparation of testosterone and epitestosterone that's applied transdermally) and "The Clear" (liquid drops of tetrahydrogestrinone – or, for short, THG – that are applied sublingually) which gained considerable notoriety during the federal investigation of Victor Conte and his Bay Area Laboratory Co-Operative (BALCO) that began in 2002.

ARE STEROIDS EFFECTIVE?

Up to the mid-1970s or so, the scientific and medical communities clung firmly to the belief that steroids didn't necessarily work. This was because at that point in time – despite more than two decades' worth of anecdotal evidence to the contrary – early studies offered no firm evidence that steroids were effective. For example, in its 1977 position statement that was "based on a comprehensive survey of the world literature," the American College of Sports Medicine (ACSM) cited 15 studies of which seven reported no increases in strength, lean-body mass and/or bodyweight from steroids "in amounts up to twice those normally prescribed for medical use." In addition, the ACSM statement noted that some of the increases in strength that were found in many studies "seem likely" due to the placebo effect.

Meanwhile, researchers in East Germany must have found the belief that steroids weren't effective to be quite amusing since their own secret studies and experiments – unpublished and unknown to the rest of the world – clearly showed otherwise (though using much higher doses than what was normally prescribed). Also undoubtedly amused by the belief that steroids weren't effective were untold numbers of coaches and athletes in the United States and elsewhere who had first-hand knowledge of and experience with the effectiveness of steroids, particularly in sports that placed a premium on strength, speed and power.

Later studies of steroids were better designed (meaning that the studies were randomized, double blind and placebo-controlled); used subjects who had a history of exercising; and employed doses that were more representative of the amounts that were actually being taken by athletes. These studies consistently showed that steroids were effective. In 1984, a revised ACSM position stand that was "based on a comprehensive literature survey" concluded that steroids "can often increase strength gains beyond those seen with training and diet alone." The position stand appeared to downplay those findings, however, adding that "this positive effect on strength is usually small and obviously is not exhibited by all individuals." The ACSM did acknowledge that small increases in strength "can be important in athletic competition."

It's now widely accepted that steroids increase strength, lean-body mass and bodyweight. These effects are amplified when steroids are taken in conjunction with strength training. Upon termination of steroid use, the drug-induced improvements in strength and size gradually diminish. There's no scientific evidence that steroids decrease fat mass. As a result, body composition is improved but mainly through an increase in lean-body mass. There's also no scientific evidence that steroids increase endurance or expedite recovery between workouts.

ARE STEROIDS SAFE?

A multitude of adverse effects from the use of steroids have been documented in the scientific and medical literature. It must be noted that for ethical reasons, studies often use relatively small doses of steroids and for short periods of time. In "real life," though, steroids are usually taken in much higher doses – which could be 100 times the therapeutic dose – and for longer periods of time thus presenting a much greater risk. So, if anything, research grossly *underestimates* the true extent of the adverse effects.

Keep in mind that what follows are *potential* adverse effects; there's a great deal of variability based on the type of steroid, dosing regimen and duration of use as well as individual sensitivity. Also worth mentioning is that while some adverse effects are reversible with cessation of use, others are not.

These adverse effects from steroid use are well-documented in the scientific and medical literature:

Liver

The second-largest organ in the body is the liver. (In case you're wondering, the largest organ is the skin.) The liver is highly vulnerable to steroid use. The most serious complications are peliosis hepatis (which results in the formation of blood-filled cysts throughout the liver) and liver tumors (both benign and malignant). These two conditions are considered life-threatening and irreversible.

Some researchers speculate that peliosis hepatis may be a pre-tumorous lesion that can become malignant with prolonged steroid use. Rupture of the blood-filled cysts or liver failure resulting from peliosis hepatis has often been fatal.

Numerous reports have been published that link the use of steroids with liver tumors. Moderate to heavy use of steroids in otherwise healthy individuals can cause liver cancer and even death over time. The period between the initial stages of liver cancer to the full-blown clinical expression may be more than five years. In other words, steroid users may have cancers growing in their livers but the symptoms have yet to reveal themselves.

The use of steroids in relatively low doses can also impair the excretory function of the liver and result in jaundice – a possible sign of liver disease or disorder – which gives the eyes and skin a yellowish tint. Finally, higher doses of steroids appear to increase the incidence of liver dysfunction.

Kidneys

Another organ of concern is the kidneys. The use of steroids increases the possibility of kidney stones, kidney dysfunction and kidney failure. Wilms' tumor – a rare kidney cancer that mostly affects children – has been associated with steroid use and can be fatal.

Cardiovascular System

There are also significant risks to the cardiovascular system. Steroids have been linked with high blood pressure (hypertension) and high cholesterol. These are two major risk factors for cardiovascular disease.

In regards to cholesterol, steroids increase low-density lipoprotein (LDL; the "bad" cholesterol) and decrease high-density lipoprotein (HDL; the "good" cholesterol). A "near ideal" range for LDL is 100 to 129 milligrams per deciliter (mg/dl) with 190 mg/dl and above considered very high; a good range for HDL is 50 to 59 mg/dl with 40 mg/dl and below considered poor. One steroid user, age 22, had an LDL of 596 and HDL of 14. Within one month of discontinuing steroids, his levels improved to an LDL of 220 and HDL of 35.

Additionally, steroids are associated with several heart conditions. This includes a thickening of the left ventricular wall which makes it more difficult for the ventricular chamber to fill and pump blood. Steroids are also linked with an increased risk of acute myocardial infarction (heart attack), cardiac arrhythmia (an irregular heartbeat) and sudden cardiac death.

One of the most graphic examples of the adverse effects that steroids have on the cardiovascular (circulatory) system was experienced by Steve Courson who began using steroids in college at the age of 18 and then throughout his eight-year career as a professional football player; he continued to use steroids even

Steroids have been linked with high blood pressure (hypertension).

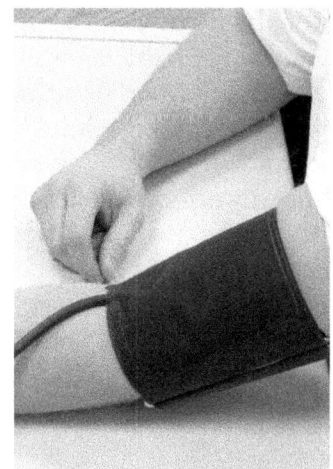

333

after his retirement in 1985. Courson – who was one of the first professional football players to acknowledge steroid use – encountered many adverse effects, including tachycardia (an accelerated heart rate). In 1984, his *resting* heart rate was as high as 160 beats per minute (bpm). When Courson checked himself into a hospital in 1988, his *resting* heart rate was 200 bpm. His medical problems forced him to seek a heart transplant . . . *at the age of 33.*

In 1989, Dr. Robert Malinowski, the Ashtabula County (Ohio) coroner who examined the body of Benji Ramirez, a high school football player, stated that steroids were a contributing factor in the 17-year-old's heart attack. This marked the first time that steroids had been officially linked to a death in the United States.

Reproductive System

Without question, steroids pose an enormous threat to the male and female reproductive systems. Essentially, steroids produce feminizing effects in men and masculinizing effects in women.

When a man introduces exogenous (external) testosterone into his system, his body reacts and reduces its production of endogenous (internal) testosterone in order to maintain a relatively stable internal environment (referred to as homeostasis). If too much foreign testosterone is added, his body will no longer produce its own supply.

This biochemical balancing act results in a number of adverse effects that are chilling. For instance, a decreased sperm count has been well-documented. One study found that the sperm count of 15 athletes was reduced by an average of 73% after two months of steroid use. Another well-documented adverse effect related to this hormonal irony is gynecomastia which is the appearance of female-like breasts on the male physique (which often requires corrective surgery). Other male-specific effects are prostate enlargement, sterility, functional impotency, testicular atrophy, difficult or painful urination and a high-pitched voice. (Given the high potential for sterility, it's no real shocker that testosterone has been investigated as a male contraceptive.)

When a woman introduces exogenous testosterone into her system, she experiences its androgenic effects and becomes more masculine. Some of these physical changes are irreversible, including enlargement of the clitoris, decreased breast size, hirsutism (an increase in facial and body hair), alopecia (a loss of scalp hair) and a deepening of the voice. Other adverse effects are an increased risk of breast cancer, uterine atrophy and menstrual irregularities (such as amenorrhea).

These adverse effects and others were noted in a study that involved 10 female steroid users. In this study, all 10 women reported a lowering of the voice; nine had increased facial hair; eight experienced enlargement of the clitoris, increased libido, increased aggressiveness and irritability and acne on the face and back; and five noticed a decrease in breast size and menstrual diminution or cessation.

Women who use steroids also increase their risk of bearing children with birth defects. When taken by pregnant women, steroids can cause masculinization of the fetus. The degree of masculinization is related to the amount of steroids being taken and the age of the fetus during the steroid use.

Psyche and Behavior

Steroids have the potential to produce a wide array of adverse effects that have a profound impact on psyche and behavior. This includes anxiety, euphoria, depression, extreme mood swings, irritability, schizophrenia, paranoia, auditory hallucinations, delusions of grandeur, sleep disturbances and an increased or a decreased libido.

In one study, researchers interviewed 41 bodybuilders and football players who had used steroids. Five of the subjects met the criteria for psychotic symptoms during periods in which they used steroids. None of the subjects had psychotic symptoms when they weren't using steroids. Of the five subjects who had psychotic symptoms, one had auditory hallucinations of voices and the other four developed various delusions. Another five subjects met the criteria for a manic episode during steroid exposure. One of these subjects bought an old car and deliberately drove it into a tree at 40 miles per hour while a friend videotaped him.

Perhaps the one psychiatric adverse effect that's most frequently discussed and displayed is commonly referred to as 'roid rage. In one study, 'roid rage was described as "a sudden and exaggerated aggressive response to a minimal provocation." Because of the high potential for impaired behavior, steroids jeopardize the safety of others. A classic example of 'roid rage was demonstrated by one individual whose steroid-amplified aggression involved him in numerous brawls and created violent thoughts like "crushing people to death" and "tearing off their limbs." Another steroid user – annoyed by a traffic delay – damaged three cars (with drivers inside) using his fists and a metal bar.

Speaking of behavior, one study found an association between steroids and criminality in that the initiation of steroid use led to an increase in criminal activity. And in a study of prisoners, those who tested positive for steroids were more likely to be convicted of a weapons offense than those who tested negative.

Research has shown that about 30% of the individuals who use steroids develop a dependence on the drug. The dependency can lead to classic symptoms of withdrawal – including depression and fatigue – when steroids are discontinued.

Linked to the psychological dependency on steroids is a condition known as muscle dysmorphia, a term that was coined by Dr. Harrison Pope and his colleagues in a 1997 issue of *Psychosomatics*. Individuals who have muscle dysmorphia are dissatisfied with their body, have low self-esteem and are preoccupied with their muscularity. Originally, the condition was referred to as reverse anorexia. With anorexia – which is more prevalent in females – no matter how much weight that a woman loses, she still sees herself as too big; with muscle dysmorphia – which is more prevalent in males – no matter how much weight that a man gains, he still sees himself as too small.

Many people who do strength training have the desire to increase their muscular size. But with muscle dysmorphia, this desire becomes pathological. In one review and meta-analysis, researchers pooled data from 31 studies that involved 5,880 subjects. They found an association between muscle dysmorphia and a number of psychological disorders, including anxiety, social physique anxiety, depression, neuroticism, perfectionism and low self-esteem. As might be suspected, the condition is more common among bodybuilders than others who simply do strength training.

Sidebar: Adding to body dissatisfaction are cultural ideals of the male physique that are sometimes well beyond the limits of mere mortals. For example, researchers measured the waist, chest and biceps of several action figures. When they scaled the measurements of a GI Joe Extreme to a 5'10" man, they found that he would have a 54.8" chest, 36.5" waist and 26.8" biceps. But wait: When they scaled the measurements of a Wolverine – a Marvel superhero – to a 5'10" man, they found that he would have a 62.0" chest, 33.0" waist and 32.0" biceps. Not to be outdone, researchers measured the chest, waist and hips of five Barbie dolls. When they scaled the average measurements to a 5'4" woman, they found that she would have a 30.9" chest, 15.3" waist and 27.3" hips.

Miscellaneous Adverse Effects

There are a variety of additional adverse effects as well. Steroid users are predisposed to connective tissue injuries. A study of 142 male bodybuilders found that steroid users had a risk of tendon rupture that was *nine times greater* than non-users. Moreover, all of the 19 steroid users who had ruptured a tendon incurred the injury only after they began using steroids. One theory is that steroids weaken connective tissue by inhibiting the formation of collagen, cellular proteins that provide structural support. To date, however, this has been shown in studies of animals but not humans. Another theory is that connective tissue doesn't respond to steroids to the same degree as muscle tissue. In other words, because of steroids, muscle tissue can improve

335

its strength and size at an accelerated rate. But connective tissue might not be able to adapt quickly enough to keep pace with the growing demands that are imposed on it from progressively heavier weights thereby increasing the possibility of serious tendon, ligament, fascia and meniscus injuries. This can be likened to installing a more powerful engine (muscle) in a car while retaining the transmission (tendon). Eventually, the increased torque that's generated by the stronger engine (muscle) would overpower the original transmission (tendon) and tear it to bits.

In one study, more than 14% of steroid users reported injection practices that were unsafe. This included reusing needles and sharing multi-dose vials and needles with others. Those who inject steroids run the risk of infection, blood poisoning and the spread of communicable diseases – such as hepatitis and human immunodeficiency virus (HIV) – from contaminated needles along with neural dysfunction as a result of improperly placed needles.

Adolescents who use steroids may experience a pre-mature fusing of their epiphyseal (or growth) plates which are cartilaginous discs that reside at each end of a long bone (such as the humerus and femur). A pre-mature closure of these structures could impede the longitudinal growth of a bone which isn't reversible.

There's strong evidence that the use of steroids leads to the use of other drugs. This, of course, represents a big problem and manifests itself in many ways.

One study found that 77% of self-reported steroid users also took at least one other illicit or nonmedical drug during the previous year. For instance, steroid users were almost 12 times more likely than non-users to take cocaine. Furthermore, studies have shown that steroid use is associated with opiate use – such as morphine and heroine – and a higher prevalence of alcohol use. In one study, 21 of 227 heroin addicts at a treatment facility were first introduced to opiate use through steroid use. In fact, 17 of those 21 individuals first purchased opiates from the same drug dealer who sold them steroids.

Individuals who use steroids also tend to employ other appearance- and/or performance-enhancing drugs such as human growth hormone and insulin. In addition, they may employ other drugs in an attempt to control the unwanted effects of steroids. For example, they may take amphetamines to combat depression; sedatives to overcome insomnia; diuretics to avoid fluid retention and reduce blood pressure; tamoxifen to prevent gynecomastia; and Human Chorionic Gonadrotropin (HCG; mainly prescribed to treat female infertility) to reverse or prevent testicular atrophy. (Diuretics and HCG are also used to mask the appearance of steroids in a drug test.)

The use of steroids can trigger an increase in oil production by the sebaceous glands of the skin and cause acne to develop anywhere on the body (though usually on the back). Additional adverse effects include fluid retention, alopecia, unprovoked nose bleeds, stretch marks and peptic ulcers.

TESTING FOR STEROIDS

In 1980, Dr. Manfred Donike – a West German biochemist who twice competed in the Tour de France – developed a technique for identifying abnormal levels of testosterone in the urine. His method – which continues to be the most common way of testing for steroids – looks at the ratio of testosterone to epitestosterone or, for short, the T/E ratio. Since the levels of epitestosterone in the body remain stable, testosterone from an outside source will elevate the T/E ratio.

A T/E ratio of 1:1 is normal with men having a slightly higher ratio and women a slightly lower ratio. Some people have a ratio of 2:1. A ratio of 3:1 is rare. In 1983, the International Olympic Committee – then recognized as the governing body in sports – employed a T/E ratio of 6:1 as the threshold (limit) for a positive test for steroids. In 2005, the World Anti-Doping Agency lowered the threshold to a T/E ratio of 4:1. Think of a 4:1 threshold like a speed limit of, say, 55 miles per hour. Staying at or below a speed of 55 miles per hour is legal while anything above it is illegal;

staying at or below a T/E ratio of 4:1 is legal while anything above it is illegal.

Since the 1980s, anti-doping laboratories have tested thousands of athletes. About 90% of them have a T/E ratio of 1:1. More than 99% are less than 5:1. Testing of 31,740 males and 15,841 females – most of whom were athletes – shows that among men, 99% have a T/E ratio of 4.6 or less and among women, 99% have a T/E ratio of 4.3 or less. This means, of course, that a small percentage of the population has levels of natural testosterone that are greater than the legal limit. (More on that point in a bit.)

Here's a synopsis of how the testing generally works: After giving a urine sample, the individual divides it into two bottles – an A sample and a B sample – and then seals the bottles which are sent to a laboratory for testing. If the A sample has a T/E ratio that's 4:1 or less, then the results are negative for steroids; if the A sample has a T/E ratio of more than 4:1, then the results are positive for steroids. In this case, a follow-up test is done with the B sample using a carbon isotope ratio (CIR) test. The T/E ratio only reveals the ratio of testosterone to epitestosterone; the CIR test – developed by Dr. Don Catlin – can determine if the testosterone is natural (endogenous) or artificial (exogenous). A person who fails a test for steroids has tested positive in both the T/E ratio and CIR test.

Sidebar: The first testing for steroids at an international competition was the 1974 British Commonwealth Games in Christchurch, New Zealand. The first testing for steroids at an Olympic competition was the 1976 Montreal Olympics. And the first testing for steroids that used the T/E ratio was at the 1983 Pan American Games in Caracas, Venezuela.

East Germany: Detection Deception

Unbelievably, despite the massive use of steroids by thousands of East German athletes for nearly 25 years, only two athletes – both female – ever tested positive for steroids on the international stage. The first athlete was 17-year-old Marlies Oelsner who tested positive for steroids at the 1975 European Athletics Junior Championships in Athens after finishing second

in the 100-meter dash. However, the European Association didn't leak the results of her urine test to the public. Sorry, bad pun. Later, as Marlies Göhr, she set the world record in the 100-meter dash (10.88 seconds in 1977) and won four Olympic medals (two gold and two silver).

The second athlete was Ilona Slupianek who tested positive for steroids at the 1977 European Cup in Helsinki after finishing first in the shot put. Later, Slupianek set the world record in the shot put – holding the title for a little more than four years – and won a gold medal at the 1980 Moscow Olympics in the shot put.

From that point on, no East German athlete ever tested positive for steroids. After the incident with Slupianek, to avert any future embarrassment and suspicion, East Germany began to pre-test its athletes for steroids prior to any international competition that did testing. (The East Germans referred to this as "departure control.") It's said that the Central Doping Control Laboratory in Kreischa administered about 12,000 tests per year to screen East German athletes. From years of conducting extensive research and keeping meticulous records, East German scientists were able to predict exactly how long it took for each athlete's T/E ratio to return to a level that would result in a negative test. An athlete whose T/E ratio was deemed too high to drop enough to test negative withdrew from the competition, often citing an injury or illness as the reason.

The system of screening athletes became clear after Germany was reunified in 1990 and investigators uncovered a trove of classified documents in Stasi files. Records showed the results of "in-house" tests on four East German female swimmers who had won a total of 10 Olympic gold medals. The pre-tests were done at the laboratory in Kreischa on August 9, 1989, about one week before the European Aquatics Championships in Bonn, West Germany. Testing positive on that date (T/E ratio in parentheses) were Heike Friedrich (8.8:1), Dagmar Hase (10.0:1), Daniela Hunger (12.5:1) and Kristin Otto (17.0:1). Remember, these were women. Despite their high T/E ratios, the quartet was sent to swim in the meet. They medaled in seven individual events (four gold, two silver and one bronze) and all three relays (claiming four gold medals) and helped East Germany to collect the most medals of any country in the championships. As predicted, their T/E ratios returned to a level that resulted in a negative test for steroids.

Many East German athletes often received a "counter-injection" of epitestosterone to normalize their T/E ratio in an attempt to mask the appearance of steroids. This practice is still done by athletes and, as a result, epitestosterone – which has no ergogenic value – is banned by the World Anti-Doping Agency as a masking agent.

East Germany Redux

In 2016, Dr. Grigory Rodchenkov – then the director of the anti-doping laboratory in Moscow – revealed that Russia had been engaging in a highly organized drug program that was sponsored by the government. The program – which was eerily reminiscent of that which was conducted by East Germany – was in effect from at least late 2011 to August 2015, involving more than 1,000 athletes who competed in more than 30 sports. This period of time spanned five major international competitions, including the 2012 London Olympics and 2015 International Association of Athletics Federations (IAAF) World Championships in Beijing along with three that were hosted by Russia on its home turf: the 2013 Summer Universiade (for university athletes; held in Kazan); the 2013 International Association of Athletics Federations World Championships (held in Moscow); and the 2014 Sochi Olympics.

Prior to this, many Russian athletes received drugs from coaches and physicians "in the field." The government took control of the drug program when it became evident that this "old school" method risked detection. As part of an early initiative in 2012, Dr. Rodchenkov – the whistleblower who's now hiding somewhere in the United States – developed a "cocktail" that consisted of oral-turinabol, oxandrolone and methenolone. These three steroids were dissolved in alcohol (Chivas whisky for men and vermouth wine for women). The mixture was swished in the mouth in order to be absorbed and then spit out. Dr. Rodchenkov determined that when taken in this manner, the steroids wouldn't be detectable after three to five days. (A later version used trenbolone – another steroid – in place of oral-turinabol.) The mixture of steroids was passed along to the various sports federations which, in turn, provided it to the athletes.

Implicated in the scandal were government officials in the Ministry of Sport; the Federal Security Service (aka the FSB; formerly the KGB which is similar to America's Central Intelligence Agency or CIA); and the Center of Sports Participation along with the Russian Anti-Doping Agency and its testing laboratories in Moscow and Sochi.

The wide-scale cheating was done two ways. One way was to falsify test results. If an athlete had a positive test for steroids or other performance-enhancing drugs, laboratory workers were directed to simply record the result as a negative test. From 2011 to 2015, more than 500 positive tests were falsely recorded as negative.

The other way was to swap "dirty" urine samples for "clean" urine samples. The "clean" samples had been collected from the athletes during periods in which they were "clean" – that is, they weren't using steroids or other performance-enhancing drugs – and kept in frozen storage until needed. Agents of the FSB had perfected a way to remove the bottle caps from the urine samples without leaving any visible trace of tampering. Whenever testing was done under the watchful eyes of international observers, FSB operatives were deployed to covertly exchange urine samples.

Harkening back to the tactics that were employed by East Germany, Russia pre-tested its athletes for steroids and other performance-enhancing drugs prior to any international competition that did testing. (This practice is now known as washout testing.) An athlete whose level of banned drugs was deemed too high to drop enough to test negative withdrew from the competition.

Sidebar: The vetting of Russian athletes for this purpose may have been going on for several decades prior to 2011, however. There are reports that during the 1988 Seoul Olympics, Russian athletes were pre-tested for steroids and other performance-enhancing drugs on the cruise ship *Mikhail Sholokhov* which was parked off the South Korean coast.

In the immediate aftermath of the scandal, 111 Russian athletes were banned from the 2016 Rio Olympics, including 67 of 68 track and field athletes (a female long jumper was allowed to compete), 26 of 30 rowers and all 10 weightlifters. Russia was banned from the 2016 Summer Paralympics in Rio and the 2017 IAAF World Championships in London. However, 19 of its athletes were allowed to compete in London as "authorized neutral athletes." And 169 of its athletes were allowed to compete in the 2018 PyeongChang Olympics as "Olympic Athletes from Russia."

The Athlete Biological Passport

A relatively new concept in testing for steroids – and other performance-enhancing drugs – is the Athlete Biological Passport (ABP). Introduced in 2009, the ABP examines selected biological variables of an athlete that have been collected over a period of time. In other words, the ABP is a historical record that compares an athlete's result/sample to his/her previous results/samples (rather than to a reference population).

The rationale behind using the ABP is that some people have naturally high levels of testosterone which could unfairly result in a positive test for steroids. But an individual's T/E ratio doesn't fluctuate too much from its average value; it varies less than 30% in men and up to 60% in women. Therefore, a T/E ratio that's high but consistent with an individual's baseline levels would be normal. On the other hand, an abnormal variation in or sudden spike from baseline levels of the T/E ratio – or any other marker in someone's "steroid profile" – could indicate the use of steroids. (Fast fact: The steroid that's found most often during testing of athletes is testosterone; the next most common are nandrolone, stanozolol and methandienone.)

Therapeutic Use Exemption

In certain instances, athletes are allowed to take steroids and other performance-enhancing drugs. Wait, what? An athlete who has a documented illness or medical condition can apply for what's known as a Therapeutic Use Exemption (TUE).

The governing body will grant a TUE in cases where (1) the athlete would experience a significant impairment to health if the drug was withheld; (2) the drug isn't likely to enhance performance beyond what would be expected from the athlete returning to a normal state of health; and (3) there's no reasonable alternative to using the drug.

OVERT SIGNS OF STEROID USE

Coaches, parents and employers may be interested in identifying the use of steroids. Although this is virtually impossible without testing, there are a few tell-tale signs.

Because steroids can be taken by injection or in tablet/pill form, users may have needles, syringes and/or pill bottles either hidden or in their possession. Puncture marks, bruises, scar tissue or calluses on the buttocks and/or upper thighs from injections are overt signs.

Many physical indicators of steroid use are related to the adverse effects. For example, users often have a bloated, puffy look to their faces and skin due to fluid retention. In addition, their eyes and skin may have a yellowish tint (from jaundice). A sudden and significant increase in size, weight and strength can also be a sign of steroid use. Other physical indicators are severe acne, alopecia, gynecomastia, unprovoked nosebleeds and stretch marks (likely due to the sudden and significant increase in size).

In terms of psychological signs, a sudden and exaggerated aggressive response for little or no reason is a behavior that may be an indication of steroid use. Other signs of steroid use can be severe depression and a significant change in libido.

Just because one or two of these signs are present doesn't necessarily indicate steroid use. However, if there are more than a few signs, the use of steroids becomes more likely.

TESTOSTERONE REPLACEMENT THERAPY

Steroids have a number of therapeutic uses and are prescribed by physicians to treat a number of medical conditions. This includes anemia, osteoporosis, significant weight loss and/or muscle-wasting from chronic infections (such as HIV), serious trauma, severe burn injuries and recovery from surgery or illness.

But the most common therapeutic use for steroids is in testosterone (or hormone) replacement therapy (TRT) to treat hypogonadism, a condition in which the gonads (testes) produce a level of testosterone that's below the normal range of healthy men. Signs and symptoms of hypogonadism include decreased libido, erectile dysfunction, gynecomastia, reduced muscular strength and size, increased body fat, depression, osteoporosis and diminished energy. (Fast fact: Total testosterone refers to all of the testosterone in the body, some of which isn't available to the cells; free testosterone refers to the testosterone that's available to the cells and, thus, is a better indicator of low testosterone or "low T.")

As men age, their level of testosterone gradually decreases; the decline usually begins around the age of 30. It's little surprise, then, that testosterone is heavily promoted for "anti-aging" purposes. In fact, you've probably seen commercials on television and/or advertisements in magazines for TRT. These promotions are quite effective: From 2000 to 2011, worldwide pharmaceutical sales of testosterone increased from $150 million to $1.8 billion.

The vast majority of testosterone prescriptions are written for men who are 40 and older. From 2001 to 2011, the use of TRT among men in that age group more than tripled, increasing from 0.81 to 2.91%. In 2011, 2.29% of men in their 40s and 3.75% of men in their 60s were getting some form of TRT. Men younger than 30 can experience hypogonadism but it's exceedingly rare; a leading endocrinologist stated that the incidence of hypogonadism among healthy 30-year-old men is less than 0.1% which is less than one in one thousand.

When a man with above-average levels of muscular strength and size pursues TRT, it raises an eyebrow. Indeed, how could a seemingly virile man have low testosterone? Well, remember that when exogenous testosterone enters the body, the production of endogenous testosterone is reduced to maintain a stable internal environment. Therefore, someone who has a history of steroid use may really have low testosterone and actually need TRT. (This is referred to as steroid-induced hypogonadism.) In one study, 19 male weightlifters (average age 42.7) who used steroids for a total of at least two years had significantly lower testosterone than 36 male weightlifters (average age 42.9) who never used steroids. Moreover, testosterone levels that were below the normal range of healthy men – a biochemical marker of hypogonadism – were seen in 10 of the 19 subjects (52.6%) who used steroids but only 8 of the 36 subjects (22.2%) who never used steroids.

To ensure that testosterone is prescribed by a physician for the treatment of hypogonadism – and not something else like the development of muscular strength and/or size to improve appearance and/or performance – individuals who are required to be drug tested may be asked to provide medical documentation that their level of testosterone is consistent with that of a hypogonadal man. On a related topic, athletes can apply for a TUE for TRT. However, some sports-governing bodies rarely grant TUEs for this purpose; *none* were issued by the International Olympic Committee for the 2012 London Olympics, for example. And currently, the Nevada Athletic Commission will not grant TUEs for TRT to athletes who participate in combat sports, including boxing, kickboxing and mixed martial arts.

TRT isn't without risks. The short-term risks of TRT include prostate cancer, prostate enlargement, heart disease, testicular atrophy and sterility.

At this time, the long-terms risks of TRT are unknown but one study captured the attention of the medical community. In the Testosterone in Older Men with Mobility Limitations (TOM) trial, 209 men aged 65 years or older with mobility problems and low testosterone were randomly assigned to receive either a testosterone gel or a placebo gel. The subjects who were given testosterone significantly improved their maximum strength in the leg press and chest press and power while stairclimbing with tote bags containing 20% of their bodyweight. That's the good news. The bad news is that they also had a significantly greater frequency of cardiovascular events, including heart attack, stroke, chest pain and hypertension. Specifically, adverse cardiovascular events were experienced by 23 of the 106 subjects (21.7%) who received testosterone and 5 of the 103 subjects (4.9%) who received the placebo. Because of safety concerns, the study was discontinued earlier than intended.

Sidebar: Early research investigated the effects of steroids on hypogonadism and impotency. Later research focused on performance. Interestingly, research has returned to investigating the effects of steroids on hypogonadism and impotency.

A MATTER OF ETHICS

The use of steroids in an attempt to improve physical capacity or athletic performance is contrary to the ethical principles and regulations of competitions as established by various athletic foundations and sports-governing bodies. Among the organizations are the International Association of Athletics Federations; the International Olympic Committee; and the National Collegiate Athletic Association.

Strong anti-steroid statements have also been issued by the National Strength and Conditioning Association and the American College of Sports Medicine as well as all major sport leagues, most notably the National Basketball Association, National Football League, National Hockey League and Major League Baseball.

STEROIDS AND THE LAW

Steroids can be purchased legally without a prescription in some countries. But in the United States, it's illegal to do so without a prescription. Steroids weren't regulated in this country until the Controlled Substances Act (CSA) of 1970 went into effect in 1971. The CSA – which regulates a wide range of drugs – has been amended multiple times. Three of the amendments pertain specifically to steroids: the Anabolic Steroids Control Act of 1990 (which classified 27 steroids as Schedule III controlled substances); the Anabolic Steroids Control Act of 2004 (which added more steroids to the list); and the Designer Anabolic Steroid Control Act of 2014 (which expanded the list of steroids that are regulated to include about two dozen new substances).

Sidebar: Schedule III controlled substances are those that may lead to moderate or low physical dependence or high psychological dependence. Besides steroids, the list of Schedule III controlled substances includes stimulants and depressants.

Federal law makes simple possession of steroids without a prescription punishable by up to one year in prison and/or a minimum fine of $1,000. The penalties increase for those with previous convictions for certain offenses. For first-time offenders, selling steroids or possessing them with the intent to sell is punishable by up to five years in prison and/or a $250,000 fine. Those penalties double for second-time offenders.

Federal law makes simple possession of steroids without a prescription punishable by up to one year in prison and/or a minimum fine of $1,000.

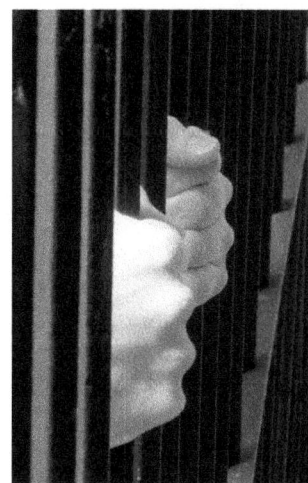

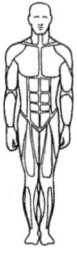

24 Evaluating the Research

How many times have you heard on the television or read in the newspaper that "a recent study found that . . ." or "new research shows that . . ."? Do you automatically accept what's reported by the media on the topics of nutrition and fitness as the gospel truth? If so, you shouldn't.

Case in point: A March 2014 article in *The New York Times* was titled "Study Doubts Saturated Fat's Link to Heart Disease." A week later, the newspaper ran an op-ed titled "Butter is Back" (in which the author urged readers to "go back to eating butter, if you haven't already"). *Time* magazine was much more emphatic a few months later. The cover of its June 23 issue carried the headline of "Eat Butter. Scientists labeled fat the enemy. Why they were wrong."

The inspiration for those periodicals was a study that appeared in the *Annals of Internal Medicine*, a publication of the American College of Physicians. The study was a review and meta-analysis that investigated the association between the intake of fat and coronary heart disease. After reviewing and analyzing 72 studies, the researchers concluded: "Current evidence does not clearly support cardiovascular guidelines that encourage high consumption of polyunsaturated fatty acids and low consumption of total saturated fats."

The meta-analysis was quickly met with a heavy barrage of sharp criticism from a phalanx of scientists, including many who referred to it as misleading and flawed along with several from the Harvard School of Public Health who cited "gross errors" and called for its retraction. (About two months later, the journal published an erratum to correct an abundance of "numerical errors" in the meta-analysis.) Among other things, the meta-analysis was flagged by the academic community for including poor studies while excluding good studies and "misrepresenting" evidence, all of which skewed the findings. The meta-analysis also failed to mention the benefit of replacing saturated fat with unsaturated fat which can significantly reduce deaths and events that are related to heart disease. In a study that looked at more than 80,000 women, for example, the researchers estimated that replacing 5% of the calories from saturated fat with calories from unsaturated fat would reduce the risk of coronary heart disease by 42%. And contrary to what was haphazardly reported by much of the media, the meta-analysis didn't determine, recommend or imply that people can eat as much saturated fat as they want without remorse.

But the damage had already been done. Without a doubt, untold numbers of people read the cover story in *Time* magazine that instructed them to "eat butter" and considered this as an open invitation to go on a feeding frenzy for fat. (Fast fact: Butter is about 0.1% carbohydrate, 0.9% protein, 81.1% fat, 15.9% water and 2.0% other nutrients; 51.4% of the fat in butter is saturated fat.)

To make a long story short, it's a good idea for you to be skeptical whenever you hear or read a media report of a study that's related to nutrition and fitness.

TERMINOLOGY

Before discussing any guidelines for evaluating research, it's important to understand some terminology that you'll likely encounter on a regular basis. Here are some terms with which you should be familiar:

An *abstract* is a brief summary of a study. It appears at the beginning of a study and usually is limited to no more than about 250 words.

The *experimental group* consists of the subjects (aka participants) who receive a treatment or an intervention. Some studies have two or more experimental groups that receive different treatments.

The *control group* consists of the subjects who didn't receive a treatment or an intervention. This group is used as a point of comparison to see if any change by the experimental group was the result of the treatment.

A *placebo* is a substance that contains no active ingredients. Often, it's a sugar pill and should be similar in appearance, taste and smell to the product that's being studied so that the subjects can't distinguish between the product and the placebo. Besides a pill, a placebo can also be a device or an item. For example, a study could compare the effects of a performance-enhancing bracelet to a fake (or "sham") bracelet that looks the same as the experimental bracelet.

A *variable* is something that can be changed. There are two types of variables: independent and dependent. Independent variables are the presumed cause and are controlled by the researchers. In a study of strength training, independent variables might be sets, repetitions, equipment or frequency of training. Dependent variables are the presumed effect and are measured by the researchers. In a study of strength training, dependent variables might be muscular strength, muscular size, peak power and percentage of body fat. To isolate the true cause of one or more effects, the researchers should manipulate only one independent variable and keep the others the same. So a study that examines the effects of repetitions on muscular strength and size should assign different repetition schemes to the experimental groups without changing the number of sets, the type of equipment, the frequency of training or any other independent variable.

Correlation refers to the association between two variables. A high correlation means that there's a strong association. However, correlation doesn't imply causation. (More on that point in a bit.)

The term *significant* appears regularly in studies (or a derivative of the word such as significantly). In normal dialogue, significant means important; in statistical dialogue, significant means probably true. It's used to describe the amount of change that's made by a group as well as the difference between two or more groups. When the amount of change is said to be significant, it means that it's probably true that the amount of change was the result of the treatment rather than pure chance. When the difference between groups is said to be significant, it means that it's probably true that the difference between groups was the result of the treatment rather than pure chance.

A *p-value* is the probability of obtaining a result and is the metric that researchers employ to determine whether the amount of change that's made by a group or the difference between groups is considered to be significant. Studies typically use a probability of 5% which is a p-value of 0.05. When $p < 0.05$, it means that there's less than a 5% probability (5 of 100) that the amount of change or the difference between groups was pure chance. Or, stated otherwise, it means that there's more than a 95% probability (95 of 100) that the amount of change or the difference between groups was the result of the treatment.

Bias is any action that distorts the true findings of a study. It's not unusual for a study to contain some degree of bias. The bias could be intentional or unintentional and can occur before, during or after the study. It manifests itself in many ways, including how the study is designed, how the data are interpreted and how the results are reported. Ironically, bias can also occur if a study *isn't* published. When studies that report negative or inconclusive findings don't get published, it's known as publication bias.

TYPES OF STUDIES

There are many different types of studies. Being able to distinguish between the types will help you to understand research and evaluate it. (Fast fact: The basic structure of an original study is summarized by the acronym IMRaD which stands for Introduction, Methods, Results and

Discussion; this is the standard format that's used in scientific publications.)

A *case study* is an in-depth review of one individual. This type of study must be interpreted with caution since the effects that are experienced by "a sample of one" (aka "an N of one") can't be extrapolated to the general population.

In an *experimental study* (aka a treatment or an intervention study), the subjects are assigned to an experimental group or a control group. As noted earlier, the experimental group receives a treatment and the control group doesn't.

In a *crossover study*, the subjects receive the experimental *and* control treatments. One group gets Treatment A followed by Treatment B while the other group gets Treatment B followed by Treatment A. The groups receive each of the assigned treatments for a designated period of time (which could be days or weeks, depending on what's being studied). In between the two treatments is a washout period that allows ample time for the first treatment to exit – or "wash out" of – the system so that there are no residual effects that might influence the second treatment. The subjects serve as their own controls in a crossover study.

A *survey* is a type of study in which quantifiable information is collected from a population or a subset of a population. Examples of surveys include questionnaires and interviews. Perhaps the most widely-known survey is the US Census.

A *cross-sectional study* is an observation of a population or a subset of a population at one specific point or "cross-section" of time. An example is measuring the body composition of a football team at the start of pre-season camp (or a subset of the team such as the offensive linemen).

A *longitudinal study* is an observation of a population or a subset of a population at several different points over a long time. An example is measuring the body composition of a football team a few times over the course of a season, perhaps at the start of pre-season camp, in the middle of the season and after the final game. A well-known longitudinal study is the Framingham Heart Study that has been going on since 1948.

A *position stand* (aka a position statement and consensus paper) is done by a panel of experts on behalf of an organization or a group. This yields a set of guidelines or "best practices" that's based on the available research that has been published on a specific topic. For instance, the Academy of Nutrition and Dietetics has a position stand on "Use of Nutritive and Non-Nutritive Sweeteners"; the American College of Sports Medicine has a position stand on "Exertional Heat Illness during Training and Competition" and the National Athletic Trainers' Association has a position stand on "Anabolic-Androgenic Steroids."

In a *literature review* (aka a systematic review), researchers conduct an exhaustive analysis of all studies of acceptable quality that examined a specific topic. A review should include all relevant studies, not just the ones that are consistent with the perspectives of the researchers who are performing the review.

A *meta-analysis* is a type of study that has been growing in popularity. Here, the results of studies that investigated the same thing are pooled together into one large study. So, for example, a meta-analysis that looks at 10 different studies with 50 subjects in each study now has a compilation of data on 500 subjects. The criteria that are used to select studies for a meta-analysis shouldn't exclude any studies that contradict the perspectives of the researchers who are performing the meta-analysis.

QUESTIONS TO ASK

The mere mention of a study makes it sound as if there's credible evidence that a product or a program is effective. But the study may be poorly designed, irrelevant or taken out of context. And that's why it's imperative for you to "study the study" whenever possible so that you can separate *science fact* from *science fiction*.

But once you get your hands on a study – the *actual* study, not just an abstract or a media report – how do you evaluate it? Here are 16 questions that you should ask to determine if a study has any credibility:

1. Was the study published in a scientific journal?

Some studies haven't been published anywhere; others appear in non-scholarly publications. In either case, it means that the study didn't go through a rigorous peer-review process in which experts in a related field (aka referees) do an impartial review of the manuscript to determine whether or not it should be published.

With very few exceptions, magazines in bookstores and on newsstands are non-scholarly publications. Any claims about the safety or effectiveness of products and programs in these types of publications are largely based on anecdotal evidence, meaning that support is rooted entirely in personal experience, not scientific research. This isn't much better than someone in the fitness center who says that after using a certain product or doing a certain program, his arm circumference increased by 1.5 inches, his sprint time in the 40-yard dash decreased by 0.2 seconds and his bench press improved by 50 pounds. Basically, his "success story" is anecdotal evidence. The individual may have gotten bigger, faster and stronger but there's no concrete proof that the changes were caused by the product or the program.

Also be wary of information that's available on the Internet where quackery abounds. Although the emergence of the Internet has given people access to an unbelievable amount of information that's literally at their fingertips, not all of it is credible. Remember, any crackpot with a keyboard can – and does – post information on the Internet.

2. Was the study properly designed?

Just because a study is published in a scientific journal doesn't guarantee that it's well designed. Consider this: A journalist submitted the same basic study of a "wonder drug" to 304 open-access journals. The study carried the names of fictitious authors and affiliations and was intentionally loaded with design flaws that

should have stuck out like a proverbial sore thumb. Yet, more than half the journals accepted the spoof study for publication. (When accepted, the study was withdrawn by the journalist so that it was never actually published.) Only 36 of the 304 journals gave review comments that the study contained design flaws. However, 16 of the 36 still accepted the study for publication.

The gold standard in clinical research is a randomized, double-blind, placebo-controlled study. What does this mean?

In a randomized study, the subjects are randomly assigned to groups – rather than selected or chosen for certain groups – in such a way that the physical/physiological profile and size of each group are roughly the same.

In a double-blind study, the researchers who are distributing the treatment and the subjects who are receiving the treatment are unaware – or "blinded" – as to who is getting what.

And in a placebo-controlled study, one group of subjects receives a treatment and another group – a control group – receives a placebo.

3. Who were the subjects in the study?

It's important to consider the subjects who were studied. For a study to be relevant, the subjects should be somewhat similar to the population of interest.

Fucoxanthin – a compound that's found in edible brown seaweed – has been promoted as a substance for losing weight/fat. In one study, 35 female subjects were fed a diet that was prepared according to the recommendations of the American Institute of Nutrition. The subjects were assigned to four experimental groups, supplementing their diets with either 0.1% fucoxanthin, 0.2% fucoxanthin, fish oil or 0.1% fucoxanthin and fish oil. (A fifth group acted as a control and didn't receive any supplement.) After just four weeks, the group that was fed the diet that included 0.2% fucoxanthin *gained 36% less bodyweight* than the group that was fed the control diet. But – and this is a really big but – the subjects in the study were mice.

Responses that are experienced by animals can't always be generalized to humans. A classic example is resveratrol, a chemical that's found in red grapes and wine that has been touted as an anti-aging substance for improving health and increasing longevity. In one study, 52-week-old mice were assigned to three experimental groups: One group was fed a standard diet; the second group was fed a high-calorie diet; and the third group was fed a high-calorie diet plus resveratrol. The group that was fed the high-calorie diet plus resveratrol experienced significantly greater improvements in lifespan – the mice lived longer – and several markers of health more than the group that was fed the high-calorie diet. There were no significant differences between the group that was fed the high-calorie diet plus resveratrol and the group that was fed the standard diet, suggesting that resveratrol offset the effects of a high-calorie diet. But to get the same relative amount of resveratrol as the mice, two scientists estimated that a human would have to consume *about 333 glasses of red wine each day*. Good luck with that.

Even if a study does involve humans, they may only be representative of a very small segment of the population. Years ago, boron was promoted as a substance for increasing muscular strength and size less than three months after the publication of a study by the US Department of Agriculture which showed that subjects who received boron increased their testosterone by as much as 268%. What wasn't emphasized about the study, however, was the fact that the subjects were 12 post-menopausal women, aged 48 to 82, whose testosterone levels were naturally low. Also, prior to taking the supplement, the women had been deprived of an adequate intake of boron for 119 days. Because post-menopausal women have a physical/physiological profile that's considerably different than the general population – or a subset of the population such as competitive athletes – it's not reasonable to expect that others will experience the same effects from boron.

4. How many subjects were in the study?

The number of subjects that are in a study is known as the sample size. Determining what constitutes an adequate number of subjects requires the use of calculations or tables but, even then, is a matter of some debate. To a degree, it depends on the type of study and what's being studied. A survey may require thousands of subjects, an experimental study may require 100 subjects and a crossover study may require even less. In general, a larger number of subjects will yield results that are more accurate and applicable. However, a study with too many subjects might not be practical, placing a strain on time, budget and personnel.

The point, though, is that a study with a very small sample size – the so-called small N – tells us little about the safety and effectiveness of a product or a program. To be clear, a study that has a small sample size doesn't necessarily mean that it's flawed or should be disregarded. But it might be a big stretch to draw a valid conclusion from a small N.

5. Was the study of sufficient duration?

There's no clear guideline as to what constitutes an adequate length of a study; like sample size, it depends on the type of study and what's being studied. And like sample size, a study that's too long might not be practical, placing a strain on resources.

When a study is too long, there's also a greater potential that some subjects will not adhere to the experimental protocol, withdraw or otherwise be "lost to follow-up" which results in missing data. What's certain, though, is that long-term studies are needed to assess the safety and effectiveness of a product or a program.

6. Was the methodology (experimental protocol) unbiased?

A graphic example of biased methodology was illustrated in a study of 34 Division III football players. In the study, the athletes were randomly assigned to two groups that did either single-set training or multiple-set and strength/power training. But besides being assigned to use different numbers of sets, the groups were also assigned to use different repetition ranges, different equipment, different exercises, different volumes of exercises and different amounts of recovery between sets. A large number of independent variables makes it impossible to compare the results of two groups and draw valid conclusions. Indeed, there's no way to tell which variable was responsible for the effect.

Also of note in this particular study is that pre- and post-testing included the hang clean, an exercise that was included in the program of the multiple-set group but not the single-set group. In effect, the multiple-set group practiced the hang clean twice per week for 14 weeks (as well as a highly related movement – a hang pull from mid-thigh – once per week) while the single-set group had no practice whatsoever. This gave the multiple-set group much greater familiarity with the hang clean and, as a result, placed the single-set group at a severe disadvantage when it came to being post-tested in that exercise.

7. Did the study account for outliers (low responders and high responders)?

An outlier is numerically distant from the rest of the data. The fact of the matter is that some individuals will be low responders and show little or no improvement from a product or a program while others will be high responders and show large improvement.

Consider the HERITAGE (HEalth, RIsk factors, exercise Training And GEnetics) Family Study. In this study, 481 individuals from 98 two-generation families did aerobic training on a stationary cycle three times per week for 20 weeks. On average, the subjects increased their oxygen intake by about 0.4 liters per minute (L/min). However, their response to training ranged from literally no change to more than 1.0 L/min which was 2.5 times the average improvement.

Also worth noting is the FAMuSS (Functional Polymorphisms Associated with Human Muscle Size and Strength) Study. In this study, 585 individuals did strength training with their non-dominant arm (biceps) for 12 weeks. On average, the subjects increased their cross-sectional area (muscle size) by 0.50 square inches (in^2), their isometric strength by 16.53 pounds and their dynamic strength by 8.60 pounds. However, their response to training in those three variables ranged from a *decrease* of 0.08 in^2 to an increase of 2.11 in^2 in cross-sectional area; a *decrease* of 35.05 pounds to an increase of 115.96 pounds in isometric strength; and *no change* to an increase of 22.49 pounds in dynamic strength.

In this study, an outlier was characterized as anyone whose response to training was at least two standard deviations away from the norm. In terms of absolute changes, the researchers identified 19 outliers (5 low responders and 14 high responders) for cross-sectional area; 24 outliers (4 low responders and 20 high responders) in isometric strength; and 17 outliers (0 low responders and 17 high responders) in dynamic strength.

Examining the relative changes that occurred in this study paints a clear picture of the variability in the response to training. Of the 585 subjects, 232 subjects increased their cross-sectional area between 15 and 25% while 36 subjects gained less than 5% and 10 subjects gained more than 40%; 119 subjects increased their isometric strength between 15 and 25% while 102 subjects gained less than 5% and 60 subjects gained more than 40%; and 232 subjects increased their dynamic strength between 40 and 60% while 12 subjects gained less than 5% and 36 subjects gained more than 100%.

The problem with outliers is that they can skew the data and produce false or misleading conclusions. For instance, suppose that a data set was comprised of 10 data points: Nine subjects had a one-repetition maximum (1-RM; the maximum weight that can be lifted one time) of 100 pounds and one subject had a 1-RM of 300 pounds. The average of those 10 data points is 120 pounds but 9 of the 10 subjects – *90% of them* – are well below the average with a 1-RM of 100 pounds. So the subject who had a 1-RM of 300 pounds – an outlier – distorted the data. Outliers can really wreak havoc on the data in studies that have a small number of subjects.

8. Did the study find significant changes?

Imagine a study in which the subjects are randomly assigned to two groups: One group receives a supplement and the other group receives a placebo. Both the supplement and the placebo could produce a significant change in some dependent variable – such as muscular strength or size – without there being a significant difference between the supplement and the placebo. So the group that received the supplement might experience a greater amount of change than the group that received the placebo but the difference between the two groups might not be large enough to conclude that the supplement is superior to the placebo; rather, the difference may be due to pure chance.

It's important to understand, too, that a change or difference can be *statistically significant* but not *clinically significant*. In other words, the change or difference may be so small that it has no practical consequence in the real world. For instance, what if a study found that after 26 weeks, the subjects who received a product lost significantly more weight – three times as much weight, in fact – as the subjects who received a placebo? At first glance, that sounds quite impressive but what if "three times as much" meant that the product produced a weight loss of three pounds while the placebo produced a weight loss of one pound? A difference of two pounds between the product and the placebo no longer sounds impressive – especially after 26 weeks – and has little relevance to people who are trying to lose weight.

9. Did the study show a true cause and effect?

An oft-stated maxim in statistics is that correlation doesn't imply causation. In other words, a correlation between two variables doesn't mean that one caused the other; it could simply be a coincidence or pure chance. Nonetheless, this shouldn't be dismissed completely since there really could be an association between the two variables.

A physician once wrote a brief article, making the case that there's a "powerful" correlation between the amount of chocolate that a country consumes per capita and the number of Nobel Prize winners that a country produces (which was used in the article as a proxy for cognitive function). His article – which was published in *The New England Journal of Medicine* – had some drawbacks. For one thing, the data used the consumption of chocolate by individual *countries*,

not individual *Nobel laureates*. Also, the data showed the consumption of chocolate over a two-year period but looked at more than 100 years of Nobel laureates.

In response to the article, researchers in Belgium pointed out that there was a high correlation between the number of Ikea® furniture stores that a country has per capita and the number of Nobel Prize winners that a country produces. And the correlation was actually *higher* than that of chocolate. So just because there's correlation doesn't mean that there's causation.

Similarly, there has been an ongoing attempt to link high fructose corn syrup (HFCS) with obesity. The roots of this movement can be traced back to researchers who noted that from 1970 to 2000, as the consumption of HFCS increased, so did the rate of obesity. They concluded that HFCS causes obesity. But again, correlation doesn't imply causation. Over the same 30 years, as property taxes increased, so did the rate of obesity. Does this mean that there's a correlation between property taxes and obesity? No more than there's a correlation between obesity and property taxes. There are far too many variables at play in the obesity epidemic to single out one variable as the dastardly villain.

So if correlation doesn't imply causation, what does? Well, the best way to show causality is through a randomized, double-blind, placebo-controlled study. In other words, it's through a study that involves an *intervention*, not an *observation*.

10. Did the study have dropouts and, if so, how were the missing data handled?

Most studies – particularly those that involve a large number of subjects and are of long duration – will have dropouts. Subjects withdraw from studies for a variety of reasons. For instance, they might experience a major change in life (such as moving away from the area or losing a job), sustain an illness or incur an injury (which could be related or unrelated to the study). Or some subjects may simply choose to no longer participate. Regardless of the reason, when subjects are "lost to follow-up," it results in missing data. And missing data can be related to the safety and effectiveness of a product or a program.

Of no small importance are dropouts that are a direct result of a treatment, something that could bias the outcome of a study and distort the conclusions. For example, if a large number of subjects withdrew from a study because they experienced an adverse effect, then this could have a major impact on the outcome and its interpretation, especially if the dropouts weren't evenly distributed among the experimental and control groups.

One literature review looked at 235 studies in which significant results were found. Dropouts were reported in 191 of the 235 studies. In most cases, the studies – which were published in five prestigious medical journals over a three-year period – had no explanation as to why the subjects were lost to follow-up. So the literature review used plausible assumptions and found that as many as 33% of the studies would no longer have significant results when the dropouts were considered. It's pretty clear, then, that dropouts can have an enormous influence on outcomes.

Researchers should note how they accounted for the missing data from the subjects. In the aforementioned literature review, 20% of the studies didn't report how the missing data were handled.

There's no standard way to account for missing data. One approach, however, is the Last Observation Carried Forward Method. As the name implies, when a subject withdraws from a study, the data that are last recorded are "carried forward" to the end of the study.

While on the topic, studies in which the number of dropouts is much less than would be expected should raise an eyebrow. In one study, 83 subjects followed a ketogenic diet for 24 weeks. Studies that investigate diets tend to have high dropout rates, especially when the intake of carbohydrates is severely restricted as is the case with a ketogenic diet. And as noted, studies that involve a large number of subjects and are of long duration are guaranteed to have

dropouts. Yet after nearly six months of following a highly restrictive diet, *none* of the 83 subjects had dropped out of the study. That's pretty much unheard of. Compare that to another study that investigated diets in which 53 women were randomly assigned to one of two experimental groups, using either a diet that was very low in carbohydrates or a diet that was moderately low in fat. By the end of six months, 11 of the 53 subjects dropped out of the study. Those numbers are about what would be expected.

11. Did the data support the conclusions?

Researchers sometimes draw conclusions that aren't supported by the data. This could be intentional or unintentional and can occur for a number of reasons. One typical reason is overgeneralizing the results. An example would be a study that found doing sets of lower repetitions of the bench press produced a significantly greater improvement in muscular strength than doing sets of higher repetitions and then broadly concluding that lower repetitions are superior to higher repetitions even though only one exercise was examined. Another example would be a study that found using a certain supplement produced greater increases in muscular size than a placebo and then broadly concluding that the supplement is safe and effective even though adverse effects weren't investigated or mentioned in the results or discussion sections.

Other reasons in which the data fail to support the conclusions have to do with the design of the study. This includes utilizing data that are inadequate (such as from having a small number of subjects) and using poor methodology (such as from having more than one independent variable).

Remember, the conclusions are where researchers have the opportunity to put their own spin on the data. As "spin doctors," they can employ data that support their position and ignore data that doesn't. Therefore, it's a good idea to review the design of the study with great care to see if the data really defend the conclusions.

12. Did the study report spectacular results?

As they say, "If it sounds too good to be true, it probably is."

According to advertisements for the Range of Motion (ROM) machine, using it for "exactly four minutes per day" will produce the "combined results" of 20 to 45 minutes of aerobic training, 45 minutes of strength training *and* 15 to 20 minutes of stretching. In other words, four minutes on the machine is supposedly the equivalent of 80 to 110 minutes of physical activity.

One study of the ROM machine was conducted in The Netherlands and carved into two poster presentations that were shown in 2007 at the 54th Annual Meeting of the American College of Sports Medicine in New Orleans. The presentations were published as two brief abstracts in *Medicine & Science in Sports & Exercise*. In the study, 16 subjects used the machine three times per week for eight weeks. Each session involved eight minutes of training, four minutes with the upper body followed by four minutes with the lower body. Over the course of eight weeks, each subject trained for a total of three hours and 12 minutes. In a cycling test to exhaustion, the subjects increased their endurance by 72%, from 14:51 to 25:31 and no, that's not a typo. This outcome is so spectacular – an average improvement in endurance of 9% per week from 24 minutes of exercise per week – that it must be interpreted with extreme caution.

An earlier study of the ROM machine was conducted in late 1994 at the University of Southern California. In this study, 24 subjects were assigned to two experimental groups: One group used the ROM machine for four minutes per day and the other group used the ROM machine for eight minutes per day. (A third group acted as a control and didn't train.) The experimental groups trained five days per week for 8.5 weeks. The subjects who exercised four minutes per day improved their maximum oxygen intake by almost 6% in about two months. These results are much more realistic. The study and its findings were summarized in a two-page letter that was sent to the company that sells the ROM machine. (The company also funded the study.) A third page supposedly contained the test results but that page is no longer with the other pages so many details are lacking. Though never published in a scientific journal – or anywhere else, for that matter – it's still mentioned on the company's website as a "scientific study." The researcher later distanced himself from the study and its findings.

13. Was there a selective reporting of the results?

To paraphrase a quote that was made in the early 1960s by Dr. Ronald Coase, a British-born economist, "if you torture the data long enough, you can make it confess to anything." Unfortunately, the selective reporting of results – a form of bias – isn't unusual. Indeed, a study that looks at enough dependent variables is bound to find one positive outcome. (Fast fact: In 1991, Dr. Coase was awarded the Nobel Prize in Economic Sciences.)

In one literature review, researchers examined selective reporting in 37 studies that were published in a prestigious medical journal. The review compared the summary protocols of the studies when they were first accepted for publication to the studies after publication. In 11 of the 37 studies, there were "major differences" in the primary outcome between the accepted version and the published version. Eight studies introduced a new primary outcome. No reasons were given for the changes.

On a related note, the same outcome can result in two conclusions that are quite similar but with vastly different messages. For instance, suppose that there was a study in which one group did slow-speed repetitions and another group did fast-speed repetitions. After 12 weeks of training, both groups significantly increased their vertical jump and there was no significant difference between groups. Based on these outcomes, a researcher who personally favors fast-speed training might conclude that doing slow-speed repetitions was no better than doing fast-speed repetitions for improving the vertical jump; a researcher who personally favors slow-speed training might conclude that doing fast-speed repetitions was no better than doing slow-speed repetitions for improving the vertical jump. Technically, both conclusions are correct and based on the same outcome yet convey different meanings.

Researchers should report *all* results, not just those in which their findings match their feelings. A selective reporting of results or ignoring/withholding unfavorable evidence – sometimes referred to as cherry picking the data – is unscientific and, frankly, unethical.

14. Did the study find any adverse effects or report any injuries?

A study might show that a product or a program lives up to its hype but it's important to know whether or not it resulted in any adverse effects or injuries.

Sodium citrate is a supplement that has been promoted for improving endurance. In one crossover study, nine elite athletes ran 3,000 meters on two separate occasions: one time after receiving sodium citrate and the other time after receiving sodium chloride (table salt). The subjects ran 3,000 meters significantly faster – by an average of about 10 seconds – after consuming sodium citrate. And don't forget, these were elite athletes so a 10-second improvement in a 3,000-meter run is pretty substantial. That's the good news. The bad news is that when using sodium citrate, eight of the nine athletes experienced gastrointestinal distress.

It's equally important to consider injuries. Maybe a study found significant improvements in, say, muscular strength and body composition. That sounds great. But what if an alarming number of subjects dropped out of the study due to injury? That doesn't sound great.

Even if study didn't find any adverse effects or report any injuries, the duration might have been too short. Long-term studies are needed to assess the safety and effectiveness of a product or a program. Remember, individuals might use a product or a program for months or years, not days or weeks. So it's all well and good if a product doesn't produce any adverse effects after four weeks but after six months, will you grow a third eye in the middle of your forehead or sprout hair on your knuckles?

Also take into account that many studies don't investigate adverse effects or injuries. In other studies, adverse effects and injuries go unreported.

Along these lines, individuals often take more than one product at a time. Combining two or more products can yield adverse effects.

15. Was the study funded and, if so, by whom?

Nowadays, reputable journals require researchers to disclose all sources of funding and professional relationships with any company or organization that may benefit from favorable outcomes . . . and for good reason.

Studies on a product are often funded by manufacturers of the same product. When a manufacturer pays to have its own product investigated, it increases the possibility that the study could be biased in some way. Needless to say, studies that are funded by manufacturers that have a direct financial interest in the outcome should be viewed with suspicion.

Industry financing has been investigated extensively and the results are unequivocal: The outcome of a study tends to favor the funder. An analysis of 206 studies found that studies with industry funding were about four to eight times more likely "to be favorable to the financial interests of the sponsoring company" than studies without industry funding. An analysis of 162 studies that were published in four psychiatric journals found that studies in which there was a conflict of interest were nearly five times more likely to have a positive outcome than studies without a conflict of interest. That's nothing: An analysis of 398 studies that were published in two medical journals found that researchers who had a conflict of interest were *10 to 20 times more likely* to present a positive outcome than those without a conflict of interest. Clearly, the funding can affect the finding.

Try to determine if any of the researchers have financial ties to the sponsor of the study. This includes being a paid employee or consultant, serving on an advisory board, receiving honoraria, owning stocks and having a patent agreement. Similarly, try to determine if any of the researchers have financial ties to a product or a program that's being studied. Remember the study on resveratrol, a substance that has been touted as having anti-aging properties? In that 2006 study, one of the researchers declared as a "competing interest" (aka a conflict of interest) that he was a co-founder of Sirtris Pharmaceuticals, "a company whose goal is to develop drugs to treat age-related diseases." (Fast fact: In 2008, Sirtris Pharmaceuticals was purchased by GlaxoSmithKline for $720 million.)

If there's a conflict of interest, you must decide whether it could have influenced (biased) the outcome of the study. Note: Just because there's a conflict of interest doesn't mean that a study is biased.

16. Were the results of the study replicated by other researchers in other laboratories?

There are instances where several studies show the same results but are conducted by the same researchers at the same laboratories. For there to be compelling evidence, similar results need to be found by different researchers at different laboratories. When different groups of researchers investigate the same topic and show

comparable results, it also adds to the body of existing evidence.

Furthermore, similar results that are produced by different researchers reduce the chance that the studies were biased toward a specific result. Otherwise, we're left to wonder, "Did the doctor 'doctor' the data?" In fact, cases of fraud are often uncovered when other laboratories are unable to replicate the results of a study.

Fraud is more prevalent in research than most people think. According to a meta-analysis that included 18 studies, nearly 2% of researchers admitted to having "fabricated, falsified or modified data or results at least once." And a little more than 14% of researchers admitted that they had "personal knowledge of a colleague who fabricated or falsified research data or who altered or modified research data." With the volume of studies that are published, those numbers are quite disturbing.

ANALYZE THIS!

It's important to stay abreast of the latest research on strength and fitness. To determine the true value of a study, its content must be fully analyzed. Having a basic understanding of terminology, the types of studies and the questions to ask will improve your ability in evaluating the research.

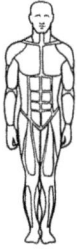

25 Strength and Conditioning FAQ

There are a number of topics that don't fit neatly into the content of the previous 24 chapters but still merit discussion. This final chapter contains 50 topics in a Q&A format that pertain to various aspects of strength and conditioning.

1. Does the position of the feet affect which part of the gastrocnemius is used during the calf raise?

Changing the position of the limbs during the performance of an exercise is believed to target different parts of a muscle. In the calf raise, for instance, some individuals change the position of their feet thinking that this will influence different parts of their calves.

Researchers randomly assigned 20 subjects to perform the standing calf raise with their feet in three different positions: neutral, internally rotated (toes pointed in) and externally rotated (toes pointed out). The subjects performed one set of 12 repetitions in each of the three positions without wearing any footwear. The calf raise was done with their forefeet elevated on a 1.5-inch block while holding a barbell across their shoulders. The weight of the barbell plus the barbell plates was equal to about 35% of their bodyweight. Testing of all three positions was done within one 30-minute session.

When their feet were externally rotated, there was significantly greater activation of the medial (inner) gastrocnemius; when their feet were internally rotated, there was significantly greater activation of the lateral (outer) gastrocnemius.

It would seem that during the calf raise, then, the position of the feet *does* target different parts of the gastrocnemius. Be that as it may, some individuals may find it uncomfortable to do the calf raise with their feet rotated excessively in one direction or the other.

2. What's the best grip width to use when doing the bench press with a barbell?

In one crossover study, 24 subjects were assigned to perform the bench press with a barbell using different grip widths on six separate occasions: two with narrow grips, two with moderate (medium) grips and two with wide grips. In each case, the subjects used the maximum weight that they could lift one time. The subjects lifted significantly more weight with the moderate grips than with the narrow and wide grips. In this study, the moderate-width grips were about 26 to 32 inches or 165 to 200% of biacromial breadth. (Fast fact: Biacromial breadth is the distance between the most lateral points on the acromion processes; the acromion process is essentially the tip of the shoulder.)

You don't have to collect this anthropometric data and calculate your ideal grip width for the bench press. Simply use a grip in which your hands are spread slightly wider than shoulder-width apart.

Think about this: If you were to get into a push-up position, you'd place your palms on the floor and almost certainly spread your hands slightly wider than shoulder-width apart. Why did you do that? You knew instinctively that this offers you more leverage than a narrow or a wide placement of your hands. So why do the bench press with a wide grip?

Different grip widths can also be used when doing the overhand lat pulldown. According to gym lore, "wide grip equals wide lats." As clever as this phrase might sound, it doesn't match reality.

In one crossover study, 15 subjects were randomly assigned to perform the overhand lat pulldown using three different grip widths: narrow, medium and wide. In each case, the subjects used the maximum weight that they could lift six times. Testing of all three grip widths was done within one session. In general, the three grips produced similar muscle activation. Though not statistically significant, the medium grip – essentially the hands spread slightly wider than shoulder-width apart – produced greater muscle activity throughout the positive (raising) and negative (lowering) phases of the repetitions. The subjects lifted 4% more weight with the narrow and medium grips than with the wide grip. In this study, the medium-width grip was 150% of biacromial breadth (which, again, is your hands spread slightly wider than shoulder-width apart).

An advantage of using a wide grip in the bench press and overhand lat pulldown is that the weight moves a shorter distance. However, a disadvantage of using a wide grip is that it results in a loss of leverage. So there's a trade-off. And the advantage of moving the weight a shorter distance isn't enough to overcome the disadvantage of a loss in leverage.

Plus, in using a wide grip in these and other multiple-joint movements, your joints are exercised throughout a much shorter range of motion than using a moderate/medium grip. In effect, when using a wide grip, you're doing partial repetitions which means that you're stimulating *part* of the muscle, not *all* of the muscle.

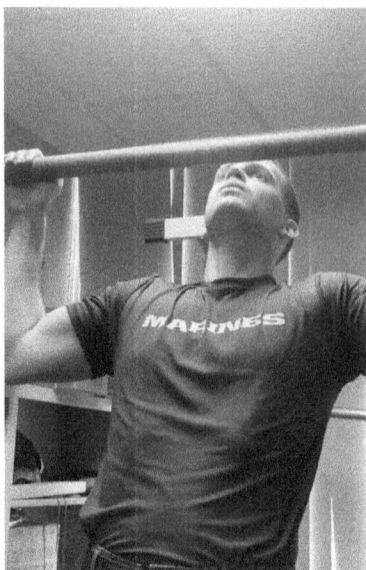

Doing pull-ups in a smooth, controlled manner and throughout a full range of motion is far more effective than doing kip-ups. (Photo provided by the US Marine Corps.)

3. Is a kipping pull-up safe and effective?

Essentially, a kipping pull-up is characterized by wildly swinging the legs, aggressively snapping/yanking the shoulders and elbows and then barely sneaking the tip of the chin over the bar. An "advanced" version of it is the butterfly kipping pull-up which is similar except that the body moves continuously in a rapid, elliptical motion. Ugh.

It's important to understand that a kipping pull-up isn't the same thing as a standard pull-up so let's not even call it a pull-up. Let's call it a kip-up.

The only branch of the US Armed Forces that incorporates pull-ups in its Physical Fitness Test (PFT) is the Marine Corps. In its PFT, "whipping, kicking or kipping of the body or legs, or any leg movement used to assist in the vertical progression of the pull-up is not authorized." In civilian-speak, this means that someone could do 50 kip-ups and not one would be counted as a legitimate pull-up. Not one. (On a related note, people who brag that they can do 50 pull-ups probably did 50 kip-ups. Big difference.)

It's often argued that the kip-up is more "functional" than the pull-up in "real life." For example, it's pointed out that if you were ever hanging from a ledge in "real life," you wouldn't pull yourself up and over it with strict form. Agreed. But you wouldn't pull yourself up and over it with a kipping motion, either. Do that and you'll almost certainly lose your grip on the ledge. Remember, you can't wrap your fingers and opposable thumbs around a ledge like you can around a pull-up bar. And if the ledge is too close to the structure, you won't have enough space to kip. Besides, how often have you found yourself hanging from a ledge in "real life"? And seriously, if you're hanging from a ledge, then you're probably up to no good.

Doing pull-ups in a smooth, controlled manner and throughout a full range of motion – upper chest to the bar at the top and arms fully extended at the bottom – is far more effective than doing kip-ups. It's not even close. Kip-ups involve an enormous amount of momentum that's initiated by swinging the legs which significantly reduces the involvement of the muscles that would otherwise be strengthened in that exercise. To be clear: Relative to the pull-up, the kip-up is useless for increasing the strength of your upper back, biceps and forearms.

The inherent dangers of kip-ups have been voiced by many professionals in the sportsmedical community. For one thing, kipping produces high forces that must be absorbed by the body. All of the force that's created by whipping the legs gets transmitted right up the body, from the legs to the hips to the lower back to the shoulders to the elbows. In particular, the shoulder and elbow joints get yanked pretty good.

Another risk of kip-ups lies in the forced hyperflexion of the shoulder. When initiating the kip, the upper arms move past the head which basically puts the shoulder joint in the same precarious position as the behind-the-neck/head lat pulldown and behind-the-neck/head shoulder press, two exercises that have long been avoided due to a heightened risk of shoulder injury. When done for high repetitions, kipping increases the risk of injury to the rotator cuff as well as what's known as a SLAP tear or lesion. (SLAP stands for superior labrum anterior posterior.)

Not to be forgotten is the forced hyperextension of the lumbar spine while kipping. This makes the lower back vulnerable to injury, especially when kip-ups are done for high repetitions.

In looking at this in terms of risks and rewards, kip-ups carry high risks and *no* rewards. Enough said.

Bottom line: Stay strict and skip the kip.

4. Why is it easier to do a chin-up than it is to do a pull-up?

Regardless of how you position your hands, just about any type of multiple-joint movement for your torso that involves a pulling motion targets the same muscles, namely your upper back, biceps and forearms. However, there are differences in your biomechanical leverage based on the grip that you use. For example, doing a chin-up with an underhand grip (palms facing

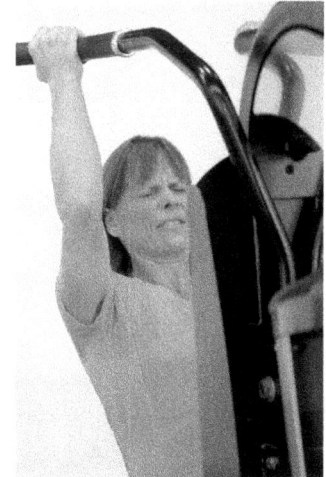

Doing a chin-up with an underhand grip is more biomechanically efficient than doing a pull-up with an overhand grip. (Photo provided by Luke Carlson.)

toward the body) is more biomechanically efficient than doing a pull-up with an overhand grip (palms facing away from the body). With an underhand grip, the radius and ulna – the bones in the lower arms – run parallel to one another; with an overhand grip, the radius crosses over the ulna forming an X. In this position, the bicep tendon gets wrapped around the lower portion of the radius, creating a biomechanical disadvantage and a loss in leverage. As a result, it's more difficult to do a pull-up than it is to do a chin-up.

This is also true when comparing underhand (supinated) and overhand (pronated) grips during other pulling and rowing movements; the same muscles are used but with varying degrees of biomechanical leverage. (Fast fact: With a parallel grip – in which the palms are facing each other – the bones in the lower arms don't cross, either; therefore, a parallel grip is also more efficient than an overhand grip.)

5. Is rotating the torso while holding a stick across the shoulders an effective exercise?

To train their obliques, many individuals sit on a bench, place a wooden stick (or similar object; sometimes a barbell) across their shoulders and rotate their torso. Or, they hold a medicine ball with their arms straight and parallel to the floor and rotate their torso in the same manner. But these exercises do little, if anything, for the obliques.

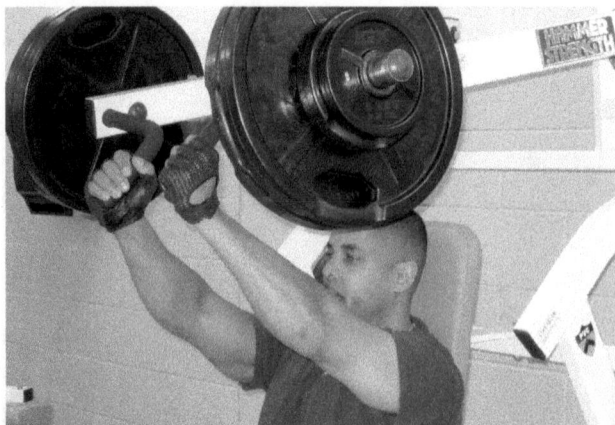

Studies have shown that there are no significant differences in the development of strength when comparing groups that used free weights and groups that used machines.

In order for an exercise to be as effective as possible, you must apply a force that opposes the resistance by 180 degrees. In other words, the application of the force must be *exactly opposite* the direction of the resistance. If the resistance is from the south, the force must be applied to the north; if the resistance is from the east, the force must be applied to the west.

Gravity is a force that always pulls straight down. Because of the effects of gravity, the force that's applied to any "dead weight" – such as a barbell or dumbbell – must be straight up. When you push or pull a barbell or dumbbell – or something similar – straight up while gravity acts straight down, the application of the force is absolutely perfect: It's 180 degrees out of sync with the resistance.

From this, it can be seen that rotating the torso with a stick (or similar object) that's placed across the shoulders is an incorrect – and ineffective – application of force. No matter how much the object weighs, the resistance is always straight down. Therefore, the force needs to be applied straight up or *perpendicular* to the floor, not *parallel* to it.

The most effective way to do torso rotation is on a machine. Here, the application of the force is congruent with the direction of the resistance.

6. Are free weights better than machines for increasing strength?

Studies have shown that there are no significant differences in the development of strength when comparing groups that used free weights and groups that used machines. The fact is that the use of *any* equipment that can expose the muscles to progressively greater demands will stimulate improvements in strength (and size, for that matter).

In one study, 22 subjects were randomly assigned to two groups: One group did the bench press and shoulder press with free weights; the other group did similar exercises with machines. Both groups used the same training protocol (three sets of six repetitions done three times per week). After five weeks, the subjects in the free-weight group increased the strength of their elbow extensors by about 22% and shoulder flexors by about 12%; the subjects in the machine group increased the strength of their elbow extensors by about 24% and shoulder flexors by about 13%. There were no significant differences between the two groups.

This isn't much of a bombshell because the same exercises that are done with barbells and machines activate the same muscles. In one study, 12 subjects were randomly assigned to perform three exercises – the bench press, shoulder press and close-grip bench press – with a barbell and a Smith machine. The researchers found that doing the three exercises with a barbell and a Smith machine using a 10-repetition maximum – the maximum weight that can be lifted 10 times – produced no significant differences in muscle activity of the pectoralis major, anterior deltoid, triceps and biceps. In other words, the involvement of the chest, shoulders and upper arms was similar regardless of whether the exercises were done with a barbell or a machine.

Since a muscle doesn't have the ability to think or see, it can't possibly "know" whether the source of resistance is a barbell, a machine or a cinder block. The sole factors that determine your response from strength training are your genetics and effort, not the equipment that you employ. To quote Dan Riley, who served as a strength coach in the National Football League for 27 years and at the collegiate level for eight years: "The equipment used is not the key to maximum gains. It's how you use the equipment."

7. To avoid injury, don't warm-up sets have to be done prior to a set that's taken to the point of muscular fatigue?

Warm-up sets aren't necessarily needed for your muscles to receive a proper warm-up. If you do a relatively high number of repetitions and lift the weight in a smooth, controlled manner without any explosive or jerking movements, then you'll actually warm up as you perform the set. Think about it: If you do a set of 10 repetitions with a speed of movement that's roughly six seconds per repetition, you'll have exercised your muscles for about one minute before you reach the point of muscular fatigue. After one minute of exercising, there's little doubt that you'll be adequately warmed up and prepared – both physiologically and psychologically – to reach muscular fatigue in a safe manner.

An exception to this would be individuals who do low-repetition sets such as competitive weightlifters. In this case, they should perform warm-up sets prior to their low-repetition efforts to reduce their risk of injury.

8. Do high repetitions tone muscles and low repetitions bulk them?

For decades, it has been thought that doing high repetitions will increase muscular definition ("tone") and low repetitions will increase muscular size ("bulk"). However, the vast majority of scientific research fails to support this contention.

In one study, 44 subjects were randomly assigned to three experimental groups. (Six subjects withdrew from the study for personal reasons; the remaining 38 subjects were used for data analysis.) One group did four sets of 3 to 5 repetitions; the second group did four sets of 13 to 15 repetitions; and the third group did four sets of 23 to 25 repetitions. (A fourth group acted as a control and didn't train.) The experimental

The vast majority of research fails to support the belief that doing high repetitions will increase muscular definition and low repetitions will increase muscular size. (Photo by Pillar Martinez.)

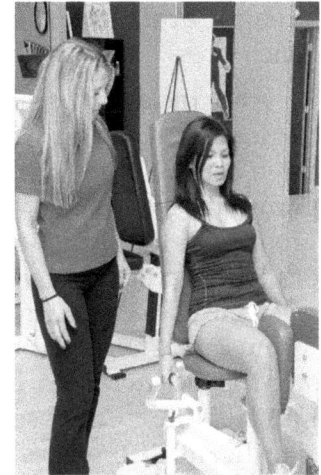

groups did one exercise for the lower body (the barbell squat) and trained three times per week for seven weeks. Each set was done to the point of muscular fatigue. All three protocols generated significant improvements in quadriceps thickness. The groups that did moderate (13 to 15) repetitions and high (23 to 25) repetitions increased thigh circumference more than the group that did low (3 to 5) repetitions which, interestingly enough, is *the exact opposite* of the prevailing notion. None of the protocols produced a significant increase in bodyweight or hamstring thickness. The researchers didn't compare the differences between groups in any of the measures.

In another study, 18 subjects were randomly assigned to two groups: One group did three sets of 8 to 12 repetitions and the other group did three sets of 25 to 35 repetitions. The groups did total-body workouts that consisted of seven exercises for all of the major muscles and trained three times per week for eight weeks. Each set was done to the point of muscular fatigue. Both protocols generated significant increases in the size of the biceps, triceps and quadriceps with no significant differences between groups. In other words, low repetitions and high repetitions increased muscular size to the same degree. As would be expected, high repetitions produced greater improvements in muscular endurance in the bench press with 50% of a one-repetition maximum (1-RM; the maximum weight that can be lifted one time). Low repetitions produced significantly greater improvements in muscular strength in the 1-RM squat but not the 1-RM bench press.

And in another study, 49 subjects were randomly assigned to two groups: One group did three sets of 8 to 12 repetitions and the other group did three sets of 20 to 25 repetitions. The groups did five exercises in each workout for all of the major muscles and trained four times per week for 12 weeks. Each set was done to the point of muscular fatigue. Both protocols generated significant increases in lean-body mass and muscle fiber cross-sectional area with no significant differences between groups. Here again, this means that low repetitions and high repetitions increased muscular size to the same degree. Both protocols generated significant increases in 1-RM strength in the leg press, bench press, leg extension and shoulder press with the only significant difference between protocols being in the bench press where low repetitions improved 1-RM strength more than high repetitions. Both protocols the size of the biceps, triceps and quadriceps with no significant differences between groups.

Each individual inherits a unique genetic profile with a unique potential for achieving muscular definition and muscular size. Some people are predisposed toward developing highly defined physiques while others are predisposed toward developing heavily muscled physiques. Whether sets consist of high repetitions or low repetitions (or intermediate repetitions), you'll still develop according to your genetics (provided that the sets are done with similar levels of intensity).

9. Are high repetitions as effective as low repetitions for increasing muscular strength?

Muscular endurance and muscular strength are directly related. If you increase your muscular endurance, you'll also increase your muscular strength.

One way to measure muscular strength is to do one repetition with a maximum weight (known as a one-repetition maximum or 1-RM); one way to measure muscular endurance is to do as many repetitions as possible with a sub-maximum weight. Now, suppose that your 1-RM in the bench press is 100 pounds (your muscular strength) and your 12-RM (the maximum weight that you can lift 12 times) is 70 pounds (your muscular endurance). And after several months of training with fairly high repetitions – say, using a range of about 8 to 12 – suppose that you've progressed to the point where your 12-RM is 85 pounds. Given the fact that you increased your 12-RM by about 20% – from 70 to 85 pounds – it's likely that your 1-RM will now be greater than your previous effort of 100 pounds. So even though you trained with fairly high repetitions, you increased your muscular strength.

By the way, it works the other way as well. If you increase your muscular strength, you'll also increase your muscular endurance. Here's why: As you get stronger, you need fewer muscle fibers to sustain a sub-maximum effort (muscular endurance). This also means that you have a greater reserve of muscle fibers available to extend the sub-maximum effort.

10. Shouldn't eccentric exercise/activity be avoided or since it's associated with extreme muscle damage and soreness?

Eccentric exercise/activity has been viewed with much apprehension for decades. It's widely believed that eccentric exercise/activity produces an extreme amount of muscle damage and soreness. But most of the studies on this topic have employed protocols that were extreme and not representative of the protocols that are done in the real world. This includes doing 100 consecutive eccentric contractions or more and running on a decline (downhill) for 30 minutes or more. Plus, the subjects that are involved in these studies often have little or no experience with eccentric exercise/activity. Is it any surprise that such protocols produce extreme muscle damage and soreness? For the uninitiated individual, doing 100 consecutive *concentric* contractions or more or running on *an incline* (uphill) for 30 minutes or more would also produce extreme muscle damage and soreness. The point is that an extreme protocol is an open invitation to extreme muscle damage and soreness.

Moreover, it has been shown that eccentric exercise/activity produces what's known as a repeated-bout (or protective) effect. This means that a prior bout of eccentric exercise/activity will protect a muscle from damage and soreness in subsequent bouts of eccentric exercise/activity. (Fast fact: The repeated-bout effect was first demonstrated in 1983 by Dr. Jan Fridén and his colleagues at the University of Umeå and the Karolinska Institute in Sweden; however, the term repeated-bout effect didn't appear in print until a 1987 study by Dr. Priscilla Clarkson and her colleagues at the University of Massachusetts, Amherst.)

In one study, for example, 10 subjects were randomly assigned to two groups: One group did 100 consecutive maximum eccentric repetitions on the leg extension with their dominant leg (using a Biodex dynamometer). The other group acted as a control and didn't do this training. Two weeks later, both groups ran five intervals on a treadmill at a 10% decline for eight minutes per interval – a total of 40 minutes of eccentric activity – at a speed that corresponded to 80% of the age-predicted maximum heart rate. (Two minutes of recovery were given between each of the five intervals.) The subjects had no prior experience with eccentric exercise/activity.

Both groups experienced significant increases in a biochemical marker for muscle damage and muscle tenderness. However, the group that did 100 consecutive maximum eccentric repetitions (a prior bout of eccentric exercise) had significantly less muscle damage and tenderness after running on a decline (a subsequent bout of eccentric activity) in comparison to the group that hadn't done the eccentric repetitions. Also recall that the subjects who performed 100 eccentric repetitions did so with their dominant leg. In the subsequent bout of eccentric activity (running on a decline), their dominant (exercised) leg had less tenderness than their non-dominant (non-exercised) leg which is additional evidence of a repeated-bout effect.

Keep in mind, too, that when lifting weights, the negative (lowering) phase of a repetition involves a relatively brief period of eccentric loading. If you lower a weight in about three to four seconds per repetition, for instance, then the eccentric loading that occurs during a set of 15 repetitions only lasts about 45 to 60 seconds. Even when this amount of time is extrapolated over the course of an entire workout, it's a far cry from the amount of eccentric loading that's used in many studies.

In short, eccentric exercise/activity is safe and productive as long as it isn't performed to an extreme. As your muscles become more familiar with eccentric exercise/activity, any amount of muscle damage and soreness that you may experience will be greatly reduced. Furthermore, the risk of muscle damage and soreness can be virtually eliminated by exercising with an appropriate level of intensity, using a reasonable volume of training and making steady and systematic increases in the workload.

Sidebar: In 1900, Dr. Theodore Hough – an American physician – described two types of muscular soreness which have since become known as acute and delayed onset. Acute muscular soreness refers to the pain and discomfort that occurs *during and immediately after* exercise/activity. It's thought that this soreness results from the accumulation of metabolic waste products – such as lactic acid – which irritates nerve endings. Delayed-onset

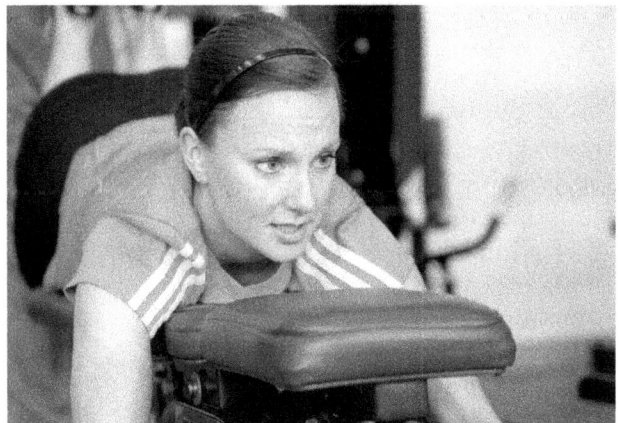

When lifting weights, the negative (lowering) phase of a repetition involves a relatively brief period of eccentric loading. (Photo provided by Luke Carlson.)

muscular soreness (DOMS) refers to the pain and discomfort that occurs *24 to 48 hours after* an exercise/activity, especially after an exercise/ activity that's extreme and/or unfamiliar. Here, the muscle may be "sore to the touch" and feel as if it's bruised. The exact cause of DOMS is unknown. It's thought that this soreness results from cellular damage to muscle fibers and/or connective tissues (such as tendons). This doesn't make sense, though, since doing exercise/activity when the muscles are sore tends to reduce some of the pain and discomfort. If the soreness was due to cellular damage, then any subsequent training should *exacerbate* the pain, not *alleviate* it.

11. What's the correct way to breathe when lifting weights?

The traditional recommendation for breathing is to exhale as you raise the weight (the positive phase) and inhale as you lower it (the negative phase). A training tip for this advice is "exhale on effort." However, doing the reverse – inhale as you raise the weight and exhale as you lower it – may have an important implication for those who suffer from hypertension.

Researchers had 20 male subjects do three sets of the leg extension and bicep curl, alternating back and forth between the two exercises while using the maximum weight that they could lift 10 times. The subjects performed each of the three sets with a different breathing technique: (1) exhaling as they raised the weight and inhaling as they lowered it; (2) inhaling as they raised the weight and exhaling as they lowered it; and (3) holding their breath as they raised the weight for the first two-thirds of the positive phase and exhaling for the remainder of the positive phase and as they lowered it. The study showed that blood pressure increased the least when the subjects inhaled as they raised the weight and exhaled as they lowered it (although it wasn't significantly different than when the subjects exhaled as they raised the weight and inhaled as they lowered it).

Aside from that, it doesn't seem to matter too much whether you inhale as you raise the weight and exhale as you lower it or do the opposite. As it turns out, inhaling and exhaling naturally fosters appropriate breathing. This is fortunate since it may be difficult for some individuals to maintain a set pattern of breathing when lifting weights, especially when training with a high level of intensity and/or employing slower repetition speeds.

One thing that must be avoided when strength training, though, is holding the breath for a prolonged period of time while straining. Forcefully exhaling against a closed glottis (airway) produces what's known as the Valsalva maneuver.

Did you ever try to clear or "pop" your ears by closing your mouth, pinching your nose and trying to exhale? If so, you employed a version of the Valsalva maneuver. Doing it while strength training is an entirely different matter, however.

The Valsalva maneuver increases the pressure in the abdominal and thoracic (chest) cavities which interferes with the return of blood to the heart. This may deprive the brain of blood and trigger a loss of consciousness. Some research refers to this as weightlifters' blackout. Use of the Valsalva maneuver may be impossible to prevent while straining to do a repetition. However, any breath holding that might occur shouldn't last for more than about three seconds.

It's thought by some that the Valsalva maneuver is advantageous during strength training but there's no scientific evidence to validate this belief. And even if that was true, the risk of prolonged breath holding outweighs any reward. (Fast fact: In 1704, Antonio Maria Valsalva – an Italian anatomist, physician and surgeon – described the "manoeuvre" that bears his name; he also coined the term Eustachian tube which was named in honor of Bartolomeo Eustachi.)

12. What's the bilateral deficit?

The term bilateral deficit refers to the fact that the sum of the force produced by two limbs separately (unilaterally) is greater than the force produced by the same two limbs simultaneously (bilaterally). Consider the leg extension, for example. If you produce 50 pounds of force with one leg and 50 pounds of force with the other, it adds up to 100 pounds of force. It seems logical to think that you should be able to produce at least 100 pounds of force when you do the exercise with both legs at the same time. But you can't because of the bilateral deficit.

There's no consensus among researchers as to why this phenomenon occurs. Theories include neural inhibition and a reduced utilization of fast-twitch fibers. In any event, studies have shown that the bilateral deficit is about 85%. So in the aforementioned example, if you produced 50 pounds of force with each leg separately – a sum of 100 pounds – you'd be able to produce about 85 pounds of force with both legs simultaneously. Strange but true.

13. What's the best way to stimulate fast-twitch fibers in the fitness center when strength training?

To answer this question, it's important to understand how muscle fibers are recruited. Under normal circumstances, the nervous system innervates (or stimulates) muscle fibers in an orderly fashion according to the *intensity* of the exercise, not the *speed* of the exercise. Slow-twitch fibers are recruited when the intensity – the demands – of the exercise are low. Intermediate ("hybrid") fibers are recruited when the slow-twitch fibers become fatigued and are no longer able to produce enough force to meet the demands of the exercise. Fast-twitch fibers are recruited only when the other fibers become fatigued and are no longer able to produce enough force to meet the demands of the exercise. The orderly recruitment pattern remains the same regardless of whether the repetition speed was fast or slow; it has *nothing to do with speed* and *everything to do with need*.

This pattern is consistent with the size principle of recruitment that was proposed by Dr. Elwood Henneman in the 1950s. He described the experimental basis of his principle in 18 related articles that were published in the *Journal of Neurophysiology* over the course of 25 years. According to this principle – which is widely regarded as one of the most important advances *ever* in the field of motor control – motoneurons

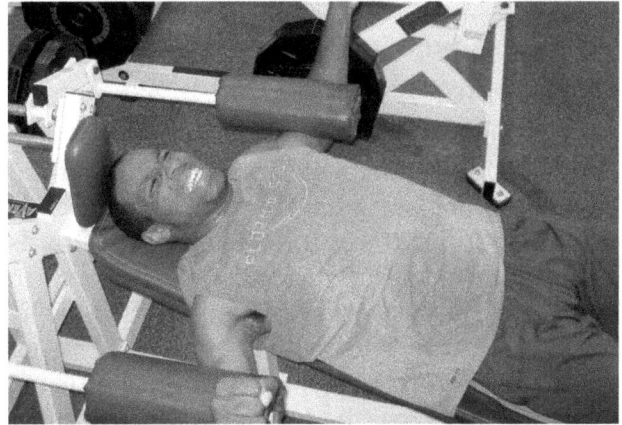

If you want to stimulate as many fast-twitch fibers as possible when strength training, you must train with a high level of intensity. (Photo by Michael Bradley.)

are recruited based on increasing size: The motor unit with the smallest motoneuron is recruited first and the motor unit with the largest motoneuron is recruited last. (A motor unit consists of a motoneuron and all the muscle fibers that it innervates.) In general, the smallest motoneurons innervate slow-twitch fibers and the largest motoneurons innervate fast-twitch fibers. Therefore, slow-twitch fibers are recruited first and fast-twitch fibers are recruited last.

This means that if you want to stimulate as many fast-twitch fibers as possible when strength training, you must train with a high level of intensity. Specifically, you must train to the point of muscular fatigue (or at least approach that point).

Sidebar: An exception to the size principle of recruitment is when a muscle is made to contract by electrical stimulation. It was once thought that doing this reverses the order of recruitment such that fast-twitch fibers are recruited first and slow-twitch fibers are recruited last. However, it now appears that during electrical muscle stimulation, the order of recruitment is non-selective/random with no specific pattern or regard for fiber type.

14. Can isometrics increase strength?

Basically, isometrics are exercises in which an individual pushes or pulls against an immovable resistance. The popularity of isometrics increased tremendously – albeit briefly – in the middle of the 20th century primarily because of two events.

First, in 1953, research by Drs. Erich Müller and Theodor Hettinger of West Germany showed that doing one six-second isometric contraction using an effort that was equal to about two-thirds of maximum could produce an increase in strength. (The increase was first reported as 5% per week but in later publications as 1.8% per week.) By the late 1950s, news of their research made its way across the Atlantic where a number of studies on isometrics were initiated, most of which also found favorable results.

Second, in 1961, Bob Hoffman – who was the founder of the York Barbell Company and coach of the US Olympic Weightlifting Team from 1948 to 1964 – authored an article in *Strength & Health* magazine in which he declared that isometrics were "the greatest system of strength and muscle building the world has ever seen." This was the first in a series of articles that was written by Hoffman about isometrics; in 1962, he also penned a book called *Functional Isometric Contraction*. Hoffman was widely credited with devising this system of isometrics but it was actually developed by Dr. John Ziegler. Regardless, the use of isometrics quickly spread across the United States "like wildfire" – to quote Hoffman – being adopted by high schools, colleges and professional teams. Fanning the flames was an article in an October 1961 issue of *Sports Illustrated* which mentioned that isometrics were being used by the San Francisco 49ers, the Pittsburgh Steelers and the Notre Dame football team.

According to Hoffman, doing functional isometric contractions for one minute a day – one maximum contraction in five different exercises that lasted 12 seconds per contraction – was an adequate stimulus for increasing strength. He promoted a number of other protocols for isometrics. An "advanced" version was referred to as an isometric-isotonic contraction. (The term isotonic is used to describe a muscular contraction that produces movement; it can refer to either a concentric or an eccentric contraction.) With an isometric-isotonic protocol, you raised a barbell – which, unlike a functional isometric contraction, was loaded with weight — a few inches (the isotonic part) then held it in one position (the isometric part). This was done within the confines of a power rack, raising the barbell from two resting pins and then holding it against two restraining pins that prevented any further movement. An isometric-isotonic contraction was performed in three positions along the range of motion. In a shoulder press, for example, you'd raise the barbell and hold it a bit higher than chest level, a bit higher than your head and a bit lower than the point where your arms are almost completely straight.

Hoffman claimed that isometrics were mainly responsible for the outstanding performances that were made by two of his weightlifters, Bill March and Louis Riecke. Hoffman's claims were later discredited when it was discovered that while performing isometrics, the two weightlifters had also taken steroids (which were provided by Dr. Ziegler). By the mid-1960s, isometrics had become yet another passing fad.

Sidebar: Doing functional isometric and isometric-isotonic contractions as outlined by Hoffman required a power rack which was, conveniently enough, manufactured and sold by Hoffman's York Barbell Company. Although the power rack had been used in the 1930s or earlier, its rise in status as a training tool didn't occur until the early 1960s during the era of isometrics.

Can isometric contractions increase strength? Absolutely. But an isometric contraction has several disadvantages. For one thing, an isometric contraction increases blood pressure beyond what would normally be encountered when strength training with conventional methods. Also, an isometric contraction is difficult to do without holding the breath which can produce the Valsalva maneuver, potentially depriving the brain of blood and triggering a loss of consciousness. Another disadvantage of an isometric contraction is that it's impossible to quantify the effort that's employed. In addition, when an isometric contraction is done at one position, improvements in strength will only occur at or near the training angle. Moreover, an isometric contraction doesn't allow the muscles to be stretched which means that after a while, an individual will likely lose flexibility. Finally, isometric contractions can quickly become monotonous and unchallenging. (Fast fact: Dr. Adolf Fick – a German physician and physiologist – first used the term isometric in 1882.)

15. What's a good equation for estimating a one-repetition maximum?

Over the years, a number of prediction equations have been developed and used to estimate a one-repetition maximum (1-RM) based on the relationship between muscular strength and muscular endurance. By using a prediction equation, a 1-RM can be estimated in a safe and practical manner without having to "max out."

Two of the most popular equations are the Brzycki equation and the Epley equation. Both equations – which have been around for more than 25 years – can be used to predict a 1-RM based on the number of repetitions that are done to muscular fatigue.

The Brzycki equation was developed by this author in 1993 when he was the strength coach and health fitness coordinator at Princeton University. The equation is as follows (where X equals the number of repetitions performed):

$$\text{weight lifted} \div (1.0278 - 0.0278X)$$

As an example, suppose that you were able to do 8 repetitions to the point of muscular fatigue with 150 pounds. Inserting these values into the equation yields a predicted 1-RM of about 186.2 pounds [0.0278 x 8 = 0.2224; 1.0278 - 0.2224 = 0.8054; 150 ÷ 0.8054 = 186.24].

The Epley equation was developed by Boyd Epley in 1985 when he was the strength coach at the University of Nebraska. The equation is as follows (where X equals the number of repetitions performed):

$$(0.033X) \text{ x (weight lifted)} + \text{weight lifted}$$

Let's use the same example of doing 8 repetitions to the point of muscular fatigue with 150 pounds. Inserting these values into the equation yields a predicted 1-RM of about 189.6 pounds [0.033 x 8 = 0.264; 0.264 x 150 = 39.6; 39.6 + 150 = 189.6].

As you can see, both equations yield roughly the same result which is consistent with research findings. In one study, 65 football players at Sacramento State University were tested in the 1-RM, 3-RM and 5-RM in the barbell squat. (The 3-RM and 5-RM are the maximum weight that can be lifted three times and five times, respectively.) The study found that when three repetitions are done to muscular fatigue, the Epley equation is more accurate in predicting a 1-RM; and when five repetitions are done to muscular fatigue, the Brzycki equation is more accurate in predicting a 1-RM.

Because genetic factors – particularly muscle fiber types – play a major role in muscular endurance, prediction equations aren't accurate for everyone. However, these equations are still a very practical and useful way to predict a 1-RM for much of the population.

16. How effective is it to do exercises on a stability ball?

Despite the core-training craze, people have trained their cores (essentially, their mid-sections) for years. Nowadays, one of the most popular items to use for core training is the stability ball.

Researchers randomly assigned 10 subjects to perform the bench press in two conditions: stable (on a bench) and unstable (on a Swiss ball). The study found that the force exerted during the unstable condition was *59.6% less* than during the stable condition. In other words, when exercising in an unstable condition, the subjects couldn't produce as much force. This is consistent with other studies that showed decreased force output with decreased stability. In this particular study, there were no significant differences in muscle activation between the stable and unstable conditions. However, a number of other studies have shown that exercising in an unstable condition results in much less muscle activation. Needless to say, producing less force and generating less muscle activity aren't desirable when it comes to strength training.

On a related note, the use of stability balls has been shown to improve performance in arbitrary tests of core stability but not athletic performance. A study that involved collegiate swimmers found that training on a stability ball improved performance in tests of core stability but not performance in swimming; a study that involved high-school athletes found that training on a stability ball improved performance in tests of core stability but not maximum oxygen intake, running economy or running posture. (Core stability, in itself, is an ambiguous term that's subject to different interpretations.) According to Dr. Jeffrey Willardson, then an assistant professor in the Physical Education Department at Eastern Illinois University, ". . . research has failed to demonstrate a significant relationship or improvement in sports performance consequent to performing exercises on unstable surfaces."

And to date, there's no scientific evidence to support the contention that instability training – on balls or other unstable objects (such as balance discs and wobble boards) – improves neuromuscular coordination or balance in another activity that requires some degree of balance. What about certain practices such as squatting while balancing on a stability ball or jumping from one stability ball to another? To quote the researchers in one study: "Whether some of these circus-type maneuvers provide specific crossover training adaptations to sport is still under debate and demands further investigation."

Not to be ignored is the potential for injury when exercising on a stability ball while holding weights. Two of these injuries made national news. In September 2005, Peter Royal broke both wrists and one forearm and injured both shoulders when an "anti-burst" stability ball burst as he was about to do the bench press with a pair of 75-pound dumbbells. He incurred five surgeries and more than $100,000 in medical bills. About two years after the accident, he and his wife filed lawsuits against the YMCA of Florida's First Coast (contending that the gym failed to maintain safe conditions) and the manufacturer of the stability ball. (A personal trainer at the YMCA had shown Royal how to do the bench press on a stability ball.) In October 2009, Francisco Garcia, a guard-forward for the

Sacramento Kings, broke his right forearm when a "burst resistant" stability ball burst while he was doing the bench press with a pair of 90-pound dumbbells. He missed 57 games that year and 24 the next. Garcia and the Kings filed lawsuits against the manufacturer of the stability ball.

These aren't isolated cases; the Federal Trade Commission's Bureau of Consumer Protection estimates that from about 2004 to 2008, more than 870 individuals were injured using stability balls. Not all of these injuries can be blamed on the manufacturer; some of these injuries are because the user did – or the trainer prescribed – an activity that was risky. Doing the bench press or any other exercise on a stability ball with heavy weights is an accident that's waiting to happen. Key point: Anti-burst and burst resistant don't mean burst proof.

When safe and sane activities are prescribed, the use of stability balls can provide variety to workouts. But when unsafe and insane activities are prescribed – or outlandish claims are made – then the use of stability balls is getting just a bit unstable.

17. What's blood flow occlusion training?

Restricting the flow of blood to exercising muscles is known as blood flow occlusion training. This type of training has its roots in Japan, where it's referred as KAATSU Training. Credit for its development has been given to Yoshiaki Sato who received the "inspiration" for KAATSU Training in 1966 and went public with the idea in 1983.

Blood flow is occluded via restrictive straps or pressurized cuffs with sensors. For the most part, the application of pressure is limited to the proximal areas of the arms, thighs and calves.

Research has shown that blood flow occlusion, using as little as 20% of a one-repetition maximum, can improve strength and size. Anecdotal reports have been made that are nothing short of miraculous, including an older wheelchair-bound man who supposedly regained the use of his legs.

But is it safe? Well, let's think about this for a minute. A restrictive strap or pressurized cuff is used to obstruct blood flow to a muscle. (Gee, that sure sounds an awful lot like a tourniquet.) This restricts the oxygen that's delivered to the muscle and the waste products that are removed from the muscle. An exercise is done that targets the muscle. When doing the exercise, there's a greater demand for blood flow to the muscle because there's a greater need to deliver oxygen and remove waste products. But blood flow to the muscle is obstructed. This means that oxygen isn't getting delivered and waste products aren't getting removed. What could possibly go wrong?

In a survey of 12,642 individuals in Japan who had received KAATSU Training, 1,651 (13.1%) sustained a subcutaneous hemorrhage. That's a pretty significant number of people. Another 164 (1.3%) experienced numbness and 35 (0.3%) cerebral anemia. There's also the potential for blood clots, muscle cell damage and necrosis. Sato, himself, was hospitalized with severe numbness in his leg due to, in his words, "reckless KAATSU Training."

Restricting your blood flow isn't normally a good thing. And it can be even more problematic when done while exercising.

18. Is vibration training effective?

A relatively new method of training is whole-body vibration (WBV). The use of WBV is becoming increasingly popular among a wide range of populations from the athletic to the elderly.

WBV has two main elements: One is the vibration that comes from a vibration device or platform; the other is the exercise/activity. WBV can be done using a single leg or both legs; static or dynamic contractions; and unloaded or loaded conditions (with additional weight).

It's touted as an effective way to prevent and treat osteoporosis and muscle atrophy as well as improve "muscle performance," "athletic power" and "body balance." As with most methods of training, however, anecdotal reports are one thing and scientific studies are another.

Most of the long-term studies (12 to 24 weeks) that used one or more comparison groups found that WBV wasn't significantly better than strength training in improving strength, vertical jump, speed of movement and fat-free mass. The acute (immediate) effects from WBV – most notably increases in vertical jump and flexibility – have led some to view WBV as a potential warm-up procedure rather than a recommended training protocol.

When administered for up to 24 weeks at 26 to 45 Hertz, WBV appears to be safe with very few adverse effects reported in the scientific literature. Nevertheless, the effects of long-term exposure to vibration are unknown.

19. Do lifting belts reduce the risk of injury or improve performance?

The use of lifting belts is fairly widespread. According to one survey, lifting belts were worn by 27% of the members of a fitness center. Moreover, 90% of the individuals who wore lifting belts said that they did so to prevent injury; 22% wore lifting belts to improve performance.

To date, no studies have looked at the effect of lifting belts on the incidence of injuries during strength/fitness applications. However, several studies have shown that doing the barbell squat and deadlift while wearing a lifting belt increases inter-abdominal pressure (IAP). An increased IAP is thought to stabilize the spine and decrease compressive forces. In addition, one study found that the use of lifting belts produced less spinal shrinkage when performing the deadlift (although the study used a protocol of eight sets of 20 repetitions with 22 pounds which is totally unrealistic).

Interestingly, no studies have looked at the effect of lifting belts on performance during strength/fitness applications. As a result, there's no scientific evidence to support the notion that the use of lifting belts improves performance.

20. Does grunting help someone lift more weight?

Walk into most fitness centers and you'll hear a cacophony of sounds, including a wide assortment of grunts and other guttural noises. In 2006, reports quickly spread across the country about a man who was escorted from Planet Fitness – a commercial fitness center – by local police for grunting which was a violation of the club's policy. In fact, the story was deemed so newsworthy that it made the front page of *The New York Times*.

Among other things, the incident triggered intense debate about whether or not a fitness center should have a no-grunting rule. Lost in the shuffle, though, was whether or not there's any merit to grunting while lifting weights.

In one study, 31 subjects were randomly assigned to do six maximum efforts of an isometric deadlift. Three efforts were done with a grunt and three without a grunt. The researchers measured and averaged the maximum decibel level of the three grunts. In order to be characterized as a grunt, the decibel level had to be more than 90% of maximum; a non-grunt was less than 25% of maximum. The study found that grunting produced an improvement in peak force but not significantly more than non-grunting. So it seems as if grunting might help but not too much.

21. What's exertional rhabdomyolysis?

Rhabdomyolysis is a condition in which muscle fibers are broken down in such an extreme manner that the cell membranes are destroyed. This releases or "leaks" intracellular contents into the bloodstream in concentrations so high that it can have dire consequences. Complications include cardiac arrhythmia (an irregular heartbeat), cardiac arrest (a sudden loss of heart function), compartment syndrome and renal (kidney) failure.

The most common risk factors for rhabdomyolysis are drug abuse, alcohol abuse, bacterial and viral infections, blunt trauma and crush injuries. Rhabdomyolysis can also result from severe exertion. Here, it's referred to as exertional rhabdomyolysis or exercise-induced rhabdomyolysis.

Many cases of exertional rhabdomyolysis involve military and law-enforcement personnel, often recruits/trainees. During 2016, for example, there were 525 cases of exertional rhabdomyolysis that were reported in the US military – a 46.2% increase since 2013 – including 211 that required hospitalization. (Of the 525 cases, 73 involved recruits.) However, there are growing reports of exertional rhabdomyolysis that was sustained by individuals who pushed themselves too hard or were pushed too hard by others such as a coach or trainer.

Factors that increase the risk of exertional rhabdomyolysis are a sudden increase in physical activity; exercises that are severe, repetitive and unfamiliar; workouts that overemphasize one or two muscles; and a hot, humid environment, especially when coupled with inadequate hydration. It's also important to know that those with sickle cell trait - which occurs in about 7 to 9% of those with African ancestry - are prone to developing exertional rhabdomyolysis.

Make no mistake about it: Rhabdomyolysis is a medical emergency. Early recognition and action are extremely critical in decreasing the possibility of long-term complications. Local signs and symptoms include muscle pain, tenderness, swelling, bruising and weakness. Systemic signs and symptoms include fever, nausea, confusion, agitation and tea-colored urine (which is often the first and perhaps most tell-tale sign of rhabdomyolysis; the dark color is due to the high urinary concentration of myoglobin, a muscle protein).

Sidebar: As noted, a complication of rhabdomyolysis is compartment syndrome. A muscle compartment is an enclosed space that contains muscle tissue, nerves and blood vessels. Though extremely rare, compartment syndrome is characterized by swelling that increases pressure in this space. The pressure can restrict or block the flow of blood to the compartment. This is a medical emergency that may require surgery to relieve the pressure. Left untreated, compart-ment syndrome can result in permanent injury to the muscle and nerves; necrosis ("death" of tissue) is a real possibility.

22. What can be done to avoid headaches that are caused by lifting weights?

Exercise-related headaches are somewhat common. These headaches are triggered by many activities, including running and weightlifting. Since most of the headaches are benign and relate to exertion, they're referred to as benign exertional headaches.

During a six-month period, a group of physicians reported that their emergency department diagnosed four patients with headaches that were related to lifting weights. The headaches were described as persistent and severe: One patient said that the pain was so severe that he felt as if he was "going to pass out"; another said that it was "the worst headache" of his life. In all four patients, the onset of the pain was sudden. The location of the headache varied, although most were in the occipital (posterior and lower) area of the head.

To avoid this type of headache, it's important for you to employ proper breathing (no breath holding) and proper technique (no excessive straining). Any activity that aggravates the condition should be avoided.

Keep in mind that headaches could be indicative of something more serious. It's a good idea, then, for those who experience this condition to seek medical attention.

23. How many calories are used during strength training and in the recovery period that follows strength training?

Estimates of caloric expenditure during and following strength training are highly variable because of many factors. This includes the amount of muscle mass that's engaged in the exercises, the effort that's used to perform the exercises and the recovery interval between exercises as well as an individual's size and body composition.

In one study, 15 women (who weighed an average of 139.7 pounds) did one set of nine exercises to muscular fatigue in an average of 21.3 minutes. During this workout, they used an average of about 56.07 calories above their baseline values or about 2.63 calories per minute.

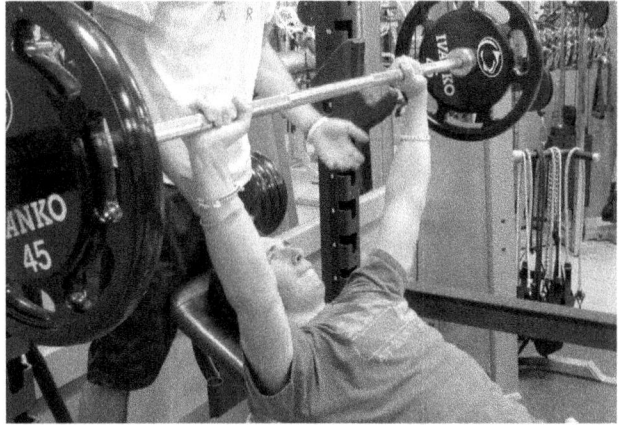

To avoid exercise-related headaches, it's important for you to employ proper breathing and proper technique. (Photo by Stevie Harrison.)

In the two hours post-exercise, the women used about 22.4 calories above their baseline values. Or look at it this way: During the two hours post-exercise, the "afterburn" was about 1.05 calories per minute of activity. (Fast fact: The technical term for afterburn is excess post-exercise oxygen consumption or EPOC.)

In the same study, the 15 women did three sets of nine exercises to muscular fatigue (à la circuit training) in an average of 63.1 minute. In this workout, they used an average of about 158.14 calories above their baseline values or about 2.51 calories per minute. In the two hours post-exercise, the women used about 22.6 calories above their baseline values. So during the two hours post-exercise, the afterburn was about 0.36 calories per minute of activity.

In another study, seven men (who weighed an average of 161.9 pounds) did six sets of 10 exercises to muscular fatigue in 90 minutes. It was estimated that in the two hours post-exercise, the men used 33.60 calories above their baseline values. During the two hours post-exercise, then, the afterburn was about 0.35 calories per minute of activity.

As part of the same study, six men (who weighed an average of 181.1 pounds) did five sets of 10 exercises to muscular fatigue in 96 minutes. It was estimated that in the two hours post-exercise, the men used 34.56 calories above their baseline values. During the two hours post-exercise, then, the afterburn was about 0.36 calories per minute of activity.

So, the afterburn that was produced by the two multiple-set protocols in the study that involved a total of 13 men was strikingly similar to the afterburn that was produced by the multiple-set protocol in the study that involved 15 women, ranging from 0.35 to 0.36 calories per minute of activity.

In the study of men, the researchers didn't determine the number of calories that were used during the workouts. Prior to the study, however, the researchers estimated the caloric expenditure for two of the men who performed five sets of 10 exercises to muscular fatigue in 96 minutes. During the workout, one man (who weighed 154 pounds) used 534 calories above his baseline value or about 5.56 calories per minute; the other man (who weighed 199 pounds) used 695 calories above his baseline value or about 7.24 calories per minute.

Sidebar: The study that involved 15 women is actually an interesting comparison of a one-set protocol to a three-set protocol in terms of caloric expenditure. Intuitively, it would seem that a greater number of calories are used when doing multiple sets of each exercise than when doing one set of each exercise. And that's true but there's another side to the story that's revealed when drilling down below the surface. In the one-set protocol, the subjects did an average of 100.7 repetitions in 21.3 minutes; in the three-set protocol, the subjects did an average

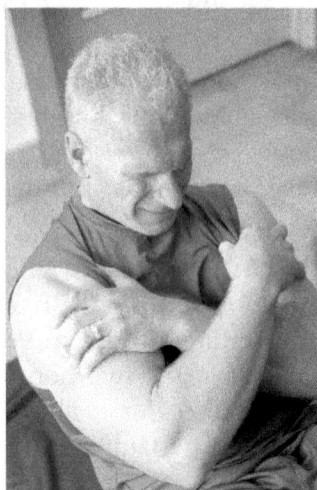

Abdominal exercises have no preferential effect on abdominal fat. (Photo provided by Luke Carlson.)

of 269.1 repetitions in 63.1 minutes. The total caloric expenditure during the three-set protocol was significantly greater than that of the one-set protocol. This is no surprise, of course, since the duration and volume of the three-set protocol was about three times as much as the one-set protocol. But here's the thing: During the first 20 minutes of the workout, the caloric expenditure of the two protocols was nearly identical. And when the total caloric expenditure was divided by the number of minutes in the workout, the one-set protocol had a slightly higher rate of caloric expenditure than the three-set protocol (2.63 calories per minute versus 2.51 calories per minute).

24. What's the best way to trim fat from the abdominal area?

The abdominal area probably gets more attention than any other body part. Many people perform countless repetitions of abdominal crunches, knee-ups and other abdominal exercises – sometimes more than once per day – with the belief that this will give them a highly prized set of "washboard abs."

In exercise science, the belief that exercise can produce a localized loss of body fat is known as spot reduction. A litmus test for evaluating spot reduction is to determine whether a significantly greater change occurs in an active (or exercised) muscle compared to an inactive (or unexercised) muscle. Spot reduction has been investigated since at least 1962. The research shows that spot reduction isn't possible.

In a classic study, 19 subjects were assigned to two groups. One group performed a sit-up program for 27 days, amounting to 5,004 sit-ups per subject (with their legs bent at a 90-degree angle, hands interlocked behind the head and no foot support). The other group acted as a control and didn't do any abdominal training. The experimental group significantly decreased the diameter of the fat cells in their abdominals, subscapular and gluteals. However, there was no significant difference between the three sites with respect to the rate of change in the diameter of the fat cells. In addition, after doing 5,004 sit-ups over the course of 27 days, the abdominal skinfold was unchanged; in fact, *it was exactly the same.* This means that exercising the abdominals didn't preferentially affect the fat in the abdominal area more than the subscapular or gluteal areas.

In a more recent study, 24 subjects were randomly assigned to two groups. One group performed seven abdominal exercises for two sets of 10 repetitions five days per week for six weeks, amounting to 4,200 repetitions per subject. The other group acted as a control and didn't do any abdominal training. The experimental group increased their abdominal endurance more than those who did no abdominal exercises. However, there were no significant differences between the two groups in decreasing any measure of abdominal fat, including android fat (the fat around the abdomen and torso), waist circumference and abdominal skinfold. This means that exercising the abdominals didn't preferentially affect the fat in the abdominal area more than not exercising the abdominals.

Why isn't spot reduction possible? Well, when you exercise, fat (and carbohydrates) is mobilized from throughout your body as a source of energy, not just from one specific area. Abdominal exercises certainly involve the abdominal muscles. But abdominal exercises have no preferential effect on abdominal fat. So although you can "spot train" muscle, you can't "spot reduce" fat. For that reason, you can do abdominal exercises until you pass out but these Olympian efforts will not automatically trim your abdomen.

By the way, there's no scientific evidence that spot reduction can occur in other areas of the body, either. One study involved a group of 20 male and female tennis players. These athletes had used one side of their body much more than the other for at least six hours per week for at least two years. As expected, their upper and lower arms on their preferred side were larger than on their non-preferred side. Among men, for example, the difference in the circumference of their lower arms was about 0.89 inches; with their upper arms, the difference was 0.37 inches. But there was no significant difference in the thickness of the subcutaneous fat over the

muscles of the arm. So, exposing one arm to considerably more activity over a fairly lengthy period of time resulted in an increase in size . . . without any preferential loss of fat.

25. Does electrical muscle stimulation increase size and strength?

Electrical muscle stimulation (EMS) has been used for years to rehabilitate muscles after injury or surgery. Because of its success in those applications, EMS has been proposed as an alternative or adjunct for healthy individuals who want to increase their size and strength.

Understand that EMS devices aren't anything new. Introduced in 1949, the Relaxacisor was perhaps the first EMS device peddled to the general public. More than 400,000 units were sold before the Food and Drug Administration stepped in and pulled the proverbial plug on the device in 1970 for being "ineffective and dangerous." Since then, not much has changed.

In one study, 27 subjects were randomly assigned to two groups: One group received stimulation from an over-the-counter EMS device according to the manufacturer's recommendations and the other group received sham stimulation from a device that looked identical to the EMS device but was modified by the researchers so that it didn't transmit any electrical current. (The subjects in the latter group were told that they'd receive a lower current that "should be less noticeable.") After eight weeks, there were no significant differences between the two groups in terms of size and strength (or in skinfold measurements). And here's a real, ahem, shocker: When piloting the procedure, at least one of the researchers received a small superficial burn from the electrode.

While previous research found that EMS is effective for increasing size and strength, the studies used high-quality, medical-grade devices which, of course, aren't available for general use. Plus, the studies typically examined one or two muscles which is much different from a comprehensive strength program.

Be advised that over-the-counter EMS devices have several drawbacks. For one thing, the devices may be wildly inaccurate and of very poor quality. Also, the electrical current may be too uncomfortable for many individuals.

26. Does a sauna belt help someone lose weight and melt fat?

A product that has been popularized in a number of infomercials is the so-called sauna belt. And like EMS devices, it's not a new idea. Sauna belts were introduced as early as the 1960s. Back then, it was simply a rubber wrap that secured around the waist. Today's high-tech version plugs into a wall socket and produces heat.

Promoters claim that the sauna belt melts fat. Can fat melt? Yes. But in order to do so, your body temperature would be so high that your brain would boil and your blood would probably coagulate. Other claims with no scientific basis are that the sauna belt can "flush out and eliminate toxins" and "enhance metabolism." But perhaps the most outrageous claim is that a belt uses "600 calories in 30 minutes." To get the same caloric expenditure, a 165-pound individual would have to run about 4.65 miles in 30 minutes, a pace of about 9.3 miles per hour. Since the only physical effort is to put on the belt and plug it in, a caloric expenditure that high is simply impossible.

A sauna belt will make you sweat and, theoretically, this could produce a small amount of weight loss. But the weight loss is from water and water has no calories. And when people are instructed to set the belt to as much as 176 degrees to supposedly promote fat loss, is anyone surprised that there are countless reports from consumers who burned their skin?

A sauna belt is basically a glorified heating pad. And an overpriced one at that.

27. Can wearing certain bracelets enhance balance and strength?

Nowadays, many individuals wear bracelets that supposedly improve a wide range of physical abilities. However, these products and other "performance jewelry" don't live up to their hype.

In one crossover study, 42 collegiate athletes were randomly assigned to do tests of flexibility, balance, strength and power while wearing either a bracelet that was marketed as performance jewelry and or while wearing a placebo bracelet. Neither the athletes nor the examiners knew which bracelet was being worn during which trial. The researchers found no significant differences between the performance jewelry and the placebo jewelry in any of the measures. Interestingly, the athletes always did significantly better in the second trial regardless of which bracelet they wore. It's likely that the increased performance in the second trial was the result of what amounts to practicing the tests in the first trial.

Bottom line: Research shows that performance bling improves nothing.

28. Can wearing certain shoes tone the hips and legs?

One of the latest products that supposedly tones and firms the muscles of the hips and legs is walking shoes. It's also claimed that the shoes can promote weight loss and improve posture.

The basic premise of the shoes is to provide instability through various designs – such as rocker-like soles and air pockets built into the soles – which make it more challenging for the wearer to maintain balance. Conceptually, this is similar to the difficulty that's encountered when trying to maintain balance on an unstable object such as a wobble board.

Promoters often point to a study in which five women walked for five minutes on a treadmill three different ways: wearing the toning shoes, wearing regular walking shoes and barefoot. It was found that the toning shoes produced significantly greater muscle activity in the gluteals, hamstrings and calves.

However, the study had severe limitations that cast a shadow of doubt on its findings: The study was short duration (involving only 500 steps), had a small number of subjects (five) and wasn't published in a peer-reviewed journal. Also raising an eyebrow is the fact that the study was funded by a manufacturer of the shoes.

Your best bet is to walk away from footwear that purports to tone your muscles.

29. Does exercising while wearing a hypoxic mask really work?

Many highly competitive athletes elect to do some of their training at elevations above 5,000 feet. At higher altitudes, the oxygen content of the air is the same as at lower altitudes – about 21% – but the partial pressure of oxygen is less. And it's this lower pressure that improves the oxygen-carrying capacity of the blood. It's thought that training at higher altitudes gives athletes a physiological advantage when training and competing at lower altitudes, especially in sports and activities that require endurance.

Higher altitudes can be simulated in altitude (or hypoxic) tents/rooms and hypobaric chambers. In an attempt to accomplish the same thing, some individuals perform exercises/activities while wearing what's known as a hypoxic (or an elevation) training mask which resembles a gas mask.

Although wearing one of these masks while exercising will certainly make it more difficult to breathe, the mask doesn't replicate the partial pressure of oxygen that would be found at higher altitudes. In addition, exercising with the mask for short periods of time can't compare to actually training at higher altitudes for days or weeks. Instead, any improvements in performance that might occur are because the mask acts as a resistive-breathing device.

In one study, 24 subjects were ranked based on their oxygen intake and then randomly assigned to two groups that did high-intensity interval training (HIIT) on a stationary cycle. Both groups did a 30-minute workout twice per week for six weeks. Each workout included a five-minute warm-up, 20 minutes of HIIT and a five-minute cooldown. One group trained with an altitude mask and the other group didn't. Subjects in both groups significantly improved their oxygen intake and peak power output in similar amounts. However, the subjects who wore the mask significantly improved their ventilatory threshold and several other markers of endurance while the other group didn't.

In one crossover study, 20 subjects performed the barbell squat and bench press (six sets of 10

repetitions and one set to muscular fatigue) along with a 25-second sprint test (maximum effort while running on a non-motorized treadmill) on two separate occasions: one time with an altitude mask and the other time without a mask. There were no significant differences between wearing a mask and not wearing a mask in the number of repetitions that were done and the workload that was used in the squat and bench press. There was no significant difference between wearing a mask and not wearing a mask in average velocity during the sprint test but the peak velocity was significantly lower while wearing the mask. It's important to note that the study began with 25 subjects. Three of them reported adverse effects from exercising with the mask – including lightheadedness, anxiety and discomfort – and didn't complete the testing. (Two others dropped out of the study for reasons that were unrelated to the mask.) The 20 subjects who completed the study reported that wearing the mask while exercising produced significantly lower ratings of alertness and focus.

These adverse effects are no surprise, really. During expiration, you exhale carbon dioxide; during inhalation, you inhale oxygen. While wearing a breathing mask, however, you exhale carbon dioxide and inhale – rebreathe – carbon dioxide. Suffice to say, this is potentially dangerous.

Bottom line: Masks should be worn for trick-or-treating, not training.

30. What are some recommendations for individuals who have exercise-induced asthma?

Exercise-induced asthma (EIA; aka exercise-induced bronchospasm or EIB) is a transient narrowing of the airways that, as the name suggests, is triggered by exercise. Classic symptoms include chest tightness, coughing, wheezing, excess production of phlegm, sore throat and shortness of breath during or after exercise.

The condition is much more prevalent than you might think; it's estimated that 12 to 15% of Americans have EIA. Moreover, the condition presents itself in recreational athletes as well as elite athletes. In one study, 39 of 170 American athletes (23%) who competed in seven sports at the 1998 Nagano Winter Olympics had EIA. The highest prevalence was cross-country skiing in which four of the seven women (57%) and three of the seven men (43%) had EIA. In another study, 42 of 107 athletes (39%) at Ohio State were found to have EIA. An estimated 70 to 90% of all individuals with chronic asthma experience EIA.

The symptoms of EIA are more likely – and more severe – during efforts that are intense or prolonged. So, those who suffer from EIA should adjust the level of their intensity and the duration of their effort accordingly. A warm-up consisting of low-intensity efforts can reduce the symptoms of EIA.

Cold, dry air can exacerbate symptoms. Here, an effective tactic is to cover the nose and mouth when exercising outdoors in cold weather. A basic, lightweight surgical mask (or dust mask) can be used as a barrier against cold air. Warm, humidified air lessens the degree of bronchospasm which suggests that swimming is an excellent activity (provided, of course, that the surrounding air isn't cold and dry).

Finally, anyone who suffers from EIA should seek the advice of a physician who may prescribe medication in the form of a bronchodilator (such as albuterol) to be taken prior to exercise/activity as a preventive measure.

31. What's a "stitch in the side"?

At one time or another, you've probably experienced a "stitch in the side" when exercising. Technically referred to as exercise-related transient abdominal pain, its cause is subject to some debate. In the opinion of most authorities, however, it's due to a restricted supply of blood to the diaphragm – the main muscle that's used in respiration – and spasm.

The pain is localized in the abdominal area. When severe, the pain is sharp; when less severe, the pain is more like a cramp, an ache or a pull.

It's related to activities that involve repetitive movements of the torso such as running and swimming. The condition is fairly common: One study reported that nearly 20% of runners experienced a stitch in the side during the previous year.

The good news is that the pain often subsides quickly. A few words of advice, though: Having a pain in the side of the abdomen doesn't automatically mean that it's a stitch in the side. The pain could be related to an abdominal strain, for example. Or it could be something that's far worse. To be on the safe side, then, it's important to consult with a physician.

32. Is it okay to exercise when sick?

The best guide for deciding whether or not to exercise when you're sick is the location of the symptoms. More specifically, are the symptoms located above or below your neck?

When the symptoms are above your neck – such as a stuffy or runny nose, headache, sore throat or sneezing – the illness is relatively mild and probably will not worsen with exercise. Sometimes, in fact, the symptoms may temporarily improve while exercising. For example, exercise may unclog a stuffy nose.

But when the symptoms are below your neck – such as a chest cold, hacking cough, muscle aches, fever, chills, nausea or vomiting – the illness is more severe and probably will worsen with exercise. In this case, rest is needed.

If the illness is mild and you choose to exercise, you should employ a level of intensity that's below normal. Symptoms that worsen during exercise are a clear indication to stop.

A related issue that often gets ignored is whether or not the illness can spread to others in the fitness center. Something like this shouldn't be taken lightly as the health of others is now at stake.

When in doubt, hold off on exercising until you're healthy. And, of course, seek medical advice.

33. Are there differences in the energy requirements between running outdoors on a road and running indoors on a treadmill?

Assuming that "running outdoors on a road" is done in a relatively calm environment – meaning that the wind doesn't offer any substantial amount of air resistance – not really. In one study, eight subjects – who were runners – ran on a track and a treadmill at three different speeds (in series): 6.7, 7.8 and 9.7 miles per hour. The researchers found that there was no significant difference in the energy requirements between running on a track and a treadmill.

This finding is in general agreement with other studies that showed little to no difference between track running and treadmill running. In fact, one study determined that equality between the two activities could be achieved by simply increasing the incline of the treadmill by a mere one percent.

So if inclement weather doesn't make it feasible to run outside on a road, you can still simulate your outdoor efforts – and obtain other health and fitness benefits – with a run inside on a treadmill.

34. Is it better to run with or without shoes?

Running without shoes is one of the latest movements afoot (pun clearly intended). Proponents of barefoot running point out that before the arrival of running shoes, humans had run barefoot or with minimal footwear since breaking ranks with apes millions of years ago.

Studies have compared the foot strike patterns of running with and without shoes. It has been shown that those who usually run with shoes tend to land on the back of their foot while those who usually run without shoes tend to land on the front of their foot *then* the back of their foot. In addition, barefoot runners who land on the front of their foot produce lower impact forces than shod runners who land on the back of their foot. This may reduce the risk of impact-related injuries but scientific evidence is lacking.

So don't shuck your shoes just yet. Besides, running outside without shoes is a risky venture.

The odds of stepping on a sharp pebble, nail or shard of glass are high. And to prevent the spread of fungal infection, it's not a good idea to run barefoot on a treadmill in a commercial setting.

35. Is there any significance as to how quickly the heart rate recovers after exercise?

Few would argue about the importance of the resting heart rate and exercising heart rate with respect to fitness. But often overlooked is the recovery heart rate following exercise.

Recovery heart rate is actually a fairly good indicator of fitness. Indeed, those who recover more quickly from exercise are most likely in better shape than those who recover less quickly. Here's something that has even greater significance, however: Several studies have found that recovery heart rate is an indicator of longevity.

In one of those studies, researchers at the Cleveland Clinic Foundation followed 2,428 patients for six years. The subjects were referred to the clinic for exercise testing (which was done on a treadmill). Their recovery heart rates were taken during a cool-down period one minute after completion of the test. In this study, an abnormal recovery heart rate was considered to be a reduction of 12 beats per minute or less; a normal recovery heart rate was a reduction of 13 beats per minute or more.

Of the 639 patients who had an abnormal recovery heart rate, there were 120 deaths from all causes (18.8%); of the 1,789 patients who had a normal recovery heart rate, there were 93 deaths from all causes (5.2%). The study found that having a heart rate that takes a long time to return to resting levels following exercise is "a powerful predictor of overall mortality."

36. Is the Body-Mass Index a valid indicator of being overweight or obese?

The Body-Mass Index (BMI) is simply a ratio of someone's weight to height. It's used as a quick and handy way to estimate if a person is underweight or overweight.

The equation for calculating BMI is to divide bodyweight (in pounds) by height (in inches squared) and multiply by 703. It has an interesting backstory that's worth mentioning.

The statistical construct that underlies the BMI was first proposed as an index of relative bodyweight by Dr. Adolphe Quetelet – a Belgian mathematician, astronomer and statistician – in 1842 in his book, *A Treatise on Man and the Development of his Faculties*. Over the years, the equation has gone by many names, including the index of weight relative to stature; index of build; weight-height index; and Quetelet Index. Dr. Ancel Keys – an American physiologist – along with his co-workers thoroughly examined the equation and first used the term Body Mass Index in an article that was published in 1972. That name, of course, stuck. (Fast fact: Besides analyzing and popularizing the BMI, Dr. Keys is known for identifying several risk factors for coronary heart disease; discovering and promoting the health benefits of the Mediterranean Diet; suggesting a link between saturated fat and heart disease; and inventing the iconic K-Rations – named in honor of Dr. Keys – that were eaten in the field by US Army soldiers during World War II.)

To calculate your BMI, follow these three steps:

• Take your height in inches and square it (multiply it by itself).

• Divide that number into your bodyweight in pounds.

• Multiply that number by 703.

If you're 6'0" and weigh 180 pounds, for example, your BMI is about 24.4 [72 x 72 = 5,184; 180 ÷ 5,184 = 0.0347; 0.0347 x 703 = 24.39]. For adults, a normal BMI is considered 18.5 to 25.0, overweight is 25.0 to 30.0 and obese is 30.0 or more.

Remember, the BMI is *an estimate*. A potential pitfall of relying on the BMI is that it doesn't distinguish fat mass from muscle/bone mass. Two people of the same height and weight would have the same BMI but it's quite conceivable that they could have markedly different levels of body fat. So even though their BMI is identical, one individual can have an excessive amount of body fat while the other can have an acceptable amount.

This is a major consideration when dealing with athletic populations. Consider this: As part of one study, researchers looked at the body composition of 165 Swedish women of which 100 were Olympic athletes and 65 were matched controls. There was no significant difference between groups in regards to BMI (athletes: 21.8; controls: 22.3). In other words, both groups had roughly the same BMI. However, there was a significant difference in body fat: The athletes were 18.4% and the controls were 31.7%.

The fact of the matter is that people who are more muscular than average – and/or have "big bones" – could be mistakenly categorized as overweight or even obese. Take football players, for example. Researchers compared the BMI and percentage of body fat of 1,958 athletes who participated in the National Football League Combine from 2010 to 2016. Based on BMI, 53.4% were considered obese. But based on percentage of body fat, only 8.9% were considered obese.

One last example: An individual who's 6'2" and weighs 240 pounds has a BMI of about 30.8 which is considered obese. But this happens to be the listed height and "competitive weight" of Arnold Schwarzenegger when he was a professional bodybuilder. Obviously, he wasn't anywhere near being obese. In reality, his percentage of body fat was in the single digits.

The bottom line is that the BMI must be interpreted with caution. If anything, the BMI should be supplemented with another measure such as body composition.

37. Does caffeine improve performance when exercising?

Caffeine – a stimulant of the central nervous system – is perhaps the most widely used drug in the world. It's a component of tea, coffee, chocolate and soda as well as pills to lose weight and combat drowsiness. It has no significant nutritional value.

Interest in the use of caffeine as an ergogenic aid (or performance enhancer) was mainly inspired by two studies that were published in the late 1970s. In those studies, caffeine produced significant improvements in endurance (in cycling). To date, numerous studies done in a laboratory have shown that caffeine increases performance in cycling and running for durations of roughly 5 to 20 minutes. But studies done outside a laboratory have found mixed results. At this time, for example, it doesn't appear as if caffeine improves sprint performance (inside or outside a laboratory).

The use of caffeine doesn't seem to improve strength or muscular endurance, either. In one study, 14 men were randomly assigned to groups that received either caffeine or a placebo one hour prior to strength training (four sets of four exercises to muscular fatigue with 70 to 80% of their 1-RM). Compared to the placebo, caffeine produced a small improvement in the number of repetitions that were done on the leg press but no improvement on the three exercises for the torso. There were no significant differences between caffeine and the placebo in the amount of weight that was lifted in any of the exercises.

In low doses, caffeine doesn't pose any serious risks for healthy individuals; when consumed in high doses, caffeine has the potential for many adverse effects such as anxiety, jitters, tremors, inability to focus, gastrointestinal distress, diarrhea, insomnia, irritability and "withdrawal headache." Since caffeine is a potent diuretic which increases the production of urine – there has been some concern that it can increase the risk of dehydration, a major fear during physical activity, especially in a hot, humid environment.

38. Is there any scientific basis for advocating "cheat meals"?

As the name implies, a cheat meal is one in which you cheat on your eating plan. Cheat meals are consumed one day per week – on "cheat day" – and are characterized by an undisciplined and unrestricted intake of food that's a "reward" for a disciplined and restricted intake of food on the other six days of the week.

These meals almost always take the form of foods that are dense with calories and the antithesis of what most people consider to be healthy; favorite options for cheat meals are burgers, fries, pizza and ice cream. Eating these foods isn't necessarily bad if done in moderation. But with cheat meals, the foods are consumed once per week in massive quantities.

Despite the seemingly widespread popularity of using cheat meals in an effort to somehow boost metabolism – and an enormous amount of online content and advice – there's no scientific support for this practice.

If anything, the use of cheat meals has raised concern in the clinical community since it meets certain criteria for being classified as an eating disorder. For example, as defined by the American Psychiatric Association, cheat meals are similar to binge-eating disorder and bulimia nervosa.

39. Should water intake be limited when exercising?

In 2005, a front-page article in *The New York Times* was ominously titled "Study Cautions Runners to Limit Intake of Water." The article quickly sparked nationwide concern about the intake of water when exercising. Much of the article was based on a study that appeared in *The New England Journal of Medicine*. The study examined 488 runners who provided blood samples and completed a questionnaire after finishing the 2002 Boston Marathon. The researchers found that 62 of the 488 runners (13%) had hyponatremia, a condition that's characterized by a low concentration of sodium in the blood. Three of the runners had critical hyponatremia.

The primary risk factor for hyponatremia is thought to be an excessive intake of fluids (which is why hyponatremia is sometimes referred to as water intoxication). This dilutes the level of sodium in the blood, creating an electrolyte imbalance that impairs neural and muscular function. Most importantly, hyponatremia can be life-threatening.

According to the study, 168 of the 488 runners – more than one third of them – drank so much fluid that they actually *gained weight during the marathon*. One individual was *nine pounds heavier* at the end of the race. Do you know how much fluid that someone would have to drink in order to gain even one pound after running for several hours let alone nine pounds? The short answer is "a lot." To gain nine pounds, an individual would have to drink a little more than a gallon of fluid and that's in addition to replacing the weight that was lost from running for a few hours. What put those runners at risk for hyponatremia wasn't drinking fluids; it was drinking *excessive amount of fluids*. (It's important to note that the study had several shortcomings that weren't mentioned by the writer of the newspaper article, including a small sample size and reliance on self-reported data. Plus, imagine being asked to fill out a questionnaire immediately after running 26.2 miles.)

While overhydration during exercise is certainly a concern, the take-home message of the newspaper article was that people should limit their intake of water when exercising. Many individuals, however, were likely frightened into the extreme, thinking that they should refrain from drinking fluids altogether.

Certainly, endurance athletes should be aware of the potential for overhydration. But for the average person, overhydration is extremely rare. In hot, humid weather, proper hydration is absolutely critical. It's recommended that you weigh yourself before and after activity and adjust your fluid intake as needed.

Sidebar: It's often said that you should drink at least eight eight-ounce glasses of water on a daily basis (aka the 8x8 Rule). However, there's no scientific evidence for this. The volume of water that's needed can vary greatly from one person to the next based on such factors as age, size, level of fitness and the duration and intensity of the activity as well as the environment. (Cold, heat, humidity and altitude all increase the need for water.) Clearly, it's important to consume an adequate amount of fluid but the 8x8 Rule doesn't hold any water.

40. Is bottled water significantly better than tap water?

Everyone assumes that bottled water is more pure than tap water. After all, it costs much more. But is it really much better?

One study compared the fluoride levels and bacterial content of commercially bottled water to that of tap water in Cleveland. The researchers examined 57 samples of five categories of bottled water that were purchased from local stores. (The five categories were spring, artesian, purified, distilled and drinking.) They also examined 16 samples of tap water that were collected from four local water-processing plants. (Four samples were taken from each plant on unannounced visits.)

Only three samples (5%) of bottled water contained fluoride levels that were in the recommended range for drinking water as required by the state of Ohio. Meanwhile, 100% of the samples of tap water were in the recommended range. In terms of bacterial count, 15 samples (26%) of bottled water had significantly more bacteria than tap water. Compared to the average bacterial count of the tap water, six samples (11%) of bottled water had at least 1,000 times the bacteria of tap water. One sample of bottled water contained *nearly 2,000 times that of the most contaminated sample of tap water*.

But what about taste? Surely bottled water must taste better. In a survey of 2,800 people in England, 60% couldn't tell the difference between bottled water and tap water. It's also interesting to note that the Natural Resources Defense Council tested more than 1,000 samples of 103 brands of bottled water and found that "an estimated 25 percent or more of bottled water is really just tap water in a bottle."

41. Is there anything wrong with eating energy bars in place of a meal?

First, keep in mind that the use of the term energy can be misleading. Numerous products use the word energy in their names. This suggests that the product will improve your stamina or make you more energetic. In truth, calories provide you with energy and three nutrients provide you with calories: carbohydrates, protein and fat. In short, people get energy from food. Technically, then, a can of non-diet soda is an energy drink, a hot dog is an energy roll, a pad of butter is an energy square, a slice of bacon is an energy strip, a chocolate-chip cookie is an energy disc and an ice-cream sandwich is an energy bar.

That being said, there's nothing inherently wrong with most of the products that have been dubbed energy bars. So you can eat an energy bar, especially when it's more convenient because of time constraints. But you shouldn't make a habit of eating energy bars in lieu of regular foods and meals. Remember, there's nothing wrong with energy bars . . . but there's nothing magical about them, either.

While on the subject, some energy bars are made to taste like candy bars. As they say, if something smells like a fish it's probably a fish. So if an energy bar tastes like a candy bar, it's probably a candy bar. Or at best, it's a glorified and an expensive one. When considering an energy bar, it's always a good idea to check the Nutrition Facts panel and the ingredients on the food label.

42. Do energy drinks give you energy?

Countless numbers of beverages have been marketed as energy drinks. These beverages have fueled a multi-billion dollar industry. In 2014, global sales were $49.9 billion, including sales in the United States of $9.73 billion.

The implication is that energy drinks will give you energy. As just noted, it's important to realize that energy is derived from calories. *Any* drink that has calories gives you energy so, technically speaking, orange juice, iced tea, non-diet soda and wine are energy drinks.

Of course, what's being marketed to consumers as energy drinks is a completely different story altogether. Standard ingredients of these beverages usually include sugar as well as various vitamins (such as vitamins B_6 and B_{12}), amino acids (such as taurine) and herbs (such as ginseng). But the real buzz often comes from a hefty dose of caffeine.

Energy is derived from calories so any drink that has calories gives you energy.

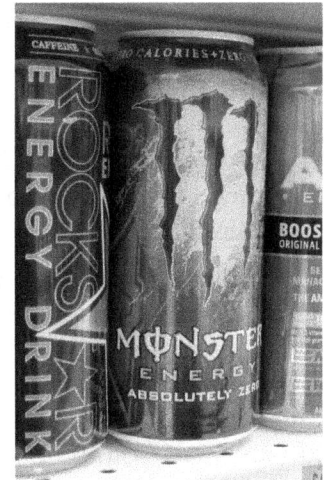

In cola-type beverages, the Food and Drug Administration considers that caffeine is "generally recognized as safe" when the amount is less than about 70 milligrams per 12 ounces. As a point of reference, a 12-ounce can of Coca-Cola® has about 35 milligrams of caffeine. Since caffeine isn't a nutrient, products aren't required to show the exact amount on the Nutrition Facts panel and, in fact, energy drinks rarely offer this information. ALRI Hypershot, though, lists *500 milligrams of caffeine in a two-ounce bottle*, a concentration that's *more than 40 times greater* than what's generally recognized as safe for a cola-type beverage.

Concerns about the consumption of too much caffeine via energy drinks shouldn't be taken lightly. In a three-year period, 265 cases of "caffeine abuse" were reported to the Illinois Poison Center (Chicago) of which 37 were from dietary supplements and 41 were from "caffeine-enhanced beverages." In nearly 12% of the 265 cases, the patients were hospitalized for medical complications from caffeine.

43. Do thermogenic products really increase metabolism?

In an effort to lose weight, many individuals take thermogenic products. It's thought that these pills and drinks increase resting energy expenditure (REE).

Researchers randomly assigned 18 subjects to groups that received either three capsules of a commercially available thermogenic product

(MET-Rx® Xtreme Amped Up Energy) or a placebo. Those who consumed the thermogenic product increased their REE by 17.3%, 19.6% and 15.3% after one, two and three hours post ingestion, respectively. Meanwhile, those who consumed the placebo decreased their REE at the same time points.

But how many more calories were used as a result of the product? Well, the REE increased by an average of about 11.46 calories during the first hour, 13.54 calories during the second hour and 10.42 calories during the third hour. This amounts to about 35.42 calories over the course of three hours. That's right, *a little more than 35 calories in three hours*.

Losing one pound of fat (3,500 calories), then, requires roughly 300 capsules of this particular product. At $39.99 for 90 capsules, that's an investment of *about $133.30 per pound of fat*.

Moreover, taking these products does absolutely nothing to improve your health and fitness or teach you good nutritional habits. It would be far better – and much cheaper – for you to lose weight by consuming less calories (eating less) and expending more calories (exercising more).

44. Does fortified water offer any advantages or benefits?

Fortified (or "enhanced") water contains vitamins but each bottle costs more than a dollar. For less than a dime, you can get pretty much the same thing by washing down a multi-vitamin/mineral supplement with a glass of water. Also of note is that fortified water usually contains more sugar – and more calories – than might be expected. An eight-ounce serving of one popular "water beverage," for example, has 13 grams of sugar. So, someone who drinks a 20-ounce bottle gets 32.5 grams of sugar (130 calories). For those who are trying to maintain or lose weight, these calories only add to their caloric budget.

Individuals who eat a balanced diet have no need to drink water that's fortified with vitamins. Remember, the best way to get vitamins (and minerals) is by eating fruits, vegetables and other wholesome foods. And the best way to get fluids is by drinking plain, old-fashioned water.

Additional "water beverages" offer an alluring array of other enhancements, including amino acids, antioxidants, herbs and minerals. None of the products live up to their advance billing.

Speaking of fortified beverages, several companies have introduced soda that has been fortified with vitamins (such as vitamins B_3, B_6, B_{12} and E) and minerals (such as chromium, magnesium and zinc). This is largely in response to consumer outcry that's directed at soda as being a major factor in the obesity epidemic along with the hope of reversing the trend of dwindling soda sales as consumers gobble up bottled water, teas, juices and sports drinks.

Yes, fortified soda is *healthier* than regular soda but that doesn't mean that it's *healthy* (or, in the words of one company's chief executive, a "health and wellness brand"). Promoting soda as "sparkling" rather than "carbonated" may be a good public relations ploy but, as they say, "A horse by any other name is still a horse." So, let's not be fooled: Candy that's fortified with vitamins and minerals is still candy. And soda – liquid candy – that's fortified with vitamins and minerals is still soda.

45. Is it true that a person doesn't start using fat as an energy source until after 20 minutes of exercise?

The main source of energy that's used during an activity depends on the *level* of effort, not the

You don't have to exercise for 20 minutes before using fat as a source of energy. (Photo by Luke Carlson.)

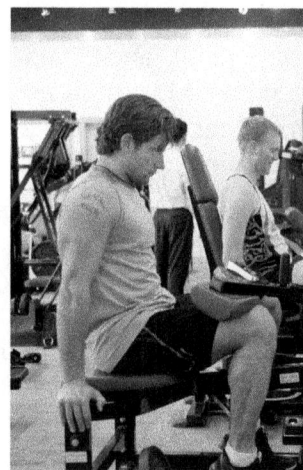

length of effort. At rest, your body primarily uses fat as an energy source. As your level of effort increases, there's a greater reliance on carbohydrates to provide energy.

Therefore, you don't have to exercise for 20 minutes before using fat as a source of energy. In fact, as you read this book, your body is primarily using fat as an energy source. Besides, it's absurd to think that your body automatically switches to fat as an energy source at exactly the 20-minute mark.

46. Does eating after 6:00pm cause someone to gain weight?

Simply because you consume calories after a certain time doesn't mean that it will result in weight gain. The most important thing that determines whether or not you gain (or lose) weight is the number of calories that you consume and expend, not the time of day.

Does it makes sense that it would be okay to eat up until 6:00pm but doing so one minute later would result in weight gain? And think about this: Suppose that you're in Georgia a few feet from its border with Alabama. Georgia is in the Eastern Time Zone and Alabama is in the Central Time Zone. So if you're in Georgia and it's 6:00pm, you're not supposed to eat or you'll gain weight. But if you quickly step across the border into Alabama where it's 5:00pm, is it now suddenly okay for you to eat without fear of gaining weight?

47. Are organic foods more nutritious than conventional foods?

Even though organic foods are more expensive than conventional foods, many people don't seem to mind paying a higher price for foods that they feel are healthier and more nutritious. But organic foods aren't really better than conventional foods when it comes to nutritional value.

British researchers examined 55 studies that were deemed to be of satisfactory quality. The studies analyzed 100 different foods and presented data on 455 nutrients and relevant substances that the researchers grouped into 98

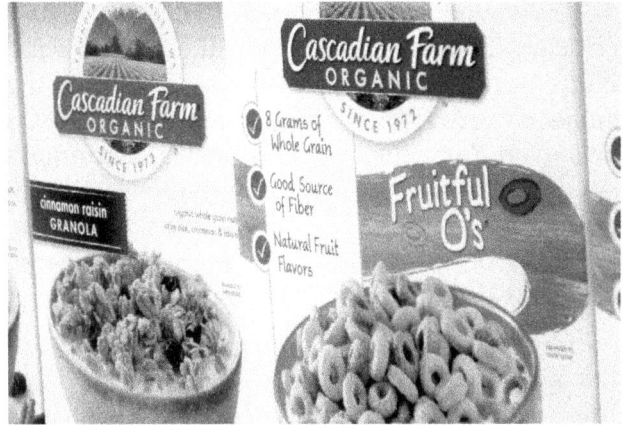

Research has found that conventional foods are just as nutritious as organic foods.

nutrient categories. It was found that organic and conventional foods are comparable in their nutrient content. In other words, conventional foods are just as nutritious as organic foods.

Not to be overlooked, however, is the fact that organic foods control the use of chemicals in crop production (such as herbicides and pesticides) and medicines in animal production (such as antibiotics and growth hormones).

48. Is weight gain associated with high fructose corn syrup?

High fructose corn syrup (HFCS) is a synthetic sweetener that was created in the late 1960s. The manufacturing process starts out with kernels of corn and ends up with a concoction of fructose and glucose. It's found in numerous foods and beverages, ranging from the fairly obvious (yogurt and sweetened beverages) to the totally unexpected (bread and tomato soup).

One study looked at the short- and long-term effects of consuming HFCS. The study consisted of two experiments. In Experiment 1, male subjects who were fed HFCS with their meals gained more weight than those who were fed sucrose (a sugar) with their meals and those who were just fed their meals for eight weeks. In Experiment 2, male and female subjects who were fed HFCS with their meals gained more weight and abdominal fat than those who were just fed their meals for six months (males) and seven months (females).

However, the study was met with heavy criticism. Some described the study as "flawed" with "inconsistent results." It was noted that the subjects were fed enormous amounts of HFCS and even then, the weight gain was extremely small ("statistically indistinguishable"). A final point is that the subjects in this study were rats. And any data collected from studies of rodents can't always be generalized to humans.

What's more, it's totally unreasonable to think that weight gain can be narrowed down to one single food or ingredient. The cause of weight gain is a function of two variables: eating too much and exercising too little.

49. Does vinegar "burn" fat?

In 2008, an article was published in *Sports Illustrated* about Jesse Chatman, who was a running back in the National Football League. The article reported on Chatman's efforts to maintain his bodyweight at an appropriate level. According to the article, the player got down to 223 pounds and then arranged a weigh-in with the trainer for the San Diego Chargers. He weighed 221 pounds "after chugging pickle juice en route to the team's facility (vinegar burns fat)."

Is this even possible? For the sake of argument, let's assume that the two-pound loss of weight came entirely from fat (especially since it's pointed out that "vinegar burns fat"). At rest – or nearly at rest such as driving a car – an individual who weighs 223 pounds uses about 1.77 calories a minute. One pound of fat has 3,500 calories. Under resting conditions, then, a 223-pound individual would "burn" two pounds of fat in roughly 3,946 minutes or about two days, 17 hours and 46 minutes. So unless the player drove to San Diego non-stop at an average speed of 60 miles per hour from somewhere like Fairbanks, Alaska, or another place that's about 3,642 miles away, it's simply impossible to "burn" two pounds of fat while driving a car.

For the record, there's absolutely nothing in vinegar that could "burn" fat. Nor is there any other substance currently known that can "burn" fat.

50. Do carbohydrates make people fat?

Contrary to what some may believe, *eating too much and exercising too little* make people fat. If anything, it's important for active individuals to consume carbohydrates to fuel their lifestyles.

Three macronutrients provide you with energy to do muscular work: carbohydrates, fat and protein. Let's talk about protein first. Protein isn't a preferred source of energy; its use is negligible while resting and minimal while exercising. That leaves carbohydrates and fat as viable options. Whether your body elects to use carbohydrates or fat for energy depends on the intensity of an activity. At low levels of effort – like walking, say – your body prefers to use a greater percentage of fat; at higher levels of effort – like jogging, running and sprinting – your body has a progressively greater reliance on carbohydrates. When your stores of carbohydrates are depleted, your body must shift its preference to your stores of fat. At first blush, this might sound like a good thing. Hey, you're using fat, right? The problem is that fat is an inefficient source of energy at higher intensities. This means that you must reduce your level of effort. If you decrease your intake of carbohydrates, there's no doubt that it will eventually have a negative impact on your endurance and stamina while training, practicing and competing.

Attached to the mistaken belief that carbohydrates make you fat is the notion that people should reduce or eliminate their intake of carbohydrates. The stigma that's associated with carbohydrates isn't anything new. In the television series *Columbo* – in an episode called "The Greenhouse Jungle" – Detective Columbo questions a woman about a kidnapping. He asks the woman if, in her opinion, a man who she knows is the kind of person who would fake a kidnapping. The woman replies, "Look, I mean I said he wasn't a very strong person. But then who is? I mean, look at me. I eat carbohydrates all the time." It's clear that the woman considers herself to be a weak person because she eats carbohydrates "all the time." The episode first aired on October 15, 1972.

Sure, those were lines from a television script that were spoken by an actress. But that perspective of carbohydrates was a sign of the times. In fact, people have viewed carbohydrates as the dastardly villain since at least the late 1960s. The relentless uprising against carbohydrates has led to a surge in low-carbohydrate diets. Like most other diets, low-carbohydrate diets have cyclical popularity, meaning that they're all the rage for a brief period of time and then fade away only to resurface again at some point in the future. An article that appeared in the American College of Sports Medicine's *Health & Fitness Journal* was called "Low-Carbohydrate Diets for Weight Loss Are Back: Do They Work Any Better This Time?" The publication date was September 1999.

In the middle of 2003, a low-carbohydrate craze began that was a craze in every sense of the word. To attract the growing number of consumers who had shunned carbohydrates, many restaurants suddenly – and sometimes comically – offered low-carbohydrate meals. (One low-carbohydrate option at Burger King® was simply a burger minus the bun.) And manufacturers hurriedly flooded supermarkets and drugstores with low-carbohydrate products (which quickly fell out of favor). That short-lived movement peaked in the early part of 2004. But the heavy criticism of carbohydrates continues.

One positive thing has come from the paranoia over carbohydrates: It brought a greater

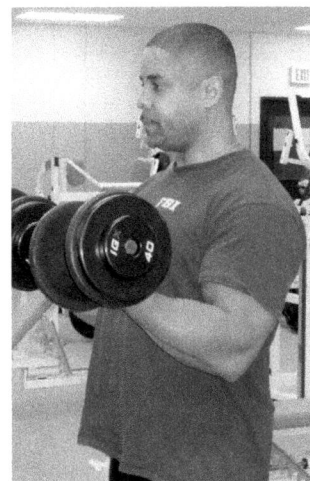

It's important for active individuals to consume carbohydrates to fuel their lifestyles.

awareness of the fact that there are different kinds of carbohydrates. An apple is high in carbohydrates . . . but so is non-diet soda. Carbohydrates that are more nutritious include fruits, vegetables and whole-grain products; they're full of vitamins and fiber. Carbohydrates that are less nutritious include processed foods such as cakes, cookies and muffins along with soft drinks and candy; they're full of "empty calories."

Anyone who tells you not to eat carbohydrates might as well tell you not to eat fruits and vegetables since these foods are mainly composed of carbohydrates.

Clearly, carbohydrates are miscast villains.

APPENDIX A: SUMMARY OF FREE-WEIGHT EXERCISES

EXERCISE	EQUIPMENT	MUSCLE(S) STRENGTHENED	REPS
Deadlift	BB DB TB	gluteus maximus, hamstrings, quadriceps, erector spinae and forearms	15-20
Ball Squat	BW DB	gluteus maximus, hamstrings, quadriceps and forearms	15-20
Lunge	BW DB	gluteus maximus, hamstrings, quadriceps and forearms	15-20
Step-Up	BW DB	gluteus maximus, hamstrings, quadriceps and forearms	15-20
Seated Calf Raise	DB	soleus	10-15
Standing Calf Raise	DB	gastrocnemius	10-15
Dorsi Flexion	DB	dorsi flexors	10-15
Bench Press	BB DB	chest, anterior deltoid and triceps	5-10
Incline Press	BB DB	chest (upper), anterior deltoid and triceps	5-10
Decline Press	BB DB	chest (lower), anterior deltoid and triceps	5-10
Dip	BW	chest (lower), anterior deltoid and triceps	5-10
Bent-Arm Fly	DB	chest and anterior deltoid	5-10
Bench Row	DB	upper back, biceps and forearms	5-10
Bent-Over Row	DB	upper back, biceps and forearms	5-10
Chin-Up	BW	upper back, biceps and forearms	5-10
Pull-Up	BW	upper back, biceps and forearms	5-10
Pullover	BB DB EZ	upper back	5-10
Shoulder Press	BB DB	anterior deltoid and triceps	5-10
Lateral Raise	DB	middle deltoid and trapezius (upper and lower)	5-10
Front Raise	DB	anterior deltoid	5-10
Bent-Over Raise	DB	posterior deltoid, trapezius (middle and lower) and rhomboids	5-10
Internal Rotation	DB RB	internal rotators	8-10
External Rotation	DB RB	external rotators	8-10
Upright Row	BB DB	trapezius (upper and lower), biceps and forearms	5-10
Shoulder Shrug	BB DB TB	trapezius (upper and lower) and forearms	8-10
Scapulae Adduction	DB	trapezius (middle and lower), rhomboids and forearms	8-10
Bicep Curl	BB DB EZ	biceps and forearms	5-10
Tricep Extension	BB DB EZ	triceps	5-10
Wrist Flexion	BB DB	wrist flexors	8-10
Wrist Extension	DB	wrist extensors	8-10
Finger Flexion	BB DB	finger flexors	8-10
Abdominal Crunch	BW	rectus abdominis	8-10
Knee-Up	BW	iliopsoas and rectus abdomninis (lower)	8-10
Side Bend	DB	obliques, erector spinae and forearms	8-10
Back Extension	BW	erector spinae, gluteus maximus and hamstrings	10-15
Stiff-Leg Deadlift	BB DB	erector spinae, gluteus maximus, hamstrings and forearms	10-15

EQUIPMENT CODES: BB = Barbell; BW = Bodyweight; DB = Dumbbells; EZ = EZ Curl Bar; RB = Resistance Band; TB = Trap Bar

NOTE: If two or more muscles are involved in an exercise, the first one listed is the prime mover. For example, the bench press involves the chest, anterior deltoid and triceps but it's considered to be a chest exercise.

APPENDIX B: SUMMARY OF MACHINE EXERCISES

EXERCISE	EQUIPMENT	MUSCLE(S) STRENGTHENED	REPS
Leg Press	PM SM	gluteus maximus, quadriceps and hamstrings	15-20
Hip Extension	SM	gluteus maximus and hamstrings	10-15
Hip Flexion	SM	iliopsoas	10-15
Hip Abduction	PM SM	gluteus medius and gluteus minimus	10-15
Hip Adduction	PM SM	hip adductors	10-15
Prone Leg Curl	PM SM	hamstrings	10-15
Seated Leg Curl	PM SM	hamstrings	10-15
Leg Extension	PM SM	quadriceps	10-15
Seated Calf Raise	PM	soleus	10-15
Calf Extension	SM	gastrocnemius	10-15
Dorsi Flexion	PM	dorsi flexors	10-15
Chest Press	PM SM	chest, anterior deltoid and triceps	5-10
Seated Dip	PM SM	chest (lower), anterior deltoid and triceps	5-10
Pec Fly	PM SM	chest and anterior deltoid	5-10
Seated Row	PM SM	upper back, biceps and forearms	5-10
Underhand Lat Pulldown	PM SM	upper back, biceps and forearms	5-10
Overhand Lat Pulldown	PM SM	upper back, biceps and forearms	5-10
Pullover	PM SM	upper back	5-10
Shoulder Press	PM SM	anterior deltoid and triceps	5-10
Lateral Raise	PM SM	middle deltoid and trapezius (upper and lower)	5-10
Rear Deltoid	PM SM	posterior deltoid, trapezius (middle and lower) and rhomboids	5-10
Internal Rotation	CC PM	internal rotators	8-10
External Rotation	CC PM	external rotators	8-10
Upright Row	CC PM	trapezius (upper and lower), biceps and forearms	5-10
Scapulae Adduction	PM SM	trapezius (middle and lower), rhomboids and forearms	8-10
Bicep Curl	CC PM SM	biceps and forearms	5-10
Tricep Extension	CC SM	triceps	5-10
Wrist Flexion	CC	wrist flexors	8-10
Wrist Extension	CC	wrist extensors	8-10
Abdominal Crunch	PM SM	rectus abdominis	8-10
Side Bend	CC	obliques and erector spinae	8-10
Torso Rotation	SM	obliques and erector spinae	8-10
Back Extension	SM	erector spinae, gluteus maximus and hamstrings	10-15
Neck Flexion	PM SM	sternocleidomastoideus	8-10
Neck Extension	PM SM	neck extensors and trapezius (upper)	8-10
Neck Lateral Flexion	PM SM	sternocleidomastoideus	8-10

EQUIPMENT CODES: CC = Cable Column; PM = Plate-loaded Machine; SM = Selectorized Machine

NOTE: If two or more muscles are involved in an exercise, the first one listed is the prime mover. For example, the seated row involves the upper back, biceps and forearms but it's considered to be an upper-back exercise.

APPENDIX C: SUMMARY OF MANUAL-RESISTANCE EXERCISES

EXERCISE	MUSCLE(S) STRENGTHENED	REPS
Hip Abduction	gluteus medius and gluteus minimus	10-15
Hip Adduction	hip adductors	10-15
Prone Leg Curl	hamstrings	10-15
Seated Leg Curl	hamstrings	10-15
Leg Extension	quadriceps	10-15
Dorsi Flexion	dorsi flexors	10-15
Push-Up	chest, anterior deltoid and triceps	5-10
Bent-Arm Fly	chest and anterior deltoid	5-10
Bent-Over Row	upper back	5-10
Seated Row	upper back, biceps and forearms	5-10
Lat Pulldown	upper back	5-10
Shoulder Press	anterior deltoid and triceps	5-10
Lateral Raise	middle deltoid and trapezius (upper and lower)	5-10
Front Raise	anterior deltoid	5-10
Bent-Over Raise	posterior deltoid, trapezius (middle and lower) and rhomboids	5-10
Internal Rotation	internal rotators	8-10
External Rotation	external rotators	8-10
Bicep Curl	biceps and forearms	5-10
Tricep Extension	triceps	5-10
Wrist Pronation	wrist pronators	8-10
Wrist Supination	wrist supinators	8-10
Abdominal Crunch	rectus abdominis	8-10
Neck Flexion	sternocleidomastoideus	8-10
Neck Extension	neck extensors and trapezius (upper)	8-10

NOTE: If two or more muscles are involved in an exercise, the first one listed is the prime mover. For example, the bicep curl involves the biceps and forearms but it's considered to be a bicep exercise.

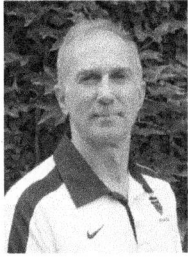

About the Author

Matt Brzycki, BS, has more than 35 years of experience at the collegiate level as an administrator, an educator and a coach. This includes work as a Health Fitness Supervisor at Princeton University (1983 to 1984); Assistant Strength and Conditioning Coach at Rutgers University (1984 to 1990); and a variety of positions at Princeton University, including Strength Coach and Health Fitness Coordinator (1990 to 1993); Coordinator of Health Fitness, Strength and Conditioning (1993 to 2001); Coordinator of Recreational Fitness and Wellness Programs (2001 to 2007); and his current role as Assistant Director of Campus Recreation, Fitness (2007 to the present).

He served in the US Marine Corps from 1975 to 1979, earning various distinctions that include the Leatherneck Award (for rifle marksmanship), meritorious promotion to the rank of sergeant, Meritorious Mast, Good Conduct Medal, Certificate of Merit, Drill Instructor Ribbon and rifle expert badge (three awards). After completing his four-year enlistment, Matt enrolled at Penn State where he earned his Bachelor of Science degree in health and physical education in 1983. In college, he was a competitive powerlifter and bodybuilder.

Matt has authored eight books, co-authored seven books and edited two books. In addition, he has authored more than 530 articles/columns on strength and fitness that have been featured in 48 different publications. Matt has given presentations throughout the United States and Canada, including the Princeton University Cross Country Camp; Princeton University Wrestling Camp; Princeton University Strength and Speed Camp; American College of Sports Medicine's Health and Fitness Summit and Exposition; Athletic Business Conference and Expo; Michigan State University Strength and Conditioning Clinic; Tampa Bay Buccaneer Strength and Conditioning Seminar; NSCA Strength and Conditioning Conference for Football; Toronto Football Clinic; FBI Law Enforcement Executive Development Seminar; and Operational Tactics National SWAT/Sniper Symposium. In addition, he has given presentations to the Central Intelligence Agency; US Customs and Border Protection; and US Secret Service Academy. He has been a guest on radio shows in Atlanta, Cincinnati and Phoenix.

He has been a part-time lecturer in the Department of Kinesiology and Health at Rutgers University (1990 to 2000 and 2012 to the present), teaching Principles of Strength and Conditioning. He taught a similar course in the Department of Health and Physical Education at The College of New Jersey (1996 to 1999). Matt has co-developed two certification courses: the SWAT (Special Weapons and Tactics) Fitness Specialist certification (2003) and the Youth Fitness Instructor/Trainer (YouthFIT™) certification (2010).

Matt served on the Alumni Society Board of Directors for the College of Health and Human Development at Penn State from 2001 to 2007, chairing its Awards Committee during his final two years. He was appointed by the governor to serve on the New Jersey Council on Physical Fitness and Sports as well as the New Jersey Obesity Prevention Task Force.

He won the 2012 and 2013 USATF-NJ Track and Field Grand Prix in the sprint events for men aged 50 to 59. In 2014, his time of 1:05.72 in the 400 (age 57) was below the qualifying standard of 1:06.40 for the 2015 National Senior Games and ranked him #73 in the United States, #86 in North America and #176 in the world among men aged 55 to 59.